Medical Coding in the Real World

AHIMA PRESS

Medical Coding in the Real World

Elizabeth Roberts

MA Ed, CPC

AHIMA PRESS

Brief Table of Contents

Detailed Table of

Part II	Coding In the Real World 157

About the Author

Elizabeth Roberts, MA Ed, CPC, has worked in the healthcare industry for over 15 years and is an AHIMA-Approved ICD-10 CM/PCS Trainer. Mrs. Roberts has a master's degree in Education and extensive experience in healthcare reimbursement and medical coding. In addition to serving as the lead instructor for the Medical Billing and Coding Department for Virginia College in Austin, Texas, she also spent three years as the senior director of content for ImplementHIT, a healthcare information technology company specializing in bite-sized educational modules for medical providers and clinical staff. An experienced consultant in medical coding and reimbursement, including practice management, HIPAA, compliance, insurance regulations, and medical coding (CPT, ICD-10, HCPCS), she enjoys helping billers, coders, clinical staff, and providers unweave the complicated tangle of coding and billing, in order to optimize healthcare reimbursement.

Preface

Job opportunities within the fields of medical billing, coding, and health information management (HIM) are growing. According to the Bureau of Labor Statistics (BLS), healthcare support occupations are projected to grow 23 percent from 2016 to 2026, which makes it *the* fastest growing major occupation group. The BLS further predicts that healthcare occupations will contribute about one-fifth of all new jobs by 2026. This continued demand and growth of the healthcare industry is due to many factors, including an aging population, increased life expectancy, and the growth of chronic conditions that require ongoing medical care (BLS 2017).

Although many healthcare jobs are held by healthcare professionals such as doctors, nurse practitioners, physician assistants, and other healthcare clinical support personnel such as physical therapists and medical assistants, any growth in the field of healthcare clinical workers leads to a concurrent growth of healthcare administrative support workers such as billers, coders, and healthcare information management specialists (among others).

This is great news for us, as growth in the healthcare sector over the next ten years represents potentially millions of new jobs requiring educated, certified professionals. This text will help you learn the basics of these administrative professions, and train you for the real world of medical coding.

One of the major advantages of the professions within health information management, which includes medical coding, is that there is no ceiling. You can go virtually as far as your motivation takes you! As you start out in the field, keep in mind that there are additional certifications and educational programs that can help you advance in your field of interest, and allow you to increase your earning potential through promotions or career transitions. The American Health Information Management Association (AHIMA), the premier association of health information management (HIM) professionals worldwide, offers an interactive career map, which includes dozens of job descriptions and possible career pathways at http://hicareers.com/CareerMap/ (see figure I.1).

Major coding and HIM organizations, such as AHIMA, typically conduct a periodic salary or coding survey to evaluate the world of coding from the coder's perspective, and to see how job responsibilities, salaries, and career expectations are changing.

As you go through this text and associated workbook, keep certifications and continuing education in mind, as they are the key to your success in a coding career. It is important to begin your coding education with an open mind. You might find coding tedious and difficult at first, but try to have fun with it! Once you have a solid coding education, the possibilities for your future are endless. This textbook is the first step in your goal toward a rewarding and exciting career. It contextualizes all learning within that "real-world" setting, and presents instructions on how to correctly identify, select, and apply healthcare codes from each of the major code sets (ICD-10-CM, ICD-10-PCS, CPT, and HCPCS), thus preparing you for *medical coding in the real world.*

Figure I.1. AHIMA Career Map

HEALTH INFORMATION CAREERS - CAREER MAPPING

	COMPLIANCE / RISK MANAGEMENT	EDUCATION / COMMUNICATION	INFORMATICS / DATA ANALYSIS	IT / INFRASTRUCTURE	OPERATIONS MEDICAL RECORDS ADMINISTRATION	REVENUE CYCLE MANAGEMENT CODING & BILLING
MASTER						
ADVANCED						
MID						
ENTRY						

Industry Careers: Current ○ Emerging ◇ | Promotional Path ——— Transitional Path ——— | FEATURED CAREER PATHS   VIEW FAQ

Made possible in part from philanthropic contributions from Career Step.

Source: ©AHIMA.

How to Use This Text

Hands-on medical coding in the real world is the basis for this coding textbook. It is organized into coding systems within medical specialties, as they are encountered in the real world, and teaches all necessary code sets as necessitated in a real-world setting. For example, healthcare codes pertaining to orthopedic conditions and services to treat those conditions are discussed within the context of an orthopedic healthcare practice. This means identifying and assigning all codes on the claim, not just those found in a certain section in the CPT coding manual, and includes diagnoses codes, supply codes, and various other necessary procedural codes, as necessary, per service.

Medical Coding in the Real World emphasizes the real-world of coding, and contextualizes codes so that students see their role in a healthcare practice. In this way, students learn what it is like to code in a real-world context. For example, instead of learning how to code labor and delivery services based on reading the labor and delivery chapter in the CPT coding manual, you will learn labor and delivery as if you were working in an actual obstetrician's office.

The chapters in this text are organized into medical specialties or settings, and students learn how to code within this contextualized space. Each chapter focuses on all of the various types of codes that are utilized within each specialty, including all procedural, diagnosis, and supply or service codes.

Chapters are organized in such a way as to build upon each other, so that more complicated specialties, or more complicated coding and application of coding guidelines, are discussed after the basic components of coding and coding guidelines are mastered. The basics of all outpatient professional coding is presented first, followed by chapters that are centered around a medical specialty or healthcare setting, and the ICD-10-CM, CPT, or HCPCS codes used within that specialty or setting. Inpatient facility coding (ICD-10-PCS) is presented at the end of the text. Evaluation and Management coding is taught early on in the text so that students can utilize their knowledge of E&M codes throughout the text, and apply them as necessary throughout the chapters.

Part I of this text discusses the basics of medical billing and coding. **Chapter 1, Your Coding Career**, discusses the many aspects of a job as a medical coder, including coding certifications. **Chapter 2, Healthcare Billing Basics**, includes a high overview of the basic principles of healthcare billing, such as the Health Insurance Portability and Accountability Act (HIPAA) and performance measures. **Chapter 3, Basics of Coding**, defines medical coding and medical code sets. **Chapter 4, Learning the ICD-10-CM Code Book**, defines and examines the organization of the ICD-10-CM code book, the structure of ICD-10-CM diagnosis codes, and basics on how to select ICD-10-CM codes from a diagnostic statement. **Chapter 5, Learning the CPT and HCPCS Code Books**, examines the CPT and HCPCS code sets and books.

Part II of this text discusses specific code sets, coding guidelines, and presents practice coding scenarios organized within healthcare-specialty-specific chapters. **Chapter 6, Supplies and Services**, discusses the HCPCS code set within the context of an ambulance supplier and durable medical equipment supplier. This chapter also includes a section on coding for medications administered in the healthcare setting. **Chapter 7, Behavioral Health Services**, examines the medical codes used within the specialty of behavioral health. This chapter also provides a preliminary discussion of evaluation and management coding. **Chapter 8, Primary Care Services**, examines the medical codes used within the specialty of primary care. This chapter provides a more thorough examination of evaluation and management coding and auditing. **Chapter 9, Eye and Vision Services**, examines the medical codes used in ophthalmology and optometry services. **Chapter 10, Urgent Care and Emergency Department Services**, examines the medical codes used within both the urgent care and emergency department setting. **Chapter 11, Surgical Services**, examines the medical codes used to identify and report surgical services performed by professionals within the inpatient and outpatient hospital settings. **Chapter 12, Anesthesia and Pain Management Services**, examines the codes used to identify services performed by anesthesiologists and interventional pain management specialists. **Chapter 13, Radiology and Imaging Services**, examines the codes used to identify radiology and imaging services, excluding radiation oncology. **Chapter 14, Laboratory and Pathology Services**, examines the codes used to report laboratory and pathology services. **Chapter 15, Orthopedic Services**, examines the medical codes used to report conditions and services performed within the specialty of orthopedics. **Chapter 16, Physical, Occupational, and Speech Therapy Services**, examines the codes used to report services provided by physical therapists, occupational therapists, and speech-language pathologists. **Chapter 17, Obstetrics and Gynecology Services**, examines the codes reported to identify services performed in both obstetrics (such as labor and delivery) and gynecology. **Chapter 18, Healthcare Specialist Services, Part I**, examines the codes used within three medical specialties, including hematology and oncology, neurology, and urology and nephrology. **Chapter 19, Healthcare Specialist Services, Part II**, examines the codes used within the specialties of gastroenterology and cardiology. **Chapter 20, Inpatient Hospital Services**, defines and examines the ICD-10-PCS code set and coding used to report facility services.

This text is thus best used in a linear fashion, from the earliest chapters, progressing to subsequent chapters, to ensure understanding of all materials presented. The following pedagogical items are included to enhance the learning process.

- Learning objectives to identify actionable outcomes after reading each chapter.
- Key terms to solidify healthcare and coding terminology.
- Figures and tables provide visual references for complex concepts and guidelines.
- **Key to Success** boxes call out insightful information from the perspective of a professional coder.
- **HCC Coding Corner** boxes provide detailed information about applying hierarchal condition category (HCC) coding. HCC icons also appear in the margin of applicable text.
- **MOD** boxes address additional details about appending modifiers to codes.

- **There's a Code for That** exercises appear throughout each chapter and provide practice to the immediate concepts.
- Codes and code descriptions are highlighted throughout the text.
- **Putting It All Together** is a section at the end of relevant chapters to tie key concepts together within a real-world coding scenario.
- End of chapter content provides an opportunity to practice the concepts presented in the chapter. Exercises range from true/false, matching, and multiple choice questions to fill-in-the-blank coding questions.

This book refers to the 2017 version of the Healthcare Common Procedure Coding System (HCPCS) and the 2018 versions of the following code sets.

- International Classification of Diseases, Tenth Revision, Clinical Modification (ICD-10-CM)
- International Classification of Diseases, Tenth Revision, Procedure Coding System (ICD-10-PCS)
- Current Procedural Terminology (CPT)

Student Workbook

This text is accompanied by a comprehensive student workbook designed to enhance important information addressed in each chapter, and to reinforce learning through practice. The *Medical Coding in the Real World Student Workbook* includes 20 chapters, each of which corresponds to the information presented in the textbook. Each workbook chapter includes a number of exercises that range from true/false, multiple choice, matching, and coding questions, to short answer questions and practice focused on correctly completing insurance claim forms and other related paperwork.

The student workbook is meant to be a companion to the textbook, and should be used in conjunction with the textbook, chapter by chapter. In this manner, the workbook should be used to reinforce the information learned in each chapter of the text, and to provide practice selecting, sequencing, and reporting the appropriate ICD-10-CM, CPT, HCPCS, and ICD-10-PCS codes, as necessary.

References

Bureau of Labor Statistics. October 24, 2017. *Employment Projections 2016-2026*. http://www.bls.gov/news.release/pdf/ecopro.pdf.

Health Information Careers. 2017. *Health Information Careers-Career Mapping*. http://hicareers.com/CareerMap/.

Health Information Careers. 2017. *Coding Professional*. http://hicareers.com/CareerMap/FullDescription.aspx?ID=46.

Acknowledgments

This text would not have been possible without the love and support of my family, especially my husband. Thank you also to my amazing editor, whose guidance, advice, and patience all helped this project come to fruition. And to all of my past, present, and future students of medical coding—this is for you!

Part I

Medical Billing and Coding Basics

CHAPTER

Your Coding Career

Learning Objectives

- Identify the different types of healthcare facilities and practices and how coding practices differ within each setting.
- Identify professional organizations that support health information management, and the benefits of coding certifications.

- Recognize the different types of healthcare providers, including different types of healthcare specialists.

Key Terms

Administrative personnel
Ambulatory surgical center (ASC)
American Health Information Management Association (AHIMA)
Certified Coding Specialist (CCS)
Classification system
Clinical personnel
Coding certification
Continuing education unit (CEU)
Date of service

Diagnosis
Emergency department
Encounter
Healthcare billing
Healthcare coding
Healthcare provider
Healthcare specialty
Hospital
Inpatient
Internal medicine provider
Large group practice

Mid-level provider
Outpatient
Physician
Primary care provider (PCP)
Procedure
Professional organization
Remote coding
Small group practice
Solo practice
Surgical specialist
Urgent care facility

There are so many career options in healthcare billing and coding that it may seem a little overwhelming to students entering the field. Essentially every health service that is provided must be coded and billed appropriately, which means that there are thousands of different career options on the administrative side of medicine. A coder's job and the codes that he or she bills will depend largely on the type of healthcare setting and healthcare practice in which they work. This could range from an endocrinologist's office, to a long-term care facility, or a healthcare billing company. On the other hand, a coder might choose to work in the inpatient hospital setting, an ambulatory surgical center, or chemotherapy infusion center. The future career options for coders are endless.

This chapter discusses possibilities in the profession of coding, the importance of professional organizations, and the different types of healthcare settings and healthcare specialties in order to help incoming coders understand what to expect once they find themselves in the real world of healthcare billing and coding. This chapter also briefly discusses the differences between healthcare facility coding versus professional (physician) coding. It is also important to note that this text focuses on professional physician coding and billing, which is different than facility coding in the inpatient setting. Professional coding is discussed throughout chapters 6 through 19, and inpatient coding is specifically addressed in chapter 20.

This text covers all of the major healthcare code sets, including procedure coding, diagnosis coding, and coding for supplies and services. These code sets include the International Classification of Diseases, 10th Revision, Procedure Coding System (ICD-10-PCS) and International Classification of Diseases, 10th Revision, Clinical Modification (ICD-10-CM) coding, as well as Current Procedural Terminology (CPT) codes and Healthcare Common Procedure Coding System (HCPCS).

Where Could You Work?

The type of coding in which you specialize will depend on where you work, so it is important to understand these different settings. In the world of healthcare billing and coding, there are two main work settings—a billing and coding company, or an actual healthcare practice or facility. A billing or coding company handles the billing or coding for a healthcare practice or facility, which means that the only contact you might have with patients would be communication regarding healthcare bills. A healthcare practice or facility sees and treats patients on a daily basis. A coder in a healthcare practice or facility may have job duties that require interaction with patients, such as answering phone calls, scheduling appointments, checking patients in and out, communication with patients regarding bills, or in performing other administrative duties. Your job description and daily responsibilities will change significantly, depending on in which of these settings you work.

The following sections introduce coding and discuss the differences in healthcare settings, including billing and coding companies, different types of healthcare practices, and inpatient and outpatient coding.

What Is Healthcare Coding?

Healthcare coding is the practice of assigning numeric or alphanumerical codes to identify the treatment, services, or supplies provided to a patient during a healthcare encounter, also known as the procedure. A **procedure** is an action of diagnosis or treatment of a condition by a healthcare professional. Codes are also assigned to identify the reason why the patient was provided with healthcare services, otherwise known as the diagnosis. A **diagnosis** is a word or phrase used by a physician to identify a disease from which an individual patient suffers or a condition for which the patient needs, seeks, or receives healthcare. Healthcare codes are assigned based on the healthcare provider's documentation for each **date of service**, or each specific day that the patient received healthcare services or care. When a patient receives more than one day of service, codes are sent for all procedures and diagnoses performed or treated across multiple dates of service.

Codes are a type of classification system that translates healthcare procedures or diagnoses into a set of numerical or alphanumerical codes. A **classification system** is a clinical vocabulary, terminology, or nomenclature that lists words or phrases with their meanings, provides for the proper use of clinical words as names or symbols, and facilitates mapping standardized terms to broader classifications for administrative, regulatory, oversight, and fiscal requirements.

Individual codes are compiled and organized into a number of different code books, and it is the coder's job to read through the documentation from the date of service, determine which procedures, services, or supplies were provided to the patient and the reason(s) they were provided, and then determine which code(s) appropriately identify those components of the patient visit. The coder must also be aware of the setting in which the services were provided, as codes may change depending on the healthcare setting. For example, one healthcare setting may report codes for the supplies provided to the patient during an encounter, whereas another may not.

Once the codes are selected, they are listed on a claim. A claim, used for payment for the services rendered, is a specialized form that contains information regarding the patient, responsible party for the services, healthcare provider, date of service, procedures, diagnoses, and any supplies used, as well as a number of additional details. The claim may be in a paper format, which is printed and then mailed to the responsible party; or in an electronic format, which is sent directly to the responsible party via an electronic data interchange (EDI) system that transmits data between computer systems. In the healthcare setting, the responsible party for the claim is usually a health insurance company, also called the third-party payer. The codes sent on a claim are used for both payment and reporting purposes. For example, when an insurance company receives a claim, it is analyzed and then paid as a bill would be. In this sense, coders are an inherent part of the billing process. Without coders to analyze documentation, select, and report the appropriate codes for services, then healthcare services would not be paid by insurance companies.

Healthcare billing is different than healthcare coding. **Healthcare billing** is the practice of sending a coded healthcare claim to a third-party payer or insurance company for payment (as described in chapter 2), and then following that claim until it is paid in full. This can include billing patients for any remaining balance, sending appeals to insurance companies for underpaid or unpaid claims, and sending patient accounts to outside collections agencies for nonpayment.

A correctly coded healthcare claim is required for healthcare providers to collect the correct payment for the services provided to a patient. In this sense, healthcare billers and coders work together to ensure that the healthcare services are reported accurately with codes and then billed correctly to the payer, to ensure appropriate payment for services rendered to each patient for each date of service. This text introduces the billing concepts for each healthcare specialty before discussing the coding process for each specialty. This helps student coders understand the close connection between billing and coding and ensure correct payment for healthcare services.

Billing and Coding Companies

A billing or coding company does just that—billing and coding of insurance claims for healthcare practitioners and healthcare facilities. Many healthcare practices, ranging from single-physician healthcare offices to large inpatient hospitals, outsource their billing and coding to a company that performs these functions for them. They choose not to code health records and send healthcare claims directly, but instead send the billing information and healthcare documentation to an outside company that will complete their billing and coding of healthcare insurance claims.

Outsourcing to a billing and coding company has its advantages—for example, the provider's office or healthcare facility does not have to use internal resources to code and send claims, and has access to a highly trained or certified staff capable of coding and billing expertly for their services. However, there are some disadvantages to outsourcing to a billing company. When using a billing company, the provider's office or healthcare facility has no control over the billing processes or the training of the employees at the billing company, which can lead to misunderstandings. Furthermore, there might be hidden costs or contractual misunderstandings with the billing company, which may cause frustration or heavy expenses.

The agreement between healthcare facilities and billing and coding companies varies greatly depending on the company. For example, some billing companies perform just the billing of the claims; the encounters are submitted to the company pre-coded by staff members within the healthcare practice. In this case, the codes for the encounter (procedures, supplies and services, and diagnosis codes, all of which are addressed in chapters 6 through 20 of this text), are identified and entered by staff such as the doctor, nursing or healthcare assisting staff, or coder within the healthcare practice. An **encounter** is the contact between a patient and a provider who has primary responsibility for assessing and treating the condition of the patient at a given time and who exercises independent judgment in the care of the patient. The codes from this encounter are then sent to the billing company that enters those codes on a claim form, sends the claim to the patient's insurance company, and then follows up on the claim until it is paid in full.

Other billing and coding companies provide services that are more comprehensive. In this case, the billing company receives the raw documentation from the patient's encounter from the healthcare practice or inpatient facility; identifies the correct codes for each procedure, diagnosis, or other supplies or services provided to the patient; enters these codes correctly on to the insurance claims; sends the claim to the insurance company or third-party payer; and follows up with it until it is paid in full.

The specific job responsibilities of working in a billing and coding company thus depends on the type of service that the company provides. As a coder, you may have opportunities to work in a billing and coding company. As an expert in the codes that represent medical necessity (ICD-10-CM), and the procedures, services, and supplies provided to the patient (CPT, HCPCS, ICD-10-PCS), you can decipher the complicated healthcare documentation used to support the codes selected. You may also choose to learn more about the billing side of coding and the complex world of billing regulations surrounding the correct coding and payment of healthcare claims. Either way, working in a billing or coding company is an exciting possibility. (Note that although this text does discuss billing in specific scenarios, it does not cover all billing procedures, rules, and regulations.)

Furthermore, though many billing companies are located within physical offices, other billing and coding practices are online. This means coders also have the opportunity to work on-site with a team of billing and coding specialists in an administrative setting, or in a virtual setting from a personal computer.

Virtual coding positions are often referred to as remote coding positions. A **remote coding** position is one in which the coder is not required to be physically present in the office or facility setting while completing his or her work. In this case, a remote coder can work from home, from a coffee shop, or anywhere else with Internet access. Coding remotely requires an in-depth understanding of coding, reliable access to the proper equipment, and the ability to stay on-task without getting distracted. Because of the possibility of additional confidentiality and security risks in remote coding from anywhere with an Internet connection, working remotely also requires knowledge of Health Insurance Portability and Accountability Act (HIPAA) privacy and security rules and regulations that govern patient privacy and access to confidential patient health information (discussed more in depth in chapter 2) to ensure secure access to patient information. Sometimes an employer may require a short term of coding on-site before allowing an employee to work remotely. Many online coding positions require completion of a face-to-face training or trial period before working remotely, while others may require the successful completion of a coding test and a coding certification. This ensures that the coder has a complete understanding of coding processes before he or she works remotely without direct supervision or assistance.

Remote coding positions are becoming more numerous within the world of healthcare, as employers realize the cost savings involved. Because the employee is not actually on-site, this requires less business overhead in terms of space, equipment, and materials. Large facilities, such as hospital systems, are more likely to employ remote coders who are expected to maintain a certain percentage of coding accuracy. Coding accuracy is the percentage of codes that are identified correctly for either diagnoses or procedures (or both) from health record documentation. As a remote coder for a healthcare facility, a certain coding accuracy percentage is typically required—usually around 90 to 95 percent—although some healthcare facilities may require a coding accuracy percentage of 98 percent!

Key to Success

Working in a virtual setting might sound convenient, but it is not for everyone. Working in a remote environment requires a great deal of self-discipline, time management skills, organization, diligence, and motivation. The remote environment also comes with plenty of distractions, both online (that is, social media, email, and other websites) and at home (for example, housework, family, and pets). If you are considering a remote coding position in the future, it is a good idea to list its pros and cons versus an on-site position, including all potential distractions and how you will overcome them to ensure success in your coding position.

Types of Healthcare Practices

If you choose to work at a healthcare practice, your job functions may vary and you may have more interaction among patients or healthcare practitioners. For example, you might have to assist the administrative staff and answer phones with the receptionist, schedule appointments, and interact directly with the healthcare practitioners and clinical staff daily. In the inpatient setting, it is more likely that you would have less contact with patients, as the coding and/or billing office is usually separate from other administrative offices.

Not all healthcare practices are created equal, however. The type of practice and the exact job functions that you are required to perform depend largely on the type of healthcare practice in which you work. A **solo practice** is a healthcare office that has one doctor who typically owns the practice and sees all of the patients that come into the office each day. A **small group practice** has from two to five healthcare providers, all of whom see patients each day. These doctors work together and may see each other's patients when needed, and may also rotate their schedules to share responsibilities. Typically, in any type of healthcare group practice, one or more of the doctors will own the business, as well as see patients, all within the same specialty. A **large group practice** may have anywhere from six to dozens of providers. Many times, a large group practice is made up of healthcare providers from many different healthcare specialties. For example, a large group practice in an inner-city area may provide family practice, pediatric, and obstetrics and gynecology services. Healthcare providers in any of these types of practices may also complete rounds at inpatient facilities, such as hospitals or long-term care facilities—meaning that they may leave the office throughout the day or at a certain time each day to treat patients that are in the inpatient setting. For example, an obstetrician working in a small group practice may have to leave the office if he or she is called to perform a delivery at the hospital, and then return to the office to see the rest of his or her patients once the delivery is done.

When a healthcare provider treats or performs a procedure on a patient in a facility such as a hospital, skilled nursing facility, or emergency room, he or she bills for the service for reimbursement. On the other hand, the facility itself also bills for the service to obtain reimbursement for the supplies, treatments, or other resources used during the patient's stay. For example, if the patient delivered a baby at the hospital, then the hospital would bill for the labor and delivery suite, room and board provided to the patient during her stay, and any other supplies or hospital resources used during the delivery, such as the use of an operating suite to perform a cesarean section. So the delivery of the infant in the hospital setting would require at least two claims: one for the professional physician services (the delivery procedure) and the hospital facility charge (the facility resources used during the patient's stay). If the patient received any other services, such as an anesthesia service by an anesthesiologist for pain management, then the anesthesiologist would report his or her services separately was well. Keep this division in mind (between facility and professional billing and coding) when reading through this text, as facility and professional services are often reported with different codes depending on who is reporting the service (facility or professional).

A **hospital** is a large facility that provides specialized healthcare treatments and has a large staff of healthcare providers and nurses on hand at all times. Hospitals may range from smaller, locally owned hospitals with a hundred staff members, to extensive hospital systems maintained throughout a large geographic area that employ thousands of staff members. An **ambulatory surgical center (ASC)** is a healthcare facility that provides same-day surgical services to patients on an outpatient basis. ASC procedures are minor or less invasive than surgeries performed in the inpatient hospital setting, and patients are discharged home on the same day of the surgery. An **emergency department** or **urgent care facility** may be either a standalone facility or attached to a larger facility, such as a hospital. Emergency departments and urgent care facilities provide same-day care for patients with healthcare emergencies or urgent healthcare needs. Study figure 1.1 to learn more about the differences between healthcare practices. Healthcare may also be provided in other settings as needed, such as long-term care facilities, nursing homes, hospice, or even in the patient's home.

As a general rule, the smaller the practice in which you work, the more likely you will be responsible for performing many different tasks, not just those of a biller or coder. For example, in a small single physician practice, you may have to perform all of the administrative duties within the office. On the other hand, the larger the practice is, the more likely you will be a smaller cog in the machine and have less varied

Figure 1.1. Types of healthcare practices

Types of Healthcare Practices

Solo Practice

A solo practice has one doctor, who typically owns the practice and sees all of the patients.

Small Group Practice

Small group practices have from two to five providers, who all see patients for the practice.

Large Group Practice

Large groups can range from about six to dozens of providers. They are typically multi-specialty.

Hospital

Hospitals are large facilities that provide specialized medical treatments and have a large staff of medical providers and nurses.

Ambulatory Surgical Center (ASC)

As ASC provides outpatient same-day surgeries to patients needing minor and less-invasive surgical procedures.

Emergency Dept/ Urgent Care

Either standalone or attached to a larger facility, an ED or urgent care provides care to patients with urgent or emergent medical needs.

responsibilities. For example, you may be responsible only for entering the codes on a claim or entering insurance payments.

Either way, it is important to be flexible, especially as you are starting your career. This may require working in multiple different positions within the healthcare office. For a student entering the field, this usually means beginning at an entry-level position, and then working your way up into a full-time coder position. For example, you may begin your coding career as a healthcare receptionist or appointment scheduler, or working with healthcare records. There are many different job responsibilities within the field of health information management, and it helps to learn as much as you can about every aspect of the healthcare office or facility. As you become more skilled in the field of healthcare administration and coding, you may work as a biller or coder, or in any number of other administrative positions within the healthcare office. Working in different positions can help you determine exactly where you fit best within the organization, ultimately increasing your career success in the long run. For instance, an expert-level coder within the field of health information management may become an auditor, a coding educator of a large healthcare facility or practice, or an independent coding consultant.

Inpatient and Outpatient Billing

It is key to note the difference between inpatient and outpatient healthcare settings. This is an important distinction, as not only do the job functions differ, but the codes and billing practices differ vastly between the settings.

An **inpatient** healthcare facility is also referred to as an acute-care setting. An inpatient facility is one in which the patient stays overnight or several days or more, if necessary. These facilities include inpatient hospitals, long-term care facilities such as skilled nursing facilities, and inpatient mental health facilities. Many inpatient hospitals are large facilities with several departments or units based upon the type of care provided, such as labor and delivery, orthopedics, or pediatrics. Furthermore, inpatient hospitals are staffed by hundreds of clinical personnel such as physicians, nurses, and various clinical assistants in areas such as digital laboratory, imaging services, and pharmacy. **Clinical personnel** are those who are trained as healthcare providers or practitioners—such as doctors, nurse practitioners, and physician assistants—as well as personnel like registered nurses, healthcare assistants, and clinical nursing assistants who are trained and qualified to provide assistive healthcare services. Clinical personnel are qualified to provide healthcare services, advice, and treatments.

Administrative staff within an inpatient hospital are also numerous and include staff members with the responsibilities of ensuring that the facility runs efficiently, such as registration and management staff, and staff that ensures the correct coding and prompt payment for healthcare services. **Administrative personnel** handle the daily functions of the business side of the healthcare practice, such as sending claims and billing patients. They also handle non-clinical patient services like handling healthcare records requests, registering patients, scheduling appointments, and sending referrals to healthcare specialists.

By contrast, an **outpatient** setting is one in which patients are not admitted to the healthcare facility, even though they may stay at the facility overnight. Also referred to as ambulatory care, outpatient services are provided to a patient who presents for the treatment and then returns home. Outpatient services can range from vaccinations to diagnostic screenings, mental health services, and complex surgical procedures. The main difference between inpatient and outpatient services is the fact that an outpatient is typically treated and discharged on the same date of service, although he or she may stay overnight in certain circumstances.

It is important to understand the difference between inpatient and outpatient healthcare settings because the codes used in each setting differ. This means that even though the patient may have received the same service in an inpatient facility that could have been done in an outpatient facility, it is billed differently depending on where the service was performed and which healthcare entity is reporting the service. As previously described, healthcare providers who perform services within the hospital setting still bill with outpatient codes, as they are billing for services independently of the inpatient facility. Figure 1.2 illustrates the different codes that may be used, depending on the healthcare setting.

Figure 1.2. Inpatient and outpatient code sets

Billing Type	Inpatient Setting		Outpatient Setting	
	Diagnosis	**Procedure/Supplies**	**Diagnosis**	**Procedure/Supplies**
Professional Reporting (doctor)	ICD-10-CM	CPT & HCPCS	ICD-10-CM	CPT & HCPCS
Facility Reporting (hospital)	ICD-10-CM	ICD-10-PCS	ICD-10-CM	CPT & HCPCS ICD-10-PCS

Keep in mind that because the codes used in each setting differ, it may be necessary to specialize in a certain type of coding. For example, a coder working in an inpatient facility setting should focus on ICD-10-PCS and ICD-10-CM coding, as well as CPT and HCPCS coding, which may also be used in some facilities; whereas a coder working in the professional setting should focus on ICD-10-CM, CPT, and HCPCS coding. This text provides training on all code sets.

Notice that inpatient and outpatient settings both use the ICD-10-CM code set to report diagnoses. The main difference between the codes used in these two settings are for procedures and supplies/services. Inpatient hospital services are billed using ICD-10-PCS codes. In the outpatient setting, CPT and HCPCS codes are used to bill for services provided to the patient during the outpatient encounter. Note that in figure 1.2, outpatient facility procedures (such as those provided by an outpatient hospital) may also use ICD-10-PCS codes for reporting purposes.

Key to Success

As you read through the chapters in this text, you will notice that the majority are centered around outpatient healthcare practices. This is because most healthcare services are provided in an outpatient setting, which utilizes three main code sets: ICD-10-CM, CPT, and HCPCS. Inpatient coding is discussed in chapter 20 (Inpatient Hospital Services), which covers ICD-10-PCS coding used in the inpatient setting and for facility reporting.

As a healthcare coder, it is important to be aware of the many professional organizations that help professionals within this field become further educated, maintain networking relationships, and keep up-to-date in the field, as well as offer coding certifications.

Professional Organizations and Coding Certifications

A **professional organization** is an association of individuals that is committed to furthering the interests of a particular profession. These organizations are an important part of the community of health information management professionals, as they offer not only educational training and resources, but also help define specific industry standards and job descriptions, stay abreast of changes within the industry, and offer networking and professional advice.

The **American Health Information Management Association (AHIMA)** is the premier worldwide association for health information management professionals. It is considered the leading source of knowledge within health information management and is a respected source of education and training for those within the profession (AHIMA 2017a). Belonging to a professional organization like AHIMA allows a coder to be on the cutting edge of developments in the profession and stay up to date with constantly changing code sets, coding guidelines, and important regulations that may impact the coding profession.

Becoming a member of any professional organization typically involves paying an annual or bi-annual membership fee, which allows access to the organization's many professional resources. For example, becoming a member of AHIMA allows access to the AHIMA Body of Knowledge (BoK), the *Journal of AHIMA* monthly publication, and discounts on AHIMA products such as books and certification exams. Membership also includes access to the AHIMA Engage community, an online forum where professionals can share advice, opinions, and expertise on health information management topics (AHIMA 2017b).

Certification is another important benefit offered by many professional organizations within health information management. A **coding certification** is a professional document of achievement given only to those coders who can demonstrate proficiency on a coding examination. Coding examinations range in scope, length, expense, and difficulty, but they all focus on the ability of an individual to identify and assign the correct diagnosis and/or procedure codes for coding and billing. Furthermore, many employers require certification for a coder to be eligible for certain coding positions. The **Certified Coding Specialist (CCS)** certification, offered by AHIMA, demonstrates a coder's ability to assign diagnosis and procedure codes, and knowledge of coding systems, medical terminology, disease processes, and pharmacology.

Once a credential is attained, a coder must stay up to date within his or her field of coding by attaining **continuing education units (CEUs)**. A CEU is a unit of measurement used in continuing education programs, and a certified coder must attain a certain number of CEUs each year to maintain his or her certification. For example, a coder with a CCS certification must attain 20 CEUs every two years (AHIMA 2017c). A continuing education program is any type of industry-specific training that offers specific instruction on a topic in the professional's field of expertise. It can be in the form of a short (one-hour) webinar, to a day- or weekend-long professional training conference, or even in the form of an industry newsletter or online training course. If the CEUs are not completed within the given time frame, the coder faces the risk of losing the certification. The means of obtaining a CEU can vary—from attending the annual AHIMA conference and seminars, watching webinars online, or completing quizzes on educational material. Each one of these learning experiences carries a specific amount of CEUs; for example, one CEU is achieved for a watching a coding webinar and answering a small quiz on the content. Once a CEU is earned, the learner gets a CEU certificate proving that he or she has earned the CEU. Not all certifications offered by professional health information management and billing and coding organizations are aimed specifically at coding. For example, AHIMA also offers certifications on healthcare administration, health data analysis, healthcare privacy and security, documentation improvement, healthcare technology, and healthcare informatics. This means that the opportunities within the field of healthcare are endless. Learning coding might just be one small step in the pathway to career success.

For a more comprehensive list of coding certifications and professional organizations, please refer to the appendix Coding Certifications and Professional Coding Organizations in this text.

Types of Healthcare Providers

In addition to understanding the various types of healthcare practices, it is important to understand the different types of healthcare providers. This includes the differences between healthcare providers and mid-level providers, as well as the differences between healthcare specialists and primary care physicians.

Healthcare Provider Types

A **healthcare provider** is a "physician or other qualified healthcare professional," and includes any individual "who is qualified by education, training, licensure/regulation (when applicable), and facility privileging (when applicable) who performs a professional service within his/her scope of practice and independently reports that professional service" (AMA 2018, xii). The term *healthcare practitioner* may also be used in lieu of *healthcare provider*, and the two may be used interchangeably.

The term *healthcare provider* is important to understand because it is more all-encompassing than the *physician* or *doctor*. A **physician** is a medical doctor who has completed post-doctoral medical training in his or her chosen specialty. However, physicians are not the only healthcare professionals that are qualified to provide services.

There are additional healthcare providers who are also trained, qualified, and licensed to provide healthcare services. These individuals are often referred to as **mid-level providers**, although they may prefer to be called "advanced practitioners" (Bishop 2012). Thus, a healthcare provider may be any of the provider types listed in table 1.1.

Table 1.1. Healthcare provider types

Physicians	Mid-Level Providers
Medical Doctor (MD)	Anesthesiologist Assistant (AA)
Doctor of Osteopathy (DO)	Certified Nurse Mid-Wife (CNM)
Doctor of Podiatric Medicine (DPM)	Certified Registered Nurse Anesthetist (CRNA)
Doctor of Optometry (OD)	Clinical Nurse Specialist (CNS)
Doctor of Dental Surgery (DDS)	Clinical Social Worker (CSW)
	Nurse Practitioner (NP)
	Physician Assistant (PA)
	Physical Therapist (PT)

As the healthcare industry changes, the amount of mid-level providers is increasing. As such, the healthcare setting in which you work will likely be billing for services provided by many provider types. For example, a small group practice may be comprised of two medical doctors (MDs), two nurse practitioners (NPs), and a certified nurse midwife (CNM).

Healthcare Specialists

Not only are there several types of providers and various workplace settings, there are also a great deal of different provider specialties. A **healthcare specialty** is a branch of healthcare practice in which a provider specializes after completing his or her residency after medical school. Healthcare specialties are typically divided among four possible areas: surgical or internal technique, body or organ system, diagnostic or therapeutic services, or the age of patients treated.

The first major division is between surgical versus internal medicine specialties. **Surgical specialists** treat and diagnose patients through major surgical techniques; for instance, exploratory abdominal surgery or nephrectomy (removal of a kidney). The major service performed by **internal medicine providers** is the establishment of a diagnosis and subsequent treatment without using surgical techniques, such as diagnosing strep throat and treating with antibiotics.

Other specialties are organ or body system based, as many healthcare conditions involve a specific organ or body system (for example, endocrinologists specialize in disorders of the endocrine system). Yet other specialties are centered around obtaining diagnostic information or a specific treatment method, such as physical therapy or radiation oncology. Other specialties are determined by the patient's age—typically pediatrics (patients from birth to age 18) or geriatrics (treating elderly patients). Within specialties, you will also find sub-specialties that combine two more general specialties; for example, a pediatric endocrinologist is a specialist who sees pediatric patients with disorders of the endocrine system.

This does not, however, mean that a patient can only be seen by one type of specialist. It is common for a patient to see a number of different specialists, according to his or her healthcare needs. For instance, a patient with end-stage renal failure (ESRD) who requires a kidney transplant might be managed by an internal medicine doctor, but the actual kidney transplant procedure will be completed by a surgical specialist.

Healthcare specialists are experts in their area of medicine, but may not be experts in all areas of medicine—which is why there is a distinction between healthcare specialists and general practitioners, also referred to as a **primary care provider (PCP)**. These healthcare providers are skilled in treating and diagnosing ailments of the entire body, as well as educated about parameters necessary to maintain health and procedures that measure health, such as mammograms and colonoscopies. PCPs provide preventive care and advice to patients in the form of annual physical examinations and health guidance, maintain the patient's comprehensive health record and history, and refer patients to specialists when necessary. Types of general practitioners include family practice providers, pediatricians (although these individuals treat a specific age group, they are regarded as PCPs because they treat the whole patient), and internal medicine providers. Obstetrics and gynecology (OBGYN) providers may also be considered primary care practitioners when they perform primary care services, although others may perform only specialist services. Examine table 1.2 to learn more about different specialty types.

Table 1.2. Types of healthcare specialties

	Provider Type	Description
Primary Care Providers: Provide whole healthcare, maintain patient health history, and perform preventive examinations and services	Pediatrician	Treats patients ages 0–18
	Family Practice	Treats patients from birth to elderly
	General Practitioner Adult Medicine Provider	Treats adult patients
	Internal Medicine	Specializes in the prevention and treatment of adult diseases
	Obstetrics and Gynecology Women's Health	Can act as a PCP for female patients
Specialty Providers: Specialize in a particular area of healthcare expertise, including diagnosis, management, and treatment	Holistic and Integrative Specialists	Specializes in whole-body health with an emphasis on holistic techniques, such as acupuncture
	Behavioral Health	Specializes in the mental health of patients, includes psychiatric services and addiction medicine
	Allergy/Immunology	Specializes in disorders of the immune system
	Anesthesiology and Pain Management	Specializes in anesthesia services and the treatment and management of pain
	Cardiology	Specializes in the diagnosis and treatment of the cardiovascular system; can be surgical, invasive, non-invasive, or specialize in treatment strategies
	Bariatric Surgery Burn-Trauma Surgery Cardiothoracic Surgery Colorectal Surgery General Surgery Hand Surgery Maxillofacial Surgery OB/GYN Surgery Orthopedic Surgery Orthopedics Foot and Ankle Surgery Orthopedics Hand Surgery Orthopedics Hip Surgery Orthopedics Knee Surgery Orthopedics Shoulder Surgery	Specializes in performing and developing surgical techniques for each respective body system or organ

Orthopedics Spine Surgery
Pediatric Surgery
Plastic and Reconstructive Surgery
Surgical Oncology
Thoracic Surgery
Transplant Surgery
Vascular Surgery

Therapy and Rehabilitation	Specializes in performing and developing therapeutic and rehabilitative services for patients and includes physical and occupational therapists and speech language pathologists
Laboratory and Pathology	Specializes in the testing or pathology and laboratory specimens
Obstetrics and Gynecology	Specializes in women's health, pregnancy, and childbirth and includes labor and delivery, maternal fetal medicine, fertility services, and midwife services
Neurology	Specializes in diagnosis and treatment of conditions affecting the neurological system
Orthopedics	Specializes in diagnosis and treatment of orthopedic conditions, such as fractures and osteoporosis
Dermatology	Specializes in the dermatological system (skin)
Geriatric Medicine	Specializes in geriatric medicine for elderly patients
Hematology and Oncology	Specializes in the detection, management, and treatment of blood conditions and malignancies; specialists within this field can sub-specialize in certain types of cancers and cancer treatments
Gastroenterology	Specialized in conditions affecting the gastrointestinal system
Radiology and Imaging	Specializes in the performance of either diagnostic or therapeutic radiology services, in addition to other types of imaging services such as ultrasounds or MRIs
Endocrinology	Specializes in ailments of the endocrine system, such as diabetes mellitus
Hospice and Palliative Care	Provides end-of life treatment for terminally ill patients
Infectious Disease	Specializes in the detection, treatment, and management of infectious diseases, such as HIV
Nephrology	Specializes in conditions affecting the kidneys
Ophthalmology Optometry	Specializes in the detection and treatment of eye conditions as well as vision services
Otolaryngology	Specializes in the ears, nose, and throat
Podiatry	Specializes in conditions affecting the feet
Rheumatology	Specializes in rheumatism, arthritis, and other disorders of the joints
Urology	Specializes in the urological system as well as the male reproductive system

If all healthcare providers can bill for services rendered, then why does it matter to discuss the differences between specialties and the distinction between specialists and primary care providers? The reasons are twofold. First, there are billing differences between PCPs and specialists, and usually a patient's insurance company requires a referral or a prior authorization from a PCP to a specialist before a patient can see the specialist (figure 1.3). The exact nature of this process depends on the patient's insurance company and plan, but it is important to understand this process because it will impact the ability to bill for services if you work in a healthcare specialist's office.

Figure 1.3. Healthcare referral process

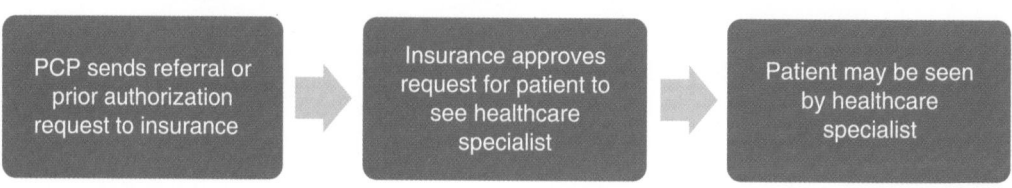

| PCP sends referral or prior authorization request to insurance | → | Insurance approves request for patient to see healthcare specialist | → | Patient may be seen by healthcare specialist |

The second reason why it is important to understand this difference is because a healthcare specialist only sees a certain set of healthcare conditions or only performs certain types of procedures, and the codes used in specialty offices are specific to that field. For example, a pediatrician sees a great number of sick patients and performs many well-being examinations and vaccinations, so coders in that pediatric office will be skilled at coding for sick visits, well-being examinations, and vaccinations. On the other hand, a cardiothoracic surgeon performs complex surgical procedures on the cardiothoracic system—such as a heart and lung transplants—so coders working in this specialty are skilled with those particular codes.

Taking this into account, this text contextualizes all coding training within a healthcare specialty. This helps beginning coders to consider a small selection of codes and begin to understand the connections between the procedure performed or service provided, as well as the reason(s) why the procedure was performed or the service was provided. For example, chapter 7 (Behavioral Health) presents the codes that are commonly reported for behavioral health services, such as psychotherapy and depression. Coding in the real world involves understanding the specific codes that are used within each specialty, understanding the unique billing circumstances or requirements for that specialty, and accurately reporting procedures and diagnoses according to coding guidelines. The subsequent chapters discuss the details of coding and billing for almost all specialty types, including primary care, durable medical equipment suppliers, ambulance suppliers, imaging centers, and laboratories.

End of Chapter Content

Instructions: Indicate whether the following statements are true or false (T or F). For false statements, rewrite the statement on the line below to make the statement true.

1. Working in different positions can help a beginning coder determine where he or she best fits within a healthcare organization.

_____

_____

2. An outpatient healthcare facility is also referred to as an acute-care setting.

_____

_____

3. An inpatient healthcare facility is also referred to as an ambulatory care setting.

_____

_____

4. Inpatient facilities include hospice, skilled nursing facilities, and rehabilitation hospitals.

_____

_____

5. Mid-level providers can bill for their services without being under the supervision of a licensed physician.

_____

_____

6. A nurse practitioner is one type of mid-level provider.

_____

_____

7. A surgical specialist treats the whole patient, including preventative medicine.

_____

_____

8. A pediatrician treats patients of all ages.

_____

_____

9. A dermatologist specializes in treating conditions of the skin.

_____

_____

10. An otolaryngologist may be referred to as an ENT (ear, nose, and throat) doctor.

_____

_____

Instructions: Choose the best answer.

1. Which of the following is an advantage of outsourcing to a billing or coding company?
   a. The provider's office must spend more money to get their claims paid.
   b. The provider's office has access to expert billers and coders.
   c. The billing and coding office is less skilled in coding than the provider's office.
   d. The provider's office must pay to have the billing company process their claims.

2. Which of the following might be one of your job responsibilities if you worked in a billing and coding company?
   a. Coding claims
   b. Taking vital signs
   c. Administering immunizations
   d. Prescribing medications

3. Which of the following types of practices has only one provider?
   a. Large group practice
   b. Ambulatory surgical center
   c. Solo practice
   d. Small group practice

4. Which of the following types of healthcare practices specializes in providing outpatient surgeries to patients?
   a. Emergency department
   b. Urgent care
   c. Inpatient hospital
   d. Ambulatory surgical center

5. Andres works in a group practice in which one third of the providers are pediatricians, one third are internal medicine doctors, and one third are cardiologists. In what type of healthcare practice does Andres work?
   a. Large single-specialty group practice
   b. Hospital
   c. Ambulatory surgical center
   d. Large multi-specialty group practice

6. Which of the following services would be provided by an outpatient healthcare practice?
   a. Vaccinations
   b. Open heart surgery
   c. Kidney transplant surgery
   d. Provider education and training

7. Which of the following codes sets is used to bill for inpatient facility procedures?
   a. ICD-10-CM
   b. ICD-10-PCS
   c. Hospital service codes
   d. CPT

8. Which of the following code sets is used to report diagnoses in both the inpatient and outpatient settings?
   a. ICD-10-CM
   b. ICD-10-PCS
   c. Hospital services codes
   d. CPT

9. Which of the following healthcare provider types is a mid-level provider?
   a. DO
   b. PA
   c. DDS
   d. DPM

10. What type of healthcare specialist would treat the patient's entire body, including providing health maintenance measures?
    a. An endocrinologist
    b. A primary care practitioner
    c. A healthcare specialist
    d. A mid-level provider

References

American Health Information Management Association. 2017a. Who We Are. http://www.ahima.org/about/aboutahima.

American Health Information Management Association. 2017b. AHIMA Engage. http://www.ahima.org/about/aboutahima.

American Health Information Management Association. 2017c. Recertification. http://www.ahima.org/certification/Recertification.

American Medical Association. 2018. *CPT 2018 Professional Edition*. Chicago: AMA.

Bishop, C. S. 2012. Advanced Practitioners Are Not Mid-Level Providers. https://www.ncbi.nlm.nih.gov/pmc/articles/PMC4093350/.

CHAPTER 2

Healthcare Billing Basics

Learning Objectives

- Examine the basic components of the Health Insurance Portability and Accountability Act (HIPAA) and their impact on healthcare operations.
- Examine the billing considerations for codes used in the healthcare setting, including different insurance and payer types and evaluate their billing rules and guidelines.

- Understand Hierarchical Condition Category (HCC) coding and its importance to the healthcare office.
- Understand performance measures and quality improvement and their importance to the healthcare office.

Key Terms

Accountable care organization
Accreditation
Administrative safeguards
Advanced beneficiary notice (ABN)
Business associates (BAs)
Capitation
Centers for Medicare and Medicaid Services (CMS)
Charge amount
Children's Health Insurance Program (CHIP)
CMS-1500
Coinsurance
Commercial insurance
Comorbidity
Complication
Computerized physician order entry (CPOE)

Confidentiality agreement
Copayment
Coverage limitations
Covered entities
Data analytics
Deductible
De-identified documentation
Electronic protected health information (e-PHI)
Employer-sponsored insurance
Encryption
Enforcement Rule
Entitlement health insurance
Fee schedule
Fee-for-service
Government-sponsored insurance
HCC coding
Health insurance exchange
Health Insurance Marketplace

Health Insurance Portability and Accountability Act (HIPAA)
Healthcare operations
Hierarchical Condition Category (HCC)
Individual insurance
Insurance policy
Insured party
Medicaid
Medical necessity
Medicare
Medigap
Minimum necessary
Noncovered services
Notice of Privacy Practices
Out-of-pocket expense
Patient Centered Medical Home (PCMH)

19

Payment

Performance measures

Per member per month (PMPM)

Physical safeguards

Premium

Prior authorization (PA)

Privacy Rule

Prospective payment system (PPS)

Protected health information (PHI)

Provider contracting

Quality improvement (QI)

Referral

Reimbursement

Risk adjustment

Risk analysis

Security Rule

Supplemental insurance

Technical safeguards

Third-party payer

Treatment

Treatment, payment, and healthcare operations (TPO)

TRICARE

UB-04

Worker's compensation insurance

In the healthcare industry, there are many rules, regulations, and guidelines that must be followed to ensure patient confidentiality, optimize insurance reimbursement, and confirm all services are documented and coded correctly. These rules and regulations are a fundamental part of ensuring that healthcare coders and billers are doing their job properly and legally. Some of these rules are governmental regulations, such as the Health Insurance Portability and Accountability Act (HIPAA); whereas others are specific to certain insurance carriers or third-party payers, such as the requirement to provide a Medicare patient with a written notice for a noncovered procedure. Yet other guidelines are built around risk adjustment, which determines the cumulative health risk of a patient population. Performance measures and quality improvement guidelines focus on a more health-centered model of patient care, rather than focusing on only the financial side of healthcare insurance reimbursement.

This chapter focuses on these regulations and guidelines, as they impact daily job functions and are a necessary part of understanding important concepts and practices within healthcare. In a billing and coding setting, these guidelines may outline the differences between how insurance claims are billed, identify nuances in coding for third-party payers, and discuss the impact of national and organizational programs in billing and coding, such as Hierarchical Condition Category (HCC) coding.

HIPAA and Confidentiality

In 1996, Congress passed the **Health Insurance Portability and Accountability Act**, otherwise known as HIPAA. HIPAA is the federal legislation enacted to provide continuity of health coverage, control fraud and abuse in healthcare, reduce healthcare costs, and guarantee the security and privacy of health information. It limits exclusion for pre-existing healthcare conditions, prohibits discrimination against employees and dependents based on health status, guarantees availability of health insurance to small employers, and guarantees renewability of insurance to all employees regardless of size. It also requires covered entities (most healthcare providers and organizations) to transmit healthcare claims in a specific format and develop, implement, and comply with the standards of the Privacy Rule and the Security Rule, as well as mandates that covered entities apply for and utilize national identifiers in HIPAA transactions (Public Law 104-191 1996).

HIPAA made sweeping changes throughout the US healthcare system. Although there was always a precedent of patient confidentiality within healthcare, HIPAA took this further by creating and enforcing strict guidelines regarding patient confidentiality. Before HIPAA was enacted, there was no federal law aimed at protecting the privacy of patients, and most confidentiality regulations were handled at a company- or state-wide level. After the implementation of HIPAA, privacy breaches or lack of patient confidentiality became punishable on a federal level. This places a great deal of emphasis on maintaining the privacy and integrity of patient information, including all healthcare and demographics information and claim data.

Healthcare practices must now proactively protect the confidentiality of their patients by following the guidelines set forth by HIPAA. However, not everyone is subject to HIPAA guidelines. Only covered entities and their business associates are held to these standards of confidentiality. These standards include the HIPAA Privacy, Security, and Enforcement Rules, as well as HIPAA confidentiality agreements.

Covered Entities and Business Associates

Before going into the specifics of HIPAA, it is important to understand what is protected under the provisions of HIPAA, as well as who is required to comply with HIPAA regulations.

HIPAA regulations specifically cover protected health information. **Protected Health Information (PHI)** is any health information that is individually identifiable, such as health records, laboratory reports, and patient healthcare history forms. PHI can be held on any type of media including paper, electronic, and orally transmitted information. This means that the Privacy Rule governs the confidentiality for all PHI that is handled in the office and includes

- Patient demographic data
- Information related to the patient's past, present, or future physical or mental health
- Information related to the provision of healthcare to the patient
- Information related to the payment (past, present, or future) for the provision of healthcare to the patient (OCR 2013a)

There are two main groups that deal with PHI, and thus must comply with HIPAA regulations—covered entities and business associates. HIPAA **covered entities (CEs)** deal directly with patient protected health information and are thus accountable for the integrity of the privacy afforded. Covered entities include healthcare plans, healthcare clearinghouses, and any healthcare provider who transmits patient health information in an electronic format.

On the other hand, **business associates (BAs)** provide services to or perform functions and activities on behalf of a covered entity, and have access to protected health information. These BAs include billing companies and entities that provide claims processing, data analysis, or utilization review. If a person or organization does *not* have access to protected health information, then they are not considered business associates and as such are not subject to HIPAA regulations.

HIPAA is composed of three rules that together keep all aspects of patient care confidential, and must be followed by covered entities and business associates. These three rules are the Privacy Rule, Security Rule, and Enforcement Rule.

HIPAA Privacy Rule

Published in December 2000, the HIPAA **Privacy Rule**—also known as the Standards for Privacy of Individually Identifiable Health Information—sets national standards for the protection of personal health information by covered entities, such as health plans and healthcare providers. This rule also enacted standards that allow individuals to understand and control how their personal health information is used. The main goal of the Privacy Rule is to secure the protection of patient health information while at the same time allowing that information to be utilized appropriately by covered entities and for public health services. In order to understand the Privacy Rule, it is essential to know what is included in PHI, such as individually identifiable health information like patient healthcare conditions, procedures performed or services provided, or patient insurance information. Privacy rules impact all staff members in the healthcare office or facility, including coders. For example, a coder working in a healthcare office accesses electronic health records via a user name and individual password, and cannot discuss patient information with anyone except other staff members in the healthcare office also involved in the patient's care.

There are many components of the HIPAA Privacy Rule that work together to safeguard the privacy of patient information and include protected health information; treatment, payment, and healthcare operations (TPO); the minimum necessary standard; and the HIPAA Notice of Privacy Practices (OCR 2013a).

Protected Health Information

Protected health information (PHI) includes common personal identifiers such as patient name, address, birth date, and Social Security Number, which are all pieces of individually identifiable information. However, records that have been properly de-identified may not be subject to strict Privacy Rule standards. In **de-identified documentation** all the aforementioned identifying characteristics have been removed. For example, an employment record with the employee's personal information— name, social security number, and date of birth—removed would be a de-identified employment record. A de-identified health record note containing patient health information but no identifying information (such as name or date of birth), is no longer considered PHI.

PHI may be released to the person who is the subject of the information, but release of this information to any other parties is strictly regulated. Included in these regulations is the treatment, payment, and healthcare operations (TPO) standard, which helps identify appropriate releases of PHI.

Treatment, Payment, and Healthcare Operations Standard

An integral component of the Privacy Rule is that some PHI must be used for certain purposes within the healthcare office and between certain parties. For example, how could an insurance company process a claim for a healthcare service if the healthcare provider was unable to release key information from the healthcare visit to them? Because of this need for specific information, the Privacy Rule allows for the use of PHI in treatment, payment, and healthcare operations.

The **treatment, payment, and healthcare operations (TPO)** standard of the Privacy Rule allows the use of protected health information for the following:

- **Treatment** refers to the provision, coordination, and management of a patient's healthcare and related services by that patient's healthcare providers. This includes consultation between providers regarding a patient and referral of the patient from one healthcare provider to another.
- **Payment** refers to the activities of the patient's health insurance plan to obtain premiums for health insurance, to determine coverage benefits, and to furnish payment for healthcare services delivered to a covered beneficiary. This also refers to the healthcare provider's activities related to obtaining payment for services rendered to the patient.
- **Healthcare operations** includes various services provided by healthcare practitioners during which patient PHI may be accessed and used. This includes case

management and coordination of care among multiple healthcare providers, participation in a heath record audit or healthcare review, evaluations of healthcare provider performance, and business planning and development.

TPO standards regulate when and to whom PHI may be shared or released, but fail to specify exactly what and how much of the health record can be released. The amount of records released is governed by the minimum necessary standard (OCR 2013a).

Minimum Necessary Standard

When a release of PHI is warranted and allowed, only the *minimum necessary* amount of PHI should be released. For example, if a general practitioner refers a patient to a plastic surgeon to revise a keloid scar, then only the parts of the health record pertaining to that scar and how it was caused should be released to the plastic surgeon. This is called the **minimum necessary** standard and it states that only the least amount of information needed for TPO may be released. Any information that is not directly related to the TPO may not be released. In this case, only the minimum necessary amount of PHI would be sent to the plastic surgeon's office because the plastic surgeon does not need to know the patient's entire health history. Rather, the plastic surgeon only needs to know about the health incidents surrounding that which he or she would be treating (in this case, records pertaining to the cause and healing status of the keloid scar).

When releasing PHI, an effective standard is to evaluate each portion of the PHI and determine if it is necessary for inclusion in the release, and to then justify the reasons why the information should be included. For example, if a health records technician is releasing the vaccination records for a patient to attend public school, then only the portion of the health record that tabulates vaccinations given to the patient should be provided. In this case, the health records technician has received a request to prove that the patient has been fully vaccinated. After searching through the health record and locating the vaccination records, she evaluates each part of the vaccination record to ensure the requested information is located on the record, such as the patient's identifying information (name and date of birth), and a list of vaccinations given to the patient and the date they were given. Any portions of this record that were not directly related to the vaccinations that the patient had been given (such as prior illness, injuries, or health encounters) would not be released. Instead of sending the entire health record, only the minimum necessary amount of information is given—in this example, *only* the one or two pages that list the vaccines the patient has received.

There are some exceptions to the minimum necessary standard, however. The minimum necessary requirement does not have to be met in the following circumstances:

- When requested by an authorized healthcare provider
- When requested by the individual who is the subject of the information, or their representative
- When disclosed to the Department of Health and Human Services for an investigation or complaint
- When required by law
- When required for compliance with HIPAA regulations (OCR 2013a)

Patients should be educated and informed regarding HIPAA regulations and when their PHI may or may not be used or released. This is accomplished using a Notice of Privacy Practices.

Notice of Privacy Practices

As a way of informing patients and other individuals about their privacy rights under HIPAA regulations, each covered entity must provide a Notice of Privacy Practices to each patient. This is a written description of the covered entity's privacy practices in regards to HIPAA, and must be signed and kept on record for each patient. Although individual covered entities are able to create their own notices, each Notice of Privacy Practices must contain certain elements as required by the Privacy Rule. Some of these items are listed as follows.

- It must inform patients of the ways in which the covered entity may use or disclose PHI.
- It must state the covered entity's duty to protect patient privacy.
- It must inform patients how to complain to the Department of Health and Human Services (HHS) if they believe that their privacy rights have been violated.
- It must include additional contact information for obtaining further information, as well as for making privacy complaints to the covered entity. (OCR 2013a)

In addition to the Privacy Rule, HIPAA also enforces two other important rules—the Security Rule and the Enforcement Rule.

Security Rule

The HIPAA Security Rule, also known as the Security Standards for the Protection of Electronic Health Information, regulates both the technical and nontechnical safeguards that organizations must put in place to keep electronic protected health information secure (OCR 2013b). Electronic protected health information (e-PHI) is essentially the same as PHI, except that it is stored or transferred in an electronic format, such as electronic health records (rather than paper health records). The Security Rule is a direct response of the transition from paper health records to electronic health records, and covers the numerous ways that electronic protected health information is put at risk. For example, healthcare providers use electronic health applications for computerized physician order entry (CPOE), or when a healthcare provider uses an electronic device (rather than paper) to record medication or treatment orders, electronic health records (EHR), and radiology, laboratory, and pharmacy applications. Healthcare insurance plans, on the other hand, provide electronic access to claims and eligibility information among other applications. While these electronic applications have the possibility to make the entire workforce more efficient, they present a number of potential security risks.

The main goal of the Security Rule is to protect e-PHI and to reduce the possibility of breaches of the information stored in e-PHI systems by creating and maintaining appropriate administrative, technical, and physical safeguards. Because healthcare organizations differ greatly in size, the Security Rule is designed to be flexible and scalable from the smallest one-physician office to a large, multi-specialty hospital or healthcare insurance plan. Covered entities can thus design security standards that are appropriate for their specific businesses, depending on their size and resources, as long as they

- Ensure the integrity, confidentiality, and availability of all their e-PHI
- Identify and protect their e-PHI against security threats
- Protect their e-PHI from unauthorized use or disclosure
- Ensure that their workforce is educated in and complies with all security standards regarding their e-PHI (OCR 2013b)

The Security Rule has three main components—administrative, physical, and technical safeguards—each of which are designed to protect the privacy and integrity of e-PHI. These safeguards require a number of different security standards, which affect coders in a number of different ways.

Administrative Safeguards

Administrative safeguards refer to the activities that a covered entity must perform in relation to the risks to e-PHI from an administrative perspective. Under HIPAA, administrative safeguards are administrative actions, policies, and procedures that manage the selection, development, implementation, and maintenance of security measures to protect e-PHI and to manage the conduct of the covered entity's or business associate's workforce in relation to the protection of that information (45 CFR 164.304). This includes risk analysis, which evaluates the likelihood of a security breach happening, and the impact that such a breach would have on the covered entity's e-PHI. Once all risks are identified and evaluated, appropriate security measures should be taken to address those risks and documentation should clearly identify all chosen security measures as well as the rationale for those measures. Furthermore, the covered entity must maintain all of its security precautions and review records on a regular basis to track and detect any e-PHI incidents, including identifying any additional new threats.

Physical Safeguards

Physical safeguards refer to physical restrictions created by the covered entity, which ensure the integrity of e-PHI. Under HIPAA, physical safeguards are Security Rule measures such as locking doors to safeguard data and various media from unauthorized access and exposures, including facility access controls, workstation use, workstation security, and device and media controls. The main provision of this is that a covered entity must limit physical access to its facility while at the same time allowing access only to authorized persons (45 CFR 164.304). For example, if the healthcare facility has an in-house server that holds all PHI, then this server should be located within a secure area that is only accessible to authorized persons. Covered entities should also implement policies and procedures for individual workstations to ensure that only authorized personnel can access and view the electronic media. These policies should also specify how e-PHI should be transferred, removed, disposed of, and reused.

Technical Safeguards

Technical safeguards refer to the policies and procedures that relate to ensuring the privacy and integrity of e-PHI from the technical side. Under HIPAA, technical safeguards are the technology and the policy and procedures for its use that protect e-PHI and control access so that only authorized persons can access the information (45 CFR 164.304). For example, a coder working in an online environment would have to log on to the company's secure system using a unique personal identifier or login name and password. Audit controls designed to record and examine access and other electronic activities within the e-PHI system must also be implemented. Integrity controls refer to policies and procedures employed to ensure that e-PHI is not improperly altered or destroyed. Finally, the covered entity must also ensure transmission security that guards against unauthorized access to e-PHI transferred over an electronic network. This is typically accomplished by using encryption, or data that has been transformed into unintelligible information that is unrecognizable without the correct key to translate the data.

The last HIPAA rule is the Enforcement Rule, which ensures that covered entities and business associates are held accountable for the provisions of HIPAA.

Enforcement Rule

The HIPAA **Enforcement Rule** contains provisions regarding compliance to HIPAA rules and regulations, investigations into breaches in privacy, and the imposition of monetary penalties for HIPAA violations. It also includes procedures for HIPAA violation hearings and the appeal process. The Enforcement Rule governs the activities of covered entities with respect to their cooperation in the enforcement process, and the actions that parties can take during compliance investigations and civil hearings and appeals (OCR 2013c). In other words, the Enforcement Rule specifies the fines and penalties that a covered entity would have to pay if a breach were to happen, and defines the legal process regarding investigations into HIPAA breaches.

HIPAA Confidentiality Agreement

Under the strict regulations put forth by HIPAA, patient confidentiality and the integrity of PHI is a forefront concern for many healthcare practices. It is important to understand all of the regulations as set forth by HIPAA, as well as the administrative, physical, and technical safeguards that are implemented by individual healthcare organizations. Coders must access the healthcare records and documentation of patient encounters with healthcare providers, as well as secured patient demographic and insurance information. As such, they are also required to be knowledgeable about HIPAA and to follow its many guidelines.

Many healthcare organizations deliver HIPAA training to their employees and have all employees sign a HIPAA **confidentiality agreement**—a legal document signed by the employee after HIPAA training that indicates the employee has been trained in aspects of HIPAA compliance and agrees to abide by the healthcare facility's measures taken to ensure HIPAA compliance. This agreement is kept on file to demonstrate HIPAA compliance and the facility's good faith measures to certify that all employees are educated in HIPAA compliance and specific measures taken by the facility to guarantee compliance.

Billing Considerations

There are more billing considerations than can be discussed in a single chapter, so this chapter includes a general overview of health insurance and discusses the basic components of how to bill a healthcare claim, including entering codes on a claim form, different types of third-party payers, varying methods of reimbursement, authorizations for services rendered, and advanced beneficiary notices. Billing considerations go hand-in-hand with coding considerations, and as such it is important to understand the different guidelines. Being a proficient coder is not just about selecting the right code; it is about understanding the many intricacies between the codes entered and the end goal of the claim, which is usually payment. Effective coding is about entering codes correctly on claims to optimize the reimbursement your practice or facility may receive from the healthcare claim.

Reimbursement, sometimes called payment, is the money that a healthcare practice or facility receives in return for providing a healthcare service to a patient. For example, reimbursement is the payment that a doctor's office receives for performing a routine physical examination, administering vaccinations, or performing a surgery. Reimbursement is also the money that a hospital receives for providing supplies and services, such as room and board, for a hospital patient. If a patient has healthcare insurance and the healthcare service provided was a covered service, then the insurance company will provide the reimbursement, minus any fees for which the patient is responsible. If the patient does not have health insurance, then he or she is responsible for all of the charges for the doctor's services and must pay the doctor's fees out of pocket (refer to chapter 1 for a discussion of health insurance).

In a real-world setting, new coders typically receive a run-down of specific best practices when abstracting and selecting codes for different insurance companies, insurance plans, and services rendered. These best practices may be printed out in the office's employee handbook, billing handbook, or simply on notes throughout the office, which are introduced to the new coder as necessary.

The first part of understanding how to correctly select codes and enter them on a claim is to learn the basics of the claim form itself. This section also discusses third-party payers, types of reimbursement for healthcare services, and authorizations, certifications, and referrals.

Healthcare Claim Forms

All codes are placed on a healthcare claim, which is then sent to the patient's health insurance company for reimbursement. A health insurance company is also referred to as a third-party payer. A **third-party payer** is a company or organization, other than the patient, that is liable for payment of the healthcare claim. The healthcare provider is the first party, and the patient is the second party. The most common third-party payer is a health insurance company. The type of claim that is used depends on where the patient was seen, either in the inpatient or the outpatient setting, as well as how the claim is billed. Although many insurance claims are now sent electronically, it is important to recognize the many different pieces of information that are included on a healthcare claim, which is best done by examining the CMS-1500 and UB-04 claim forms.

The **CMS-1500** form (figure 2.1) is the standard paper claim form to bill third-party payers in the professional, or physician outpatient setting. The CMS-1500 form was developed by CMS and is maintained by the National Uniform Claim Committee (NUCC). It was most recently updated in 2012 to include enough space for up to 12 diagnosis codes. Previously, the form only allowed enough room for four diagnosis codes. This allows healthcare offices to provide a greater amount of detail regarding the patient's diagnosis, and why the patient required treatment.

The **UB-04** form, also known as the CMS-1450 form (figure 2.2), is the standard paper claim form maintained by the National Uniform Billing Committee (NUBC) used to bill third-party payers in the facility inpatient setting. It may also be used to report services performed in the facility outpatient setting. This chapter will focus on entering codes on the CMS-1500 claim form, as the majority of this text discusses professional practitioner, supplier, and ambulance coding. Instructions on entering codes on the UB-04 claim form used for inpatient or facility billing will be found in chapter 20 (Inpatient Hospital Services).

There are three sections of the CMS-1500 claim form, which are divided by arrows pointing vertically on the right side of the page (figure 2.3). The top section is for "Carrier" information: the name of the third-party payer and the billing or claims address. The second section is "Patient and Insured Information," which contains identifying information for the patient and insured, including his or her basic demographics, and information about the insurance policy and coverage details such as insurance identification number, group number, and employer name. Other fields in this section are used to identify secondary insurance coverage and details about the claim.

For coding purposes, the most important section of the CMS-1500 claim form occupies the second half of the page, and is designated by the arrows that read "Physician

Figure 2.1. Sample CMS-1500 claim form

Source: CMS 2017b.

Figure 2.2. UB-04 claim form

Source: CMS 2017a.

Figure 2.3. Sections of the CMS-1500 form

Source: CMS 2017b.

or Supplier Information." This section of the claim form includes information that is specific to the services that were provided to the patient on the claim, such as

- Where the service was provided
- Important dates, such as hospitalization dates or dates unable to work

Figure 2.4. Box 21: Diagnosis or nature of illness or injury

21. DIAGNOSIS OR NATURE OF ILLNESS OR INJURY Relate A-L to service line below (24E)			ICD Ind.	
A. |_____	B. |_____	C. |_____	D. |_____
E. |_____	F. |_____	G. |_____	H. |_____
I. |_____	J. |_____	K. |_____	L. |_____

Source: CMS 2017b.

- ICD-10-CM diagnosis codes to represent medical necessity for the service provided
- Dates of service for the claim
- CPT and HCPCS codes to identify the actual service, procedure, or supply provided
- Modifiers to provide more information regarding the service provided
- Charges for individual services, and the number of units per service
- Provider identifying information, such as rendering provider and billing provider
- Additional service information

Each box of the CMS-1500 claim form is numbered so that individual areas may be easily referenced. Box 21 is where diagnosis codes are entered, and there is enough space for 12 individual diagnosis codes, on lines A through L (see figure 2.4). These diagnosis codes identify the medical necessity for the services provided. **Medical necessity** is the reason why a healthcare service or treatment is performed. The standards of medical necessity must be met in order for an insurance company to cover a healthcare service, so in order to be medically necessary a service must meet the accepted standards of medicine, and it must be used to prevent, treat, or diagnose an illness or injury, condition, or disease (or the symptoms thereof). In other words, a service or procedure must be medically necessary or it will not be paid for by the patient's insurance company. This medical necessity is identified by reporting up to 12 diagnosis codes on the healthcare claim.

One diagnosis code is entered per line. If there are more than 12 diagnoses for the claim, then they may be entered on additional claims forms, or only the 12 most important diagnoses are entered on the claim (and the additional diagnoses are left off of the claim). The specific diagnoses that should always be reported on the claim are the ones that are primarily responsible for the services provided, in addition to those that are required per ICD-10-CM guidelines. These 12 diagnoses should clearly identify the medical necessity for the procedures performed or the services provided. If more than 12 diagnoses are necessary, then additional claim forms may be added to include all additional diagnosis codes. Chapters 3 and 4 of this text provide additional information on how to select, assign, and sequence diagnosis codes to identify the medical necessity for a service. Additionally, diagnosis coding is discussed throughout the remaining chapters of this text within the context of specific healthcare specialties.

Procedure codes are entered in box 24.D (see figure 2.5). This box is where procedures, services, or supplies are reported (discussed in chapter 5) using the appropriate CPT/HCPCS procedure codes and up to four modifiers (introduced in chapter 5). There are six lines on the CMS-1500 claim form, so six individual procedures may be included on an individual claim form. If more than six procedures were performed, then additional claim forms may be added. This is usually done automatically by the

Figure 2.5. Box 24.A through 24.D

Source: CMS 2017b.

Figure 2.6. Box 21 through 30

Source: CMS 2017b.

billing system that is utilized to bill claims. When entering codes in the system, coders simply have to report all applicable procedure and diagnosis codes, and the system determines if an additional form is needed or not.

Each procedure code is attached to a charge so that when a procedure code is entered it includes a charge for the service rendered. When multiple procedure codes are entered, the total charge amount for all services is entered at the bottom of the claim—this is the total claim amount. On the other hand, diagnosis codes are not attached to charges, so entering additional diagnoses on the claim will not increase the charge amount for that claim.

Charges are entered in box 24.F on the CMS-1500 claim form. The total charges are entered in box 28. Figure 2.6 shows two procedure codes with charges: 99211 is attached to a $25.00 charge, and 85025 is attached to a $30.00 charge. The total for these charges together (the total claim amount) is $55.00, as listed in box 28, below the individually listed charges.

Box 24.G, to the right of box 24.F, identifies the amount of units for each charge. This is also an important component of the CMS-1500 form, as it identifies how many units of a specific procedure were performed. The example in figure 2.6, lists one unit of each performed procedure, meaning that each procedure was only performed once and is only being billed once (one unit). When an individual procedure code is billed more than once, the number of units should correspond to the number of times the procedure is being billed. For example, if the procedure identified by 85025 had been performed twice, then the number of units would be changed to two units.

Chapter 6 (Supplies and Services), chapter 7 (Behavioral Health), and chapter 10 (Urgent Care and Emergency Department Services) discuss additional areas of the

CMS-1500 claim form that are relevant to coders, such as box 24.B Place of Service, which identifies where the service was performed. As you read through this text, pay attention to these areas of the CMS-1500 form, as it is a necessary part of learning how to code. Coding is more than simply selecting the correct diagnosis and procedure codes; it is knowing how to place these codes correctly on a CMS-1500 (or UB-04) form and including all other necessary elements appropriate to bill a third-party payer.

Key to Success

As the healthcare industry changes, so does the CMS-1500 form, so do not be surprised if it changes again in the future. For example, the form used to only have enough room for four diagnosis codes; now it can hold 12! To keep abreast of changes and updates to the form, you can reference the NUCC website at http://www.nucc.org.

Third-Party Payers

A third-party payer, also known as the insurance carrier, is the party that pays for the healthcare claim when a patient has a health insurance policy. For example, if a patient who subscribes to a commercial insurance company presents to the office for treatment, then any charges for treating the patient will be sent on a healthcare claim to his or her third-party payer, the commercial insurance company. However, if the patient does not have any healthcare insurance coverage, then the claim will be paid directly by the patient. Any payments that come directly from the patient are referred to as **out-of-pocket expenses**, or patient responsibility amounts.

In its most basic form, health insurance protects high out-of-pocket costs to the patient, who pays a **premium**—a monthly charge to keep the insurance policy active for coverage—in return for the insurance company paying for any healthcare services that the patient receives. For example, a patient pays a monthly premium for health insurance, which covers the cost of healthcare services for the patient, such as a sick visit to the doctor, a surgery, an x-ray, or any laboratory or pathology tests. This is similar to automobile insurance—an individual pays a monthly amount (premium) to an auto insurance company that covers any costs incurred in the case of an accident or other expense (barring mechanical expenses). So in the same way that car insurance pays to fix a person's car if he or she gets in an accident, health insurance pays for the healthcare expenses when a patient goes to the doctor.

It is not quite this simple, however. There are many different aspects of this relationship that govern to which healthcare practitioners and facilities the patient must go, what healthcare services will be covered by the insurance, and how much the patient must also pay for the healthcare service. These differences depend on the patient's type of insurance plan, and the policy and coverage limitations. **Coverage limitations** refer to the services that an insurance plan will pay for (cover) when they are provided by a healthcare practitioner, as well as what services will not be covered and classified as the patient's out-of-pocket charges.

There are hundreds of different insurance plans, both commercial and government-sponsored, so it is impossible to address features of all policies here, but it is important to understand the basic types of insurance plans and the relationship between insurance plans and reimbursement. There are two main divisions in insurance plans—commercial and government sponsored. Nontraditional insurance is an additional insurance type, which may be used to cover healthcare expenses.

Commercial Insurance

Commercial insurance plans are run by for-profit companies, which are not government entities, and require a monthly premium in return for healthcare coverage. Examples of these companies include Blue Cross Blue Shield Association, United Healthcare, Kaiser Permanente, and Cigna.

Each health insurance company offers different insurance policies. An **insurance policy** is a formal contract between an individual and the insurance company. The **insured party**, otherwise known as the policy holder, is the individual who is the primary benefit holder on the insurance policy. This policy defines many things, including

- Covered healthcare expenses for which the insurance company will pay
- The exact terms under which the insurance will pay for a healthcare expense
- The duration of coverage
- The premium amount
- Patient out-of-pocket expenses
- Plan maximums and any other limitations

If more than just one individual is covered by the insurance policy, then this contract will also identify all others covered by the policy, as well as specific coverage and patient responsibility amounts. For example, if the insured party pays premiums for additional family members—such as spouse and children—then the health insurance policy will identify these additional benefit holders and specify how they are covered by the policy.

Premiums for commercial plans are paid in several different ways, but the two most common are employer-sponsored or individual plans. **Employer-sponsored insurance** plans are those offered by an employer to eligible employees within the organization. This results in many people signing up for the same plan so the premiums are typically lower as more people are buying into the plan, and there are fewer coverage limitations such as noncovered services or high out-of-pocket amounts (addressed in the following sections). The employer traditionally pays a portion of the health insurance premiums, which reduces the premium amount the individual must pay for coverage.

Individual insurance plans are purchased by an individual who does not go through an employer to attain coverage. In today's changing world of health insurance coverage, in addition to purchasing coverage through an employer-sponsored plan, individuals may now purchase an individual plan through a government-run health insurance exchange. This **health insurance exchange** allows insurance companies to offer health insurance plans to individuals who must pay premiums for coverage. However, if the patient does purchase health insurance coverage through an exchange, and if he or she qualifies financially, the government may provide the patient with a subsidy to help pay for the premiums. It is important to understand that even though this healthcare exchange was created and is overseen by a government agency (either by the federal or state government), it is not government-sponsored insurance. The insurance companies offering coverage on the exchanges are for-profit commercial entities, and the policies offered require patient out-of-pocket expenses and premiums paid for coverage.

Commercial insurance plans typically share costs with the patient by requiring certain out-of-pocket expenses depending on the service provided, as specified by the insurance policy. This means that they require the patient to pay for an amount of services provided, depending on the patient's policy. Usually if the patient has a plan with higher premiums, then he or she gets the benefit of lower out-of-pocket expenses.

There are four main types of patient responsibility: copayments, deductible, coinsurance, and noncovered services.

Copayment

A copayment, or copay, is an amount of money that the patient is responsible for paying to the healthcare provider before he or she may be seen. For example, if a patient has a $30 copayment on his or her policy for office services, then the patient must pay $30 to the doctor's office before being seen. Copayment amounts depend on the healthcare setting as well as the type of service provided. For example, emergency department copays are typically much larger (such as $150) because the service is expected to be more expensive. The type of service also affects the copayment amount. For example, according to federal regulations insurance companies must cover preventive services such as routine examinations and specific vaccinations at 100 percent, meaning that patients do not have to pay anything out of pocket for these services (Healthcare.gov 2017). In this case, if the patient presented to his doctor's office for a routine examination, he would not have to pay his copay amount.

Deductible

A deductible is a preset amount that must be paid in full before insurance benefits will begin. Deductibles can range from a few hundred to many thousands of dollars, depending on the insurance policy. For example, Patient A may have an employer-sponsored group insurance plan with a $750 deductible, whereas Patient B has an individual health insurance plan through a healthcare exchange with a $6,000 deductible. No matter what the amount is, no insurance benefits will be paid until the patient pays the full deductible amount (out of the patient's pocket). If Patient A is seen for any type of healthcare services, she will have to pay $750 out of her own pocket before any additional charges will be paid by her insurance company. The same goes for Patient B—even though his deductible is much larger, it still works in the same manner. He will have to pay $6,000 out of his own pocket before his insurance plan will pay for any additional charges.

Deductibles are reset at the end of each benefit year, meaning that the amount paid into the deductible each year also resets. For example, if Patient A had met her $750 deductible (meaning she had paid $750 out of pocket for services provided) in the benefit year 2018 (January 1, 2018 to December 31, 2018), then this amount would reset to $750 for the new benefit year (January 1, 2019 to December 31, 2019). She would have to pay another $750 in 2019 before any benefits would be paid by her insurance company.

Coinsurance

Coinsurance refers to a category of patient responsibility that is based on a percentage of allowed amount. An allowable amount is the amount of money that an insurance policy allows to be paid for a specific procedure code. The allowable amount and the actual charge sent by the healthcare office for the procedure (as indicated in box 24.F of the CMS-1500 form) often do not correspond. For example, a healthcare office may charge $200.00 for procedure code 10022, Fine needle aspiration, with imaging guidance, but the allowable amount is only $170.23. This means that the insurance only *allows* $170.23 to be paid for procedure code 10022, no matter how much the healthcare office charges for it.

Coinsurance amounts kick in after any copayments or deductibles have been paid, and do not have a limit nor do they reset at the end of each benefit year. They are typically referred to by their percentage amounts. For example, if a patient has an 80/20 coinsurance, then this means that the insurance company will pay for 80 percent of the allowable amount, and the patient will be responsible to pay for 20 percent of the allowable amount. If Patient A has an 80/20 coinsurance on her plan, and the allowed amount of the doctor's charges equal $100, then her insurance will pay $80 and she will have to pay $20 for the service. As previously mentioned, coinsurance amounts do not reset and there is no limit to the coinsurance like the deductible, so the amount paid will greatly depend on the charge for the service provided. If Patient A was seen in the hospital and the allowed amount added up to $10,000, then her insurance would have to pay $8,000 and she would have to pay $2,000.

It is important to understand that patients may have all three types of patient responsibility amounts on their coverage. Patient A might have a copayment for services rendered, a deductible, and a coinsurance. This means that she must pay a copay before being seen by a healthcare provider. If she has not met her deductible for that benefit year, then she must pay for all of the doctor's charges before her insurance will pay anything. Furthermore, even after she has met her deductible and paid her copay, she will still have to pay her coinsurance amount.

Noncovered Services

There is one more category of charges that falls onto patient responsibility, or out-of-pocket expenses—noncovered services. Noncovered services are services that are specifically excluded from coverage per the insurance policy. This means that the service will not be covered (paid for) by the patient's health insurance, no matter what. For example, if Patient A is seen at her physician's office and receives a vision screening, but vision services are not covered on her policy, then the insurance will not pay for the charge vision screening charge. This noncovered service will be transferred to the patient's responsibility, meaning that Patient A will have to pay for the entire cost of the vision screening. Figure 2.7 illustrates the four types of patient responsibility.

Government-Sponsored Insurance

Government-sponsored insurance is a type of entitlement health insurance coverage that is provided by the government. Government-sponsored insurance is managed at either the state or federal level or a combination of both, depending on the type of insurance. Entitlement health insurance is a type of coverage for which individuals must be eligible based on certain criteria. What this means is that government health

---

Figure 2.7. Types of patient responsibility

Types of Patient Responsibility

Copayment: A set amount of money that a patient must pay their medical provider before they may be seen

Deductible: An amount that must be paid in full before insurance benefits will begin

Coinsurance: A category of patient responsibility that is based on a percentage of allowed charges

Noncovered Service: A service that is specifically excluded from coverage per the insurance policy insurance plans are not offered to everyone; rather they are provided only to individuals who meet the eligibility criteria for coverage. Some of these plans are offered free of charge, so the insured does not have to pay premiums or out-of-pocket expenses. Others are offered with smaller premiums than commercial plans and with a varying level of patient out-of-pocket expenses.

The federal and individual state governments also run a variety of health programs including health insurance plans. These include the Veterans Health Administration (VHA) and Indian Health Services (HIS), among others. The three main types of government-sponsored entitlement health insurance plans are Medicare, Medicaid, and TRICARE.

Medicare

Medicare is a federal health insurance plan for individuals who are age 65 or older, individuals with disabilities, and those with end-stage renal disease (ESRD). Medicare is unique because it is funded by federal funds and individual plan premiums that are paid by plan enrollees. In return, Medicare health insurance plans share costs with enrollees by requiring copayments, deductibles, and coinsurance amounts that differ depending on the type of coverage the patient has. Medicare is also strict about covered versus noncovered services, as there are many healthcare supplies and services that are not covered by Medicare. These include long-term (or custodial) care, dentures and most dental care, eye examinations, and certain supplies or products such as hearing aids (Medicare.gov 2017a). When a service is likely noncovered by Medicare, it may be necessary to complete an advanced beneficiary notice, as described later in this chapter.

Medicare is managed by the Centers for Medicare and Medicaid Services (CMS), a federal organization that administers Medicare, Medicaid, the Children's Health Insurance Program (CHIP), and the Health Insurance Marketplace (the federal online health insurance exchange that allows individuals to purchase insurance plans offered by commercial companies). CMS is an important organization, as they administer both Medicare and Medicaid and in doing so set the standard for what many health insurance companies cover and consider medically necessary. The CMS website is a great resource for coders, billers, and healthcare information management professionals, as it also provides official information and education on topics that are important to the healthcare industry, such as HIPAA training (CMS 2014).

Advanced Beneficiary Notices

It is important to understand the difference between insurance companies and what they do or do not cover, as the majority of all payments in the healthcare office come from health insurance payments on claims for covered services. A coder needs to know what specific services a person's health insurance may or may not cover and ensure payment for that service. This is especially important in the case of Medicare, which may or may not cover specific services depending on coverage determinations and medical necessity.

In questionable circumstances, it may be necessary to issue an advanced beneficiary notice (ABN), a form issued to Medicare patients to inform them that a service might not be covered (that is, paid) by Medicare (see figure 2.8). An ABN is used only when a healthcare provider is furnishing an item or providing a service that is usually paid for by Medicare, but might *not* be covered in this specific instance. It also gives the patient the option of either refusing the service or agreeing to pay for the service if Medicare does not pay. The ABN is an important way of allowing patients to make an informed decision on their healthcare and the costs that may be incurred due to services performed. In

Figure 2.8. Advanced beneficiary notice (ABN)

A. Notifier:

B. Patient Name: **C. Identification Number:**

Advance Beneficiary Notice of Noncoverage (ABN)

NOTE: If Medicare doesn't pay for **D.**_____ below, you may have to pay.
Medicare does not pay for everything, even some care that you or your health care provider have good reason to think you need. We expect Medicare may not pay for the **D.**_____ below.

D.	E. Reason Medicare May Not Pay:	F. Estimated Cost

WHAT YOU NEED TO DO NOW:
- Read this notice, so you can make an informed decision about your care.
- Ask us any questions that you may have after you finish reading.
- Choose an option below about whether to receive the **D.**_____ listed above.
  Note: If you choose Option 1 or 2, we may help you to use any other insurance that you might have, but Medicare cannot require us to do this.

G. OPTIONS: Check only one box. We cannot choose a box for you.
☐ **OPTION 1.** I want the **D.**_____ listed above. You may ask to be paid now, but I also want Medicare billed for an official decision on payment, which is sent to me on a Medicare Summary Notice (MSN). I understand that if Medicare doesn't pay, I am responsible for payment, but **I can appeal to Medicare** by following the directions on the MSN. If Medicare does pay, you will refund any payments I made to you, less co-pays or deductibles.   ☐ **OPTION 2.** I want the **D.**_____ listed above, but do not bill Medicare. You may ask to be paid now as I am responsible for payment. **I cannot appeal if Medicare is not billed**.   ☐ **OPTION 3.** I don't want the **D.**_____ listed above. I understand with this choice I am **not** responsible for payment, and **I cannot appeal to see if Medicare would pay.**

H. Additional Information:

This notice gives our opinion, not an official Medicare decision. If you have other questions on this notice or Medicare billing, call **1-800-MEDICARE** (1-800-633-4227/**TTY:** 1-877-486-2048).
Signing below means that you have received and understand this notice. You also receive a copy.

I. Signature:	J. Date:

CMS does not discriminate in its programs and activities. To request this publication in an alternative format, please call: 1-800-MEDICARE or email: AltFormatRequest@cms.hhs.gov.

According to the Paperwork Reduction Act of 1995, no persons are required to respond to a collection of information unless it displays a valid OMB control number. The valid OMB control number for this information collection is 0938-0566. The time required to complete this information collection is estimated to average 7 minutes per response, including the time to review instructions, search existing data resources, gather the data needed, and complete and review the information collection. If you have comments concerning the accuracy of the time estimate or suggestions for improving this form, please write to: CMS, 7500 Security Boulevard, Attn: PRA Reports Clearance Officer, Baltimore, Maryland 21244-1850.

Form CMS-R-131 (Exp. 03/2020)   Form Approved OMB No. 0938-0566

Source: CMS 2017c.

other words, it is a way of protecting the patient from unknown healthcare expenses, as well as giving patients transparent information about their healthcare costs.

Some instances when an ABN should be issued include when

- Medicare may not pay for an item or service
- Medicare usually pays for the item or service
- Medicare is expected to deny the payment because the service or item is not considered medically reasonable and necessary

An ABN is an important part of understanding the link between properly documented, reported, and coded services and the payment for such services, because it shows how the services reported with procedure codes must match the reason why those services were rendered (as identified by the diagnosis codes). The insurance still might not pay for the service whether or not these codes align, in which case an ABN would be necessary. This is just one example of how coding cannot be removed from billing, as it is integral to ensuring payment of claims. As such, many sections of this text discuss the billing implications of coding (such as ABNs), to create a more comprehensive+ view of coding in the real world.

Medicaid

Not to be confused with Medicare, **Medicaid** is a government-sponsored entitlement health insurance program for individuals and families with little or no resources. This means that a family of four living at the poverty line can qualify for Medicaid for the entire family, which will cover healthcare expenses for all eligible individuals within the family (Medicaid.gov 2017). Medicaid eligibility requirements and specific income amounts are set by each individual state, and so they vary from state to state depending on the amount of resources allocated to the Medicaid program. Therefore, a family of four living in New Mexico may find that they are eligible for Medicaid for the entire family, including the adults, whereas that same family living in Texas may find that only the children are eligible for Medicaid coverage.

The Medicaid program is unique in that it is not necessary to pay insurance premiums in return for health insurance coverage, and there are no patient out-of-pocket expenses. It is also unique in that it is jointly funded and run by both the federal and state governments. Though what may be covered in one state may not be covered in another state, and the eligibility requirements may vary from state-to-state.

The **Children's Health Insurance Program (CHIP)** is a program that is similar to Medicaid, and covers children in families that are low income but are not low enough to qualify for Medicaid coverage. For example, if the family has a low income but not low enough for the entire family to qualify for Medicaid, then only the children (and not the adults) may be eligible for coverage under CHIP. Depending on the families' resources and income level and the state in which the individuals live, the CHIP program may require a modest premium as well as low patient out-of-pocket expenses. For example, the annual CHIP premium may be less than $50, and requires $5 to $35 copayments at the time services are rendered (Texas HHS 2017).

Key to Success

Although they sound alike, do not confuse Medic*are* with Medic*aid*. They are both government-sponsored health insurance programs administered by CMS, but Medicare is for the elderly, disabled, and those with ESRD, and Medicaid is for those with low income and few resources.

TRICARE

TRICARE is a government-sponsored entitlement health insurance plan administered by the United States Defense Health Agency (DHA). It is a federally run health insurance plan, separate from both Medicare and Medicaid. TRICARE provides health insurance coverage for individuals that are part of the US armed forces and their dependents. This includes uniformed members of the Army, Navy, Marines, Air Force, Coast Guard, Public Health Service, and the National Oceanic and Atmospheric

Administration (NOAA). Recipients of TRICARE insurance may or may not have to pay premiums for coverage and/or out-of-pocket expenses, depending on the member's type of service, status, and enrollment plan. Those in active status typically do not have to pay premiums for coverage nor out-of-pocket expenses, whereas their dependents on the insurance coverage may have to pay modest amounts for services, such as a $12 copayment. TRICARE also covers retirees of the US Armed Forces, who must pay an inexpensive annual premium as well as modest out-of-pocket expenses. For example, the annual TRICARE health insurance premium for a family of four may be less than $1,000 (TRICARE 2017).

Nontraditional Insurance

In addition to commercial and government-sponsored insurance plans, there are a few different types of insurance coverage that will cover healthcare expenses. In order to be covered by one of these plans, patients have to either pay a premium or meet some other type of eligibility requirement. Coverage for claims under the following policies varies depending on the reason for treatment and the type of coverage the patient has, as well as other factors. For example, an automobile insurance plan may cover up to $25,000 of eligible healthcare expenses. So if a car accident resulted in an injury, then the automobile insurance would cover up to $25,000 of the healthcare expenses related to that injury.

It is important to be aware of these nontraditional insurance types, as the biller needs to send the claim for healthcare services to a different insurance company and may also require additional codes on the healthcare claim to identify the extenuating circumstances surrounding the accident or injury. These extenuating circumstances are reported using external cause codes, which identify the manner in which the injury occurred, place of occurrence, activity in which the patient was engaged when the injury occurred, and the patient's status when the injury occurred (such as work, volunteer, or leisure activity status). External cause codes are diagnosis codes and are introduced in chapter 4.

These nontraditional insurance types include worker's compensation, automobile and homeowner's insurance, and supplemental insurance policies.

Worker's Compensation

Worker's compensation insurance is a type of insurance that covers injuries and illnesses that were suffered by a patient while on the job. Worker's compensation is a bit different than either commercial or government-sponsored insurance plans because the patient neither has to pay an insurance premium nor meet some sort of eligibility criteria. Worker's compensation insurance is provided to the patient by his or her employer. In this case, the employer pays the premiums to the insurance company, to cover any healthcare expenses for his or her employees.

Although it varies from state to state, company size, and number of employees, employers are required to cover the healthcare expenses for any employee that suffers a work-related illness or injury. For example, if an employee working as a construction worker was injured by a forklift while doing his job, then the healthcare expenses incurred by this injury would be covered by worker's compensation insurance. In addition to healthcare expenses, worker's compensation may also provide the patient with money to help cover the costs of being out of work because of the injury or due to any disability that may result from the injury. Furthermore, if the employee suffers a fatal accident, worker's compensation may provide financial compensation to his or her survivors. These additional disability or survivor benefits may be funded by the state in which the patient lives.

There are many required forms, healthcare examinations, and updates that are required in worker's compensation claims. Also, the type of worker's compensation coverage greatly depends on the state in which the injury occurred, the type of employer, and specifics surrounding the way in which the injury or illness occurred. Because of these complicated details, worker's compensation claims are usually managed by agencies that deal specifically with worker's compensation and they sometimes employ healthcare providers solely to provide worker's compensation examinations and evaluations.

Automobile and Homeowner's Insurance

Most people are familiar with automobile insurance. This type of insurance covers damage to your vehicle or another's vehicle in the case of a motor vehicle accident. It works similarly to health insurance, in that individuals must pay a premium in return for coverage and the insurance company shares the expenses with the individual through deductibles. Homeowner's insurance is also a familiar type of insurance, except this insurance covers damage to an individual's home. For example, if a person's home is damaged by a fire, then the homeowner's insurance will pay the owner of the policy a predetermined amount to help cover the costs of lost or damaged personal items, to repair the structure, or to purchase new appliances.

Both auto and homeowner's insurance will also cover the costs of healthcare claims in certain circumstances. For example, Patient A was driving her vehicle and texting on her cell phone when Patient B pulled out in front of her. Patient A collided with B's car, resulting in a whiplash injury for Patient B and damage to both vehicles. In this case, the motor vehicle accident (MVA) was cause by Patient A, so her auto insurance will pay for the claims to repair both vehicles, and she will have to share some of these costs by paying her deductible amount. Furthermore, the healthcare provided to Patient B will also be covered by Patient A's auto insurance. So in this case, her car insurance is paying for a healthcare claim.

Homeowner's insurance my also pay for healthcare services in certain circumstances. For example, Patient A was spending time at Patient B's house when she slipped on the stairs exiting the residence and fractured her ankle. Patient A may choose to file a claim for her injuries through Patient B's homeowner's insurance, which will pay for her healthcare claims.

Supplemental Insurance

Supplemental insurance plans are also important to understand, as they may impact the patient's ability to pay for healthcare services and healthcare administrative personnel may need to help patients by providing CMS-1500 forms for healthcare services or other proof of healthcare services rendered.

Supplemental insurance policies help patients pay the out-of-pocket expenses related to healthcare. For example, if a patient with a high-deductible health insurance plan is injured in a recreational football game accident, his healthcare expenses are covered by his regular health insurance company but he is still responsible for the charge amount sent to his deductible. In this case, if the patient had a supplemental accident insurance policy, then the supplemental insurance could help him pay for his deductible. Supplemental insurance policies differ depending on the type of insurance offered and the specifics of coverage. They range from accident coverage (as in the previous example), coverage for cancer treatments, coverage for disabilities only, or for coverage of a specific set of healthcare services or treatments. Supplemental insurance plans are typically low cost, and patients can pick and choose which type of coverage they prefer and tailor coverage to their specific needs. These plans act as an umbrella, in that they help cover the patient from the financial burdens for which he or she may be responsible in the case of a healthcare emergency or unplanned treatment.

One example of a commercial supplemental accident insurance policy is that offered by Aflac. An individual must subscribe to an Aflac policy by paying monthly premiums and, in return, Aflac reimburses the patient a specified amount of money if he or she suffers a certain type of accidental injury. For example, Patient A has an Aflac policy that covers accidental injuries, including fractures. Patient A just suffered a fractured ankle, for which Aflac will pay the patient $500. The patient sends in a claim to Aflac with information regarding the injury and Aflac sends the patient the funds that correspond to each specific injury (or service performed to treat the injury). This money can be used to cover the cost of the healthcare service as well as any other financial obligations that Patient A may have incurred due to the injury, such as out-of-pocket expenses, income lost from time out of work, or costs spent traveling to and from healthcare appointments (Aflac 2017).

Another common supplemental insurance is **Medigap**, a policy that is specifically for Medicare beneficiaries. It is designed to "fill the gap" left by patient out-of-pocket expenses such as copayments, deductibles, and coinsurance amounts. Unlike Medicare, Medigap policies are not run by the government. Instead, they are offered by commercial insurance companies specifically to cover the gaps in Medicare coverage, which result in patient balances that are not payable by Medicare. For example, if a Medicare patient also has a Medigap plan, then this plan can help pay for noncovered services such as the deductible and coinsurance amounts left over after the claim is paid by Medicare. In order to obtain Medigap coverage, individuals must pay a monthly premium to the commercial insurance company for coverage. Like all supplemental insurance plans, Medigap will not cover all fees, but only those fees and remaining amounts as specified in the Medigap policy.

Medigap and traditional supplemental insurance policies (like Aflac) differ in that Medigap is administered by an actual health insurance company, whereas Aflac is not. Healthcare claims are sent directly to Medigap policies for payment just like a regular health insurance claim (after the primary insurance pays their share), whereas Aflac only requires proof of the patient's diagnosis or treatment. In this case the healthcare office may have to provide a CMS-1500 claim form or complete an Aflac form so the patient can submit this proof to his or her supplemental insurance plan for payment. Review examples of the different types of third-party payers in figure 2.9.

Figure 2.9. Third-party payers

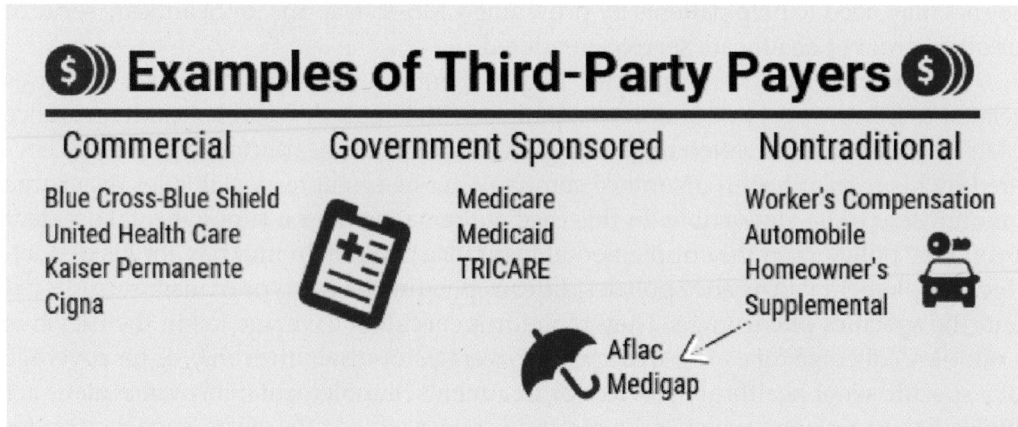

In addition to the varying kinds of insurance plans, there are forms of reimbursement for healthcare services that differ depending on a number of factors, including the healthcare setting and the way in which the healthcare provider has contracted with the insurance company. The three most common reimbursement types are fee-for-service, capitation, and prospective payment.

Reimbursement Types

As previously discussed, reimbursement for healthcare services occurs when an insurance company pays a healthcare provider for a service rendered. There are different forms of reimbursement, which vary from inpatient and outpatient settings, provider type, and ways in which the healthcare provider has contracted with the insurance company. In order for a doctor to be able to send a healthcare claim for payment to any insurance company, he or she must be fully contracted with the patient's insurance company. For example, if Dr. Alameda sees a patient with Effective Eagle Insurance, then in order for Dr. Alameda to send a claim to Effective Eagle and get paid for any healthcare services rendered to the patient, she must be contracted with Effective Eagle. **Provider contracting** is when the insurance company and the healthcare provider come into an agreement so that when the healthcare provider delivers healthcare services to patients, the insurance company will provide reimbursement for the healthcare services provided. The contract signed by both parties defines important terms, informs each party of their rights and responsibilities to each other and to the patient, and defines the payment for services performed.

In the outpatient setting, the two most common ways in which the payment can be made are either by fee-for-service or through capitation. Prospective payment systems are used in the inpatient or facility setting to determine the amount of payment before the patient receives healthcare services.

Fee-for-Service

Fee-for-service reimbursement is separately reporting and billing each procedure, treatment, or item performed by the healthcare provider (namely, one fee for each service) on the claim for the healthcare service. For example, if a primary care provider performs a sick visit examination, then he reports the sick visit examination and may choose to set the fee for that particular service at $75. On the other hand, the fee for a wart removal may be $110. Each service has a different fee, as determined by the work, risk, overhead, and skill involved in that service. The dollar amount charged for each service is referred to as the **charge amount**.

Typically, insurance companies do not pay the full charge amount. Rather, they pay the amount that is predetermined in the fee schedule agreed upon during provider contracting. A **fee schedule** is a list of dollar amounts that the insurance company will pay for services performed by the healthcare provider. This is done either with a percentage amount (such as 70 percent of all charges) or by setting individual amounts for each particular service performed. In this more common scenario, the healthcare practitioner provides the insurance company with a list of commonly performed procedure codes, the insurance company specifies fee amounts per procedure code, and the two parties negotiate on the fee amounts until they reach an agreement.

Fee-for-service is the common type of reimbursement in the outpatient setting. It is based solely on the procedure codes that were billed for the services rendered, each of which must be supported with diagnosis codes to represent the medical necessity for the service. A less commonly used form of reimbursement is capitation, which does not rely on the individual procedure codes sent for each healthcare service.

Capitation

Capitation is a reimbursement type in which an insurance company pays a healthcare provider a set dollar amount each month for each patient. This per member per month payment (PMPM)—the amount paid per patient each month—is defined in the provider contract, as well as other stipulations regarding payments and claims requirements. Capitation plans also require that the patients select and see their primary care physician, who is the recipient of the capitation plan payment.

In capitation, the insurance company makes the payment to the healthcare provider each month, whether or not the patient is seen by the provider. When the patient does present for treatment, the provider cannot bill this service for reimbursement (because he or she already got paid for it via the monthly capitation payment). This creates problems when the patient is seen an inordinate amount of times throughout the month, which might require the provider to spend more resources treating the patient than the monthly capitation payment covered. On the other hand, there will be months in which patients are not seen at all. Capitation plans thus put the focus less on the actual procedures performed, and more on efforts to keep the patient well and not requiring health treatments or other services.

Even though providers are not paid for particular services performed, it does not mean that a healthcare claim is not coded and sent to the insurance company. This claim is still sent to prove the medical necessity of the service and to describe any procedures that were performed on the patient, but the claim is not reimbursed.

The final type of reimbursement is called prospective payment, which reimburses provided services with a pre-determined, fixed amount, based on the patient's diagnosis and the services performed.

Prospective Payment Systems

A prospective payment system (PPS) is a type of reimbursement system based on preset payment levels rather than actual charges billed after the service has been provided. It is founded on predetermined payment rates or periods and linked to the anticipated intensity of services delivered as well as the patient's condition. Prospective payment systems are used for inpatient services (Inpatient Prospective Payment System or IPPS), outpatient facility services (Outpatient Prospective Payment System or OPPS), home healthcare services, and skilled nursing facility services. This does not mean that the facility must see into the future to predict the patient's health needs, but instead it groups the factors surrounding the patient's admission into a category of payment. For example, if an otherwise healthy patient with appendicitis was seen in the inpatient setting and received an appendectomy, then the payment for the inpatient services would be based on the diagnosis of appendicitis, as well as the procedure performed (appendectomy). On the other hand, if the patient had a diagnosis of appendicitis along with diabetes mellitus, hypertension, and chronic kidney disease, as well as advanced age, then the payment for this patient would be higher for the same procedure, because the additional diagnoses would categorize the patient's service into a higher payment category. These additional diagnoses are called comorbidities and complications. A comorbidity is either a medical condition that coexists with the primary cause for hospitalization and affects the patient's treatment and length of stay, or a pre-existing condition (like diabetes mellitus or hypertension) that, because of its presence with a specific diagnosis (like appendicitis), causes an increase in length of stay by at least one day in approximately 75 percent of cases. A complication is a medical condition that arises during an inpatient hospitalization (for example, a postoperative wound infection), or a condition that arises during the hospital stay that prolongs the length of stay at least one day in approximately 75 percent of the cases. The more complications or comorbidities that a patient has, the more likely the facility will have to expend greater resources on treating the patient, requiring a higher level of payment than for the same service rendered on an otherwise healthy patient.

PPS is used for services provided at acute inpatient hospitals, outpatient hospitals, home health agencies, hospice, inpatient psychiatric facilities, inpatient rehabilitation facilities, long-term care hospitals, and skilled nursing facilities. More about prospective payment systems is discussed in chapter 20 (Inpatient Hospital Services).

In certain instances, before a service can be rendered, that service must be authorized by the insurance company. These are called prior authorizations, prior certifications, or referrals.

Authorizations, Certifications, and Referrals

Just because a patient has health insurance and is seen by a doctor does not mean that the patient's insurance company will pay for anything that the healthcare provider does. Furthermore, this does not mean that the patient can see whichever doctor that he or she prefers. Because healthcare services can be costly, health insurance plans have many stipulations that must be followed in order for patients to be seen by doctors other than their primary care physicians, and also for specialized treatments such as MRIs or physical therapy services. These specialized services and treatments must be pre-authorized before health insurance will pay for them.

A **prior authorization (PA)** (sometimes called a prior certification), is permission from an insurance company for a patient to receive a healthcare service from a provider. Consider the following example.

> *Dr. Alameda sees a teenage boy in her office after an accident at his school in which he sustained a head injury during a soccer game. She would like to order a CT scan to rule out any serious injuries. Before she can send the patient to the hospital to receive the service, she must contact the patient's health insurance company and provide specific details about the incident and the patient's diagnosis, as well as her justification for sending the patient for the scan. This is the prior authorization request. If the insurance company agrees, then it will authorize the service and Dr. Alameda can then call the hospital to schedule the boy for the service.*

If the patient's insurance does not authorize the service, then it will not pay for it. In this example, if the CT scan was denied, the doctor might have to determine if a different imaging service should be performed. It may be necessary to send the request to a utilization review professional, who can determine if the service requested is indeed medically necessary and should be authorized by the insurance company. Typically, when this happens, it is handled by either the clinical staff or the healthcare provider. Once the service has been approved, the insurance company will issue an authorization number, which must be included on the claim in order to receive payment for the service. As a coder or biller, it is important to ensure that this number is included on the claim or it will not be reimbursed by the insurance company. The prior authorization number should be entered in box 23 of the paper CMS-1500 claim form (see figure 2.10).

Figure 2.10. Box 23

23. PRIOR AUTHORIZATION NUMBER

Source: CMS 2017b.

A **referral** is similar to a prior authorization. A referral is a request from one doctor—usually the patient's primary care provider—who sends (refers) the patient to another doctor, or for a service from another provider. The requirement for a referral depends on the patient's insurance policy, as some plans require referrals whenever the patient is seen by a provider other than his or her PCP, whereas other policies only require referrals for out-of-network providers (providers that are not contracted with the patient's insurance company).

Dr. Alameda sees a patient with high anxiety and feelings of depression. She wants this patient to see a psychiatrist. This patient's insurance requires a referral in order to authorize any service provided by any doctor other than the patient's primary care physician, Dr. Alameda. So Dr. Alameda must send a referral request to the insurance company, who will examine the patient's diagnoses and treatment requested and either authorize or deny the referral. Furthermore, in order for the psychiatrist to see the patient, they need the referral number, which proves that the insurance has authorized the service, and they will get reimbursed for any authorized services that they perform.

Just as in prior authorizations, if the insurance company does not authorize the referral to the psychiatrist, then it will not pay for any of the fee charged by the psychiatrist. The patient still has the option to go see the psychiatrist, but if she does then she would have to pay for any services out of pocket because the insurance did not agree to pay for the service. In these cases, it is especially important to understand the varying health insurance types, as each health insurance has different requirements regarding authorizations.

Key to Success

Prior authorizations, prior certifications, and referrals are like permission slips for patients to see another doctor or to receive a healthcare service. The request is to the insurance company, who then provides permission for the service and agrees to pay for it. Without the permission, insurance will not reimburse the healthcare providers for the nonauthorized service. The patient can still receive the service, but is responsible for paying for it out of his or her own pocket.

In addition to reimbursement, there are other factors that impact the financial side of medicine, some of which can provide either lucrative incentive bonuses or damaging penalties. These include Hierarchical Condition Category coding and risk adjustment, as well as performance measures and quality improvement.

Risk Adjustment and HCC Coding

As a way of predicting their budget for the upcoming year, insurance plans analyze their patient pool (all of the patients that are covered by each specific insurance plan), in terms of how healthy they are and how likely they are to incur expensive treatments in the following year. This is called **risk adjustment**, and is performed by insurance companies as a part of their financial analysis. Risk adjustment is a complex methodology that takes into account all known health elements of each patient that is a member of that particular health plan. Risk adjustment uses a multifaceted approach to analyze patient risk, which includes

- Patient diagnosis
- Age
- Gender
- Socioeconomic status
- Insurance type
- Specific claims data (AHIP 2016)

These components add up to a single risk score per patient, which is then used to calculate the total risk score for the group. It is important to note that this risk score is not for managing the patient's condition or to adjust payments to the healthcare provider, but only to help predict the future healthcare needs of the patient population. For example, if health plan A risk adjusts its patient base and finds that 50 percent of patients have diabetes mellitus along with another chronic condition then it can safely assume that it will result in additional and more expensive treatments than if only 25 percent of their patient base has diabetes mellitus with another chronic condition.

Because most risk adjustment data is calculated based on patient diagnosis codes and claims data, it makes sense that coders are at the forefront of risk analysis; and as risk analysis becomes more important for health plans to manage their bottom line, job opportunities are only set to increase.

The majority of risk analysis comes into play in what is called Hierarchical Condition Categories (HCC), based on individual patient diagnosis codes and correct documentation techniques. Additionally, it is important to understand accountable care organizations and their role in risk analysis.

Hierarchical Condition Categories (HCC)

The bulk of risk analysis data is in the form of patient diagnosis codes, which are taken from the claims submitted by healthcare providers for services rendered to a health plan's patients. In other words, diagnosis codes are taken from healthcare claims whenever patients are seen and used for risk adjustment purposes. These codes are tabulated into what is called a **Hierarchical Condition Category (HCC)**. Otherwise known as HCC coding, this is the practice of placing all patient diagnosis claims into groups of conditions, which are positioned strategically in order of risk from least risky to most risky. For example, diabetes mellitus is included within hierarchical condition categories, as it is a chronic condition that has a long-term impact on the patient's health. When a patient with diabetes mellitus presents for treatment, and the provider's office reports the diagnosis code for the patient's diabetes, then this code is captured by the patient's health insurance company and placed into a hierarchical condition category. Some categories (or conditions) are considered riskier than others, and thus result in a higher risk adjustment. Ultimately, the more diagnoses that fit into HCCs, the higher the risk for the patient population. This results in additional funding to the insurance company, which uses risk adjustment (by utilizing HCCs) to calculate how much money they may have to pay each year for patient healthcare services.

HCCs result in risk adjustment scores for each patient that are tallied up to complete the risk adjustment score for the entire patient population, as previously described. Usually only conditions that are costlier to manage medically are found in HCCs, and some patients can have different conditions that will place them in multiple HCCs. For example, a patient may have a liver condition as well as substance abuse, and a personal history of an amputation. Because these three conditions are all tabulated in HCC adjustments, they would add up to a higher risk adjustment score than if the patient only had one of these conditions. Some of the additional diagnoses calculated in HCCs include infections, disability status, transplant status, disease interactions, cerebrovascular diseases, psychiatric conditions, and diabetes, among others.

Therefore, HCCs are completely reliant on the diagnosis codes included on claims. In turn, diagnosis codes are completely reliant on the provider's documentation of the patient's healthcare condition and the services performed. Coders are uniquely suited to engage in HCC coding and ensure that all HCC codes are captured on all claims and supported by documentation in the health record.

HCC coding is specially focused on capturing all patient conditions that impact the hierarchical condition category, and which are fully supported by documentation in the health record. HCC coding is a growing field of healthcare coding due in part to the growth of Medicare Advantage plans, which base their payments on the relative health of the patient identified by the HCC in which the patient falls, as expressed by their diagnosis code(s) (Optum360 2017). This is different than regular coding, which is typically used for reimbursement purposes. When diagnosis coding is used only for reimbursement, the focus is on diagnoses that impact reimbursement by indicating the medical necessity for the service provided. The diagnosis code identifies the medical necessity for the service provided and the insurance company pays for the service. HCC coding is more inclusive, however, and requires reporting of all reportable diagnosis codes in order to present a complete picture of the patient's health. Consider the following example.

Wanda presented to her PCP's office for a sick visit, with a bad cough and a fever for the last few days. Wanda has a significant healthcare history, including a past history of breast cancer, diabetes mellitus type II, and she is status post an amputation of her left foot following a gangrenous foot ulcer. At her visit today, her PCP performs a basic medical examination and diagnoses Wanda with acute bronchitis, prescribes an antibiotic, and schedules a follow-up examination for her in two days to see how she is doing.

Key to Success

Note that in the given example, Wanda, the patient, is "status post" amputation of her left foot following a gangrenous foot ulcer. This means that she has had a recent amputation of the left foot. The term *status post*, sometimes abbreviated as S/P, is a common phrase in healthcare and is used to indicate that a patient has had a significant event or procedure happen in the recent past. For example, a patient who had a motor vehicle accident (MVA) one week ago may be identified in the health record as status post MVA.

In coding for reimbursement purposes only, the only diagnosis that would be required for payment purposes would be the diagnosis of bronchitis. However, this diagnosis would be insufficient for HCC coding purposes. Because acute bronchitis is not a chronic or long-lasting condition expected to impact the patient health for a long period, it is not included in HCC calculations. Therefore, if only the acute bronchitis code was included in the healthcare claim, then it would be a misrepresentation of the patient's overall health status and would not impact the risk score for the patient. HCC coding would require the reporting of all additional conditions of the patient, including the history of cancer, diabetes, and amputation status. These additional codes do impact the hierarchical condition category, and as such would allow a more accurate representation of the patient's risk than if only the acute bronchitis code was reported.

In other words, HCC coding is not only about reimbursement for healthcare services; it recognizes that diagnosis codes are used for more than just medical necessity and, in this case, helps to create a better picture of the patient's overall health.

In short, HCC coding requires coders who are skilled at understanding coding rules and HCCs, and who can correctly identify and assign all diagnosis codes from health record documentation. Because only certain diagnosis codes for healthcare conditions impact the HCC, it is important to understand these particular conditions and how they should be accurately documented in the health record in order to substantiate code selection. Because of this, throughout the rest of this text you will find HCC Coding Corners, which discuss conditions that impact HCC coding and how they should be supported by documentation in the health record.

HCC Coding Corner

HCC Coding Corners discuss conditions that impact HCC coding and how they should be supported by documentation in the health record.

Accountable Care Organizations

An **accountable care organization (ACO)** is a group of healthcare providers that coordinate to give high-quality care to their patients. This group of providers can be comprised of many different healthcare offices such as individual providers, large healthcare groups, hospitals, and other healthcare clinics. The ACO focuses on providing high-quality care, especially to patients with chronic conditions (such as those that fall into hierarchical condition categories), and ensuring that these patients have access to quality care when needed.

There are three main goals of an ACO:

- Provide better care for patients, which results in
- Better health for the Medicare advantage population, as indicated by the
- Lower cost of providing care to these patients. (CMS 2016a)

ACOs that meet these goals have the opportunity to participate in the Medicare Shared Savings Program. This program allows all of the providers grouped into the ACO to report their data for each performance year together, and share in any savings accrued by participation in the ACO. This shared savings is what makes participation in an ACO especially important to the bottom line for the participating healthcare providers. The way this process works is that the claims for a healthcare office are paid regularly for a period of time, often called the performance year. After the year is over, the claims are reviewed to see if the ACO generated losses or savings for the Medicare plan for the performance year (CMS 2016a).

This review is a complicated process initiated by the insurance company(ies), and includes an analysis to ensure that all diagnosis codes that impact HCCs were captured at least once per patient per year. If the review shows that the ACO generated savings for the Medicare program (by correctly reporting all necessary HCC codes and providing high-quality care to patients as indicated by other factors), then these savings are shared with the ACO. The healthcare offices involved in the ACO receive an additional payment, sometimes called an incentive payment, based on their performance throughout the year.

One of the last major components to understanding the basics of billing for healthcare services is knowing how healthcare providers are increasingly held accountable for the *quality* of the service that they provide to patients. These initiatives are called performance measures or quality improvement initiatives, and they serve to quantify the quality of care provided by healthcare providers.

Performance Measurement

Historically, it has been difficult to measure how effective a healthcare provider is, besides perhaps a patient questionnaire; but in today's world of data analytics, all the data generated from a healthcare office can be used to measure the performance of a healthcare service. Data analytics refers to the act of quantifying qualitative data and analyzing it to categorize it and extract patterns. This data is then used to create a measure of the quality that a healthcare practitioner provides his or her patients. This data can be analyzed from a single medical doctor, to hospitals comprising thousands of healthcare providers.

Data analytics is the complex analysis of all the information generated by a healthcare practice to determine the level of care that it provides to patients. This level of care is identified with special performance measures that rate specific desired outcomes, or procedure codes that identify extra steps the healthcare practice has taken to improve the quality of care. The process of analyzing this data and determining the quality of care provided is called performance measurement.

Key to Success

If you are interested in data analytics, AHIMA offers a specialty Certified Health Data Analyst (CHDA®) certification. For more information on this and other certifications, refer to the appendix, Coding Certifications and Professional Coding Organizations.

Performance measures are a set of predefined quality outcomes that are used to determine the level of the quality of care that is provided to patients. Performance measurement analyzes the success of a healthcare practice, facility, or other group, in meeting its predetermined performance measures. Results from the performance measurement help the healthcare practice identify areas of improvement or areas of success, which can be shared with other providers to learn from that success.

These measures can be internally created by each specific healthcare entity. For example, if a healthcare office has the goal to reduce incidence of undiagnosed postpartum depression, it may choose to create a measure that identifies all mothers who receive a postpartum depression evaluation. Measuring how many mothers receive the evaluation in terms of a percentage indicates how well the practice is accomplishing its goal of reducing undiagnosed postpartum depression. If the percentage is 50 percent, then this means that only 50 percent of women received the evaluation and that the practice needs to do a better job of administering the evaluation. On the other hand, if the score was 100 percent, then it means that all postpartum women received the evaluation and the office had met its predetermined goal. These percentages are the measures of the performance goal.

Performance measures are also set by a number of official organizations and healthcare associations that measure specific outcomes desired for specific settings, specialties, or types of providers. For example, one of the performance measures for pediatric patients is the percentage of all patients who are at least two years of age who have received all age-appropriate vaccines at the time of reporting (CMS 2012). This is a specific measure that pediatricians can use to analyze their success at administering vaccines to their patients.

Many of these measures are compiled into official groups by agencies like CMS or the National Committee for Quality Assurance (NCQA), who endorse a set of measures, all of which combine to create a well-rounded picture of performance. For example, there are numerous measures used to identify the quality of care provided to diabetic patients through comprehensive diabetes care. This group of measures for comprehensive diabetes care includes blood pressure control, performance of an eye examination, hemoglobin A1c control status and testing, and medical attention for nephropathy (NCQA 2017). These measures combine to form a more inclusive picture of the quality of care provided to diabetic patients.

Performance measures are also used for more than simply determining how good a doctor is at his or her job or how good a medical practice is. There are other reasons why performance measurement is important including quality improvement, transparency, accreditation, recognition as a medical home, and financial incentives.

Quality Improvement

Quality improvement (QI) uses the information generated from performance measurement to establish processes or programs that are aimed at improving quality scores. For example, if a healthcare practice's quality score for postpartum depression evaluations is 50 percent, then it is necessary to review the process of how the evaluation is administered, how patients are identified, and how the healthcare practice can go about improving that score. On the other hand, if the score is already 100 percent, then the healthcare practice can share their best practices with other offices to help them succeed in their performance measures.

Depending on the size of the organization and past performance measures, quality improvement may play a large role in an organization. For example, if a large hospital system has poor scores on surgical site infections or hospital-acquired conditions, then it may choose to implement a QI program that employs a number of doctors, nurses, and administrative staff to focus solely on improving performance measures throughout the organization.

Transparency

An important part of creating performance scores is about being transparent to stakeholders of the organization, such as patients and organizations that provide funding. This means that all stakeholders can clearly see the quality scores of the organization. Transparency about quality allows patients to make informed decisions regarding their healthcare services. For example, a patient may choose to go to a hospital with high quality scores and avoid a hospital with low quality scores, as these scores indicate the quality of care that the patient may receive at either organization. Scores are publicly available and searchable through Medicare resources such as Medicare Physician Compare, which permits users to search through publicly available provider data to compare performance results (Medicare.gov 2017b), as well as through individual hospital websites.

Accreditation

There are several different organizations within the healthcare industry, many of which provide accreditation of healthcare entities. Accreditation is a recognition or certification that an entity meets specific performance standards. For example, accreditation of a vocational college that offers a coding program demonstrates that the program is rigorous, meets all standards, and has positive outcomes in terms of student success. Healthcare practices and facilities can be accredited by organizations such as the Accreditation Association for Ambulatory Health Care (AAAHC), the Joint Commission, or the National Committee for Quality Assurance (NCQA). Accreditation of a healthcare facility indicates that the facility meets all standards and has consistently high-performance scores.

Recognition as a Medical Home

A medical home is an important recognition for outpatient practices. As the name indicates, a **Patient Centered Medical Home (PCMH)** is centered in the patient's primary care office (such as a primary care physician), and acts as a home for all the healthcare services that the patient needs. This does not mean that it provides all the healthcare services that a patient might need, but instead helps to coordinate care between different healthcare providers and specialists, medical treatments and prescriptions, and communicate with the patient's insurance company about patient progress, preventive examinations and screenings, and other services. Performance measures are vital to the concept of the medical home, as a medical office attains a PCMH status by maintaining solid performance measurements and implementing office policies aimed at providing quality care to its patients.

Financial Incentives

Finally, performance measurement is important because of the connection between high (or low) performance scores and financial incentives (or penalties). Financial incentive programs provide bonus payments for healthcare entities that have high performance scores. For example, in the professional physician setting, there are two important programs.

- Merit-based Incentive Payment System (MIPS), which is a program that awards a positive payment adjustment (an incentive payment) to healthcare providers who demonstrate high performance in four categories: quality of care delivered, cost of care delivered, improvement activities, and advancing care information (QPP 2017a).
- Alternative Payment Model (APM), which is an arrangement between the healthcare provider and insurance, so that practitioners who provide high-quality and cost-effective care can get added incentives for high-quality care provided to patients. APMs can focus on a specific medical condition, an episode of care, or a certain patient population within the healthcare practice (QPP 2017b).

In the hospital setting, Medicare employs three separate programs that are designed to pay hospitals for high quality scores.

- The Hospital Readmissions Reduction Program focuses on reducing the number of readmissions for high-cost or high-volume procedures. Hospitals that reduce the number of readmissions for certain identified conditions or procedures (such as hip and knee replacements or coronary artery bypass graft surgery) are eligible for incentive payments (CMS 2016b).
- The Hospital Value-Based Purchasing (VBP) Program compares the performance measures for hospitals across the country and offers incentives on each hospital's performance (CMS 2017d).

- The Hospital-Acquired Condition Reduction Program reduces payments to hospitals with high rates of hospital-acquired conditions (HACs), such as catheter-induced urinary tract infections. This program is designed to encourage hospitals to improve patient safety during hospital stays by reducing the amount of infection or other adverse safety events acquired during the hospitalization period (CMS 2017e).

Some of these incentives can be quite lucrative, ranging in the hundreds of thousands of dollars, depending on the size of the healthcare facility, so they are a huge impetus for engaging in performance measurement and trying to achieve higher performance scores. On the other hand, if the facility engages in performance measurement and the scores are low, the healthcare facility may be penalized and ordered to pay a monetary penalty, or fine, due to their poor performance scores.

End of Chapter Content

Instructions: Indicate whether the following statements are true or false (T or F). For false statements, rewrite the statement on the line below to make the statement true.

1. HIPAA made sweeping changes to the healthcare industry by introducing performance measurement.

   _____

   _____

2. PHI stands for private healthcare information.

   _____

   _____

3. The minimum necessary standard dictates that only the minimum necessary amount of PHI should be shared when a release of PHI is warranted.

   _____

   _____

4. Risk adjustment evaluates the likelihood that a security breach might happen.

   _____

   _____

5. Reimbursement, otherwise known as payment, is the money that a provider receives for healthcare services.

   _____

   _____

(Continued on next page)

(Continued)

6. The CMS-1500 claim form is used for billing services performed in the outpatient setting for professional services.

_____

_____

7. A health insurance company is also referred to as a third-party payer.

_____

_____

8. Insurance premiums are the payments that are sent to healthcare providers for services rendered.

_____

_____

9. Commercial insurance policies are run by for-profit companies.

_____

_____

10. In an employer-sponsored insurance plan, the employers pay the entire premium amount for the patient.

_____

_____

Instructions: Choose the best answer.

1. Which of the following is a covered entity under HIPAA?

   a. Healthcare provider
   b. Healthcare billing company
   c. Patient
   d. Lawyer

2. Which HIPAA rule sets national standards for the protection of PHI?

   a. Security Rule
   b. Privacy Rule
   c. PHI Rule
   d. Encryption Rule

3. What is the name of the document that informs patients about their privacy rights under HIPAA?

   a. HIPAA Confidentiality Agreement
   b. Privacy Agreement
   c. Covered Entity Notice
   d. Notice of Privacy Practices

4. Which HIPAA rule contains provisions that cover compliance to HIPAA rules and regulations, investigations into breaches in privacy, and the imposition of monetary penalties?

   a. Privacy Rule
   b. Security Rule
   c. Enforcement Rule
   d. HIPAA Confidentiality Agreement

5. Which of the following would be used to bill an insurance company for services that were performed in the inpatient facility setting?

   a. CMS-1500 claim form
   b. UB-04 claim form
   c. NUCC claim form
   d. CMS claim form

6. How many individual diagnoses can be entered on a single CMS-1500 claim form?

   a. 12
   b. 16
   c. 4
   d. 8

7. If a service is specifically excluded from coverage in an insurance policy, who must pay for the healthcare service if it is provided?

   a. The healthcare provider
   b. The insurance company
   c. The patient
   d. No one, the service is provided free of charge

8. Which of the following patient out-of-pocket expenses is a percentage of allowable amount?

   a. Copayment
   b. Deductible
   c. Coinsurance
   d. Noncovered service

9. Which of the following government-sponsored health insurance plans covers individuals who are elderly or disabled?

   a. Medicare
   b. Medicaid
   c. Entitlement health insurance
   d. TRICARE

10. Which of the following is an example of non-traditional insurance?

    a. TRICARE
    b. Commercial Blue Cross Blue Shield policy
    c. Automobile insurance
    d. Medicaid

11. Which of the following types of reimbursement pays a per member per month amount?

    a. Fee-for-service
    b. Capitation
    c. Prospective payment system
    d. Risk adjustment

12. Which of the following is an insurance process that analyzes their patient pool in terms of health risk and how likely those patients are to incur expensive treatments for the coming year?

    a. Risk adjustment
    b. Risk analysis
    c. Performance measurement
    d. Quality improvement

13. ter... pract_e Measurement 55

    a. HCC ...zing data to de-
    b. Perform... at a healthcare
    c. Risk adjus...?
    d. Risk analysis

14. Which of the follow... quantifying data and a... and extract patterns?

    a. Data referrals
    b. Prior authorization requests
    c. Data analytics
    d. Risk analysis

15. If a healthcare practice or facility receive... performance scores, which of the following might happen?

    a. They might receive financial incentives
    b. They might receive financial penalties or fines
    c. They may have to increase their efforts at quality improvement
    d. They might have to begin seeing less patients

References

45 CFR 164.304: Definitions.

Aflac. 2017. Accident Insurance. https://www.aflac.com/individuals/products/accident-insurance.aspx.

America's Health Insurance Plans. 2016. The Medicare Advantage Risk Adjustment System: What It Is and Why It's Important. https://www.ahip.org/wp-content/uploads/2016/04/Risk-Adjustment-Why-is-it-important.pdf.

Centers for Medicare and Medicaid Services. 2017a. Details for title: CMS 1450. https://www.cms.gov/Medicare/CMS-Forms/CMS-Forms/CMS-Forms-Items/CMS1196256.html.

Centers for Medicare and Medicaid Services. 2017b. Details for title: CMS 1500. https://www.cms.gov/Medicare/CMS-Forms/CMS-Forms/CMS-Forms-Items/CMS1188854.html.

Centers for Medicare and Medicaid Services. 2017c. Fee for Service Advance Beneficiary Notice of Noncoverage. https://www.cms.gov/medicare/medicare-general-information/bni/abn.html.

...rvices. 2017d. https://www.cms ...ves-Patient-Assessment ...ased-purchasing/index Centers for Hospital value-Based-Purchasing/. .gov/Medicaid Services. 2017e. -Instruction ...tion Reduction Program .html w.cms.gov/Medicare/Medicare Centers ...nent/AcuteInpatientPPS/HAC Hos...n.html. (H...

...re and Medicaid Services. 2016a. ...re Organizations: What Providers Need Cen s://www.cms.gov/Medicare/Medicare ...vice-Payment/sharedsavingsprogram ...ds/ACO_Providers_Factsheet_ICN907406.pdf.

...Medicare and Medicaid Services. 2016b. ...ssions Reduction Program (HRRP). https:// ...w.cms.gov/Medicare/Medicare-Fee-for-Service ...ayment/AcuteInpatientPPS/Readmissions-Reduction ...rogram.html.

...nters for Medicare and Medicaid Services. 2014. Medicare Program-General Information. https://www .cms.gov/Medicare/Medicare-General-Information /MedicareGenInfo/index.html.

Centers for Medicare and Medicaid Services. 2012. 2014 Clinical Quality Measures (CQMs) Pediatric Recommended Core Measures. https://www .cms.gov/Regulations-and-Guidance/Legislation /EHRIncentivePrograms/Downloads/2014_CQM _PrediatricRecommended_CoreSetTable.pdf.

Healthcare.gov. 2017. Preventive Health Services. https:// www.healthcare.gov/coverage/preventive-care -benefits/.

Medicaid.gov. 2017. Eligibility. https://www.medicaid. gov/medicaid/eligibility/index.html.

Medicare.gov. 2017a. What Part A & Part B Doesn't Cover. https://www.medicare.gov/what-medicare-covers/not -covered/item-and-services-not-covered-by-part-a -and-b.html.

Medicare.gov. 2017b. Improving Health Care Quality. https://www.medicare.gov/physiciancompare/#about /improvinghealthcarequality.

National Committee for Quality Assurance. 2017. Comprehensive Diabetes Care: This HEDIS Measure. http://www.ncqa.org/report-cards/health-plans/state -of-health-care-quality/2016-table-of-contents/diabetes -care.

Office for Civil Rights. 2013a. Summary of the HIPAA Privacy Rule. https://www.hhs.gov/hipaa/for -professionals/privacy/laws-regulations/index.html.

Office for Civil Rights. 2013b. Summary of the HIPAA Security Rule. https://www.hhs.gov/hipaa/for -professionals/security/laws-regulations/index.html.

Office for Civil Rights. 2013c. The HIPAA Enforcement Rule. http://www.hhs.gov/hipaa/for-professionals/special -topics/enforcement-rule/index.html.

Optum 360. 2016. The Three Keys to HCCs and Risk Adjustment. https://www.optum360coding.com /CodingCentralArticles/?id=1636.

Public Law 104-191. 1996. 110 Stat. 1936. Short title see 42 U.S.C. 201 note. http://uscode .house.gov/.

Quality Payment Program (QPP). 2017a. An Introduction to Group Participation in the Merit-based Incentive Payment System (MIPS) in 2017. https://www.cms .gov/Medicare/Quality-Payment-Program/Resource -Library/Group-Participation-in-MIPS-2017.pdf.

Quality Payment Program (QPP). 2017b. Medicaid and the Quality Payment Program. https://qpp.cms.gov/docs /QPP_Medicaid_All_Payer_Fact_Sheet.pdf.

Texas Health and Human Services. 2017. CHIP Children's Medicaid: Costs. https://chipmedicaid.org/en/Costs.

TRICARE. 2017. Cost and Fees Sheet. https://tricare .mil/~/media/Files/TRICARE/Publications/Misc /Costs_Sheet.pdf.

Resources

Centers for Medicare and Medicaid Services. 2017. http://www.cms.gov.

Centers for Medicare and Medicaid Services. 2017. Shared Savings Program. https://www.cms.gov /Medicare/Medicare-Fee-for-Service-Payment /sharedsavingsprogram/index.html?redirect =/sharedsavingsprogram/.

Centers for Medicare and Medicaid Services. 2015 (October). Medicare Advanced Beneficiary Notices. https:// www.cms.gov/Outreach-and-Education/Medicare -Learning-Network-MLN/MLNProducts/downloads /abn_booklet_icn006266.pdf .

Health Resources and Services Administration (HRSA). 2011. Performance Management and https://www .hrsa.gov/sites/default/files/quality/toolbox/508pdfs /performancemanagementandmeasurement.pdf.

Medicare.gov. 2017. What's Medicare Supplement Insurance (Medigap)? https://www.medicare.gov/supplement -other-insurance/medigap/whats-medigap.html.

National Quality Forum. 2017. http://www.qualityforum.org /Measuring_Performance/Measuring_Performance.aspx.

National Uniform Claim Committee. 2017. http://www .nucc.org.

Solove, D. J. 2013 (April). HIPAA turns 10: Analyzing the past, present and future impact. *Journal of AHIMA* 84(4): 22–28. http://bok.ahima.org/doc?oid=106325# .WXXeLYgrI2w.

TRICARE. 2017. http://www.tricare.mil.

CHAPTER

Basics of Coding

Learning Objectives

- Identify the types of codes, including the history of the ICD, CPT, and HCPCS code sets, and explain their uses in the healthcare setting.
- Analyze the additional uses of codes.
- Discuss future coding developments.

- Analyze the connection between code linkage and medical necessity and understand how to link codes on a healthcare claim.
- Discuss healthcare coding guidelines.

Key Terms

Clinical modification (CM)
Code linkage
Coding guidelines
Current Procedural Terminology (CPT)
Evaluation and management (E/M) service
HCPCS Level I codes

HCPCS Level II codes
Healthcare Common Procedure Coding System (HCPCS)
Healthcare codes
ICD-10-CM
ICD-10-PCS
ICD-11
ICD-9

International Classification of Diseases (ICD)
Legacy system
Medical necessity
Modifier
Procedural coding system (PCS)

Learning healthcare coding begins with learning the different types of codes, the settings in which they are used, and the many uses of codes. But knowing what a code is and what it is used for is not enough to be a proficient healthcare coder. Proficient coding involves understanding the guidelines that govern proper coding, and how to use them to correctly select, sequence, and report codes. Furthermore, it is also imperative to understand medical necessity, the connection between medical necessity and codes, and how to link the two together.

This chapter presents these basics of coding—explaining the different code sets, discussing the history and future of coding and the current uses of codes, examining and applying coding guidelines, and analyzing medical necessity and code linkage, including how to link codes on a claim to indicate medical necessity for the service provided.

What Are Healthcare Codes?

The implementation of HIPAA (discussed in chapter 2), required the Department of Health and Human Services (HHS) to adopt national standards for healthcare transactions, security, and code sets. Although they had been used prior to the implementation of HIPAA, this requirement further imbedded the use of coding into the world of healthcare and reimbursement.

Healthcare codes are the numeric or alphanumeric translations of all the services, supplies, treatments, diagnoses, conditions, and other reasons for healthcare treatments. Envision all the different procedures, services, surgeries, therapies, treatments, and supplies that could be provided to a patient in a healthcare setting. Also consider all of the different diagnoses, problems, diseases, healthcare conditions, or other reasons why a patient may need a healthcare service. There are an infinite number of possible scenarios. Now imagine how difficult it would be to report all those scenarios to a third-party payer on a single sheet of paper, or in a single electronic file. This is where codes come into play. For example, instead of describing a patient's condition, the coder translates the condition (strep throat) into a diagnosis code (J02.0, Streptococcal pharyngitis), which is entered on the healthcare claim.

Healthcare code sets are the tabulated listings of the diagnoses, procedures, diagnostic tests, and treatments, equipment, and supplies provided to patients in the healthcare setting. They are divided into specific sets, each of which identify a specific type of diagnosis, procedure, service, or supply. There are five code sets outlined in HIPAA regulations adopted for use by HHS. They include International Classification of Diseases (ICD), Healthcare Common Procedure Coding System (HCPCS), Current Procedural Terminology (CPT), Codes on Dental Procedures and Nomenclature (CDT), and National Drug Codes (NDC). For the purposes of healthcare coding, this text focuses on three code sets—ICD, CPT, and HCPCS. These three code sets are used in inpatient, outpatient, facility, and physician settings, as necessary. Each one of these codes are unique; they have a different format, number of characters or digits, and are either numeric (containing only numbers) or alphanumeric (containing both numbers and letters). Furthermore, each of these codes sets is used for a unique purpose.

International Classification of Diseases (ICD) Codes

The origins of tracking patient diagnoses can be traced back to 17th century London with the London Bills of Mortality, compiled by John Graunt, which attempted to classify all the causes of death and track childhood mortality rates. Beginning in 1837, William Farr continued to collect information on the causes of death, and also worked to secure internationally recognized classifications for the causes of death. In 1893, a statistician named Jacques Bertillon presented his Bertillon Classification of Causes of Death, which was adopted by the American Public Health Association in 1898 and recommended for use in Canada, Mexico, and the United States, with the additional recommendation that this data set be revised every 10 years (WHO 2017).

Over the next 75 years, this classification system was expanded and formalized to include not just causes of death, but also causes of morbidity (sickness), combinations of illnesses and diseases, manifestations of diseases, and other reasons for healthcare encounters. The ninth revision of the International Classification of Diseases (ICD-9) was developed in October 1975 during the International Conference for the Ninth Revision of the International Classification of Diseases, assembled by the World Health Organization (WHO). This revision included detailed code descriptions with subclassifications and extended code structure, and was divided into three different volumes. The ICD-9 code set was used in the United States from 1975 until the implementation of ICD-10 on October 1, 2015 (WHO 2017).

International Classification of Diseases (ICD) codes are now in their 10th revision, ICD-10. The World Health Organization developed the ICD-10 code set in 1993, which was revised for use in the United States through a development committee composed of CMS, the National Center for Healthcare Statistics (NCHS), the American Hospital Association (AHA), and AHIMA. On October 1, 2015, the United States replaced the ICD-9 code set by implementing ICD-10, making it the last industrialized nation in the world to transition from ICD-9 to ICD-10.

The version of ICD-10 that is now used in the United States is different than what is used by other countries and was developed specifically to coordinate with data reporting requirements and to correspond with US clinical practices. It includes two major divisions: Clinical Modification (CM) and Procedural Coding System (PCS). ICD-10 **Clinical Modification (CM)**, is the compilation of ICD-10 codes used to report diagnoses. ICD-10 **Procedural Coding System (PCS)**, is the compilation of ICD-10 codes that are used to report hospital inpatient procedures. These two divisions are unique to the US version of ICD-10. No other country uses the PCS codes, as these codes are used specifically for billing purposes to identify the procedure(s) performed in the inpatient setting. These two divisions are used for different purposes and are published as two different coding manuals, each with a different organization and format.

The format and structure of the ICD-10-CM and PCS code books are discussed in chapters 4 and 20, respectively. Furthermore, specific ICD-10-CM diagnosis codes and coding guidelines are discussed throughout chapters 6 through 19. The next sections introduce ICD-10-CM and ICD-10-PCS coding, as well as ICD-9.

International Classification of Diseases, Tenth Revision, Clinical Modification (ICD-10-CM)

ICD-10-CM codes are three- to seven-character alphanumeric codes that are used to identify a patient diagnosis or other reason for a healthcare encounter. For example, if a patient presented to a healthcare office and was diagnosed with a headache then an ICD-10-CM code for headache (R51, Headache) would be assigned on the claim. On the other hand, if the patient was not ill, but presented to the office for a flu shot, then the ICD-10-CM code assigned on the claim would indicate that the patient presented for the administration of a vaccine (Z23, Encounter for immunization). It is very common that patients have more than one diagnosis or reason for a visit. In these cases, use of more than one code is allowed. Up to 12 unique ICD-10-CM codes are allowed per outpatient claim form (using the CMS-1500 claim form). If it is necessary to include more than 12 diagnosis codes on a claim, additional codes may be sent on additional claim forms (refer to chapter 2 for the discussion on the CMS-1500 claim form). In the hospital setting, over 20 diagnosis codes may be assigned on the UB-04 claim form.

An ICD-10-CM code must be assigned for every single patient for every single healthcare encounter. This is because ICD-10-CM codes represent the medical necessity for the service performed. Remember, as discussed in chapter 2, medical necessity is the reason why a healthcare service or treatment is performed. The standards of medical necessity must be met in order for an insurance company to cover a healthcare service, so in order to be medically necessary a service must meet the accepted standards of medicine, and it must be used to prevent, treat, or diagnose an illness or injury, condition, or disease (or the symptoms thereof).

The link between ICD-10-CM codes and medical necessity is extremely important to understand, because if a healthcare treatment or procedure does not have medical necessity, then insurance will not pay for it. In other words, the diagnosis code *is* the medical necessity for the service.

Key to Success

Without a diagnosis code to indicate that a service was medically necessary, health insurance will not reimburse the healthcare provider for the procedure. Remember, the patient's diagnosis should always identify the reason why the patient is receiving healthcare services. If there is no medically necessary reason for the services, then insurance will not pay for them.

More about medical necessity and its indications for any procedures performed or supplies given to the patient is discussed later in this chapter. ICD-10-CM codes and code book are also discussed in detail in chapter 4.

International Classification of Diseases, Tenth Revision, Procedure Coding System (ICD-10-PCS)

The second division of the ICD-10 code set is known as ICD-10-PCS. ICD-10-PCS codes are seven-character alphanumeric codes that are used in hospital reporting to identify procedures that were performed in the hospital inpatient setting. As such, these codes are only used for facility billing. For example, if a patient received an appendectomy (removal of the appendix) in an inpatient hospital, then the hospital would use a PCS appendectomy code to report that the patient had an appendectomy procedure performed during his or her hospital stay. Note that PCS codes may also be used in the outpatient hospital setting for statistical purposes.

Unlike ICD-10-CM codes, PCS codes are used to report actual procedures that were performed on patients, such as surgeries, deliveries, or radiologic examinations. Also unlike ICD-10-CM codes, PCS codes do not identify any medical necessity for the service performed. Rather, they simply identify the actual service that was performed. However, procedures represented by PCS codes must still be supported with medical necessity, which means that both ICD-10-CM and PCS codes may be reported on the same claim. For example, the PCS code for a rhinoplasty (090K0ZZ, Alteration of Nasal Mucosa and Soft Tissue, Open Approach), would be reported in addition to the ICD-10-CM code that represent the medical necessity for the rhinoplasty (M95.0, Acquired deformity of nose).

Keep in mind that PCS codes are only used for inpatient facility billing purposes, such as inpatient hospital services. Because ICD-10-PCS codes are used primarily in the inpatient setting, this text focuses on them in chapter 20 (Inpatient Hospital Services). The remaining chapters of this text discuss outpatient coding, which utilizes ICD-10-CM, CPT, and HCPCS codes.

Key to Success

Do not get confused by the differences between ICD-10-*CM* and ICD-10-*PCS* codes. CM stands for Clinical Modification, which is used for diagnostic coding. PCS stands for Procedural Coding System, which is the section of ICD-10 codes that represent procedures and other services performed. CM = diagnosis; PCS = procedure.

International Classification of Diseases, Ninth Revision (ICD-9)

ICD-9 codes are the International Classification of Diseases codes that were used prior to the implementation of ICD-10 codes. The ICD-9 code set is composed of three volumes, all published in the same code book: Volumes one and two are the index and tabular listings for diagnosis codes, and volume three contains procedure codes. Volume three of the ICD-9 code set was replaced by the ICD-10-PCS code set, which is used in essentially the same manner, but has greatly expanded the specificity for reporting inpatient procedures.

ICD-9 diagnosis codes are three- to five-digit numeric or alphanumeric codes that serve essentially the same purpose as ICD-10-CM, as they are used to report patient diagnoses of other reasons for a patient encounter. However, they were out of date clinically and allowed little room for including critical elements in diagnosis reporting, such as the laterality of a condition (whether a condition occurred on the right, left, or on both sides of the body). Thus, the code set was changed to the more inclusive ICD-10 code set, which allowed greater expansion to contain more detail regarding patient conditions, updated the codes to include relevant clinical and encounter information, and include more functionality for reporting combinations of healthcare conditions.

Even though ICD-9 codes are no longer mandated for use by CMS through HIPAA, this does not mean that they are irrelevant. This means that the ICD-9 code set is no longer maintained by any governing committee, nor is it updated on an annual basis (as the other code sets are). Only HIPAA-covered entities had to switch from the ICD-9 to ICD-10-CM code set on October 1, 2015. This means that there are a few entities that did not have to make the change, such as automobile insurance carriers; so in some very rare instances ICD-9 codes may be required to bill a nontraditional insurance claim. More importantly, keep in mind that every HIPAA-covered entity used ICD-9 before October 1, 2015. This means that all old accounts receivable, data collection and reporting, and patient records contain ICD-9 codes rather than ICD-10-CM. Therefore, it is important to understand ICD-9 coding as a legacy system—an older and outdated coding system that has been replaced by a more clinically accurate, up-to-date coding system (ICD-10-CM).

Healthcare Common Procedure Coding System (HCPCS) Codes

Healthcare Common Procedure Coding System (HCPCS) codes have a shorter history than either ICD or CPT, but this does not mean that they are any less important. In the early 1980s, CMS developed a code set—HCPCS codes—for the purpose of identifying services, products, or supplies that were not included within the CPT code set. In 1983, CMS required that a HCPCS code must be reported for reimbursement

Figure 3.1. HCPCS code set divisions

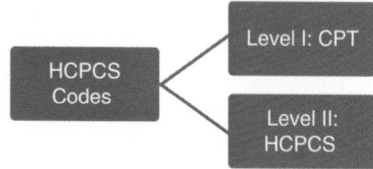

on Medicare claims (CMS 2017b). Although this standard only set the requirement for Medicare claims, third-party payers followed suit and HCPCS codes quickly became a standardized code set for all claims.

The adoption of HCPCS was due in part to the need for a standard code set to be recognized by all insurance payers, facilitating the submission of claims for reimbursement. The HCPCS code set included additional services and supplies, which were not included in the CPT code set, such as durable medical equipment and medicinal agents administered in the health setting. However, HCPCS did not include all surgical and healthcare procedures and treatments that were included in the CPT code set. Because the HCPCS coding system is not as extensive as the CPT code set, the CPT code set was adopted as part of the HCPCS codes. This meant that although CPT codes are developed and maintained as a separate code set by the AMA, they are still included within the HCPCS code set, separated as two different levels of codes. This created two levels within the HCPCS code set: Level I and Level II codes (figure 3.1).

- **HCPCS Level I codes** (commonly referred to as CPT) are the CPT codes that are developed, maintained, and copyrighted by the AMA. They represent the healthcare procedure, treatment, or service provided at the healthcare encounter.

- **HCPCS Level II codes** (commonly referred to as simply HCPCS or Level II codes) are the HCPCS codes that are developed, maintained, and published by CMS. They represent the supply, service, or other treatment provided to the patient. They also include ambulance services (CMS 2017b).

Both Level I and Level II codes are used for professional reporting for reimbursement purposes. They are published in separate code books, but may be used concurrently to bill for services provided.

Key to Success

Although CPT (Level I) codes are technically part of the HCPCS code set, they are usually referred to as simply CPT codes. HCPCS codes, however, are still sometimes referred to as Level II codes. Remember, Level II codes are the same as HCPCS codes (see figure 3.1).

HCPCS Level I: Current Procedural Terminology (CPT) Codes

The history of CPT coding is not nearly as extensive as ICD coding, but it is an important part of understanding how the codes are used today. In 1965, the Health Care Financing Administration (HCFA), now known as CMS, passed Medicare and Medicaid (discussed in chapter 2), which made it necessary to implement a standardized system of reporting procedures for reimbursement. Before that time, most patients paid out of pocket for healthcare services and were later reimbursed by their insurance company. The passage of Medicaid and Medicare changed this dynamic and it became necessary to create a standardized set of codes that could be used for billing purposes. HCFA appointed the American Medical Association (AMA) to create a set of codes for use in billing procedures, which became the Current Procedural Terminology code set first published in 1966. These codes have been updated annually since 1970 (Beck 2007). The current version, CPT-4, is still in use today and is referred to as simply CPT.

Current Procedural Terminology (CPT) codes are five-digit numeric or alphanumeric codes used to report procedures, treatments, and diagnostic and therapeutic services that were performed in the outpatient setting. Unlike the other code sets discussed in this text, which are in part developed by CMS, the CPT code set is developed, maintained, and copyrighted by the American Medical Association (AMA).

Similar to ICD-10-PCS codes in purpose, CPT codes are used to report the procedures performed on patients and are used for reimbursement purposes. However, ICD-10-PCS codes are used in the hospital inpatient setting, whereas CPT codes are used in all outpatient settings and for reporting inpatient services performed by professional healthcare providers. For example, if a physician treated a fracture and placed a cast on a fractured arm, then this service would be reported with a CPT code (24500, Closed treatment of humeral shaft fracture; without manipulation), and there would be a specific dollar amount charged for that specific CPT code (determined by the healthcare provider's office) that corresponds to the work, risk, and skill required to perform the service. In this way, healthcare providers can charge and get paid more for procedures that are riskier, or require more skill, more overhead, or more work than other procedures. For example, if a doctor performed a low-level sick visit that required 10 minutes of face-to-face time, he would charge less than if he performed a high-level face-to-face visit that required an hour of his time.

CPT codes encompass any type of procedure, treatment, diagnostic test, or other service that a healthcare provider could perform. These include office visits and evaluations, anesthesia services, surgical procedures, radiologic studies and treatments, laboratory and pathology procedures, and miscellaneous healthcare procedures such as hearing evaluations or chiropractic adjustments. Because they are reimbursed by insurance companies, medical necessity s required and indicated by an ICD-10-CM code placed on the same claim. Without an ICD-10-CM code to identify the medical necessity for the procedure performed, the procedure code will not be reimbursed. For example, if an orthopedist manipulated a fracture and placed a cast on a patient's arm, then he would include the CPT code for the procedure, attached to a charge for that specific procedure. He would also need to identify the medical necessity for the service by including an ICD-10-CM code for the diagnosis (fracture), indicating that the service was medically necessary.

CPT codes may also be appended with a **modifier** that identifies any additional information regarding the service provided or modifies the code description. CPT modifiers are developed and maintained by the AMA, and are published in an appendix to the CPT code book. This appendix also lists a small amount of HCPCS modifiers, published and maintained by CMS, that are also included in the HCPCS code book. Modifiers can alter the code description or provide more information regarding the service, and typically impact payment of the codes themselves. For instance, modifier -53, Discontinued procedure, indicates that the service was discontinued. If this modifier is appended (placed at the end) of a procedure code, then the payment for the procedure will likely be reduced, because the procedure was discontinued and was not performed in full. For example, a bronchoscopy was discontinued in the middle of the service because the patient went into respiratory distress. On the other hand, modifier -22, Increased procedural services indicates that a procedure required more work, time, or effort to complete. For example, a bronchoscopy was especially difficult due to obstructions in the bronchi. In this case, then, the insurance would reimburse the provider at a higher rate than usual because the procedure was increased in terms of difficulty, time, or effort.

HCPCS Level II: HCPCS Codes

HCPCS codes are five-character alphanumeric codes that are used to report supplies, services, and miscellaneous procedures that are performed or supplied in the outpatient setting that are not described by CPT codes. They are commonly used in conjunction with CPT codes, and are accepted by all third-party payers.

The majority of HCPCS codes represent any additional supplies that may be used in the outpatient setting, or any supplies that may be provided to the patient for take-home use. For example, if a patient presents to the healthcare office and requires a nebulizer breathing treatment, and the office provided the patient with a nebulizer machine, oxygen mask, and oxygen tubing, then HCPCS codes would be used to identify these items, with an appropriate charge attached to each item. Services such as ambulance transportation are also included in the HCPCS code set, as well as drugs or other medications that are administered in the healthcare setting, such as a shot of antibiotics for an extremely sick patient. They are not required for every claim, but instead are only used when provided to the patient, as medically necessary. More about HCPCS coding and coding for supplies provided to the patient in the office setting is discussed in chapter 6.

HCPCS codes must also be supported with a diagnosis code to identify the medical necessity for the service or item supplied to the patient. For example, if a patient was given a nebulizer machine in the office so they could continue breathing treatments at home, then the diagnosis code included on the claim would have to indicate the medical necessity for the supply, such as asthma or pneumonia. For an ambulance service provided to a patient who had suffered a laceration in a work-related accident, then the diagnosis code would have to identify the patient's injuries that required the ambulance transportation.

There are many codes within the HCPCS code set that are used specifically for Medicare beneficiaries. Because CMS maintains and develops the HCPCS Level II codes, many of these codes have been developed specifically for use on Medicare and Medicaid claims. For example, cervical and prostate cancer screenings provided to Medicare patients would be reported with the appropriate HCPCS codes, rather than the equivalent CPT code(s). If services are provided to a Medicare patient, it is always necessary to check for the appropriate HCPCS code before using a CPT code. Refer to the discussion of billing considerations in chapter 2, and the many ways in which the patient's insurance company impacts the codes that are reported.

Modifiers may also be appended to HCPCS codes to alter the meaning of the HCPCS supply or service. HCPCS modifiers are developed and maintained by CMS, and are published in the HCPCS code book. They work in essentially the same way as CPT modifiers, by providing more information regarding a service or supply. For example, modifiers -AE, Registered dietician and -AH, Clinical psychologist identify the type of provider that provided the service; and modifiers -T6, Right foot, second digit and -LM, Left main coronary artery identify the exact anatomical location of the procedure. Modifiers are always two characters, are either numeric or alphanumeric, and are always placed at the end of outpatient procedure codes (CPT or HCPCS). They are never used in conjunction with diagnosis codes (ICD-10-CM or ICD-9) or inpatient procedure codes (ICD-10-PCS).

Key to Success

Do not confuse ICD-10-PCS codes with CPT codes. PCS codes are used by a facility to identify the procedures that were performed on a patient and they are not attached to charges on claims. CPT codes, however, are attached to charges for procedures that were performed by individual healthcare professionals, which may have been provided in an inpatient or outpatient setting such as office or clinic visits, surgical procedures, or diagnostic studies.

Updates to the Code Sets

Each code set is updated at least on an annual basis. This means that every year it is necessary to purchase new code books, review changes to the codes, and update any coding strategies as necessary. Updates to the ICD-10 system are implemented on October 1st of every year, and updates to the CPT codes are implemented on January 1st of each year. Changes to the HCPCS code set are made on a quarterly basis (every three months), but new books are published only at the beginning of each year and are effective in January (see figure 3.2). HCPCS code changes are also published through CMS provider bulletins that are published on the CMS website when available.

Note that usually only a handful of changes are made each year, as necessitated by advancements in medicine, new clinical treatments, and changes in clinical discourse. This means that coders do not have to learn all new codes every year. Instead, it is important to review new codes and code changes to make any necessary changes in daily coding practices and update healthcare practice management and EHR systems.

Figure 3.2. Code updates schedule

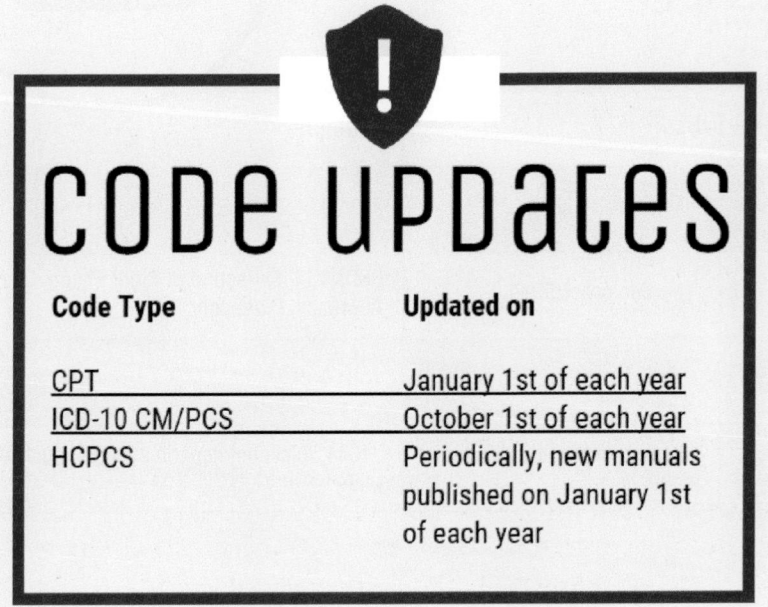

CODE UPDATES

Code Type	Updated on
CPT	January 1st of each year
ICD-10 CM/PCS	October 1st of each year
HCPCS	Periodically, new manuals published on January 1st of each year

Putting the Codes Together

There are two parts—diagnosis and procedure—to every claim, either professional physician (submitted on the CMS-1500 claim form) or facility inpatient (submitted on the UB-04 claim form). The diagnosis codes (ICD-10-CM) identify the medical necessity for the procedure or the supply provided (ICD-10-PCS, CPT, HCPCS), and each must be included on every claim sent. At a minimum, one procedure code (either CPT, HCPCS) must be submitted with one diagnosis code (ICD-10-CM) for professional or physician encounters. For facility or inpatient claims, at least one diagnosis code must be reported (ICD-10-CM) depending on whether or not a procedure was performed on the patient during his or her stay. If a procedure was performed, then procedure code(s) would be necessary to identify the service(s) performed (ICD-10-PCS codes). It is important to understand that all of these codes are used in conjunction with one another and they cannot be separated. Refer to chapter 2 to review the CMS-1500 claim form; the UB-04 claim form is discussed in greater detail in chapter 20.

Therefore, the majority of this text requires the learner to identify both the procedure (ICD-10-PCS, CPT, or HCPCS) codes as well as the diagnosis (ICD-10-CM or ICD-9) codes for practice exercises, as would be required in a real-world setting. Although this approach is more difficult at first—especially when learning how to use each of the code sets and without having experience in coding—it is ultimately more representative of the actual job of a coder. Examine figure 3.3, to review the types of codes and their uses.

Figure 3.3. Healthcare codes and their uses

Code	Reported by	Use	Example
ICD-10-CM	facility and professional	medical necessity	J03.90, Acute tonsillitis, unspecified
ICD-10-PCS	facility (inpatient and outpatient)	reporting procedures	0BDN0ZX, Extraction of Right Pleura, Open Approach, Diagnostic
CPT	professional and outpatient facility	reporting procedures, charging for services	33050, Resection of pericardial cyst or tumor
HCPCS	professional and outpatient facility	reporting procedures, charging for services	J1644, Injection, heparin sodium, per 1000 units

Distinguishing between Diagnoses and Procedures

ICD-10-CM codes are used to identify the reason why a patient received healthcare services, which is usually some sort of medical diagnosis. CPT codes are used to report the procedures, services, or treatments that were performed by the healthcare provider. It is easy for beginning coders to get confused when first learning about procedural coding, especially when trying to keep procedural coding and diagnostic coding separate. Procedures are the *verbs*; that is, a procedure is what the healthcare provider *did* to the patient. Diagnoses are the reasons *why* those procedures were performed. If confused, it can be helpful to ask the following questions, especially when coding for complicated procedures.

What did the doctor do? = Procedure code (CPT)

Why did the doctor do it? = Diagnosis code (ICD-10-CM)

It is important to clearly understand this distinction before moving forward with coding. Read the following vignette for help understanding the differences between diagnostic and procedural coding.

Rudy is a beginning coder and is having a hard time learning the differences between diagnostic and procedural coding. She knows that diagnosis codes are ICD-10-CM codes and that procedure codes are CPT codes, but she is still having problems understanding the two when she is faced with complicated medical documentation. She is currently working on a health record for a patient who came in for a screening colonoscopy, which is a preventive service. During the colonoscopy, the doctor encountered a number of small polyps in the sigmoid colon. The doctor then did a biopsy of three of the polyps during the colonoscopy.

Rudy must code for both the diagnosis and the procedure on the claim, but is having difficulty starting. Her coding supervisor suggested that to help, she ask herself the following questions: What did the doctor do? and, Why did the doctor do it? The answers to those questions will help her abstract the documentation and differentiate between the diagnosis and the procedure, which she can then look up in her code books.

First, she asks herself: What did the doctor do? Searching through the documentation, she pulls out the word that identifies the procedure—colonoscopy. The doctor also did a biopsy because he found multiple polyps during the colonoscopy, so the procedure was a colonoscopy with biopsy of three polyps. Now that she has the procedure, Rudy asks herself the other question: Why did the doctor do it? In this case, the patient came in for a screening colonoscopy, which is a preventive examination. But then the doctor found multiple polyps and performed a biopsy. So, in this case, the reason why the doctor did the biopsy was because of the polyps. If there had not been any abnormalities encountered during the colonoscopy, then she would have to use the diagnosis code for a screening colonoscopy.

Now that Rudy has her answers, she can begin to search for the codes in the code books. She knows that the procedure was a colonoscopy with biopsy of three polyps, which she will look up in the CPT code book; and the diagnosis was polyps of the sigmoid colon, which she will look up in the ICD-10-CM code book.

For practice asking and answering these two questions, complete the exercises in There's a Code for That 3.1.

3.1

There's a Code for That

Determining the procedure versus the diagnosis

Using the two questions *What did the doctor do?* and *Why did the doctor do it?*, identify the procedures and diagnoses from the following statements. (Only identify the diagnosis and procedure, do not look up the codes for either.)

1. Frank presented to the office of his psychiatrist to begin treatment for depression. After psychoanalysis and a physical examination, his psychiatrist prescribed an antidepressant.

   Procedure: _____

   Diagnosis: _____

2. A patient presented to the emergency room complaining of severe abdominal pain, fever, and vomiting. After evaluation, it is determined that she has a ruptured appendix. She is rushed into emergency appendectomy surgery to remove the ruptured appendix.

   Procedure: _____

   Diagnosis: _____

3. A 15-year-old male presented to the office of his PCP for a refill of his asthma prescription. After brief evaluation and management service, the physician assistant refilled his asthma prescription.

   Procedure: _____

   Diagnosis: _____

4. A 15-year-old male presented to the office of his PCP with wheezing and trouble breathing due to his asthma. After an extended evaluation and management service and a nebulizer breathing treatment, the physician diagnosed the patient with asthma with acute exacerbation (asthma attack), and prescribed a rescue inhaler.

   Procedure: _____

   Diagnosis: _____

5. 45-year-old with suspected pneumonia received a chest x-ray. X-ray confirms pneumonia in the lower left lobe of the lung.

   Procedure: _____

   Diagnosis: _____

In addition to reporting diagnoses and procedures, codes have multiple other uses. From risk adjustment to performance measures (discussed in chapter 2), as the uses of codes become more varied, job opportunities for coders increase and become more diverse.

Additional Uses of Healthcare Codes

In addition to identifying the medical necessity for a service or identifying the procedure performed or supply provided, there are numerous other uses of codes. These range from simple internal tracking to nationwide (and international) reporting of diseases. They include the following.

- *Public health and tracking of disease.* The billions of diagnoses reported by health providers each year are tracked and analyzed by official organizations, such as the Centers for Disease Control (CDC). This information is used for public health purposes (CDC 2015). For example, if the CDC notes an increase in the incidence of certain sexually transmitted diseases, then it might fund more research into effective reduction and treatment strategies including public health campaigns that inform the public about the dangers of unprotected sex. Healthcare conditions are also tracked in the same way on an international scale. For example, worldwide health issues like pandemics or epidemics are tracked via codes.

- *Internal tracking.* Codes are used internally by both large and small healthcare practices and facilities to evaluate their own patient population and treatment. For example, if a small healthcare practice is about to order their supply of the influenza vaccine for the coming flu shot season, then they might analyze how many influenza vaccines were given in the previous year to estimate how many vaccines they may have to administer during this flu shot season. For a large healthcare practice, such as a hospital with thousands of healthcare providers, codes may be used to identify internal facility issues, such as the number of patients who acquire a urinary tract infection due to catheterizations.

- *Performance Measurement and Quality Improvement.* Facilities also use the data generated from codes to track their performance on certain performance measures, and to implement quality improvement programs when necessary.

- *Risk adjustment.* Risk adjustment and HCC coding (discussed in chapter 2) are important to many practices and facilities, the data for which is calculated from patient diagnosis codes. HCC coding can impact the bottom line for both insurance companies and individual practices, and is an increasing area of concern for many healthcare providers.

- *Research and funding.* The information compiled from the analysis of codes is also used in research and funding. If a certain type of cancer is becoming more prevalent, for example, then additional research or funding may be allocated toward that specific type of cancer, its causes, and its treatment. This is an important use of codes, as it helps identify future public health needs as well as the efficacy of healthcare treatments.

- *Evaluate the utilization of healthcare facilities.* The use of procedure codes can help support decisions for new healthcare equipment or other utilization of healthcare facilities. For example, procedure codes may be used to track the number of patients whose operations used robotic assistance, or who received care in a pediatric critical care unit. For example, if a large hospital facility just purchased a $250,000 full-body x-ray machine, they can evaluate how many patients are served using that machine to help justify the cost. On the other hand, utilization tracking might result in the closure of a certain area of the hospital or specialized service that is costing more money than it generates.

Codes have been in use for over 100 years, and their usage has evolved into this multifaceted approach to analyze, predict, and track healthcare conditions, procedures, and facility usage, as well as to charge for services provided and analyze funding for a year's worth of services from an insurance perspective. It is important to briefly examine the future directions of codes.

The Future of Healthcare Coding

The healthcare industry changes rapidly, and just as codes have evolved over the last 100 years, they will continue to evolve into new formations with new uses and new meanings. It is important to briefly look into the future of coding to see what may lie on the horizon.

The World Health Organization released the ICD-10 code set in 1993, and even though the United States has only recently transitioned to ICD-10, the release of a completely new, updated diagnosis coding system is in development. The International Classification of Diseases, 11th revision (ICD-11), is currently in development and is expected to be implemented after 2018 (WHO 2015). This version is being developed by WHO and, once completed, will be systematically implemented throughout the world just as ICD-10 was. However, the actual implementation of the ICD-11 code set is dependent on each country adopting it.

As part of the natural progression of diagnosis codes and the conditions they represent, the ICD code set is being revised to ICD-11 to better reflect progresses in healthcare practice and clinical study, as well as to be used with electronic practice management systems and health applications. Some of the features included within the ICD-11 codes, which are either completely new or build upon the foundations of ICD-10 will be

- Available in multiple languages
- Enabling collaboration and revision by peers and interested parties to ensure accuracy and relevance
- Structured in such a way that definitions, signs, symptoms, and other related information may be recorded more accurately
- Compatible with electronic health record systems (WHO 2015)

It is important to understand that the ICD-11 code set is still in development by the World Health Organization and has yet to be finalized or released. Even after it is released, it is unlikely that the United States will adopt the ICD-11 codes immediately. It took more than 20 years for the United States to transition to the ICD-10 codes set once it was released, so any update to ICD-11 will likely happen years in the future.

This chapter has previously discussed medical necessity, but it is necessary to go one step further and detail how to identify the medical necessity for specific procedures by linking them together. This is called code linkage.

Code Linkage and Medical Necessity

As previously discussed, medical necessity is indicated using ICD-10-CM codes that identify and justify the reason why a procedure was performed. For example, if a patient had an appendectomy, then the ICD-10-CM code should indicate the reason why the patient had the appendectomy, normally appendicitis. In other words, the diagnosis code must match the procedure. If the codes do not match (if there is no medical necessity for the procedure provided), then the procedure performed will not be paid.

Code linkage is linking the diagnosis and procedure code together to identify the medical necessity for specific procedures. Note that code linkage is only necessary for reported professional services provided by a qualified healthcare practitioner, and reported on the CMD-1500 claim form. Inpatient facility claims billed on the UB-04 form do not utilize the code linkage concept. This is especially important in the case of claims that have more than one procedure or diagnosis code. Consider the following example.

Dr. Alameda has just seen Benjamin for a sick visit encounter. He is an avid swimmer and has been experiencing severe ear pain for the last few days. During the encounter, Dr. Alameda diagnoses Benjamin with otitis externa (swimmer's ear) of the left ear and prescribes an antibiotic. She also noted a small common wart (verruca vulgaris) on the bottom of his left palm that has been causing him some discomfort. After obtaining approval from the patient, she freezes the wart and covers it with a bandage and tells Benjamin that the wart should fall off and he should return to the office if he has any further problems with it.

In this example, the patient has two diagnoses: left sided swimmer's ear (H60.332, Swimmer's ear, left ear), and verruca vulgaris (B07.9, Viral wart, unspecified). There were also two procedures performed: an office evaluation and management service to identify the encounter with the doctor (99213, Office or other outpatient visit, established patient, level 3), and the freezing of the wart (17000, Destruction, premalignant lesions; first lesion). An **evaluation and management (E/M)** service is a patient encounter with a healthcare professional in which the patient receives assessment, counseling, or routine health services. In other words, the healthcare provider evaluates the patient's healthcare needs or condition, and then manages said needs or condition. E/M services, otherwise known as "patient encounters" or "office visits" are a common component of many healthcare services. (Coding for evaluation and management services is discussed in detail in chapters 7 and 8 of this text). In the previous example, there were two unrelated procedures that were performed (an E/M service and the freezing of a wart) for two unrelated diagnoses (swimmer's ear and viral wart). Therefore it is necessary to link each diagnosis code with the procedure code that it supports (code linkage).

In this scenario, the diagnosis of swimmer's ear would be linked to the office evaluation and management service, and the diagnosis of the wart would be linked to the cryosurgery for the removal of the wart. The linkage identifies the medical necessity for each service. The cryosurgery was performed because of the wart and the office evaluation was performed because of the swimmer's ear (see figure 3.4)

Actually linking the codes together is done in the software that the healthcare office uses to report codes and send claims. This is done in different ways depending on the type of system used by the coder, but it typically involves identifying the specific diagnosis codes for each procedure. For example, if the swimmer's ear diagnosis was assigned as the first diagnosis on the claim, then it is assigned diagnosis number 1 or letter A. The wart diagnosis would be assigned as diagnosis number 2 or letter B.

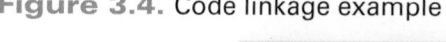

Figure 3.4. Code linkage example

Figure 3.5. Code linkage

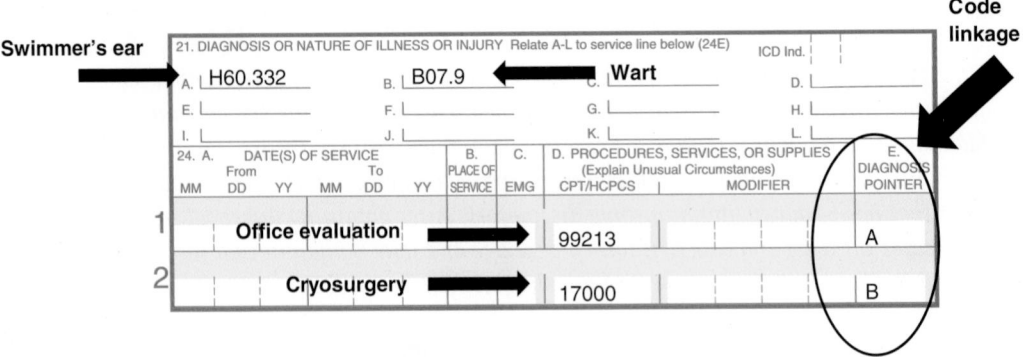

Source: CMS 2017a.

Because the office evaluation procedure code is listed as the primary procedure on the claim, then it is linked to diagnosis A. The secondary procedure, the cryosurgery, would be linked to diagnosis B. Up to 12 individual ICD-10-CM diagnosis codes may be included on a CMS-1500 paper claim, and as many procedure codes as necessary are also included, so it is important to take great care during the code linkage process. However, it is essential to ensure accurate reimbursement for the procedures performed and all of the charges billed.

On the CMS-1500 claim form, it is easy to see the code linkage to ensure that all codes are linked together properly. Review figure 3.5, which illustrates the properly linked codes from the previous example. There are 12 lines on which to enter individual diagnosis codes (box 21.A through 21.L). The letter of the diagnosis corresponds to the procedure code that it supports, as indicated in each line (lines 1 and 2). Box 24.E is the Diagnosis Pointer box, in which the letter of the diagnosis code is entered onto the line for the procedure to which it corresponds. So in this example, diagnosis A is linked to procedure 1, and diagnosis B is linked to procedure 2.

Remember that each procedure provided or item supplied, whether inpatient or outpatient, must be linked to diagnosis code to identify the medical necessity for the service. This means that CPT and HCPCS codes should all be supported with medical necessity in the form of ICD-10-CM codes.

Besides knowing the different types of codes, the history of their development, and how to link them together to indicate medical necessity, a coder needs to know the rules for their usage. Rules that govern coding are called guidelines and each set of codes has its own guidelines. It is important to be able to accurately locate, read, and use applicable guidelines to be a successful coder.

Coding Guidelines

Finding the correct codes is only one part of being a skilled coder. Coders must also know how to report identified codes appropriately. There are several rules that help coders locate, select, and sequence codes. Otherwise known as **coding guidelines**, these are the rules that specify which codes to use in given situations, how to sequence them, which modifiers to use, and how to combine them with other codes. These guidelines also often refer to the documentation of the healthcare encounter and how specific details need to be documented in order to select specific codes.

Official coding guidelines exist for both CPT codes, ICD-10-CM codes, and ICD-10-PCS codes, and are published on an annual basis with the code books for reference. Depending on the publisher and the edition of the code book being used, these official coding guidelines may or may not be included within the code book itself. Specific coding guidelines and where to find them are discussed in chapter 4 (ICD-10-CM coding), chapter 5 (CPT and HCPCS coding), and chapter 20 (ICD-10-PCS coding) of this text, and specific coding guidelines are discussed contextually throughout this text.

Key to Success

Additional coding guidelines and resources to help interpret coding guidelines are available through other publications, such as CPT Assistant and the American Hospital Association (AHA) Coding Clinic. Professional organizations, such as AHIMA, also offer coding advice and interpretations of coding guidance for coding professionals.

The Importance of Documentation

The importance of accurate, appropriate documentation cannot be overstated. Not only does it provide the information to help substantiate a code, but it is the record of everything that occurred in the healthcare setting. Without documentation to support code selection, it is not only impossible but unethical and illegal to select codes arbitrarily. Remember:

If it's not documented, it never happened!

What this means is that even if the patient came into the office with a certain condition and the physician performed several procedures, if that physician failed to document the encounter in the health record, then it cannot be coded.

Every code that is selected from a patient encounter must be substantiated by documentation in the health record. To select a code, coders must first review the documentation, extract the necessary information, and select the right code. Once the correct code(s) are selected, then the coder must review any guidelines or other rules before sequencing these codes on the claim and requires the following characteristics.

- *Complete:* Documentation for each encounter must be complete and signed by the healthcare provider. The healthcare provider's credential must also be clearly noted.
- *Detailed:* Documentation must include sufficient detail needed to support code selection. This text discusses the necessary details for code selection at length, but it is important to remember that all necessary details must be included in the provider's documentation in order to select a code. For example, the detail of laterality (which side a condition occurred) must be included in the documentation if a coder is to select a diagnosis code that indicates the laterality.
- *Legible:* In the days of paper health records, legibility was a huge burden in appropriate documentation. Now the majority of healthcare providers have transitioned to electronic health records, so legibility is not as big of an issue. However, if using paper records all documentation must be fully legible. Illegible handwriting is just as erroneous as incomplete documentation. Code selection is impossible if you cannot read the provider's handwriting and illegible handwriting cannot support the selection of a code.

- *Contain all necessary patient identifiers:* When paper health records are used in any form (even if it is simply a questionnaire that is later scanned into an electronic health records system), it must contain at least two patient identifiers. Usually, the patient's name and date of birth are the two patient identifiers that are the easiest to include on patient health records.
- *Formatted:* Specific encounter types are typically formatted into the same template. This eases codes selection, as well as helps with understanding when reviewing the documentation of the health encounter. Some examples of formatted records would be problem-oriented visit templates, vaccine administration records, surgical notation templates, anesthesia records, and laboratory results. Many of these templates and formats are illustrated in their respective sections throughout this text.

Not only does incomplete documentation cause problems logistically by not allowing for correct code selection, but it can also create problems in the long run in the case of audits or insurance chart reviews. Proper documentation, on the other hand, supports code selection, adheres to documentation standards, and allows a coder to most effectively utilize coding guidelines. For coders interested in documentation improvement, AHIMA offers the Certified Documentation Improvement Practitioner (CDIP®) certification (see the appendix Coding Certifications and Professional Coding Organizations in this text).

Guidelines for Code Sets

Each code set has its own unique set of guidelines, or rules, that are used to help identify, select, and sequence the correct codes. In addition to official guidelines, many insurance plans have specific guidelines on how codes should be listed on claims. So coders may find that even though the official coding guidelines offer one direction, an insurance company requires the coder to code something differently.

For example, ICD-10-CM coding guidelines might require the coder to sequence a pain code after the code for the acute condition, whereas the insurance requires the acute condition to be placed before the pain code. This is a very common scenario. Ultimately, the real world is more complicated than following the rules in a code book, and as long as the coder does not code for anything fraudulently, unethically, or for something that is not supported by the documentation, the best course of action is usually to code the encounter as indicated by the patient's health insurance. That being said, follow the coding guidelines as best as possible in every situation. This is especially true in coding certification exams, which often specifically test a coder's ability to utilize the coding guidelines.

Whether or not a code book actually contains guidelines or coding advice depends on the publisher as well as the edition of the code book that a coder is using. For example, the CPT Standard edition does not contain the same coding guidelines and advice as that of the CPT Professional edition, which contains additional guidelines, anatomical drawings, and notations throughout the book. As a new coder, it is a good idea to purchase the best code books possible, or even additional specialty coding reference guides. When learning coding for the first time, or in your first position as a coder, purchasing high-quality manuals is a solid investment to help you in your journey to becoming an expert coder.

Specific coding guidelines are discussed throughout this text, when applicable. Additionally, how to locate and use the coding guidelines is discussed in chapter 4 (Learning the ICD-10-CM Code Book) and chapter 5 (Learning the CPT and HCPCS

Code Books). When coding throughout the rest of this text and in the real world, remember to use the coding guidelines—they are the rules that help you figure out how to correctly select, sequence, and assign codes.

End of Chapter Content

Instructions: Indicate whether the following statements are true or false (T or F). For false statements, rewrite the statement on the line below to make the statement true.

1. HIPAA standardized the use of five different code sets.

_____

_____

2. Inpatient and outpatient coding consists of the three main code sets: ICD, CPT, and HCPCS.

_____

_____

3. The two divisions of the ICD code set are CM and CPT.

_____

_____

4. The CM at the end of ICD-10-CM stands for classifications of morbidity.

_____

_____

5. For professional claims, medical necessity is identified by code linkage.

_____

_____

6. ICD-9 codes were implemented on October 1, 2015.

_____

_____

7. The CPT code set is published by CMS.

_____

_____

(Continued on next page)

(Continued)

8. Codes may be used to evaluate the utilization of facility resources.

_____

_____

9. Procedural classifications were first developed in the 17th century.

_____

_____

10. HCPCS codes may also be referred to as Level II codes.

_____

_____

Instructions: Choose the best answer.

1. What are the alphanumeric translations of services, supplies, and diagnoses?
   a. Healthcare codes
   b. Healthcare transcriptions
   c. Translations of healthcare diagnoses
   d. International Classification of Diseases

2. Codes are either numeric or:
   a. Seven characters
   b. Alphanumeric
   c. Six digits
   d. They are only numeric

3. Which of the following ICD code set revisions is currently in use?
   a. ICD-9
   b. ICD-10
   c. ICD-11
   d. CPT-4

4. Which of the following code sets is used to report hospital or facility inpatient procedures?
   a. ICD-10-CM
   b. HCPCS
   c. CPT
   d. ICD-10-PCS

5. What is the reason why a healthcare procedure was performed?
   a. Medically unnecessary
   b. CPT codes
   c. Medical necessity
   d. Personal reasons

6. What is code linkage?
   a. Linking diagnosis codes with other diagnosis codes to identify medical necessity for a procedure
   b. Linking HCPCS codes with CPT codes to identify medical necessity for a procedure
   c. Linking ICD-10-PCS codes with HCPCS codes to identify the medical necessity for a procedure
   d. Linking ICD-10-CM codes with a procedure code to identify the medical necessity for the procedure

7. In which of the following situations might you use an ICD-9 code?
   a. For a claim with a date of service before 10/01/2015
   b. For a claim with a date of service after 10/01/2015
   c. For all claims no matter what the date of service
   d. For hospital inpatient claims only

8. Which of the following is a five-digit numeric code that is used to report procedures?

 a. ICD-10

 b. HCPCS

 c. CPT

 d. ICD-9

9. Which of the following code sets is used to report diagnoses or supplies rather than procedures?

 a. CPT

 b. ICD-10-CM

 c. ICD-10-PCS

 d. HCPCS

10. Which of the following code sets evolved over the course of hundreds of years and began as a registry system for the causes of mortality?

 a. ICD

 b. CPT

 c. HCPCS

 d. NDC

11. Which of the following are the two divisions of the ICD-10 code set?

 a. CM and CPT

 b. PCS and HCPCS

 c. PCS and CM

 d. CPT and PCS

12. The HCPCS code set is divided into two Levels. Level II codes are commonly referred to as which of the following?

 a. HCPCS

 b. CPT

 c. ICD-10-PCS

 d. ICD-10-CM

13. What is linking the diagnosis and procedure code together called?

 a. Code necessity

 b. Medical necessity

 c. Code linkage

 d. Medical linkage

14. On the CMS-1500 form, in which box are the diagnosis pointers located?

 a. Box 24.A

 b. Box 21.E

 c. Box 24.E

 d. Box 24.D

15. Finish the following sentence: If it's not documented, it _____.

 a. Always happens

 b. Doesn't matter

 c. Can be coded

 d. Never happened

References

Beck, D. E. and D. A. Margolin. 2007 (Spring). Physician Coding and Reimbursement. *Ochsner J* 7(1): 8–15. https://www.ncbi.nlm.nih.gov/pmc/articles/PMC3096340/.

Centers for Disease Control and Prevention. 2015 (November 6). International Classification of Diseases, (ICD-10-CM/PCS) Transition–Background. https://www.cdc.gov/nchs/icd/icd10cm_pcs_background.htm.

Centers for Medicare and Medicaid Services. 2017. Details for title: CMS 1500. https://www.cms.gov/Medicare/CMS-Forms/CMS-Forms/CMS-Forms-Items/CMS1188854.html.

Centers for Medicare and Medicaid Services. 2017 (July 25). HCPCS - General Information. https://www.cms.gov/Medicare/Coding/MedHCPCSGenInfo/index.html?redirect=/medhcpcsgeninfo.

World Health Organization. 2017. History of the Development of the ICD. http://www.who.int/classifications/icd/en/HistoryOfICD.pdf.

World Health Organization. 2015 (April 14). Report of ICD-11 Revision Review. http://www.who.int/classifications/icd/reportoftheicd11review14april2015.pdf?ua=1.

Resources

Centers for Medicare and Medicaid Services. 2017 (July 26). Code Sets Overview. https://www.cms.gov/Regulations-and-Guidance/Administrative-Simplification/Code-Sets/index.html.

National Center for Health Statistics. 2017. International Classification of Diseases, Tenth Revision, Clinical Modification (ICD-10-CM). https://www.cdc.gov/nchs/icd/icd10cm.htm.

World Health Organization. 2016. Classifications. http://www.who.int/classifications/icd/en/.

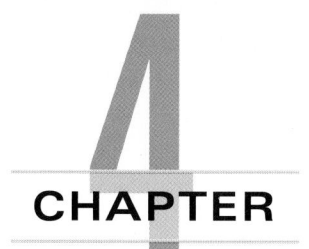

CHAPTER 4

Learning the ICD-10-CM Code Book

Learning Objectives

- Examine the organization, format, notations, and conventions used in the ICD-10-CM code book.
- Recognize and utilize general coding guidelines for ICD-10-CM codes.
- Examine the structure of ICD-10-CM codes.

Key Terms

Accidental intent
Activity
Acute conditions
Adverse effect
Assault
Benign neoplasm
Bilateral
Billable code
Carcinoma in situ
Chronic condition
Code first
Combination code
Cross-reference
Definitive diagnosis
Episode of care
Essential modifier
Etiology
Excludes notes
Excludes1
Excludes2
External cause codes
External Causes of Injury Index
First-listed diagnosis

Histologic type
Includes notes
Inclusion terms
Index to Diseases and Injury
Initial encounter
Injury mechanism
Intent
Intentional self-harm
Invalid code
Laterality
Main term
Malignant neoplasm
Manifestation
Metastasis
Morphology
Neoplasm
Neoplasm of uncertain behavior
Nonessential modifier
Not elsewhere classifiable (NEC)
Not otherwise specified (NOS)
Official Guidelines for Coding and Reporting (OGCR)

Patient status
Place of occurrence
Placeholder X
Primary neoplasm
Secondary neoplasm
See also
See condition
Sequela
Sequencing
Seventh character extension
Signs
Specificity
Subsequent encounter
Subterm
Symptoms
Table of Drugs and Chemicals
Table of Neoplasms
Tabular List
Toxic effect
Underdosing
Undetermined intent
Use additional code

Each of the codes sets—ICD-10-CM, CPT, HCPCS, and ICD-10-PCS—have a different intended use, format, and number of characters or digits. They are also published in separate code books, each of which has a different organization, conventions, and guidelines. Therefore, it is necessary to spend some time getting to know the varying code structures, organization of the book, and format and symbols used in each code book, as well as how to find and use the guidelines, and how to use each code book to identify and assign the appropriate codes. This chapter focuses on the many intricacies of the ICD-10-CM code book and code set, which is used for diagnostic coding. Chapter 5 (Learning the CPT and HCPCS Code Books) focuses on learning the procedural coding books.

Please note that because ICD-10-PCS coding is mostly used in the inpatient setting, the format of ICD-10-PCS codes and the organization of the PCS code book is discussed in chapter 20 (Inpatient Hospital Services).

ICD-10-CM Organization and Format

The ICD-10 code set is a national creation of codes used to identify diagnoses and inpatient procedures, and is a publicly available resource. Unlike CPT codes (discussed in detail in chapter 5), which are created, maintained, and copyrighted by the American Medical Association (AMA), ICD-10 codes may be compiled and published into a code book by any party. This means that ICD-10 code books vary greatly, depending on the publisher of the code book. However, even though certain ICD-10-CM code books may have more information such as guidelines, color-coding, or references, the ICD-10-CM codes and code descriptions are all the same. This text refers to the AHIMA ICD-10-CM code book.

However, the organization, format of the sections, the codes and code descriptions, and the conventions used throughout the book are the same, no matter the publisher. This ensures consistency and appropriate code selection across all ICD-10 code books.

ICD-10-CM codes are some of the longest healthcare codes and require a strict attention to detail, as each character added to the code identifies a specific detail about the patient's healthcare condition. It is important to always code to the highest level of specificity to ensure each and every detail of the patient's condition is reflected in the code.

Key to Success

Before getting into specifics of the ICD-10-CM organization and format, look at the outer edge of the pages of the ICD-10-CM code book. Though it may vary by publisher, the majority of ICD-10-CM code books have a colored outer edge or indented tabs on the side of the page opposite the binding. These colors or tabs identify different sections of the ICD-10-CM book. As you learn how to use the ICD-10-CM code book, these colors or tabs can help you locate and access certain sections within the book.

The ICD-10-CM code book is divided into two major sections: the Index and the Tabular List. Each of these sections is further divided into additional subsections and chapters.

The Index

The Index to the ICD-10-CM code book is comprised of four different sections. Each of these sections is designed to allow coders to find the main term of the condition, disease, or other reason for a healthcare encounter, and direct the coder to the code for that condition. For example, if a coder is looking for the code for pharyngitis (sore throat), then he can access the index to find the term *pharyngitis*, which will direct him to the code J02.9, Acute pharyngitis, unspecified.

The four individual subsections of the Index each allow the user to look up different types of conditions or reasons for an encounter. They are: the Index to Diseases and Injury, the Table of Neoplasms, the Table of Drugs and Chemicals, and the External Cause of Injuries Index.

Index to Diseases and Injury

The **Index to Diseases and Injury** (often referred to as the Main Index), is the main index to the ICD-10-CM code book. This is the largest index of the ICD-10-CM code book, and allows coders to look up any condition coded with an ICD-10-CM code in alphabetical order, with the exception of the majority of neoplasms, poisonings and adverse effects, and external causes (discussed later in this chapter).

The following steps should be followed when searching for a code using the Main Index.

The first step is to find the main term for the condition, disease, or other reason for the encounter. Then, check for cross-references, subterms, and nonessential modifiers. Finally, locate the code and then verify it in the Tabular List (the alphanumerical listing of all ICD-10-CM codes, discussed as follows). See figure 4.1 for a reminder of the steps to using the Main Index.

Find the Main Term

The coder first needs to find the main term for the condition, disease, or other reason for the encounter. The main term is the noun that describes the patient's diagnosis or

Figure 4.1. Steps to using the Index to Diseases and Injury (Main Index)

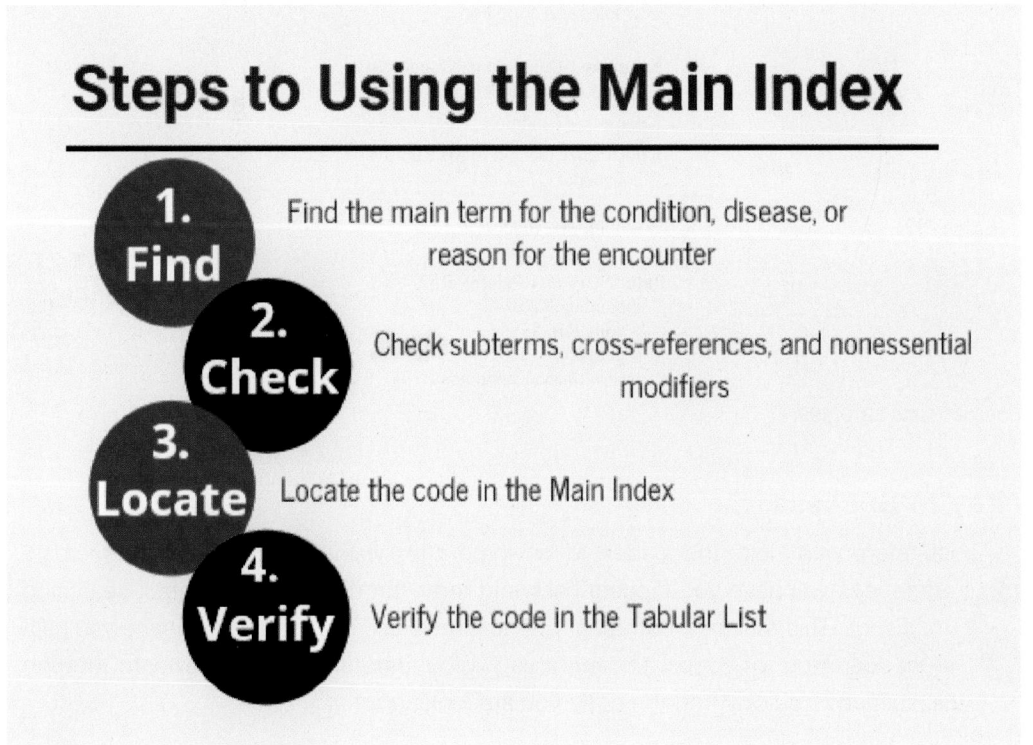

Steps to Using the Main Index

1. Find — Find the main term for the condition, disease, or reason for the encounter

2. Check — Check subterms, cross-references, and nonessential modifiers

3. Locate — Locate the code in the Main Index

4. Verify — Verify the code in the Tabular List

reason for encounter, such as the term *pharyngitis*. The main terms should be abstracted from the documentation for the encounter. So the coder needs to read through the provider's documentation of the encounter carefully, extract the diagnoses, conditions, or other reasons for the encounter, and then locate the codes for those reasons and assign them on the claim. The rest of the chapters in this text will help guide the coder through this process until it becomes second nature. Once the main term is located in the Main Index, then any cross-references, subterms, or nonessential modifiers must be checked before confirming code selection.

Check Cross-References, Subterms, and Modifiers

Once the main term is located in the Main Index, there may be a cross-reference that informs the coder to "*see* condition." This is a **cross-reference**, which instructs the coder to look elsewhere for a code. In this case the "*see* condition" cross reference tells the coder to search for the code by looking up the condition, rather than the term he or she initially located. The "*see* condition" cross-reference is very common when looking up diagnoses that are located at specific anatomical sites. For example, Smith is a beginning coder and needs to find the code for knee pain. He chooses to look up the term *knee* in the Index. Once he locates the term *knee* he notes that he cannot find *knee pain*; instead, there is a cross-reference that instructs him to "*see* condition." Instead of looking up the word *condition*, Smith must look up the condition of the knee; the knee is in pain, so he looks up the term *pain*. Once Smith looks up the word *pain*, he notes that this entry also contains a cross-reference, which instructs the coder to "*see also* painful." The "*see also*" cross-reference instructs the coder to look elsewhere for a code if the precise condition cannot be found in the current index entry. In this case, Smith should *see also* painful if he cannot locate the code for knee pain within the *pain* entry in the Main Index (figure 4.2a and 4.2b).

Figure 4.2a. ICD-10-CM Main Index example 1

Example: *see* condition

Klumpke (-Déjerine) palsy, paralysis (birth) (newborn) P14.1
Knee —*see* condition
Knock knee (acquired) M21.06-
    congenital Q74.1

Example: *see also*

Pain(s) (*see also* Painful) R52
    abdominal R10.9
        colic R10.83
        generalized R10.84
            with acute abdomen R10.0

Source: Casto 2018, 199.

Key to Success

Cross-references help the coder to navigate the Main Index. Sometimes cross-references will have you flipping back and forth through the Main Index searching for a code. This may be frustrating, but don't give up! The more experience you gain from searching for codes, the more you will understand how to navigate through this section to quickly find the code you are looking for.

Figure 4.2b. ICD-10-CM Main Index example 1 (continued)

Example: subterm (essential modifier)

```
joint M25.50
     ankle M25.57-
     elbow M25.52-
     finger M25.54-
     foot M25.57-
     hand M25.54-
     hip M25.55-
     knee M25.56-
     shoulder M25.51-
     toe M25.57-
     wrist M25.53-
```

Source: Casto 2018, 239.

After Smith notes the cross-references, he notices there are many subterms under the main term *pain*. **Subterms** are indented under the main term to indicate that they pertain to the main term, and to identify variations of the main term. For example, there are many different types and sites of pain, so the subterms indented beneath the main entry *pain* describe various types or sites of pain. Smith notes that under the main term *pain*, there are quite a few columns of subterms. He searches for the subterm *knee*, but notes that he cannot find it. In this case, he must first locate the term *joint*, and then find the specific joint *knee* as a subterm.

Key to Success

Sometimes the subterms are listed in a complex manner. When searching for a condition in which there are numerous subterms in the Main Index, it is a good idea to scan the entire list of subterms to understand how they are listed. When Smith was searching for this term, he had to navigate through multiple subterms, and subterms of subterms. Because of the complexity of ICD-10-CM codes, many publishers include lines down each column of the Index to help coders navigate through the many different subterms. It may also be helpful to use a ruler or straightedge when maneuvering through the Index to keep track of subterms.

Subterms are considered **essential modifiers** because they impact the code that is selected. The location of the pain is an essential modifier that leads the coder to assign a code different than the code for an alternate site of pain. **Nonessential modifiers** are words located in parentheses next to the main term or a subterm within the Index. They offer more information, but do not impact code selection. For example, Smith now needs to find the code for pain due to intestinal gas. He now knows to look up the condition—in this case *pain*—and then the type or site of the pain, *intestinal gas pain*. Smith notes that the subterm *intestinal* is not listed in the subterms, but the word *gas* is. Next to the word *gas* is the nonessential modifier *intestinal* in parentheses (see figure 4.3). In this case, the word *intestinal* offers more information about the gas pain,

Figure 4.3. ICD-10-CM Main Index example 2

Example: nonessential modifier

```
gallbladder K82.9
gas (intestinal) R14.1
gastric —see Pain, abdominal
```

Source: Casto 2018, 239.

but does not impact the code selection. In other words, it does not change the code that is selected in the way that *knee* did for *knee pain*. Sometimes several nonessential modifiers may be listed next to a main term or subterm in the Index. These just provide more information and help with code selection.

Locate and Verify the Code

Once the main term or subterm has been located and any nonessential modifiers and cross-references have been noted, the coder should look to the right of the term to find the ICD-10-CM code. For example, if Smith is looking for the code for knee pain, and has maneuvered through the index to find the entry *pain, joint, knee*, then he finds the code M25.56- to the right of the word *knee* (see figure 4.2b). But he is not done yet. Smith now must verify that this is the correct code, especially because the code is listed with a hyphen (-) at the end of it. This means that the code needs an additional digit that must be selected when referencing the Tabular List. If Smith were to assign the code M25.56 without the required sixth character, then he would be assigning an invalid code. The additional character that should be assigned to the code M25.56- is found in the Tabular List and, in this case, the code needs one additional digit to identify the laterality of the pain (which knee is in pain—the right or the left). The diagnosis description does not state the laterality, so the correct code is M25.569, Pain in unspecified knee. This information is found within the Tabular List.

The Tabular List is the alphanumerical listing of all ICD-10-CM codes. Not only is it necessary to check the Tabular List to verify the code selected and assign all necessary characters to the code, as in the previous example, but it also contains important information about code selection, sequencing, and guidelines that govern appropriate code selection. The Tabular List and additional characters are discussed in detail in the next section of this chapter.

Key to Success

Default codes are the code for the unspecified version of a condition, and can be easy to overlook. For example, if a coder is looking for the code *pain, unspecified*, then it is not necessary to look any further than the first entry in the Index: Pain(s) (*see also* painful) R52. The code R52 should be assigned for unspecified pain. Default codes are always listed next to the main term in the Main Index, and represent the least specified version of that condition.

For practice identifying the main term, identifying essential and nonessential modifiers, and using the Main Index, complete the exercises in There's a Code for That 4.1, 4.2, and 4.3.

There's a Code for That

4.1

Identify the main term

Using the ICD-10-CM-CM code book, identify the main terms for the following diagnostic statements.

1. Knee pain.

Main term: _____

2. Reactive airway disease.

   Main term: _____

3. Difficulty swallowing.

   Main term: _____

4. Intervertebral disc degeneration.

   Main term: _____

5. Inguinal hernia.

   Main term: _____

Essential versus nonessential modifiers

4.2

There's a Code for That

Look up the following terms in the Main Index and identify if the modifier listed is either essential or nonessential (the first one has been completed for you).

	Main term	Modifier	Essential or nonessential
Example	Pachyonychia	congenital	*nonessential*
1.	Strain	back	
2.	Entropion	eyelid	
3.	Cholesterolemia	pure	
4.	Thrush	vaginal	

Using the Main Index

4.3

There's a Code for That

Using the Main Index, identify the code for the following diagnostic statements. For this exercise, only locate the code from the Main Index, you do not need to verify the code in the Tabular List.

1. Pneumococcal pneumonia.

   ICD-10-CM code: _____

2. Diaper rash.

   ICD-10-CM code: _____

3. Oropharyngeal dysphagia.

   ICD-10-CM code: _____

4. Echolalia.

   ICD-10-CM code: _____

5. Muckle-Wells syndrome.

   ICD-10-CM code: _____

6. Congenital gastrointestinal tract anomaly.

   ICD-10-CM code: _____

In the Index, the Table of Neoplasms follows the Index to Diseases and Injury and is used to locate ICD-10-CM codes for neoplasms such as benign moles and various cancers.

Table of Neoplasms

Also referred to as the neoplasm table, the **Table of Neoplasms** is an index that allows coders to identify codes for neoplastic conditions such as malignant tumors and diseases, and benign growths. A **neoplasm** is an abnormal growth of tissue and can be fast-growing and invasive, such as malignant cancer, or a benign mass or tumor. The neoplasm table is divided first by the anatomic site of the neoplasm, and then the behavior of the neoplasm. There are four different neoplasm behaviors: benign, malignant, carcinoma in situ, or uncertain behavior.

Benign neoplasms are noncancerous growths of tissue, such as a mole or uterine fibroid. They may be problematic and need excision (or removal), but they are not invasive and will not spread to other tissues.

Malignant neoplasms are commonly referred to as cancer. These neoplasms invade surrounding tissues and destroy them, and can be fatal. Malignant neoplasms can metastasize—or spread—throughout the body, creating **metastases** (or mets), which are offshoots of the original cancer. Metastases, or metastatic growths, are known as **secondary neoplasms**, or the site of the metastatic growth. The **primary neoplasm** is the where the growth originated. For example, a malignant melanoma of the skin may metastasize to the liver and brain. In this case, the primary neoplasm would be the melanoma, and the secondary neoplasms would be the liver and the brain. Note that even though there are three cancers present (skin, liver, and brain), the metastases are still only referred to as secondary sites (rather than secondary and tertiary). No matter how many metastases are present, they are still referred to as secondary neoplasms because they are secondary to the primary neoplasm.

Carcinoma in situ (abbreviated as ca in situ) neoplasms are growths of tissue that are potentially cancerous. These growths are not invading other tissues at the time of diagnosis, but may invade other tissues in the future.

Neoplasms of uncertain behavior are neoplasms that have not yet been confirmed as any of the other three types (benign, malignant, or ca in situ). These neoplasms require further evaluation and testing before their behavior can be determined.

It is important to understand the different behaviors of neoplasms because code selection varies depending on the neoplasm behavior. For example, the code for a benign neoplasm of the appendix (D12.1, Benign neoplasm of appendix) differs from the code for a malignant neoplasm of the appendix (C18.1, Malignant neoplasm of appendix). Furthermore, the Table of Neoplasms is divided in such a way as to guide the coder to the correct code based on both the site and behavior of the neoplasm.

The Table of Neoplasms is organized alphabetically by site, and then by the neoplasm behavior. For each site, there are six columns, each of which identify the behavior of the neoplasm. These six columns are: malignant primary, malignant secondary, ca in situ, benign, uncertain behavior, and unspecified behavior (see figure 4.4). A neoplasm of unspecified behavior is one that has not definitively been determined to be either malignant or benign. It is commonly used when a provider is testing the neoplasm to determine its behavior.

To find the code for a neoplasm using the Table of Neoplasms, it is necessary to identify the site of the neoplasm and then the behavior. However, if the coder knows the histologic type of the neoplasm, then it can be located by finding the histologic type of the neoplasm in the Main Index. The **histologic type** of the neoplasm is the specific type of microscopic structure of the growth, such as carcinoma, myeloma, or

Figure 4.4. Neoplasm table

	Malignant Primary	Malignant Secondary	Ca in situ	Benign	Uncertain Behavior	Unspecified Behavior
Neoplasm, neoplastic	C80.1	C79.9	D09.9	D36.9	D48.9	D49.9
A						
abdomen, abdominal	C76.2	C79.8-	D09.8	D36.7	D48.7	D49.89
cavity	C76.2	C79.8-	D09.8	D36.7	D48.7	D49.89
organ	C76.2	C79.8-	D09.8	D36.7	D48.7	D49.89
viscera	C76.2	C79.8-	D09.8	D36.7	D48.7	D49.89
wall—see also Neoplasm, abdomen, wall, skin	C44.509	C79.2	D04.5	D23.5	D48.5	D49.2
connective tissue	C49.4	C79.8-	-	D21.4	D48.1	D49.2
skin	C44.509					
basal cell carcinoma	C44.519	-	-	-	-	-
specified type NEC	C44.599	-	-	-	-	-
squamous cell carcinoma	C44.529	-	-	-	-	-

Source: Casto 2018, 324.

sarcoma. The histology of the neoplasm is also referred to as the **morphology** of the neoplasm, or morphological type of neoplasm. If the morphology of the neoplasm is not known, then it is necessary to refer to the Table of Neoplasms. Often the entry for the morphology or histologic type of the neoplasm in the Main Index refers the coder to the neoplasm table.

Follow these steps below to look up a code in the neoplasm table.

1. Identify the morphological type of the neoplasm and look it up in the Main Index. This often leads the coder to the Table of Neoplasms, although this is not always the case. When the morphological type of the neoplasm is an entry in the Main Index, it will lead the coder directly to the code for the neoplasm without having to refer to the neoplasm table. If this is the case, then it is still necessary to verify the code in the Tabular List. For example, Marion is looking for the code for right-sided renal cell adenocarcinoma (a cancer of the kidney). She looks up the morphological type of the cancer—*adenocarcinoma*—in the Main Index, then locates the subterm *renal cell*, which leads her to the code C64-. She then verifies this code in the Tabular List and adds the required fourth character, leading her to select the code C64.1, Malignant neoplasm of the right kidney, except renal pelvis. In this example, the Main Index led Marion directly to the code she was searching for. A detailed description of finding codes in the ICD-10 code book is discussed later in this chapter.

2. When the morphological type of the neoplasm is not known or not specified, the coder must reference the neoplasm table and search for the site of the neoplasm. For example, Marion is looking up the code for a malignant neoplasm of the right kidney. Because the morphological type is not specified, she must go directly to the Table of Neoplasms and find the entry for *kidney*. Next to the word *kidney* is a nonessential modifier, *parenchymal*, and there are also a few subterms. Just like the Main Index, the nonessential modifiers in parentheses simply provide more

information. The subterms are different—more specific sites—so the coder should scan the subterms to ensure that he or she has the correct site located.

Key to Success

When locating neoplasms of the skin in the neoplasm table, note that the entry for skin neoplasms is very large and it is easy to get lost within this section of the table. Also, it is important to differentiate between neoplasms of the skin versus neoplasms of deeper tissues or structures. For example, a neoplasm can be in the breast or on the skin of the breast. If the neoplasm is on the skin of the breast, then the coder should reference the entry for *skin*, and then find the subterm for *breast*.

3. Identify the behavior of the neoplasm and select a code. Once the site is found in the neoplasm table, identify the behavior of the neoplasm and select the code for the appropriate behavior. For example, Marion is looking for the code for a malignant neoplasm of the right kidney and locates the columns for malignant neoplasms. At this point, Marion has two options—malignant primary or malignant secondary. Remember that a secondary neoplasm is a growth, or metastasis of the primary neoplasm. Marion's code description does not mention that it is a secondary neoplasm or that it is a metastasis, so she selects the code for the primary neoplasm, C64-.

4. Verify the code in the Tabular List. Once the code has been located it is necessary to verify the code in the Tabular List. For example, now that Marion has located code C64-, she must verify the code in the Tabular List and add the fourth character (to represent the laterality of the neoplasm in this case). This leads her to select code C64.1, Malignant neoplasm of right kidney, except renal pelvis. See figure 4.5 for a reminder of the steps to looking up a neoplasm.

The next section of the Index is the Table of Drugs and Chemicals, which allows coders to find codes for toxic effects of chemicals, medicines, and other substances.

Table of Drugs and Chemicals

The third section of the Main Index of the ICD-10-CM code book is the **Table of Drugs and Chemicals** (also referred to as the table of drugs), which lists the toxic effects of drugs, chemicals, and other substances. A **toxic effect** is the result of a toxin—such as a chemical, medicinal, or other substance—on the body. For example, the toxic effect of a chemical may be a burn of the skin. Toxic effect codes are unique because they do not identify the effect of the poisoning, like loss of consciousness or confusion, but rather the substance that caused the toxic effect, the intent of the poisoning, and the encounter. If additional signs, symptoms, or manifestations of the poisoning are present, then they should be coded in addition to the code for the toxic effect code.

Follow these steps to locate and assign a code for a toxic effect.

1. Identify the substance that caused the toxic effect. The Table of Drugs and Chemicals is arranged alphabetically by the name of the substance that caused the toxic effect, so the first step in finding the code for a toxic effect is to identify the substance and find the entry for that substance in the table of drugs. For example, Jamie works in a family practice clinic and she is coding for a patient who had an allergic reaction (rash) to amoxicillin that was prescribed to treat a strep throat

Figure 4.5. Steps to looking up a neoplasm

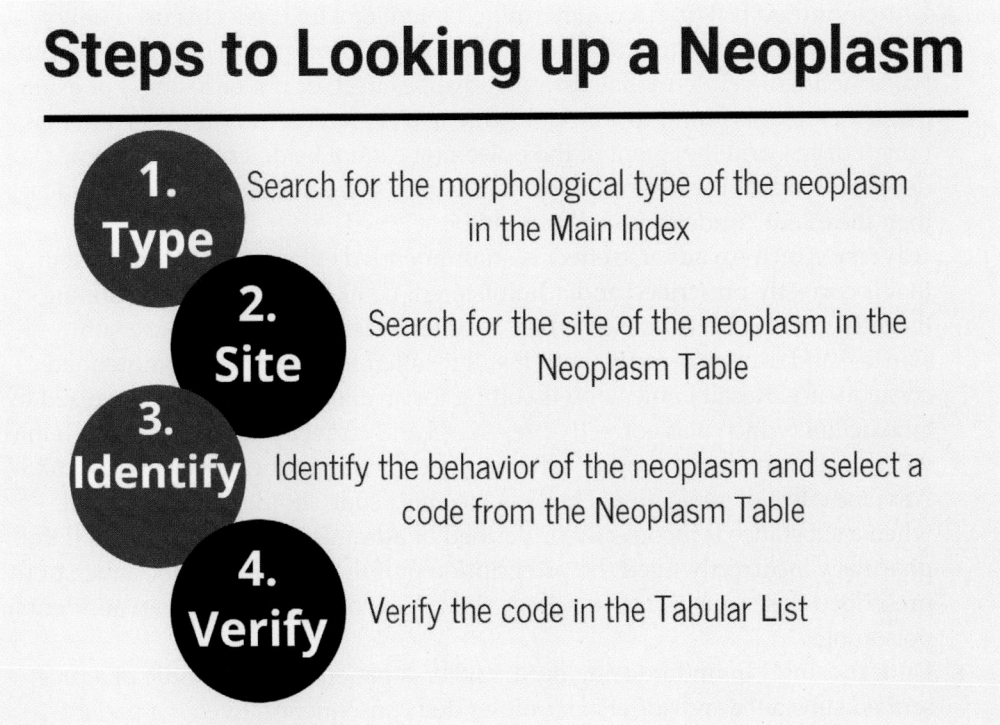

infection. This is the first time this patient has been seen for this problem. In this example, the amoxicillin caused the allergic reaction (toxic effect), so Jamie finds the entry for *amoxicillin* in the table of drugs. Note that most drugs are listed by their generic names, although this depends on the publisher of the ICD-10-CM code book. There are also subterms and nonessential modifiers for the substances listed in the table of drugs, just like the other indices in the ICD-10-CM code book.

2. Identify the intent of the toxic effect. After the substance has been located, the next step is to identify the intent. The **intent** of the toxic effect is the reason why the toxic effect happened. In ICD-10-CM, there are six different intentions that may be identified for a toxic effect code: accidental intent, intentional self-harm, assault, undetermined intent, adverse effect, and underdosing. The code for each intent is located in one of the six corresponding columns.

   a. **Accidental intent.** An accidental toxic effect is an unintentional effect of a substance that was either taken inadvertently or in excess. For example, nausea and vomiting are accidental side effects of excessive alcohol consumption. The accidental intent is the default for toxic effects that cannot be identified as intentional, assault, an adverse effect, or underdosing.

   b. **Intentional self-harm.** A toxic effect resulting from intentional self-harm is due to a substance that is taken deliberately as an act of hurting one's self. For example, if a patient consumed an entire bottle of hydrocodone on purpose in an attempted suicide, then this overdose would be intentional self-harm.

   c. **Assault.** A toxic effect that occurs due to assault is one that was purposefully inflicted upon one person by another person, with the intent of hurting the recipient of the substance. For example, if a person spikes someone's drink with

Rohypnol (the date-rape drug) to cause a toxic effect, then the intent of this poisoning is assault.

d. **Undetermined intent.** An undetermined intent of a toxic effect is used only when the intention of the toxic effect cannot be determined to be any of the other types: accidental, intentional, assault, adverse effect, or underdosing. For example, if a patient is found unconscious due to a poisoning caused by a combination of drugs, and the intent of the poisoning cannot be determined to be accidental, intentional self-harm, due to assault, an adverse effect, or an underdose, then the intent "undetermined" should be selected.

e. **Adverse effect.** An adverse effect is an unintended effect caused by a substance that is correctly prescribed and administered. Unlike an accidental poisoning, this adverse effect was caused when a patient was supposed to take a substance—and did so correctly—but it still resulted in some sort of unintended consequence. Recall Jamie, who is coding for an allergic rash that was caused by amoxicillin (which was correctly prescribed and correctly administered)—Jamie will select the code the for the "adverse effect" intent of the poisoning, T36.0X5-, Adverse effect of penicillins. The adverse effect code should not be selected when a substance is incorrectly prescribed or administered. For example, if the pharmacy incorrectly filled the prescription or if the patient took too much of the prescribed dose causing a toxic effect, then this would be coded as an accidental poisoning.

f. **Underdosing.** An underdosing occurs when a patient takes too little of a prescribed substance and suffers an unintended consequence. Even if a patient purposefully underdoses and causes a reaction or negative consequence, it is not coded as intentional self-harm unless the patient underdosed specifically as an act of self-harm. For example, if a 76-year-old male patient did not take his entire dose of insulin because he either could not afford it or if he simply calculated the dose wrong, then this would be coded with underdosing intent.

3. Verify the code and add the seventh character extension (discussed in detail later in this chapter) for the episode of care. After the intent of the toxic effect has been determined, the next step is correctly identifying a code from the Table of Drugs and Chemicals is to add the seventh character extension to identify the encounter. Note that the seventh characters are *not* listed in the table of drugs. The encounter (in this case initial encounter) identifies where the patient is in the timeline of care for their condition. To select the correct encounter, the coder must verify the code in the Tabular List and add the correct seventh character. For example, Jamie is coding for the first time the patient has been seen with this allergic reaction to the amoxicillin prescription, so she should select the seventh character "A" for initial encounter. Her code is now complete, T36.0X5A, Adverse effect of penicillins, initial encounter. Encounters are discussed in full later in this chapter.

4. Check for additional codes and sequencing. After the correct code has been identified, additional codes may be needed to identify the manifestations of the poisoning. The **manifestation** of the poisoning is the sign or symptom that occurred because of the poisoning. These include the signs, symptoms, related conditions, or other manifestations that were caused by exposure to the substance. For example, Jamie found the code for the amoxicillin adverse effect, but she still needs to select a code for the manifestation of the adverse effect—the rash. To do this, she looks up the manifestation in the Main Index, and finds the code R21, Rash and other nonspecific skin eruption. Because Jamie now has two codes, she must pay attention to the sequencing of the codes. **Sequencing**, or placing the multiple

Figure 4.6. Steps to using the Table of Drugs and Chemicals

Steps to Using the Table of Drugs

1. Substance Identify the substance that caused the toxic effect

2. Intent Identify the intent of the toxic effect

3. Locate Locate the code in the table of drugs, according to the substance and intent

4. Verify Verify the code in the Tabular List, and add the seventh character for the encounter

5. Check Check for additional codes and sequencing instructions in the Tabular List

diagnosis codes in the correct order, plays an important part in the coding of toxic effects. Sequencing instructions are listed in the Tabular List section of ICD-10-CM, and depend on the intent of the poisoning. Specific sequencing instructions are discussed later in this chapter. See figure 4.6 for a reminder of the steps to using the Table of Drugs and Chemicals.

The last section of the Index is the External Causes of Injury Index, which lists codes that describe the circumstances surrounding an injury.

External Causes of Injury Index

At times it is necessary to identify the extenuating circumstances surrounding an injury or other healthcare condition. In these instances, one or more codes identifying the external cause of the injury or illness, listed in the **External Causes of Injury Index**, must be included. For example, if a patient suffered a fractured ankle, then the external cause codes would identify how the patient fractured the ankle, the activity the patient was engaged in and where he or she was when the injury happened, and the patient's status at the time of the injury.

External cause codes are useful in providing more information regarding injuries. They are also used for data analytics purposes, to identify trends, and to track injuries caused by certain activities like skateboarding or skydiving, or animal bites. Note, however, that these codes are never used as primary diagnosis codes; they are always sequenced after any actual medical diagnoses. For example, if a patient was bitten by a dog and suffered a wound to the hand, then the diagnosis code for the hand wound would be sequenced first, followed by the external cause code for the dog bite.

Reporting external cause codes varies from state to state. For example, in some states reporting all external causes for all injuries is required, whereas in other states it is not required and some insurance plans may outright reject external cause codes. External cause codes may be required on claims that deal with motor vehicle accidents or workplace injuries, so they may be necessary in these circumstances even in states that do not require the reporting of external cause codes. For the purposes of this text, external cause codes are required whenever known and applicable to describe the extenuating circumstances surrounding an injury.

Key to Success

There are many different types of external cause codes and maneuvering through the Index to External Causes requires thoughtful consideration of exactly what you are searching for. When searching, it is imperative to focus on the type of external cause code—the injury mechanism, place of occurrence, activity, or patient status—and look up each code separately.

Follow these steps to find external cause codes using the External Causes of Injury Index.

1. Identify the extenuating circumstances surrounding the injury. There are four possible codes that may be included to fully describe the external causes of an injury. If each of these circumstances is known, then one code should be assigned for each, for a total of four codes. Once the four components of the external causes have been identified, look up each one in the external cause index and find the individual codes for each component. These four components are the injury mechanism, patient activity, place of occurrence, and patient status.

    a. The **injury mechanism** is the way an injury happened. For example, if a patient fell off a ladder and fractured his ankle, then the injury mechanism is the fall from the ladder.

    b. The patient's activity should also be identified. The **activity** is what the patient was doing when the injury occurred. For example, if the patient was painting the outside of a building when he fell from the ladder and fractured his ankle, then the activity is painting.

    c. The **place of occurrence** is where the patient was when the injury occurred. This should be as detailed as possible to describe the specifics of the location. For example, if the patient was painting the outside of his house, then the code may describe the type of house, such as single-family home or multi-family housing unit. In this example, the place of occurrence would the yard of a single-family house. The work status of the patient at the time the event occurred

    d. The **patient status** identifies the patient's work context during the accident by identifying if the patient's injury was related to employment, volunteer work, or military status. For example, if the patient was painting the outside of his home during a time when he was not employed and at his leisure, then the patient status would be leisure status.

2. Look up the external causes using the External Cause of Injury Index. This index works very similarly to the Main Index, with cross-references and subterms listed under the main terms. Finding each of the four components can be tricky,

however, so it is helpful to know the following tips. For the injury mechanism, it is helpful to search for the main cause or item involved in the injury, such as the term *fall*, and then what the patient fell from: *from, ladder*. When looking up the patient activity, find the word *activity*, and then check the subterms to find the appropriate activity. When looking up the place of occurrence, search for the term *place of occurrence*, and check the subterms for the correct location. Finally, to find the correct code for the patient status, search for the term *status of external cause* and find the correct patient status in the subterms.

Key to Success

Familiarize yourself with the External Causes of Injury Index by scanning the main terms. This will help when learning how to use the index to find your codes. Start at the beginning of the Index and read through or quickly scan the main terms in each column on each page. Make a note of how the causes are organized so that you can find them easily when you are coding for external causes.

3. Verify the codes in the Tabular List and add the seventh character episode of care when appropriate. Coders must always verify the codes found in the index by checking the Tabular List. This is also important with injury mechanism codes as they require a seventh character extension to identify the episode of care for the injury. For example, if the patient is still in active treatment for the fractured ankle due to the fall from the ladder, then the episode of care selected for the injury mechanism code would be "A" for initial encounter (discussed in detail later in this chapter). Read through the following example to find the appropriate codes for this patient's injury. Refer to figure 4.7 for a reminder of the steps to

Figure 4.7. Steps to using the External Causes of Injury Index

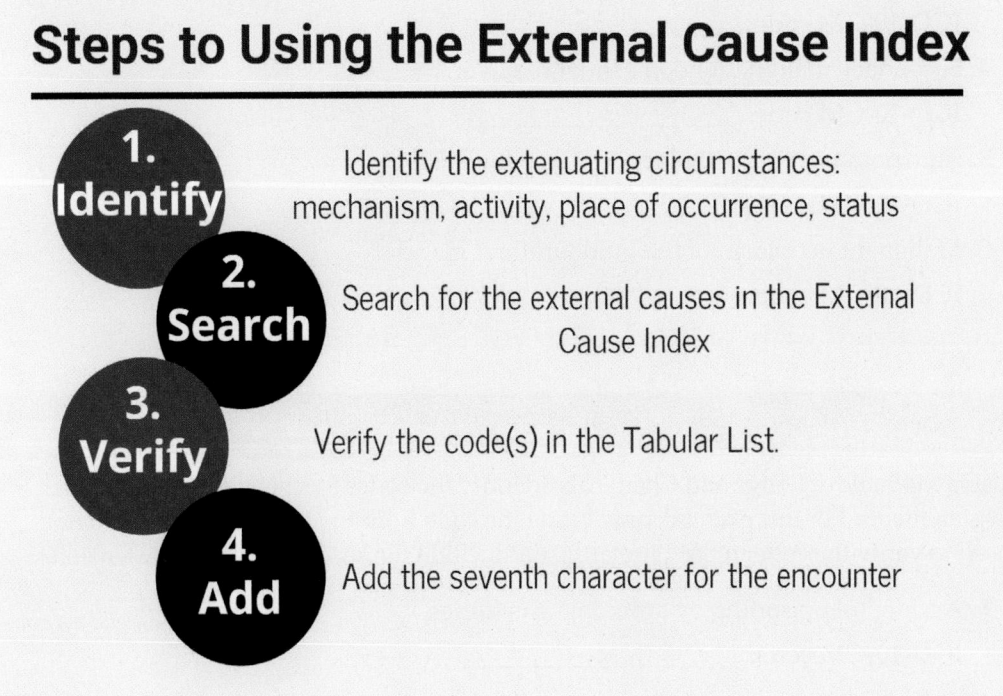

Steps to Using the External Cause Index

1. Identify — Identify the extenuating circumstances: mechanism, activity, place of occurrence, status

2. Search — Search for the external causes in the External Cause Index

3. Verify — Verify the code(s) in the Tabular List.

4. Add — Add the seventh character for the encounter

Figure 4.8. External cause codes example

Terrence was in the yard of his single-family home painting the outside of the building during his weekend leisure time, when he fell off his ladder and fractured his left ankle.

Primary injury code: S82.892A, Other fracture of left lower leg, initial encounter

Injury mechanism code: W11.XXXA, Fall on and from ladder, initial encounter

Activity: Y93.H9, Activity, other involving exterior property and land maintenance, building, and construction (*painting outside of building*)

Place of occurrence: Y92.017, Garden or yard in single-family (private) house as the place of occurrence of the external cause

Patient status: Y99.8, Other external cause status (*leisure activity*)

using the External Causes of Injury Index and figure 4.8 for an example of how to assign external cause codes.

For practice using the Table of Neoplasms, the Table of Drugs and Chemicals, and the External Causes of Injury Index, complete the exercises in There's a Code for That 4.4, 4.5, and 4.6.

4.4

There's a Code for That

Using the Table of Neoplasms

Using the Table of Neoplasms, identify the codes for the following diagnostic statements. For this exercise, only locate the code from the Index, you do not need to verify the code in the Tabular List.

1. Benign neoplasm of the ascending colon.

   ICD-10-CM code: _____

2. Basal cell carcinoma of the skin of the neck.

   ICD-10-CM code: _____

3. Primary malignant neoplasm of the vermillion border of the upper lip.

   ICD-10-CM code: _____

4. Secondary malignant neoplasm of the liver.

   ICD-10-CM code: _____

5. Carcinoma in situ of the neck of the pancreas.

   ICD-10-CM code: _____

6. Malignant neoplasm of the bulbourethral gland.

   ICD-10-CM code: _____

4.5

There's a Code for That

Using the Table of Drugs and Chemicals

Using the Table of Drugs and Chemicals, identify the codes for the following diagnostic statements. For this exercise, only locate the code from the Main Index, you do not need to verify the code in the Tabular List or include the seventh character extension.

1. Accidental poisoning by ammonia gas fumes.

   ICD-10-CM code: _____

2. Adverse effect of MAO inhibitor.

ICD-10-CM code: _____

3. Patient was admitted for ingestion of noxious mushrooms as a suicide attempt.

ICD-10-CM code: _____

4. Patient was admitted to the ICU for acute poisoning by chlorinated insecticide. Patient was applying the insecticide to the outside of his house when the wind blew the substance into his face causing ingestion of the substance.

ICD-10-CM code: _____

5. Code for ricin poisoning as an assault attempt.

ICD-10-CM code: _____

6. Poisoning by Hycodan, undetermined intent.

ICD-10-CM code: _____

Using the External Causes of Injury Index

4.6

There's a Code for That

Read the following scenario that describes the external causes of in injury. Using the External Causes of Injury Index, identify the codes for the external causes. For this exercise, only locate the code from the Main Index, you do not need to verify the code in the Tabular List or include the seventh character extension.

Carter, a 15-year-old high school student, was playing soccer on a public soccer field after school when he was struck by the soccer ball in the face and suffered a broken nose.

1. What is the injury mechanism and for Carter's injury and the ICD-10-CM code for the injury mechanism?

Injury mechanism: _____

ICD-10-CM code: _____

2. What is the place of occurrence and the ICD-10-CM code for the place of occurrence?

Place of occurrence: _____

ICD-10-CM code: _____

3. What was the patient's activity when the injury occurred and the ICD-10-CM code for the activity?

Activity: _____

ICD-10-CM code: _____

4. What is the patient's status and the ICD-10-CM code for the patient's status at the time of injury?

Patient status: _____

ICD-10-CM code: _____

The Tabular List follows the four sections of the Index. This is the largest section of the ICD-10-CM code book, and lists all of the actual ICD-10-CM codes and includes instructions and guidelines for the use of selected codes.

Tabular List

The Tabular List of the ICD-10-CM code book is the structured list of ICD-10-CM codes, organized alphanumerically, and divided into chapters based on body system or condition. The Tabular List includes more than simply a list of ICD-10-CM codes. It employs a specific format to help coders identify valid codes, includes references to guidelines to help with code selection, and employs various symbols, notes, and other conventions to help lead coders to their correct code. The Tabular List is first divided into 21 chapters and each chapter includes a selection of ICD-10-CM codes. Each chapter is formatted similarly, and contains the same symbols and other conventions to help coders select the correct code. Finally, there are important guidelines that pertain to using the Tabular List. Depending on the publisher of the ICD-10-CM code book, each chapter may also include the Official Guidelines for Coding and Reporting, which also govern appropriate code selection.

Chapters of the Tabular List

There are 21 chapters in the ICD-10-CM Tabular List. Each chapter is divided based on a specific body system or condition. Several of the individual chapters begin with a new letter of the alphabet, although this is not always the case. Some chapters contain codes from two or more letters of the alphabet, and other chapters contain codes that start with the same letter of the alphabet. Study the list of ICD-10-CM chapters in figure 4.9, paying close attention to the range of codes that are within each chapter.

Figure 4.9. Table of contents of the Tabular List

Table of Contents

1. Certain infectious and parasitic diseases (A00-B99)
2. Neoplasms (C00-D49)
3. Diseases of the blood and blood-forming organs and certain disorders involving the immune mechanism (D50-D89)
4. Endocrine, nutritional and metabolic diseases (E00-E89)
5. Mental, Behavioral and Neurodevelopmental disorders (F01-F99)
6. Diseases of the nervous system (G00-G99)
7. Diseases of the eye and adnexa (H00-H59)
8. Diseases of the ear and mastoid process (H60-H95)
9. Diseases of the circulatory system (I00-I99)
10. Diseases of the respiratory system (J00-J99)
11. Diseases of the digestive system (K00-K95)
12. Diseases of the skin and subcutaneous tissue (L00-L99)
13. Diseases of the musculoskeletal system and connective tissue (M00-M99)
14. Diseases of the genitourinary system (N00-N99)
15. Pregnancy, childbirth and the puerperium (O00-O9A)
16. Certain conditions originating in the perinatal period (P00-P96)
17. Congenital malformations, deformations and chromosomal abnormalities (Q00-Q99)
18. Symptoms, signs and abnormal clinical and laboratory findings, not elsewhere classified (R00-R99)
19. Injury, poisoning and certain other consequences of external causes (S00-T88)
20. External causes of morbidity (V00-Y99)
21. Factors influencing health status and contact with health services (Z00-Z99)

Source: Casto 2018, 459.

Key to Success

It is useful, both as a beginner and as an experienced coder, to place tabs at the beginning of each chapter and on codes commonly used in your specialty, to make code location easier. Also, many coding books include a different colored or shaded edge for each chapter that helps to locate codes more quickly.

Key to Success

The letter at the beginning of the codes does not correspond to the type of condition or body area, although it may be helpful to make up letter associations for certain code groups. For example, codes from chapter 15: Pregnancy, childbirth, and the puerperium, all start with the letter *O*. You may choose to associate *O* codes with *obstetric* conditions.

Formatting and Conventions of the Tabular List

All of the chapters in the Tabular List are formatted similarly, so that coders can easily locate and select the appropriate code. Furthermore, the Tabular List also contains a number of conventions that help coders select the correct code and identify if the code chosen is reportable for a certain type of setting, patient, or billing or coding purpose. These include the abbreviations NOS (not otherwise specified) and NEC (not elsewhere classifiable), special highlighting, and symbols on each page to alert the coder to nuances of the codes.

Format of the Tabular List and Specificity

The Tabular List is formatted and organized based on sections, categories, subcategories, and codes. Each chapter is composed of one or more sections, combining conditions that are similar in nature. Sections may include codes from many different categories and all categories are three characters. If a three-character category is not further subdivided, then it is considered a code. As discussed later in the chapter, subcategories can extend codes to four, five, six, or seven characters. Each time a new subcategory is added, it adds more detail to the code (with the exception of placeholders). Three-character categories are listed the left of the columns, with subcategories and codes indented beneath the category and any additional subcategories.

For a code to be reportable, or valid, it must be extended to the full amount of characters possible. In figure 4.10 it would be incorrect to code E08.0 because there is a more specific code indented beneath it. In this case, the coder should select E08.00, Diabetes mellitus due to underlying condition with hyperosmolarity without nonketotic hyperglycemic-hyperosmolar coma (NKHHC), which is a valid code. There may be as many indentions underneath a category needed to create up to a six-character code.

However, not all individual codes are fully listed within the Tabular List. To save space, the ICD-10-CM code book does not include the seventh character extensions with each code. Instead, the seventh character extension options are listed in a box within the category, and an instructional notation is included within the Tabular List to inform the coder that a seventh character is necessary. This notation differs, depending

Figure 4.10. Section, category, subcategory, and code

Diabetes mellitus (E08-E13)

Review coding guideline C.4.a

category ➡ **E08   Diabetes mellitus due to underlying condition**

Code first the underlying condition, such as:
congenital rubella (P35.0)
Cushing's syndrome (E24.-)
cystic fibrosis (E84.-)
malignant neoplasm (C00-C96)
malnutrition (E40-E46)
pancreatitis and other diseases of the pancreas (K85-K86.-)

Use additional code to identify control using:
insulin (Z79.4)
oral antidiabetic drugs (Z79.84)
oral hypoglycemic drugs (Z79.84)

Excludes1: *drug or chemical induced diabetes mellitus (E09.-)*
gestational diabetes (O24.4-)
neonatal diabetes mellitus (P70.2)
postpancreatectomy diabetes mellitus (E13.-)
postprocedural diabetes mellitus (E13.-)
secondary diabetes mellitus NEC (E13.-)
type 1 diabetes mellitus (E10.-)
type 2 diabetes mellitus (E11.-)

Review coding guideline C.4.a.6.a

subcategory ➡ **+ E08.0   Diabetes mellitus due to underlying condition with hyperosmolarity**

MCC **E08.00   Diabetes mellitus due to underlying condition with hyperosmolarity without nonketotic hyperglycemic-hyperosmolar coma (NKHHC)**

code   MCC Exclusion see Appendix A PDX collection 0518
HAC   see Appendix B for HAC conditional logic

Source: Casto 2018, 860.

on the publisher of the ICD-10-CM code book, so it may be a small red dot, check mark, stop sign, or a plus (+) symbol. If the code is not extended to the required number of characters, it is considered an invalid code and cannot be reported on a claim form. A code that has been extended to the full amount of required characters is considered a **billable code**, as it may be reported for billing purposes. Study figure 4.11 to see how this symbol instructs the coder to add more characters to the code.

In figure 4.11, code S04.0 has a plus symbol to the left of it, which indicates that the coder needs to add an additional code, indented below. Code S04.01 also has a plus symbol located to the left of it, which means that an additional character needs is needed and the codes are indented below. The next indented code, S04.011, has a plus symbol as well as the "7th" sign, indicating that an additional character is needed, but there are no more codes indented below. Instead, the coder must refer to the top of the category to find the seventh character extension options, which are usually listed in a box at the beginning of the code category or subcategory. (Note that the formatting of the seventh character options depends on the publisher of the ICD-10 code book. In the AHIMA ICD-10-CM code book, the seventh character options are located in a gray box). In this case, the coder would have to select one of the seventh character extension options and add it to the code to create a valid code, such as S04.011A, Injury of optic nerve, right eye, initial encounter; S04.011D, Injury of optic nerve, right eye, subsequent encounter; or S04.011S Injury of optic nerve, right eye, sequela.

Reporting the code with the most possible characters is referred to as coding to the highest level of specificity. **Specificity** is the amount of detail included within a code description. In other words, the more characters a code has, the more specific it is. Coders must report the code that has the most possible characters.

Figure 4.11. Seventh character additions

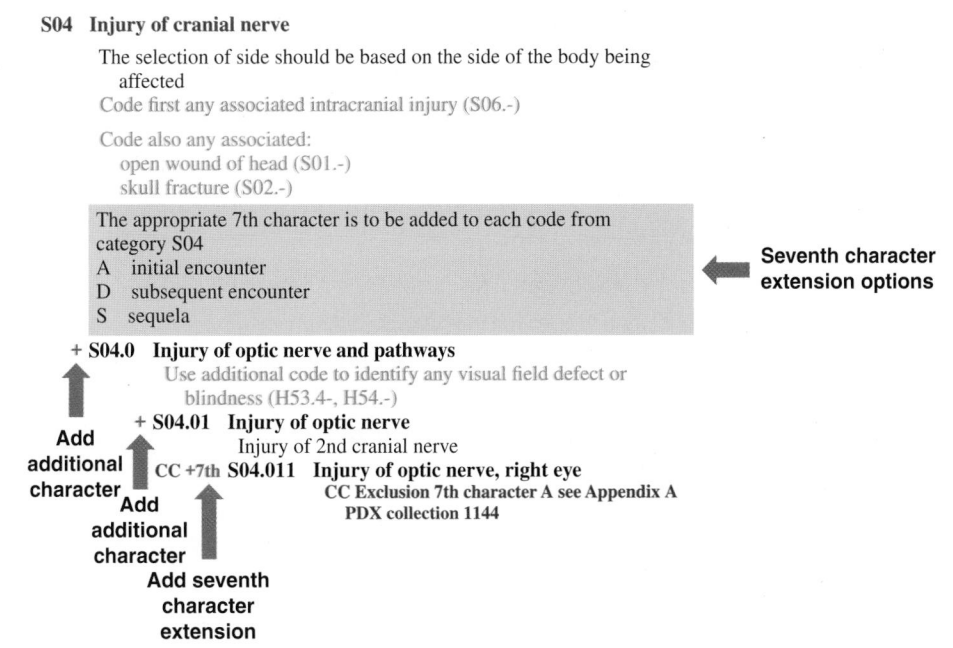

Source: Casto 2018, 950.

Key to Success

An easy way to check if the code needs more characters to add specificity is to look for the plus symbol to the left of the code. Remember that this sign also depends on the publisher of the ICD-10 code book. Instead of a plus sign, you might find a small red stop sign, a check mark, or other notation indicating that an additional character is necessary. If the additional character symbol is present, then you must descend to the next level and add another character. If there is no additional character symbol next to the code, then it is a valid code and it may be reported on a claim. Valid codes are also referred to as billable codes, as they are valid for claims and billing purposes.

Abbreviations NOS and NEC

One of the conventions within the Tabular List is the use of two very common and important abbreviations— NOS and NEC. NOS stands for **not otherwise specified**, which means that the healthcare provider's documentation was not specific enough to select a more specific, or detailed, code. For example, if the provider's documentation stated that the condition was dysphagia, NOS, then the coder would select the unspecified version of the code for dysphagia, R13.10, Dysphagia, unspecified. The Tabular List may include the abbreviation NOS within the code description to help coders identify unspecified codes.

NEC stands for **not elsewhere classifiable**, and indicates that no code exists for a specified condition. In other words, the condition that the coder is searching for does not have a specific code, so the "other" option must be selected. For example, if the provider's documentation specifies that the patient has neurogenic dysphagia, the coder would check the term *dysphagia*, and then look for a code for neurogenic dysphagia specifically. However, no code for neurogenic dysphagia exists. The coder should not select the unspecified version of the condition, because it *was* specified—in this case there is no code for it. The coder should select the code to indicate that the condition is not elsewhere classifiable under a different code, and report code R13.19, Other dysphagia.

When searching for NOS codes in the Tabular List, they may be listed as either NOS or unspecified. NEC codes may be referred to as "other" or "other specified type." Remember: NOS = Unspecified; NEC = Other. Note also that both abbreviations may also be found in the ICD-10-CM Index.

Key to Success

Be careful when using unspecified codes. The thousands of specific ICD-10-CM specific codes make it easy to find a code for the exact condition. Therefore, unspecified codes should be reported rarely, as the overuse of unspecified codes can trigger an audit. However, there are many times that unspecified codes are necessary and thus they are still commonly used in the healthcare office. Reporting unspecified diagnoses is discussed further in chapter 8 (Primary Care).

Special Highlighting and Symbols

Many publishers of the ICD-10-CM code book include special highlighting and symbols throughout the Tabular List to help coders identify nuances of the codes displayed on the page.

Highlighting is added to help the coder take note of particular guidelines, notations, and special instructions regarding the codes. Highlighting is consistent throughout the code book so that coders can visually pick out the important aspects of the codes and apply that information to help them report the codes correctly. For example, there are instructional guidelines within many codes that have *Includes* and *Excludes* notes (these are discussed later in this chapter). To help coders note these guidelines, they may be highlighted in different colors to help them stand out (see figure 4.12). Note that the Includes note is highlighted in gray, the Excludes1 note is highlighted in yellow, and the Excludes2 note is highlighted in green.

Codes and terms may be highlighted throughout the Tabular List to indicate that they may be included within a specific set of codes, such as HCC (Hierarchical Condition Category) codes, or codes that are included within performance measures sets, like hospital-acquired conditions (HAC), both discussed in chapter 2. Additionally, manifestation codes are commonly highlighted, as well as codes that are unacceptable to report as a primary diagnosis (PDX), both discussed later in this chapter.

Figure 4.12. Example of highlighting in the Tabular List

K72 Hepatic failure, not elsewhere classified
Includes: fulminant hepatitis NEC, with hepatic failure
hepatic encephalopathy NOS
liver (cell) necrosis with hepatic failure
malignant hepatitis NEC, with hepatic failure
yellow liver atrophy or dystrophy
Excludes1: *alcoholic hepatic failure (K70.4)*
hepatic failure with toxic liver disease (K71.1-)
icterus of newborn (P55-P59)
postprocedural hepatic failure (K91.82)
Excludes2: *hepatic failure complicating abortion or ectopic or molar*
pregnancy (O00-O07, O08.8)
hepatic failure complicating pregnancy, childbirth and the
puerperium (O26.6-)
viral hepatitis with hepatic coma (B15-B19)

Source: Casto 2018, 722.

There are also symbols or letters that are strategically placed on the pages of the Tabular List. They are commonly placed directly to the right or left of a code, and provide more information about that code. They function just like footnotes, in that they refer the coder to additional information about that code, located on the bottom edge of the page. Depending on the publisher of the code book, the symbol may be a bullet point, such as a pink dot, or a small letter M to indicate that the code is for use on maternal claims only. On the other hand, a green bullet or small letter N indicates that the code is for use on newborn records only. Other symbols identify codes for a specific age group, such as pediatric or adult patients, or for a certain gender, either male or female. For example, in figure 4.13, the codes located in this section all have a small pink dot, as well as a small female gender sign next to them. Note that according to the information at the bottom of the page, the pink dot means that this code is applicable for a maternity condition. The gender symbol means that the condition should be used for female patients. Thus, the code book indicates that these codes should only be used on maternal records, for female patients.

As a coder, it is important to always pay attention to each and every detail on the page, as it was put there for a reason. Success as a coder depends on the coder's ability to pay attention to these small details, understand what they mean, and then use the information to select the most appropriate code. These notes at the bottom of the page provide helpful information, and can help coders determine when a code may or may not be appropriate to report.

Figure 4.13. Notations within the Tabular List

Source: Casto 2018, 860.

Key to Success

As you learn how to use the Tabular List, make a note of the highlighted terms and symbols within the code book you are using. When you begin using your code book for the first time, note the line of footnotes at the bottom of each page in the Tabular List. These notes help coders to recognize what the highlighting means, in addition to other symbols used in the Tabular List. When in doubt, always refer to the bottom of the page to check what the symbol or highlighting means.

Coding conventions—standards and rules that govern how to use the codes within the ICD-10-CM code book—are also found throughout the Tabular List.

Conventions in the Tabular List

In addition to the format, punctuation, and symbols used within the Tabular List, this section also includes conventions for the use of ICD-10-CM codes. Coding conventions are found in the guidelines at the beginning of nearly all ICD-10-CM code books. Some publishers also include chapter-specific guidelines at the beginning of each chapter.

In order to understand guidelines a little better, it is important to discuss the **Official Guidelines for Coding and Reporting (OGCR)**. The OGCR is the set of official guidelines for the use of the ICD-10-CM code set, published by the set of four organizations that make up the Cooperating Parties for ICD-10: AHA, AHIMA, CMS, and NCHS (CMS 2018). So, in addition to creating and maintaining the code set, this group also creates the rules that govern how to use it. The OGCR includes general rules that are for use throughout the code set, as well as a large section of chapter-specific guidelines that are applicable to codes specific to certain chapters. Many ICD-10-CM code books include the guidelines in full at the beginning of the code book, and others include the full OCGR at the beginning of the code book, as well as the chapter-specific guidelines at the beginning of each chapter. Yet other code books may omit the OCGR completely. The full version of the current year's OGCR can be found on the CMS website, at www.cms.gov.

As the rules on how to use codes, this text commonly refers to the OGCR, or guidelines, within the ICD-10-CM code book. When a guideline is especially important for coding purposes, they are included in the text for reference (see figure 4.14).

Conventions are certain guidelines that are applicable to the entire Tabular List, which should be understood before diving into ICD-10-CM coding. Listed as the first section of the OGCR, conventions are general rules for the use of the ICD-10 code book. Some of these conventions have already been discussed in this chapter—such as the abbreviations NEC and NOS, and the use of "other" and "unspecified" codes. Additional important conventions are Includes notes, Excludes notes, "and," "with," "code also," and sequencing instructions, and etiology and manifestation notations.

Figure 4.14. OGCR I.C.1.c. Infections resistant to antibiotics

c. Infections resistant to antibiotics

Many bacterial infections are resistant to current antibiotics. It is necessary to identify all infections documented as antibiotic resistant. Assign a code from category Z16, Resistance to antimicrobial drugs, following the infection code only if the infection code does not identify drug resistance.

Source: CMS 2018.

Key to success

The coder needs to know how to locate and use the OGCR, so it is important to understand the configuration of the ICD-10-CM code book you are using, and know where to find the OCGR—both the full set and the chapter-specific guidelines.

Includes Notes

Includes notes appear directly underneath a three-character category to further define and give examples of the content that is included within the category. For example, in figure 4.12 the Includes note lists a number of conditions that are included in the category of K72. This means that the conditions listed in the Includes notes may be coded with codes starting with K72.

Inclusion terms are also common throughout the Tabular List. These work similarly to Includes notes, but instead pertain to specific codes rather than a category of codes. Inclusion terms may be synonyms for the condition or a list of various conditions assigned to a specific code. For example, in figure 4.15 the inclusion terms indicate that cholangitic, hematogenic, lymphogenic, and pylephlebitic liver abscesses are all included within the code K75.0, Abscess of liver. Note that the lists of inclusion terms are not exhaustive—so if a term does not appear in the list of inclusion terms, but the condition still fits within the code description, it is still acceptable to assign the code.

Excludes Notes

Excludes notes are the opposite of Includes notes, as they identify conditions that are similar but independent of each other. The ICD-10-CM code set has two types of Excludes notes—Excludes1 and Excludes2. The Excludes1 note is a pure Excludes note, meaning that the condition listed under the Excludes1 note and the coded condition are mutually exclusive and should never be coded together. For example, a congenital form and an acquired form of a condition. Looking at figure 4.15, *cholangitis without liver abscess (K83.0)* is listed as an Excludes1 condition, which means that coders should not code K75.0, Abscess of liver with K83.0, Cholangitis without liver abscess. In this case, the coder would have to select *either* K75.0 *or* K83.0, not both.

Excludes2 notes identify conditions that are "not included here." This means that if the patient had the condition located under the Excludes2 note, then they should code for that condition elsewhere. If the patient has both the condition within the Excludes2

Figure 4.15. Inclusion terms, Excludes1 notes, and Excludes2 notes

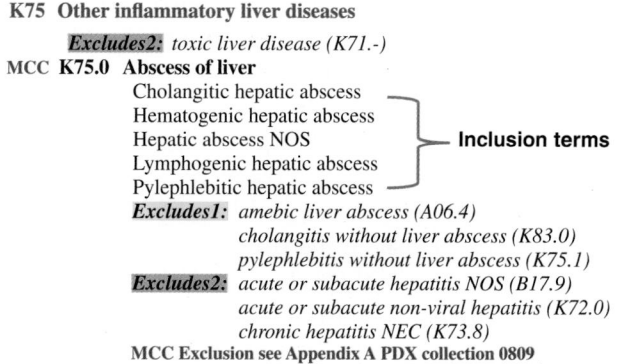

Source: Casto 2018, 723.

note *as well as* the coded condition, then both of the codes may be reported together, as appropriate. Looking at figure 4.15, *acute or subacute hepatitis NOS (B17.9)* is listed as an Excludes2 note under the K75.0 code. So if a patient had both an abscess of the liver and unspecified acute or subacute hepatitis, then it would be appropriate for the coder to identify each of the conditions with an individual code: K75.0, Abscess of Liver, and B17.9, Acute or subacute hepatitis NOS.

There is an important exception to Excludes1 notes. Coders may code for both conditions if they are unrelated to each other. The reason for this is that sometimes a diagnosis code is a general code for a condition that can manifest in multiple ways. For example, code F45.8, Other somatoform disorders, includes many different conditions, from teeth grinding to psychogenic dysmenorrhea. Thus, the initial code is for G47.63, Sleep related teeth grinding—which contains an Excludes1 note for *other somatoform disorders (F45.8)*—and then it would be acceptable to code G47.63 *with* F45.8 only if the condition coded for by F45.8 is unrelated to the sleep-related teeth grinding, such as psychogenic dysmenorrhea (teeth grinding and dysmenorrhea are unrelated conditions). Whenever there is confusion regarding whether or not two conditions are related, the coder should query the provider to verify the diagnoses and obtain more information.

And, With, Code Also, *and Sequencing Instructions*

Sequencing, or placing the codes in a particular order, is an important part of ICD-10-CM coding. When sequenced correctly, the diagnosis codes should tell the story of why the patient presented for treatment. Typically, when a patient has more than one healthcare condition, the diagnosis code primarily responsible for the services provided is sequenced before any others. If the patient has two or more diagnoses, each of which requiring the same amount of treatment or management, then either of the diagnoses should be sequenced first. However, there are a few conventions within the Tabular List of the ICD-10-CM that instruct coders how to sequence certain conditions, and whether or not to include other codes to identify additional healthcare conditions. These are *and*, *with*, *code also*, and sequencing instructions.

When referencing the Tabular List to verify code selection, coders will encounter the term *and*, which should be interpreted to mean *and* or *or*. For example, the code A18.0-, Tuberculosis of bones and joints, can include tuberculosis of the bones, tuberculosis of the joints, or tuberculosis of the bones and joints.

When the term *with* appears in the Tabular, it should be interpreted to mean *associated with* or *due to*. This term presumes a causal relationship between the two conditions linked by the word *with*. For example, K71.1-, Toxic liver disease with hepatic necrosis, codes for hepatic failure *due to* drugs, as indicated by the word *with*.

The *code also* note informs the coder that two codes may be necessary to fully describe a condition. For example, H35.0-, Background retinopathy and retinal vascular changes, includes the note Code also any associated hypertension (I10). This means that if the patient has a condition classifiable to a code beginning with H35.0-, as well as associated hypertension, then the coder should include a code for both conditions. However, this note does not include sequencing instructions regarding which code should be listed first, so the coder must determine the sequencing of the two codes. To determine the code that should be sequenced first, the coder must read through the provider's documentation of the healthcare encounter and identify the primary diagnosis code. Additional instruction on how to assign the primary diagnosis code is provided later in this chapter as well as in chapter 8 of this text.

Sequencing instructions are listed in the Tabular List of the ICD-10-CM code book in the same way that *code also* notes are included. There are located beneath a section, category, or subsection, and give coders more information on how to sequence two or more codes. The following are sequencing instructions found in the Tabular List.

- *Code first* instructions list conditions that should be coded before the code identified. For example, there is a *code first* note under J18, Pneumonia, unspecified organism that instructs the coder to Code first associated influenza, if applicable (J09.X1, J10.0-, J11.0-). If the patient had both pneumonia due to unspecified organism and influenza, then the coder would code for each condition with the influenza code first and the pneumonia code second: J11.00, Influenza due to unidentified influenza virus with unspecified type of pneumonia, then J18.9, Pneumonia, unspecified organism.

- *Use additional code* instructions list conditions that should be coded after the identified code. For example, there is a *use additional code* note under D57, Sickle-cell disorders, instructs the coder to Use additional code for any associated fever (R50.81). If the patient had both a sickle cell disorder coded under category D57 and an associated fever, then the fever would be coded in addition to the sickle-cell disorder, ordered as follows: D57.- Sickle-cell disorders, then R50.81, Fever presenting with conditions classified elsewhere.

Etiology and Manifestation

The **etiology** of a disease is the cause of that disease, and the manifestation is the signs and symptoms of the disease (as discussed previously in the chapter). For example, the etiology of streptococcal sore throat is the streptococcal bacteria, whereas the manifestation of the disease is the sore throat and perhaps another symptom like fever. Refer to figure 4.16 for the OGCR related to etiology and manifestation coding.

Figure 4.16. OGCR I.A.13 Etiology/Manifestation Convention

13. **Etiology/Manifestation Convention ("Code first", "Use additional code" and "In Diseases Classified Elsewhere" Notes)**

Certain conditions have both an underlying etiology and multiple body system manifestations due to the underlying etiology. For such conditions, the ICD-10-CM has a coding convention that requires the underlying condition be sequenced first, if applicable, followed by the manifestation. Wherever such a combination exists, there is a "use additional code" note at the etiology code, and a "code first" note at the manifestation code. These instructional notes indicate the proper sequencing order of the codes, etiology followed by manifestation.

In most cases the manifestation codes will have in the code title, "in diseases classified elsewhere." Codes with this title are a component of the etiology/manifestation convention. The code title indicates that it is a manifestation code. "In diseases classified elsewhere" codes are never permitted to be used as first-listed or principal diagnosis codes. They must be used in conjunction with an underlying condition code and they must be listed following the underlying condition. See category F02, Dementia in other diseases classified elsewhere, for an example of this convention.

There are manifestation codes that do not have "in diseases classified elsewhere" in the title. For such codes, there is a "use additional code" note at the etiology code and a "code first" note at the manifestation code and the rules for sequencing apply.

In addition to the notes in the Tabular List, these conditions also have a specific Alphabetic Index entry structure. In the Alphabetic Index both conditions are listed together with the etiology code first followed by the manifestation codes in brackets. The code in brackets is always to be sequenced second.

An example of the etiology/manifestation convention is dementia in Parkinson's disease. In the Alphabetic Index, code G20 is listed first, followed by code F02.80 or F02.81 in brackets. Code G20 represents the underlying etiology, Parkinson's disease, and must be sequenced first, whereas codes F02.80 and F02.81 represent the manifestation of dementia in diseases classified elsewhere, with or without behavioral disturbance.

"Code first" and "Use additional code" notes are also used as sequencing rules in the classification for certain codes that are not part of an etiology/ manifestation combination.

See Section I.B. 7. Multiple coding for a single condition.

Source: CMS 2018.

In ICD-10-CM coding, occasionally the etiology and manifestation of a disease are reported using a **combination code**—one code for both etiology and manifestation. The ICD-10-CM code set contains numerous combination codes, such as diabetes mellitus codes that combine the etiology (diabetes) with the manifestation (diabetic retinopathy). So for a patient with diabetes mellitus type II with diabetic retinopathy, only code E11.319, Type 2 diabetes mellitus with unspecified diabetic retinopathy without macular edema would need to be coded.

When the etiology and manifestation are coded separately using two different codes, coders must pay close attention to sequencing guidelines to ensure the correct sequencing of the codes. This is common when a condition is caused by an infectious organism. Although some combination codes do exist, it is often necessary to include both manifestation code and the etiology code for conditions caused by known infectious organisms. For example, category J04 Acute laryngitis and tracheitis requires that the coder Use additional code (B95 to B97) to identify the infectious agent. If the infectious agent is known, then it would be coded after the J04 code, as follows: J04.0, Acute laryngitis, then the code for the infectious agent, B95.0, Streptococcus, group A, as the cause of diseases classified elsewhere.

In addition to coding conventions, there are applicable coding guidelines throughout the ICD-10-CM code book that are not chapter specific. That is, they do not apply to only one chapter, but rather to all codes in the book.

OGCR General Coding Guidelines

The ICD-10-CM code book includes general coding guidelines for use with all of the codes in the ICD-10-CM code set. It is important to understand these guidelines, as they govern the way that codes are selected, sequenced, and reported on claims. Note that some guidelines pertain specifically to outpatient (professional) services, and others pertain to the inpatient (facility) setting. Professional outpatient guidelines are discussed here, with inpatient facility guidelines discussed in chapter 20 of this text.

Several of these instructions have already been discussed throughout this chapter, but a few remain. Namely, the guidelines on when to code for signs and symptoms versus a definitive diagnosis; sequencing of acute and chronic conditions; laterality; and primary diagnosis. There are additional important guidelines, however, it more useful to discuss these guidelines within the context of actual coding examples. The remaining chapters of this text include a discussion of the relevant guidelines when applicable.

Signs and Symptoms versus Definitive Diagnosis

Signs and symptoms are acceptable for reporting purposes only when the definitive diagnosis has not been confirmed by the healthcare provider (see figure 4.17). **Signs** of a disease or disease process are objective evidence that can be observed or detected by someone other than the individual affected by the condition. For example, a fever would be a sign of a disease process. **Symptoms**, on the other hand, are subjective evidence of a disease or a disease process experienced by the individual affected by the condition. For example, a headache, lethargy, and nausea would all be symptoms of a disease.

Coders should only report signs and symptoms when a definitive diagnosis has not been determined by the healthcare provider. A **definitive diagnosis** is the condition or disease confirmed to be the cause of the signs or symptoms. For example, if a patient presents to the office with the signs and symptoms of fever, headache, lethargy, and nausea, and the doctor determines that the patient has influenza, then influenza is the definitive diagnosis.

Figure 4.17. OGCR I.B.4, I.B.5, I.B.6

---

4. Signs and Symptoms

Codes that describe symptoms and signs, as opposed to diagnoses, are acceptable for reporting purposes when a related definitive diagnosis has not been established (confirmed) by the provider. Chapter 18 of ICD-10-CM, Symptoms, Signs, and Abnormal Clinical and Laboratory Findings, Not Elsewhere Classified (codes R00.0–R99) contains many, but not all codes for symptoms.

See Section I.B.18 Use of Signs/Symptom/Unspecified Codes

5. Conditions that are an Integral Part of a Disease Process

Signs and symptoms that are associated routinely with a disease process should not be assigned as additional codes, unless otherwise instructed by the classification.

6. Conditions that are not an Integral Part of a Disease Process

Additional signs and symptoms that may not be associated routinely with a disease process should be coded when present.

Source: CMS 2018.

When a definitive diagnosis has been identified, it is not acceptable to report the signs and symptoms that are commonly included within the disease process. As these signs and symptoms are integral to a disease process, they are already included within the code description. In this case, only the influenza diagnosis code would be reported. It is not necessary to report the signs and symptoms of fever, headache, lethargy, and nausea, as these are an integral part of the disease process of influenza.

It is acceptable to code for the signs and symptoms when:

- A definitive diagnosis has not yet been determined. It may take several encounters before a definitive diagnosis is confirmed, and it is common that patients may not return for a definitive diagnosis. In these cases, code for the signs and symptoms.
- Signs and symptoms that are *not* an integral part of a disease process may be reported when present. For example, if the patient also had swelling of the hand and the signs and symptoms of influenza, then the sign of swelling would be reported in addition to the definitive diagnosis of influenza. (CMS 2018)

Acute and Chronic Conditions

Acute conditions have a severe and sudden onset; that is, they occur quickly and are serious in nature. For example, acute bronchitis is typically caused by an infectious organism, producing severe symptoms of coughing that occurs rapidly. A chronic condition, on the other hand, is a syndrome or condition that has been in development for a long period of time, and is a constant disease state. For example, chronic bronchitis is a constant state of bronchial inflammation that causes a persistent cough. Some conditions may also be referred to as subacute, and others may present with an acute exacerbation of a chronic condition. These may be referred to as "acute and chronic" or "acute on chronic."

It is important to make the distinction between acute and chronic conditions, as the acuity of the condition impacts the sequencing. Acute conditions are sequenced first. For example, if a patient with chronic bronchitis presents to the healthcare office for treatment of an acute exacerbation, or worsening, of his bronchitis, then it would be appropriate to code for both the acute bronchitis and the chronic bronchitis. In this case, the code for the acute condition would be sequenced before the code for the chronic condition.

Occasionally, there is a combination code that includes both the acute and chronic versions of a condition. If a combination code is available, then it should be used instead of individual codes for the acute and chronic conditions (see figure 4.18).

Laterality

Laterality refers to the side on which a condition appears. The human body has several symmetrical organs. Other than the internal organs, there are two different sides to most of the rest of the human body. ICD-10-CM diagnosis codes capture the side affected by a condition by including the laterality within the code description. Codes exist for right, left, and bilateral (affecting both right and left sides) conditions. If the condition does present bilaterally, but there is not a bilateral option available, then coders should assign the codes for both the right and left sides. When the documentation does not specify the laterality of the condition, it is acceptable to report the code option with unspecified laterality (see figure 4.19).

First-Listed Diagnosis

All diagnosis codes must be supported by documentation from the patient's health record. Once all codes have been identified, it is then necessary to determine the primary reason for the encounter and sequence the codes according to the primary reason for the encounter by using chapter-specific coding guidelines. The first-listed diagnosis in outpatient coding is the first diagnosis code listed on a claim when more than one diagnosis code is applicable. It may also be referred to as the primary diagnosis. As previously mentioned, sequencing of diagnosis codes is important, as they tell the

Figure 4.18. OGCR I.B.8, I.B.9

---

8. Acute and Chronic Conditions

If the same condition is described as both acute (subacute) and chronic, and separate subentries exist in the Alphabetic Index at the same indentation level, code both and sequence the acute (subacute) code first.

9. Combination Code

A combination code is a single code used to classify:

- Two diagnoses, or
- A diagnosis with an associated secondary process (manifestation)
- A diagnosis with an associated complication

Combination codes are identified by referring to subterm entries in the Alphabetic Index and by reading the inclusion and exclusion notes in the Tabular List.

Assign only the combination code when that code fully identifies the diagnostic conditions involved or when the Alphabetic Index so directs. Multiple coding should not be used when the classification provides a combination code that clearly identifies all of the elements documented in the diagnosis. When the combination code lacks necessary specificity in describing the manifestation or complication, an additional code should be used as a secondary code.

Source: CMS 2018.

Figure 4.19. OGCR I.B.13

---

13. Laterality

Some ICD-10-CM codes indicate laterality, specifying whether the condition occurs on the left, right or is bilateral. If no bilateral code is provided and the condition is bilateral, assign separate codes for both the left and right side. If the side is not identified in the medical record, assign the code for the unspecified side.

When a patient has a bilateral condition and each side is treated during separate encounters, assign the "bilateral" code (as the conditions still exists on both sides), including for the encounter to treat the first side. For the second encounter for treatment after one side has previously been treated and the condition no longer exists on that side, assign the appropriate unilateral code for the side where the conditions still exists (e.g., cataract surgery performed on each eye in separate encounters). The bilateral code would not be assigned for the subsequent encounter, as the patient no longer has the condition in the previously-treated site. If the treatment on the first side did not completely resolve the condition, then the bilateral code would still be appropriate.

Source: CMS 2018.

story of why the patient presented for treatment in the outpatient setting. Please note that inpatient coding guidelines are different for determining the first-listed condition (called the principal diagnosis in inpatient coding). The guidelines discussed here are for outpatient coding purposes only.

The first-listed diagnosis should be the one chiefly responsible for the healthcare services provided. Any additional coexisting conditions, pertinent patient history or status codes, or diagnoses should be sequenced after the first-listed diagnosis (see figure 4.20). For example, if a patient with diabetes mellitus type II presented to the office for treatment of an acute upper respiratory infection, then the first-listed diagnosis would be the one that was primarily responsible for the services provided on that day, with additional conditions sequenced subsequently. In this case: J06.9, Acute upper respiratory infection, unspecified, then E11.9, Type 2 diabetes mellitus without complications. The patient came in for treatment of the respiratory infection, so the respiratory infection code is sequenced first, followed by the diabetes code. Again, note that this guideline is for the professional outpatient setting, and inpatient facility guidelines may differ (refer to chapter 20).

Sometimes the definitive diagnosis is not known, but the provider has an idea of what it might be. Conditions that are documented as "suspected," "rule out," "probable," or "questionable," should not be coded as they are not confirmed by the healthcare

Figure 4.20. OGCR III, III.A

Section III. Reporting Additional Diagnoses

GENERAL RULES FOR OTHER (ADDITIONAL) DIAGNOSES

For reporting purposes the definition for "other diagnoses" is interpreted as additional conditions that affect patient care in terms of requiring:

- clinical evaluation; or
- therapeutic treatment; or
- diagnostic procedures; or
- extended length of hospital stay; or
- increased nursing care and/or
- monitoring

The UHDDS item #11-b defines Other Diagnoses as "all conditions that coexist at the time of admission, that develop subsequently, or that affect the treatment received and/or the length of stay. Diagnoses that relate to an earlier episode which have no bearing on the current hospital stay are to be excluded." UHDDS definitions apply to inpatients in acute-care, short-term, long term care and psychiatric hospital setting. The UHDDS definitions are used by acute-care shortterm hospitals to report inpatient data elements in a standardized manner. These data elements and their definitions can be found in the July 31, 1985, *Federal Register* (Vol. 50, No, 147), pp. 31038–40.

Since that time the application of the UHDDS definitions has been expanded to include all nonoutpatient settings (acute-care, short-term, long-term care and psychiatric hospitals; home health agencies; rehab facilities; nursing homes, etc). The UHDDS definitions also apply to hospice services (all levels of care).

The following guidelines are to be applied in designating "other diagnoses" when neither the Alphabetic Index nor the Tabular List in ICD-10-CM provide direction. The listing of the diagnoses in the patient record is the responsibility of the attending provider.

A. Previous Conditions

If the provider has included a diagnosis in the final diagnostic statement, such as the discharge summary or the face sheet, it should ordinarily be coded. Some providers include in the diagnostic statement resolved conditions or diagnoses and status-post procedures from previous admission that have no bearing on the current stay. Such conditions are not to be reported and are coded only if required by hospital policy.

However, history codes (categories Z80–Z87) may be used as secondary codes if the historical condition or family history has an impact on current care or influences treatment.

provider. If a condition is "suspected" but not confirmed, then code only for the signs and symptoms present at the time of the encounter (see figure 4.21). For example, a provider may evaluate a patient with low energy, joint pain, and depression, and suspect that she has hypothyroidism. However, the coder cannot assign the code for hypothyroidism until the provider is certain that it is the patient's definitive diagnosis.

Code all documented conditions that coexist at the time of the encounter and that require or affect patient care, management, or treatment (see figure 4.22). For example, it may be necessary to include a relevant family history code, if that family history has an impact on the current care of the patient. This guideline is especially important in HCC coding (discussed in chapter 2), which requires that coders report all coexisting conditions for risk adjustment purposes. Remember that HCC coding involves identifying and reporting codes that give a full and clear picture of a patient's health. This is more than simply what is required for the payment of a claim, but also includes codes that identify aspects of a patient's health—pertinent personal medical history and status codes, and all other conditions present at the time of the encounter, even if they are not related to the treatment provided that day. Chronic or ongoing diseases may be reported as many times as necessary to report the treatment and care for the ongoing condition.

Figure 4.21. OGCR IV.H

> **H. Uncertain Diagnosis**
>
> Do not code diagnoses documented as "probable", "suspected," "questionable," "rule out," or "working diagnosis" or other similar terms indicating uncertainty. Rather, code the condition(s) to the highest degree of certainty for that encounter/visit, such as symptoms, signs, abnormal test results, or other reason for the visit.
>
> *Note:* This differs from the coding practices used by short-term, acute-care, long-term care and psychiatric hospitals.

Source: CMS 2018.

Figure 4.22. OGCR IV.J

> **J.   Code All Documented Conditions that Coexist**
>
> Code all documented conditions that coexist at the time of the encounter/visit, and require or affect patient care treatment or management. Do not code conditions that were previously treated and no longer exist. However, history codes (categories Z80–Z87) may be used as secondary codes if the historical condition or family history has an impact on current care or influences treatment.

Source: CMS 2018.

ICD-10-CM Code Structure

The structure of ICD-10-CM codes is unique from any other code set. Unlike CPT, HCPCS, or even ICD-10-PCS codes, ICD-10-CM codes vary in length, ranging from three to seven characters and are alphanumeric. Also unique to ICD-10-CM codes is the use of a placeholder X, which keeps the place of a character so that the code can be extended fully to the required amount of characters. And, finally, some ICD-10-CM codes use a character to identify the episode of care, extending the code to the full seven characters. When learning how to use the ICD-10-CM code book, a coder should first examine each of these unique features before looking at the features of the code book itself, or how to locate and assign an ICD-10-CM code.

Code Structure and Format

ICD-10-CM codes range from three to seven characters in length. This length is determined by the requirements for each code and, typically, longer codes (seven characters) contain more detail than shorter codes (three characters), as each additional character adds more detail to the code description. No matter the code length, a decimal point is always placed after the third character in the code and additional characters are placed after the decimal point. Add as many additional characters as needed in order to code to the full extent, as determined by the ICD-10-CM guidelines.

ICD-10-CM codes are alphanumeric, as follows (see figure 4.23):

- The first character is always a letter
- The second character is always a number
- Characters three through seven may be either numbers or letters
- All letters of the alphabet are used with the exception of U, which has been reserved for future expansion or updates of the ICD-10-CM code set.

Figure 4.23. ICD-10-CM code structure

ICD-10-CM Code Structure	Examples
• Three to seven characters • First character is always alpha • Second digit is always numeric • Characters three through seven are either alpha or numeric • All letters are utilized (except for U)	• R12, Heartburn • J91.0, Malignant pleural effusion • C72.21, Malignant neoplasm of right olfactory nerve • Z3A.20, 20 weeks gestation of pregnancy • H02.821, Cysts of right upper eyelid • S09.21XA, Traumatic rupture of right ear drum, initial encounter

The ICD-10-CM code format is based on a possible length of seven characters total. This does not mean that each code has seven characters. ICD-10-CM codes range from three to seven characters total (see figure 4.24). The first three characters of an ICD-10-CM code are referred to as the category. Codes that start with the same three characters are within the same category. For example, category I11 stands for hypertensive heart disease, so each code that starts with I11 is a type of hypertensive heart disease. In the same manner, I12 stands for hypertensive chronic kidney disease, so each code that begins with I12 is a type of hypertensive chronic kidney disease (see table 4.1).

The category is followed by a decimal point and a varying number of characters. Note that ICD-10-CM codes range from three to seven codes. This means that there are a number of three-character category codes, such as I10, Essential (primary) hypertension. This code is not further divided as it has no additional characters or details. This is rare, however, as most ICD-10-CM codes do contain additional characters after the decimal point, each of which add further information to the code.

Figure 4.24. ICD-10-CM code format

ICD-10 Code Format:

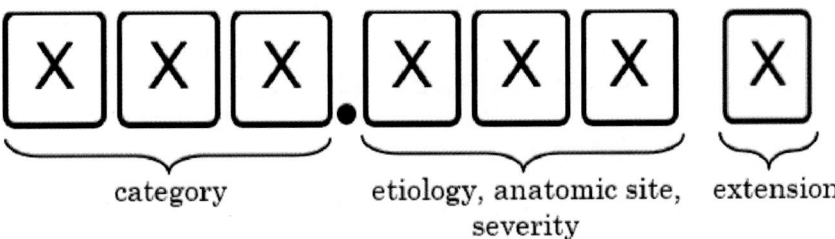

Source: Adapted from DeVault et. al 2014.

Table 4.1. Categories I10 and I12

I10 Essential (primary) hypertension	I10 Essential (primary) hypertension
I11 Hypertensive heart disease	**I11**.0 **Hypertensive heart disease** with heart failure **I11**.9 **Hypertensive heart disease** without heart failure
I12 Hypertensive chronic kidney disease	**I12**.0 **Hypertensive chronic kidney disease** with stage 5 chronic kidney disease or end-stage renal disease **I12**.9 **Hypertensive chronic kidney disease** with stage 1 through stage 4 chronic kidney disease, or unspecified chronic kidney disease

I13 Hypertensive heart and chronic kidney disease	**I13**.0 **Hypertensive heart and chronic kidney disease** with heart failure and stage 1 through stage 4 chronic kidney disease, or unspecified chronic kidney disease
	I13.1 **Hypertensive heart and chronic kidney disease** without heart failure
	    I13.10 ...... with stage 1 through stage 4 chronic kidney disease, or unspecified chronic kidney disease
	    I13.11 ...... with stage 5 chronic kidney disease, or end-stage renal disease
	I13.2 **Hypertensive heart and chronic kidney disease** with heart failure and with stage 5 chronic kidney disease, or end-stage renal disease

There are four additional characters that may be added to an ICD-10-CM code after the decimal point. Characters four, five, and six each add further detail to the code description, including the etiology (the cause of a disease), anatomic site, and severity of the condition. The meanings of these three characters vary. For example, in table 4.1, the fourth character for category I12 indicates if the hypertensive heart disease presents with or without heart failure. For category I13, the fourth character identifies the stage of chronic kidney disease. For category I13, codes within the subcategory I13.1 each have an additional number that identifies the stage of chronic kidney disease for hypertensive heart and chronic kidney disease without heart failure. Again, these characters have different meanings for each specific category of codes, so it is important to read through each code description and take note of the ways codes change depending on the characters added.

Up to three additional characters may be added after the decimal point, each of which provides more detail to the code. The last possible character— in the seventh location—is referred to as the seventh character extension, discussed in detail later in this chapter. This character is always placed in the seventh and last location, and usually represents the episode of care for the encounter. The episode of care identifies the patient's place within the care continuum. For example, the episode of care may identify that the patient is still in active treatment status, or is coming in for a subsequent encounter after the active treatment phase has passed.

Seventh Character Extensions and Episode of Care

Each character added to an ICD-10-CM code provides an additional detail, each of which makes the code more specific (see figure 4.25).

Normally, codes that are extended to the seventh character contain a seventh character episode of care identifier. In the majority of cases, the seventh character identifies the episode of care but there are exceptions to this—in rare instances, the seventh

Figure 4.25. ICD-10-CM seven-character code example

S62.512A

Displaced fracture of proximal phalanx of left thumb, initial encounter for closed fracture

S62 –Fracture at wrist and hand level
    S62.**5** –fracture of thumb
        S62.5**1** –proximal phalanx
            S62.51**2** –displaced
                S62.512**A** –initial encounter for closed fracture

Character	1	2	3	4	5	6	7
Code	S	6	2	5	1	2	A
Description	Fracture at wrist and hand level			Thumb	Proximal	Displaced	Initial, Closed

CC +7th **S62.512** **Displaced fracture of proximal phalanx of left thumb**
    CC Exclusion 7th character B see Appendix A PDX collection 1285
    CC Exclusion 7th characters K & P see Appendix A PDX collection 0897
    HAC 7th character B see Appendix B for HAC conditional logic

character may be used to identify a detail other than the episode of care. If the seventh character is not added to the code, then it is considered an invalid code and will not be accepted on a claim.

A seventh character extension is always placed in the last position (the seventh character) of an ICD-10-CM code, and includes more information about the condition or the episode of care for that condition. Although the seventh character most commonly identifies the episode of care, it is also used in obstetrics coding and a few other places within the ICD-10-CM code book. Note that the seventh character extension is not always a letter. In obstetrics coding, the seventh character may be a number, used to identify the fetus in a multiple gestation pregnancy. Seventh character extensions other than the episode of care are discussed when necessary throughout the remainder of this text.

Commonly the seventh character extension identifies the episode of care and for certain conditions, such as fractures, there are up to 16 episodes of care possible. These are discussed in detail in chapter 15 (Orthopedic Services). The three most common episode of care characters found throughout the ICD-10-CM code book are represented by the letters A, D, and S.

- **A- Initial Encounter.** This episode of care is used during the active treatment phase of a condition, or when the patient is still receiving treatment for a condition. Note that this does not mean *only* the first time that patient is seen. Episode of care letter A may be used multiple times, as long as the patient is still receiving active treatment; for example, if a patient receives wound treatments every day for a complicated wound that requires extensive observation.

- **D- Subsequent encounter.** This episode of care is used when the patient is seen during the healing phase of the encounter and is no longer receiving active treatment for the condition. For example, when a patient presents for cast removal after the healing phase of a fracture is completed.

- **S- Sequela**. A sequela is a condition that is the consequence of a previous disease or injury. Formerly referred to as a late effect, this letter should be used when a patient is seen for a complication of the condition after the healing phase has been completed. For example, the patient has residual pain in the hip after a hip fracture three years ago.

Review the following examples to see how the encounter affects the episode of care for the patient.

Billy, a five-year-old boy, was playing at a local park feeding the squirrels when he was bit on his left forearm by a squirrel. He presents to the urgent care clinic for cleaning and evaluation of the injury. He is diagnosed with a 1cm puncture wound without foreign body on the left forearm due to the squirrel bite. The urgent care doctor cleaned the wound and placed two stitches, prescribed an oral antibiotic, and ordered the patient to see his PCP the next day.

The diagnosis code assigned by the urgent care doctor would be S51.832-, Puncture wound without foreign body of left forearm. This code is not complete, as it requires a seventh character to identify the episode of care for the visit. In this case, the patient is in the active phase of treatment, so the letter A for initial care would be added to the end of the code: S51.832A, Puncture wound without foreign body of left forearm, *initial encounter.*

The next day, Billy presents to his PCP's office for an evaluation of his injury as ordered by the urgent care doctor. His PCP examines the wound and determines that is it healing well at this point, and that Billy should continue to monitor the wound and return to the office in two weeks for removal of his stitches, or sooner if any signs of infection are present.

The diagnosis code assigned by the patient's PCP for this visit would be the same as that assigned by the urgent care doctor: S51.832A, Puncture wound without foreign body of left forearm, *initial encounter.* Notice that even though this is the second time that the patient has been seen for the same wound, he is still in the active phase of treatment. Because of this, the seventh character "A" indicating active care is added to the end of the code.

Three days after Billy was seen by his PCP, his mother brings him into the office because the wound is red, painful, and there is a small amount of pus coming out of the puncture site. After evaluation of the fluid, the doctor prescribes a different antibiotic, cleans the wound, and replaces the stitches. He then orders the patient to return in two weeks or sooner if necessary.

In this case, the diagnosis code is the same for the wound of the arm: S51.832A, Puncture wound without foreign body of left forearm, initial encounter. At this point, the child has been seen three times for the same injury, and each service has been some sort of active care for the patient's injury, so the seventh character "A" for initial encounter is assigned for all three.

Billy presents to the office of his PCP two weeks after the initial injury for removal of stitches and evaluation of the healing status of his wound. His PCP examines the wound, which is well-healed at this point, but is notable for a large scar that has begun to form at the site of the wound. The PCP then removes the two stitches and informs the patient that he no longer has to be seen for this injury.

The diagnosis code for this case would be the same that has been used for the same injury previously, with the exception that the episode of care is different. In this case, the patient is in the healing phase of the injury, and is no longer receiving active treatment for the wound. Thus, the seventh character D, for subsequent care, replaces the A at the end of the code. The code assigned would be as follows: S51.832D, Puncture wound without foreign body of left forearm, subsequent encounter.

Three months after the initial injury, Billy's mother returns with him to the office because of a large keloid scar that has formed at the initial injury site. The scar is painful and irritating, and the mother would like to have the PCP evaluate the scar to see if there is anything that they can do. The PCP examines the wound site and diagnoses Billy with a keloid scar due to the initial squirrel bite injury.

For this visit, the PCP assigns a code for the keloid scar that is a sequela of the previous injury, the puncture wound. So two codes are necessary: one to identify the keloid scar and one to identify the previous injury, the puncture wound. The puncture wound diagnosis will be the same as those used previously for the same injury, but since the episode of care is different the seventh character extension will be changed to S to recognize that the patient is coming in for a sequela of the injury: S51.832S, Puncture wound without foreign body of left forearm, sequela. Refer to table 4.2 for a simplified timeline of these visits.

Table 4.2. Example of episodes of care for an injury

Date	Encounter	Episode of Care
Day 1	Urgent Care for initial injury	A-Initial
Day 2	PCP office for follow-up	A-Initial
Day 5	PCP office for wound infection	A-Initial
Day 22	PCP office for follow-up and suture removal	D-Subsequent
Month 3	PCP office for evaluation of scar	S-Sequela

Key to Success

Rather than thinking of the episode of care letter A as the first time a patient is seen, think of it as "Active Care." A = Active Care. The letter A should be used for any visit in which the patient is undergoing active care, not necessarily the first time that the patient is seen.

The appropriate episode of care letter should be added to the end of the ICD-10-CM code depending on where the patient presents on their timeline of care. Note that although A, D, and S, are the three most common episode of care identifiers, they are not the only ones. Some fractures have up to 16 different seventh character extensions, each identified with a letter, which identify the type of fracture, episode of care, and healing status (these are discussed in detail in chapter 15, Orthopedic Services).

Episode of care extensions are most commonly used with injury codes, such as fractures, burns, open wounds, and such. They are also used with external cause codes. **External cause codes** identify the circumstances surrounding an injury, poisoning, or adverse event, such as the activity that the patient was engaged in when the injury occurred, where the patient was when the injury took place, and the injury mechanism (how the injury happened).

For practice identifying the seventh character extension, complete the exercises in There's a Code for That 4.7.

4.7

There's a Code for That

Identify the seventh character extension options

Using the Tabular List, identify the possible seventh character extensions for the following codes by locating the seventh character extension options.

1. What are the seventh character extension options for S03.01, Dislocation of jaw, right side?

   Seventh character options: _____

2. What are the seventh character extension options for S12.030, Displaced posterior arch fracture of first cervical vertebra?

   Seventh character options: _____

3. What are the seventh character extension options for H40.221, Chronic angle-closure glaucoma, right eye?

   Seventh character options: _____

4. What are the seventh character extension options for O32.1, Maternal care for breech presentation?

   Seventh character options: _____

When assigning seventh character extensions, pay close attention to the guidelines outlined in the ICD-10-CM code book, as they will specify which extensions to use and their definitions. Sometimes an ICD-10-CM code is not yet extended to six characters, but a seventh character is still required. In these cases, a placeholder X must be used to extend the code to six characters, so that a seventh character may be added.

Placeholder X

In some cases, an ICD-10-CM code requires the use of a seventh character extension to identify the episode of care, but that code is not yet extended to six characters. For example, code S02.91-, Unspecified fracture of skull, requires the addition of a seventh character to identify the episode of care for the visit. However, this code is only five characters long (see figure 4.26).

This means that the code must be extended to six characters, so that the seventh character may be added. In this case, it is necessary to insert the placeholder X as the sixth character, in order to add the seventh character. **Placeholder X** is used to extend a code to the required number of characters so that a seventh character extension may be placed. In this example, the letter X is placed in the sixth location, and the correct episode of care letter (A, D, or S) is placed in the seventh location (see figure 4.27).

Figure 4.26. Incomplete code example (5 out of 7 characters assigned)

Character	1	2	3	4	5	6	7
Code	S	0	2	9	1		

Figure 4.27. Complete code example (7 out of 7 characters assigned)

Character	1	2	3	4	5	6	7
Code	S	0	2	9	1	X	A

Figure 4.28. Complete code example with three placeholders (characters 4, 5, and 6)

Character	1	2	3	4	5	6	7
Code	W	5	2	X	X	X	A

The correct code to an unspecified fracture of the skull for an initial encounter would be S02.91XA, Unspecified fracture of the skull, initial encounter. If the code is not extended to seven characters, it is an invalid code. An **invalid code** is not coded to the full extent and may not be used for coding or billing purposes. For example, if an invalid code was sent on a claim for insurance payment purposes, then the insurance company would not pay the claim. It is extremely important to ensure that only valid codes are assigned.

Sometimes, multiple placeholders must be placed to extend a code to the required amount of characters in order to add a seventh character extension. For example, code W52, Crushed, pushed or stepped on by crowd or human stampede, only has three characters. However, a seventh character extension must be added to identify the episode of care for this encounter. In this case, *three* placeholders must be added to extend the code to the correct number of characters, so that the episode of care may be placed in the seventh location (see figure 4.28).

In this example, the correct code for an initial episode of care would be W52.XXXA, Crushed, pushed or stepped on by crowd or human stampede, initial encounter.

The ICD-10-CM code book has conventions and symbols that help coders identify when a seventh character extension is necessary, what the seventh characters are, and when a placeholder is needed. The code book is also carefully organized into a standardized format so coders can locate and assign codes correctly. It is important to go over the organization, format, conventions, and guidelines located within the ICD-10-CM code book to learn how to assign codes correctly.

For practice adding the seventh character extensions and placeholders, complete the exercises in There's a Code for That 4.8 and 4.9.

Seventh character extensions

4.8

There's a Code for That

Using your understanding of the seventh character extensions A, D, and S, answer the following questions (A-initial, D-subsequent, S-sequela)

1. Melinda was seen for a fracture of her wrist after falling on the sidewalk. This is the first time she has been seen for this injury. What is the episode of care for this encounter?

   Seventh character: _____

(Continued on next page)

4.8

Continued

2. A patient returned to the orthopedist's office for the removal of a cast on her lower left leg. The fracture was well-healed and the cast was removed. What is the episode of care for this encounter?

Seventh character: _____

3. Sheila suffered a fracture of her hip five years ago and now presents for treatment of arthritis of her hip due to the fracture five years ago. What is the episode of care for this injury?

Seventh character: _____

4. After initial treatment at the ER, a male patient returned to his primary care physician's office for treatment of a wound infection. What is the episode of care for this injury?

Seventh character: _____

4.9

There's a Code for That

Placeholder X

Using your understanding of the purpose and function of the placeholder X, answer the following questions.

1. The ICD code for parachutist entangled in object is V97.21-, Parachutist entangled in object, which requires a seventh character to identify the episode of care for this encounter. Which of the following would be the correct way to code for "Parachutist entangled in object, initial encounter"?
   a. V97.21A
   b. V97.XXXA
   c. V97.21XA
   d. V97.21AX

2. Complete the following code for: W54.0-, Bitten by dog, initial encounter

   ICD-10-CM code: _____

3. Complete the following code for: S60.00-, Contusion of unspecified finger without damage to nail, subsequent encounter.

   ICD-10-CM code: _____

4. Complete the following code for: W35.- Explosion and rupture of boiler, initial encounter.

   ICD-10-CM code: _____

End of Chapter Content

Instructions: Indicate whether the following statements are true or false (T or F). For false statements, rewrite the statement on the line below to make the statement true.

1. All ICD-10-CM codes begin with a letter.

_____

_____

2. The first three characters of an ICD-10-CM code are referred to as the subcategory.

_____

_____

3. The maximum amount of characters that an ICD-10-CM code can have is seven.

_____

_____

4. The seventh character of an ICD-10-CM code typically identifies the episode of care.

_____

_____

5. The seventh character A may only be used once for any given injury.

_____

_____

6. The two major divisions of the ICD-10-CM code book are the Index and the Tabular List.

_____

_____

7. Main terms are indented under the subterms to indicate that they pertain to the subterm.

_____

_____

8. Nonessential modifiers impact the code selected from the Main Index.

_____

_____

(Continued on next page)

(Continued)

9. Once the code is located in the Main Index, it is not important to verify the code in the Tabular List.

_____

_____

10. An adverse effect occurs when a substance that is correctly prescribed and administered causes a toxic effect.

_____

_____

Instructions: Choose the best answer.

1. Which of the following is not true regarding ICD-10-CM codes?

   a. The first character may be either a letter or a number
   b. They range from three to seven characters
   c. All letters of the alphabet are used except for the letter U
   d. The second character is always a number

2. Which of the following codes would be a valid ICD-10-CM code?

   a. 460.9
   b. Z3A.20.Z
   c. J91.0
   d. P09.X6594

3. What is the purpose of the additional characters after the three-character category code?

   a. They add more detail to the code description
   b. They make the procedure more complicated
   c. They make the ICD-10-CM code more difficult to look up
   d. There are never any characters added to three-character category codes

4. The episode of care extension A, for initial encounter should be used when?

   a. When the patient is receiving follow-up care after an injury has healed
   b. When the patient is pregnant with more than one fetus
   c. When the patient is receiving care for a sequela of an initial condition
   d. When the patient is in the active treatment phase for an injury

5. What is used to extend a code to the required number of characters so that a seventh character extension may be placed at the end of a code?

   a. External cause
   b. Placeholder X
   c. Seventh character extension
   d. A, for initial encounter

6. In which Index would you find the codes for a cancerous tumor?

   a. Main Index
   b. Neoplasm Table
   c. Table of Drugs
   d. External Cause Index

7. In which Index would you find the codes for the mechanism of an injury, as well as the place of occurrence for an injury?

   a. Main Index
   b. Neoplasm Table
   c. Table of Drugs
   d. External Cause Index

8. What is the noun that described the patient's diagnosis or reason for encounter?

   a. External cause
   b. Main term
   c. Subterm
   d. Excludes1 note

9. Which cross-reference in the Main Index instructs coders to look elsewhere for a code if the precise condition cannot be found in the current entry?

   a. See also
   b. See condition
   c. Code first
   d. Use additional code

10. Which of the following neoplasm behaviors indicates a cancerous tumor?

    a. Benign
    b. Unspecified
    c. Uncertain behavior
    d. Malignant

11. Which of the following is the structured list of ICD-10-CM codes, organized alphanumerically and divided into chapters based on body system or condition?

    a. Main Index
    b. Tabular List
    c. Table of Drugs and Chemicals
    d. External Cause of Injury Index

12. A three-digit code is referred to as a:

    a. Category
    b. Subcategory
    c. Section
    d. Subclassification

13. Which note is a pure Excludes note that means two conditions are mutually exclusive of each other?

    a. Excludes1
    b. Excludes2
    c. Includes
    d. Essential modifier

14. Which of the following sequencing instructions tells the coder to place the additional code *after* the current code selected?

    a. Code first
    b. See also
    c. Use additional code
    d. Code also

15. Which of the following is the cause of a disease?

    a. Etiology
    b. Manifestation
    c. Combination code
    d. Underlying infection code

16. In the absence of a definitive diagnosis, what does a coder report?

    a. Suspected conditions
    b. Probable conditions
    c. Integral conditions
    d. Signs and symptoms

17. When a patient has both the acute and chronic versions of the same condition, which is sequenced first?

    a. Acute
    b. Chronic
    c. The combination code
    d. Neither

18. When a condition affects both sides of the body it is:

    a. Lateral
    b. Bilateral
    c. Combination
    d. Acute

19. What is the term for the primary diagnosis listed on outpatient claims?

    a. First-listed diagnosis
    b. Principal diagnosis
    c. Secondary diagnosis
    d. Sequenced diagnosis

References

Casto, A.B., ed. 2018. *ICD-10-CM Code Book*. Chicago: AHIMA.

Centers for Medicare and Medicaid Services. 2018. ICD-10-CM Official Guidelines for Coding and Reporting FY 2018. https://www.cms.gov/Medicare /Coding/ICD10/Downloads/2018-ICD-10-CM-Coding -Guidelines.pdf.

DeVault, K., A. Barta, and M. Endicott. 2014. *ICD-10-CM Coder Training Manual*. Chicago: AHIMA.

CHAPTER

Learning the CPT and HCPCS Code Books

Learning Objectives

- Understand the structure and purpose of CPT codes.
- Examine the organization and format of the CPT code book.
- Recognize and utilize the symbols, conventions, and coding guidelines for CPT codes.

- Understand the structure and purpose of HCPCS codes.
- Examine the organization, format, symbols, and conventions used in the HCPCS code book.

Key Terms

Add-on code

Anesthesia section

Category I code

Category II code

Category III code

Eponym

Evaluation and Management
    Services section

Indented code

Medicine section

Modifying term

Parenthetical note

Pathology and Laboratory section

Radiology section

Resequenced code

Separate procedure

Special report

Standalone code

Surgery section

Synonym

Table of Drugs

Telemedicine service

Unlisted procedure codes

Diagnostic coding is the first half of coding and the second is coding for any procedures performed—reporting the actual services, treatments, and procedures performed by the healthcare provider. There are three code books that include procedure codes: ICD-10-PCS, CPT and HCPCS. ICD-10-PCS codes are for procedures performed in the facility inpatient setting. As such, the PCS code book is discussed in chapter 20 (Inpatient Hospital Services) and is not included in this chapter.

As noted in chapter 3 (Basics of Coding), both CPT and HCPCS code sets have been adopted for use by the Centers for Medicare and Medicaid Services (CMS) and are known collectively as HCPCS codes. CPT codes are considered Level I codes, and HCPCS codes are considered Level II codes. They are published, created, and maintained by different organizations so it is important to learn the basics of each code book separately, as they differ greatly from each other.

This chapter focuses on the basics of CPT—the CPT guidelines and codes, including CPT code structure and purpose, and the format and organization of the CPT code book. It then focuses on HCPCS, including HCPCS code structure and purpose, and the format and organization of the HCPCS code book.

CPT Code Structure and Purpose

CPT codes are five characters in length, beginning with at least four numbers and ending with either a letter or a number. The majority of CPT codes are all numeric. Unlike ICD-10-CM codes, CPT codes never change in length. They always remain five characters, no matter how detailed the reported healthcare procedure.

Each CPT code identifies a specific procedure or service that was performed by the healthcare provider. For example, code 40808, Biopsy, vestibule of mouth identifies a surgical procedure in which a tissue sample was taken from the inside of the cheek for examination. This code reports the specific surgical procedure performed by the healthcare provider, and that will be reported to the insurance company (along with an ICD-10-CM code to identify the medical necessity for the biopsy).

There are CPT codes for thousands of healthcare procedures, ranging from office visits, anesthesia services, and surgeries, to radiological services and laboratory procedures, in addition to new and emerging technological advancements in medical and surgical procedures and performance measures. The different types of healthcare services or procedures are divided into three categories, and assigned numerical codes that are similar in value. Refer to table 5.1 to see the different code ranges for different procedure types.

Table 5.1. CPT code ranges by procedure type

Category Type	Procedure Type	Code Range
Category I	Evaluation and Management	99201–99499
	Anesthesiology	00100–01999, 99100–99140
	Surgery	10021–69990
	Radiology	70010–79999
	Pathology and Laboratory	80047–89398
	Medicine (except Anesthesiology)	90281–99199, 99500–99607
Category II	Supplemental Tracking Measures	0001F–9007F
Category III	New and Emerging Technologies	0042T–0504

CPT codes are organized with similar procedures grouped together numerically, so that similar procedures or procedures performed on the same body system all begin with the same number. For example, all evaluation and management codes begin with the same two numbers—99—such as 99381, Initial comprehensive preventive medicine evaluation and management of an individual; infant (age younger than 1 year); and all radiology services begin with the number 7, such as 71048, Radiologic examination, chest, 4 or more views. As coders learn more about the intricacies of the CPT coding system, these similarities will become more apparent. Experienced coders may be so familiar with the CPT code structure that they can simply look at a code and identify the procedure or know on which body system the procedure was performed.

When assigning CPT codes for services, coders should select the name of the procedure that most accurately describes the service performed, and not one that is simply like the code being described. Many times, healthcare procedures vary by only a small detail, such as the time involved in performing the procedure, or in the approach to a surgical procedure. CPT coding relies heavily on a close reading of the healthcare provider's documentation of the service performed. Any further procedures performed at the same time are reported with additional CPT codes. For example, if a provider performed a biopsy of the vestibule of the mouth and the incision and drainage of a simple pilonidal cyst, then each of these two services would be reported with the appropriate CPT code: 40808, Biopsy, vestibule of mouth, and 10080, Incision and drainage of pilonidal cyst; simple. However, in some instances multiple procedures are bundled into one code (this is discussed fully in chapter 11).

Note also that according to CPT guidelines, inclusion of a code in the CPT code set does not indicate the procedure or service will be reimbursed, nor does it indicate endorsement by the AMA (AMA 2017). So although a code may exist for a procedure or procedure(s), health insurance coverage is not guaranteed for each code, and reporting a CPT code does not ensure payment for the service.

The CPT Code Book

The American Medical Association (AMA) publishes the CPT code book on an annual basis and maintains the code set. The two most common versions published by AMA each year are the *CPT Standard Edition,* which is a basic manual that lists the CPT codes, and the *CPT Professional Edition,* a more enhanced version of the CPT code book that includes anatomical drawings, extended guidelines, and a three-color format. It is important for first-time coders to have the best code book available; this text recommends using the *CPT Professional Edition* while learning to code. This version of the CPT code book includes more information, guidelines, and notes throughout, which helps beginning coders understand the many intricacies of CPT coding.

Like the ICD-10-CM code book, the CPT code book includes a Tabular List of all CPT codes as well as an index and a number of appendices. CPT codes are divided into three categories, described as follows, with most CPT codes falling within Category I codes (refer to table 5.1). After the tabular listing of codes (which includes Category I, II, and III codes), are 16 appendices (listed later in this chapter), followed by the index (also discussed in detail later in this chapter).

Category I codes are the largest set of codes within the CPT code book and are commonly referred to as simply CPT codes. These procedures have been approved by the Food and Drug Administration (FDA), are performed by physicians or other healthcare practitioners throughout the United States at a frequency consistent with their intended clinical use, are consistent with current clinical practice, and have a documented clinical efficacy for treating healthcare conditions (AMA 2017).

Category I CPT Codes

Category I codes are divided into six sections and make up the majority of the CPT code set. These sections group similar procedures together, such as radiology procedures or anesthesia services (see table 5.1). When learning procedural coding, it is important to keep these sections in mind, as the codes within each section are different in nature than those in the other sections. For example, the Pathology and Laboratory section only lists codes that report pathology and laboratory services, even though these services may be performed with procedures from the radiology, surgery, or medicine sections. Ultimately, the sections help coders navigate through the code book by grouping similar procedures together, but they are not exclusive of each other and coders may report procedures throughout all sections of the CPT code book as necessary.

It is also important to note that there are guidelines specific to each individual section of the CPT code book at the beginning of each section. These guidelines provide the rules on how to use the CPT codes in each of the sections, and offer additional information and advice about how to code correctly from each section, respectively. This text will continuously refer to CPT guidelines from the beginning of each of these sections as well as from within each chapter. This chapter also includes a full discussion of common CPT guidelines.

Key to Success

An easy way to see the different sections of the CPT code book is to look at the far edge from the binding, which is either shaded in a different color grey or highlighted in the colors red, green, or blue. These varying colors or shades can help you maneuver through the code book to find sections and codes more easily.

The six sections of Category I CPT codes are: Evaluation and Management, Anesthesia, Surgery, Radiology, Pathology and Laboratory, and Medicine.

Evaluation and Management

The first section of Category I codes in the CPT code book is the **Evaluation and Management Services section**, which lists codes 99201 through 99499. Evaluation and management codes are perhaps the most important codes in all professional procedural coding, making up the majority of all codes reported for professional services in either the inpatient or outpatient setting. They are commonly referred to as E/M codes, E&M codes, or EM codes. E/M codes are used to report any service in which a healthcare professional evaluates and then manages a patient, or the treatment of a patient, such as an office sick visit, hospital discharge, routine physical examination, or inpatient critical care visit. E/M codes may be used across all healthcare settings, and as such this section is divided based on the type of E/M service (such as a consultation), place of service (such as in a skilled nursing facility), and patient status (such as new or established patient). These components for E/M services are discussed in detail in chapter 7.

Because of the importance of evaluation and management services, there are a great deal of guidelines that govern E/M coding. When coding for E/M services, this text will commonly refer to these guidelines as necessary to explain the nuances of E/M coding. Furthermore, because E/M coding is used in all healthcare settings and by all types of qualified healthcare professionals, E/M services will be used constantly throughout this text. This text introduces E/M coding in chapter 7 (Behavioral Health) and includes further detail on E/M code selection in chapter 8 (Primary Care).

Key to Success

You may have noticed that the first section of the CPT code book, E/M codes, is out of numerical order. E/M codes start with the number 9, which should indicate that they come at the end of the book. The CPT code book lists E/M codes first so that they are easily accessible to coders, as they are common codes that must be constantly referenced.

Anesthesia

The Anesthesia section lists services that are performed by anesthesiologists, anesthesia assistants, or other healthcare providers, and is reported with codes 00100 through 01999. These services are performed to reduce sensation and alleviate pain, usually during surgery or invasive procedure.

There are a few different types of anesthesia services, including general anesthesia, moderate sedation, monitored anesthesia care, and regional or local nerve blocks. The anesthesia services included within this section code for services that are used to anesthetize a patient undergoing a surgical procedure, up to and including general anesthesia, such as code 00500, Anesthesia for all procedures on esophagus. Moderate (conscious) sedation, regional, and local anesthesia services codes are located in different sections of the CPT code book. For example, moderate sedation codes (99151 through 99157) are located within the Medicine section, and codes for local anesthetic injections are located within their respective surgical subsections, such as 64455, Injection(s), anesthetic agent and/or steroid; plantar common digital nerve(s). Anesthesia services, including a discussion on general anesthesia coding and coding for moderate sedation anesthesia and local anesthetic injections, are discussed in chapter 12 (Anesthesia and Pain Management Services).

Surgery

The Surgery section is the largest of all sections in the CPT code book. It lists all of the invasive procedures that may be performed to treat patients, reported with codes 10021 through 69990. The Surgery section is also divided into subsections based on body systems, each of which is further divided into anatomical regions, organs, or procedure types. These subsections are

- General (10021 to 10022)
- Integumentary (10030 to 19499)
- Musculoskeletal (20005 to 29999)
- Respiratory (30000 to 32999)
- Cardiovascular (33010 to 37799)
- Hemic and Lymphatic (38100 to 39599)
- Digestive (40490 to 49999)
- Urinary (50010 to 53899)

- Male Genital (54000 to 55899)
- Reproductive System Procedures (55920)
- Intersex Surgery (55970 to 55980)
- Female Genital (56405 to 58999)
- Maternity Care and Delivery (59000 to 59899)
- Endocrine (60000 to 60699)
- Nervous (61000 to 64999)
- Eye and Ocular Adnexa (65091 to 68899)
- Auditory (69000 to 69979)
- Operating Microscope (69990)

Healthcare providers from all different specialties may report services from the surgery section, as needed, although most providers will specialize in a certain body area or surgery type. For example, a cardiothoracic surgeon specializes in surgeries of the heart, coronary vessels, and organs within the thoracic cavity. This means that coding for a cardiothoracic surgeon requires an in-depth knowledge of the procedural codes in the cardiovascular system subsection of the CPT code book. The intricacies of these codes will be discussed in the context of healthcare specialties throughout the rest of the chapters in this text.

Radiology

The **Radiology section** lists all of the procedures that use radiant energy to diagnose medical conditions, such as x-rays, MRIs, and ultrasounds. This section also includes procedures that use radiant energy to treat medical conditions, such as radiation oncology, a special branch of medicine that uses radiation to treat cancerous tumors. Codes in this section range from 70010 to 79999.

Pathology and Laboratory

The **Pathology and Laboratory section** lists codes that represent diagnostic studies on human specimens and tissue samples, reported with codes 80047 through 89398. What is important to note about these codes is that they are for the testing of the sample only—the procurement of the sample, such as biopsy or resection of a tumor, is reported with a different code from the surgery section of the CPT code book. Pathology and laboratory (often abbreviated as path and lab) codes report just the testing of the specimen to determine its pathology. Some path and lab procedures must be performed at specialized testing facilities, whereas others may be done in a regular outpatient clinic setting. As such, this text will include pathology and laboratory codes throughout the chapters as necessary.

Medicine

The last section of Category I CPT codes is the **Medicine section**, which lists codes 90281 through 99607. This section is a miscellaneous grouping of all the procedures, treatments, studies, and tests performed on patients that do not belong elsewhere in the book. Some of the procedures are minimally invasive, such as heart catheterizations and vaccination injections, but none are as invasive as the procedures included in the Surgery section. Most of the procedures in this section are noninvasive, such as psychiatry treatments and chiropractic manipulations.

Procedures listed in the Medicine section are performed by an array of different healthcare providers, and are commonly performed in the outpatient office setting.

This text presents these procedures within the context of certain healthcare specialties, along with necessary procedure codes from throughout the rest of the CPT sections.

Key to Success

It is a good idea to place tabs on the outer edges of your code book to help you easily locate the various sections of the CPT book. Even advanced coders utilize tabs to help them quickly locate and assign commonly used codes and important guidelines.

Category II codes are listed in the CPT code book immediately after the Medicine section, which is effectively the end of Category I codes. Category II codes list supplemental tracking codes used for performance measurement.

Category II Codes

As discussed in chapter 3, performance measurement is the act of tracking a practice or facility's performance against specific measures. Category II codes are completely optional, they are not required to be reported on any claim and are not reimbursable—they will never be paid. They are intended only to facilitate data collection for performance measurement purposes. Category II codes are supplemental tracking codes that report the performance of a test, evaluation, counseling service, or other procedure that is part of a facility's performance measurement program. For example, code 0545F, Plan for follow-up care for major depressive disorder, documented (MDD ADOL), may be used to report that a practice completed a plan for follow-up care for a patient with major depressive disorder (MDD), documented in the health record. If this MDD follow-up care plan is tracked as part of that practice's performance measures, then a report can be run on how often the follow-up care plans are completed and documented, on which patients, and for which specific diagnoses.

Category II codes are five characters in length, the first four characters are numbers, and the last character is always the letter F. This is done to make the number of characters consistent with the rest of the CPT codes, but to differentiate them from Category I and Category III codes.

Category III Codes

Category III codes are a set of temporary codes used to report emerging technology, services, procedures, and service paradigms, and the use of these codes is integral to the identification and establishment of new healthcare procedures and treatments. They are composed of five characters and end with the letter T (a string of four numbers ending with the letter T).

Unlike Category I codes, these codes are for technologies and procedures that may not yet have FDA approval or proven clinical efficacy, and are not performed frequently throughout the United States. However, this does not mean that the procedures are not clinically effective or that they will never get approval. The purpose of these codes is to report them as necessary, and if it is determined that the procedures meet the criteria of a Category I code, then they will be integrated into the Category I code set. In this way, codes for emerging technologies and new procedures can be included within most CPT codes, and used by physicians across the country for reporting purposes.

Coders should be especially careful when reporting Category III codes, as they are not necessarily covered by insurance. Furthermore, it is important to understand the relationship between unlisted procedures and Category III codes. **Unlisted procedures** are useful codes that may be reported when a provider performs a medical procedure that does not have a corresponding CPT code. Unlisted procedures are found in the Category I section of codes in the CPT code book, and are not included in the Category III codes. Consider the following example.

A pediatrician commonly sees patients who have fallen in cacti, and have multiple small thorns in their extremities. These are small and delicate thorns, and she uses an effective procedure for removing them by placing a piece of sticky tape along the extremity over the thorns and quickly removing the tape, which extracts the thorns.

There is no procedure code in the CPT code set that includes the use of sticky tape to remove foreign bodies from the skin of a patient. Thus, the pediatrician may choose to use an unlisted code to report the service, but before using an unlisted code she must first check in the Category III codes section for a code that captures the procedure. If a Category III code exists, then the unlisted procedures code may not be used. Figure 5.1 illustrates this decision-making process.

Figure 5.1. Decision tree for using unlisted procedures codes

If it is determined that an unlisted procedure code should be used, then a special report should be sent with the unlisted procedure code to explain the procedure in detail and the rationale for providing the procedure to the patient. Special reports are discussed in more detail in the guidelines section later in this chapter. Review figure 5.2 for a reminder of the three categories of CPT codes, and the type of codes included within each category.

Figure 5.2. CPT code categories and sections

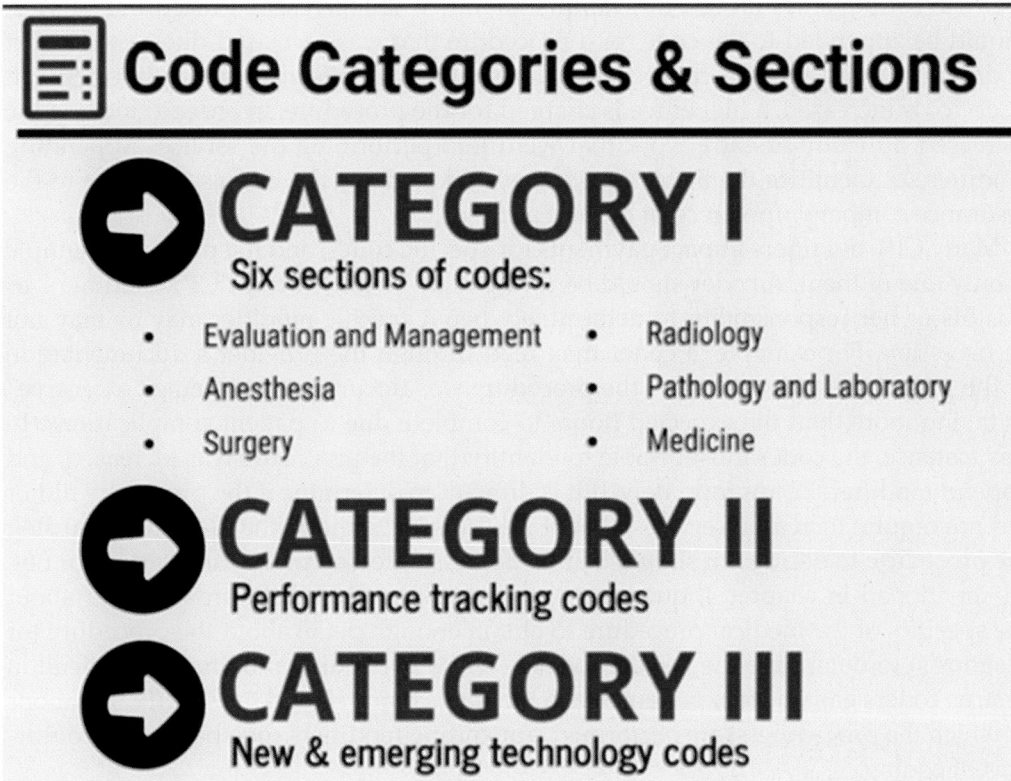

Appendices

Sixteen appendices, listed in numerical order, follow the Category III codes section, each containing additional valuable information for using CPT codes. Appendices are updated regularly and may be removed, added, or edited as needed by the American Medical Association.

Perhaps the most important appendix is Appendix A, which contains the listing and descriptions of CPT modifiers (introduced in chapter 3). The remaining appendices are useful for coding in certain specialties or for coding in specific situations.

Appendix A: Modifiers

Appendix A contains a list of all CPT modifiers, as well as a selection of commonly used HCPCS modifiers. CPT modifiers are developed by the American Medical Association as part of the CPT code set, whereas HCPCS modifiers are developed by CMS as part of the HCPCS code set. However, HCPCS modifiers may be used to identify certain situations or add further details to a procedure code, and as such are frequently used with CPT codes as well as with HCPCS codes. The list of CPT modifiers in the CPT code book is a complete list, whereas the list of HCPCS modifiers is a shortened list that includes only the most common HCPCS modifiers used with CPT codes. The full list of HCPCS modifiers is included in the HCPCS code book, discussed in detail later in this chapter.

As described in chapter 3, modifiers are used to alter the meaning of a code, such as to indicate that a procedure was discontinued after it was begun, or that it was an increased procedural service. They are two characters and added to the end of a CPT code to provide additional information to the description of the procedure or how it was performed. Sometimes, this added information may impact the way the code is paid, which makes modifiers extremely important to understanding the connection between coding and billing. For example, modifier -22, Increased Procedural Service, should be appended to the code for a procedure that was increased due to some sort of difficulty during the procedure or because of the patient's medical condition. When a service is increased, a higher fee is charged for the procedure, in order to include the increased difficulty or extra work that went into performing the service. Appending modifier -22 identifies the increased service, and explains the increased charge to the insurance company upon receipt of the claim.

Many CPT modifiers impact payments for specific codes, and the previous example is only one of them. A coder should be aware of all of the different CPT modifiers, as it is his or her responsibility to determine when a specific modifier may or may not be necessary. For example, a coder may read through the provider's documentation of the procedure and notice that the procedure was documented as being "extensive" or taking more than the expected hours to complete due to patient complications. In this instance, the coder must be able to identify that the procedure was increased, and append modifier -22 appropriately. If it is difficult to determine if the procedure did or did not require increased services, then it is necessary to query the provider regarding the procedure to decide if it should be billed as an increased procedural service or not. As mentioned in chapter 4, querying involves asking the healthcare provider about the specifics of the medical procedure to obtain enough detail about the procedure (or diagnosis) to determine the correct code(s). While appending modifiers is difficult at first, as coders gain more experience with the codes reported and the specific situations in which the procedure(s) are performed, appending modifiers soon becomes a routine part of coding.

Note that in Appendix A, modifiers are not listed with a preceding hyphen (-). However, they are commonly presented as such (like -22 rather than 22). This is because they are added to the end of a procedure code, and the hyphen is used to separate the end of the CPT code from the modifier. For example, if code 20005, Incision and drainage of soft tissue abscess, subfascial, was an increased procedural service, then it would be reported as 20005-22. In the real world, modifiers may or may not have the preceding hyphen, as some insurance payers simply tag the extra digits onto the CPT code (such as 2000522). This requires a certain amount of flexibility when identifying CPT codes and modifiers. Remember that the first five digits are always the CPT code, and the additional two digits are the modifier for the service.

Modifiers (both CPT and HCPCS), and how they may impact the payment of codes, are discussed throughout the rest of this text as necessary, in the context of coding procedures in specialty-specific healthcare offices.

MOD

There are many different modifiers and it is easy to forget that they are a necessary component of procedural coding. To help remember modifiers and their meanings, it is a good idea to create a set of flash cards with modifiers 22 through 99, as well as the HCPCS modifiers listed in Appendix A, and test yourself. Expert coders can simply read a procedural description and know when a modifier is needed, and which modifier to add to the procedure code.

Appendix B: Summary of Additions, Deletions, and Revisions

This appendix lists all of the additions, deletions, and revisions made throughout the CPT code set from the previous year's codes. The changes are made by striking out the text or symbols, or by adding new symbols alongside the codes to indicate what has been changed. This appendix is less important for new coders, who may not be familiar with the codes from the previous year. However, it will be more important for coders who are working in the field and need a quick reference guide to see what has been changed for the new year.

Appendix C: Clinical Examples

This appendix is made up of a set of clinical examples, which are useful tools in illustrating what the different levels of E/M codes look like across multiple different specialties. Documentation from actual encounters does not need to match the clinical examples. They are provided for informational use only as an aid in E/M code selection.

Appendix D: Summary of CPT Add-On Codes

Appendix D is a list of the **add-on codes** included within the CPT code set. It is provided only for informational purposes to help coders identify these add-on codes. An add-on code is a CPT code that may not be used alone; instead, it must be added to another CPT code. Add-on codes typically represent extra work, time, body area, or additional procedure that was performed in addition to the primary service. For example, code 11200, Removal of skin tags, multiple fibrocutaneous tags, any area; up to and including 15 lesions is the primary code for the removal of up to 15 skin tags. If the provider removed more than 25 skin tags, then the add-on code 11201, Removal of skin tags, multiple fibrocutaneous tags, any area; each additional 10 lesions, or part thereof, to identify the additional amount of skin tags removed by the provider. Add-on codes are identified by a plus symbol in the Tabular List, and are discussed in more detail later in this chapter.

Note that the list of add-on codes in Appendix D does not include the code descriptions. Code descriptions are included within the Tabular List.

Appendix E: Summary of Codes Exempt from Modifier -51

This appendix is a list of all codes that are exempt from the use of modifier -51 that are located within the surgical and medical sections of codes of the CPT code book. Modifier -51, Multiple Procedures, may not be appended to the codes on this list. This is a helpful list, as this modifier is one of only two (including modifier -63, Procedure Performed on Infants less than 4 kg), that may or may not be appended to specific CPT codes. Note that this list is similar to the list provided in Appendix D, and does not include any code descriptions. This is to save space by eliminating the sometimes lengthy code descriptions.

Also, this list is not an exhaustive list and does not include all modifier -51 exempt codes. This appendix only lists those modifier -51 exempt codes located within the surgical and medical code sections of the CPT code book. For example, pathology and laboratory codes, ranging from 80047 to 89398 are modifier -51 exempt, but they are not included in Appendix E (this is discussed in more depth in chapter 14, Independent Laboratory and Pathology Services). This again is to save space by eliminating a large amount of codes that are by definition exempt from this modifier.

Appendix F: Summary of CPT Codes Exempt from Modifier -63

This appendix is a list of all codes that are exempt from modifier -63. Modifier -63, Procedure Performed on Infants less than 4 kg, may not be appended to the codes on this list. Modifier -63 should be appended whenever a procedure is performed on any infant that weighs less than 4 kg, except for those procedure codes listed in this appendix. This is because certain procedures within the CPT code book are designated as being performed on infants or neonates, and as such already identify the increased complexity of the procedure performed without the need for modifier -63. Note that this list is similar to the two previous appendices, and does not include any code descriptions; code descriptions are included within the Tabular List.

Appendix J: Electrodiagnostic Medicine Listing of Sensory, Motor, and Mixed Nerves

This appendix lists nerves that apply to electrodiagnostic services, such as nerve conduction tests, electromyography, and neuromuscular junction testing. These procedures are reported with codes 95907 through 95913, and Appendix J is included within the CPT code book to enhance the appropriate reporting of these codes. It also includes a table that helps in code identification and number of units when more than one study is performed, or if more than one area is involved in the study.

Appendix K: Product Pending FDA Approval

Appendix K lists products that are currently pending FDA approval. These codes identify vaccine toxoids and are updated every year.

Appendix L: Vascular Families

Appendix L displays a diagram of the branches of vascular families, assuming that the starting point of catheterization is the aorta. This is a useful diagram to help coders assign codes according to first, second, third, or beyond third order of vascular branch, and is useful in coding catheterizations.

Appendix M: Renumbered CPT Codes–Citations Crosswalk

This appendix is a listing of crosswalked, deleted, and renumbered codes presented with the associated coding references for the deleted codes. These codes are those that were reported previously with a different CPT code, and have now been renumbered to a different CPT code. This list helps coders identify the previous code and the replacement code (like a crosswalk linking the old code to the new code).

This appendix consists of a table with the following columns: Current Code(s), Deleted/Former Code (which was replaced by the current code), Year Code Deleted, and Citations Referencing Former Code—Applicable to Current Code(s). Note that these codes were deleted in the years 2007 to 2009, and are included here for reference purposes only (if needed), as the practice of deleting and renumbering codes is no longer being used for the CPT code set.

Appendix N: Summary of Resequenced CPT Codes

Appendix N is a listing of resequenced codes. As discussed in the next section, some CPT codes are presented out of numerical order. These codes have been resequenced (out of numerical order) so that they are listed with a more appropriate section of codes (such as the same procedure type). This appendix lists these resequenced codes here for reference. As CPT codes are updated on an annual basis, they are subject to changes in description of the procedure performed, and as such may need to be included in a more appropriate selection of codes. When the code is resequenced, it is listed out of numerical order, with a pound sign next to it. These codes are discussed more in depth later in this chapter.

Note that this appendix does not include any code descriptions; code descriptions are included within the Tabular List.

Appendix O: Multianalyte Assays with Algorithmic Analyses

Appendix O lists Multianalyte Assays with Algorithmic Analyses (MAAA) services, some of which are unique to a single clinical laboratory or manufacturer. The list presented in this appendix includes the proprietary name and clinical laboratory or manufacturer, the alphanumeric procedure code, and the code descriptor. Some, but not all, of these codes are also presented in the Category I codes in the CPT code book, and not all MAAA codes are presented in this appendix. This is due to the fact that not all MAAA codes have yet been assigned a Category I CPT code. These tests are listed with a temporary four-digit number followed by the letter M, such as 0008M, for the Prosigna Breast Cancer Assay, manufactured by NanoString Technologies.

Appendix P: Codes That May Be Used for Synchronous Telemedicine Services

Appendix P, the last appendix in the CPT code book, is a listing of CPT codes that may be used to report a synchronous **telemedicine service**. A telemedicine service is one that links healthcare organizations and patients from diverse geographic locations and transmits text and images for (medical) consultation and treatment; they are also referred to as telehealth services. These procedures must be real-time and involve electronic communication using interactive telecommunications with audio and visual capabilities. They are included in this appendix for reference. Note that the list does not include any code descriptions; code descriptions are included within the Tabular List.

Removed Appendices

As previously mentioned, the CPT code set is updated every year, effective January 1st. These updates reflect changes in clinical and medical practice and coding guidelines, and may include new codes, deleted codes, and changed codes. Included in these changes are all of the additional components that constitute CPT coding including modifiers, code descriptions, and supplementary information and guidance related to the codes. Sometimes this may result in the information in an appendix becoming invalid or obsolete, and in these rare instances an appendix may be removed entirely from the CPT code book.

There are three appendices in the CPT book that have been removed from the current edition. These are Appendix G: Summary of CPT Codes That Include Moderate (Conscious) Sedation, Appendix H: Alphabetical Clinical Topics Listing, and Appendix I: Genetic Testing Code Modifiers. Appendices G and H have been removed completely from the CPT code book, whereas the information previously presented in Appendix I is now stored on the AMA website. Because of the rapid changes to genetic tests, this information is now stored electronically on the AMA website.

Complete the following practice exercises in There's a Code for That exercises 5.1 and 5.2 to test your knowledge of CPT categories and appendices.

Category I, II, and III codes — 5.1

There's a Code for That

Examine the procedure code and identify if it is a Category I, Category II, or Category III CPT code.

1. 0213T
   a. Category I
   b. Category II
   c. Category III

(Continued on next page)

5.1

Continued

2. 55400
   a. Category I
   b. Category II
   c. Category III

3. 82776
   a. Category I
   b. Category II
   c. Category III

4. 0529F
   a. Category I
   b. Category II
   c. Category III

5. 0001F
   a. Category I
   b. Category II
   c. Category III

5.2

There's a Code for That

CPT Appendices

Identify which appendix you would use to locate the following information.

1. CPT modifiers.

   Appendix: _____

2. CPT codes exempt from modifier -63.

   Appendix: _____

3. CPT codes exempt from modifier -51.

   Appendix: _____

4. Clinical examples.

   Appendix: _____

5. Summary of CPT add-on codes.

   Appendix: _____

6. CPT telemedicine codes.

   Appendix: _____

Index

The CPT Index, located directly after the appendices, is the last section of the CPT code book. This Index functions much like the ICD-10-CM Index by listing the main terms of a procedure, then referencing the coder to a CPT code or codes. This allows coders to look up the main terms for a procedure to find the correct procedure code. Once the main term is selected, then any modifying terms and cross-references are followed until a code can be selected. A more in-depth review of how to locate a CPT code is discussed later in this chapter.

Main Terms

Main terms for a procedure are different than the main terms used to find diagnostic codes. Remember, when coding for healthcare encounters, coders must identify both the diagnostic information as well as the procedural information.

To determine the procedure(s) from the documentation, the coder should ask: *What did the doctor do?* The answer to this question should identify the verbs or actions performed by the healthcare provider, such as an examination, a surgical procedure, or other healthcare treatment. To discern the diagnoses from the documentation, the coder should ask: *Why did the doctor do it?* The answer to this question should provide the reasons why the procedure(s) performed by the healthcare provider were medically necessary. Study figure 5.3 for an example of identifying the procedure(s) and diagnoses from a documentation sample.

Figure 5.3. Identifying procedures and diagnoses

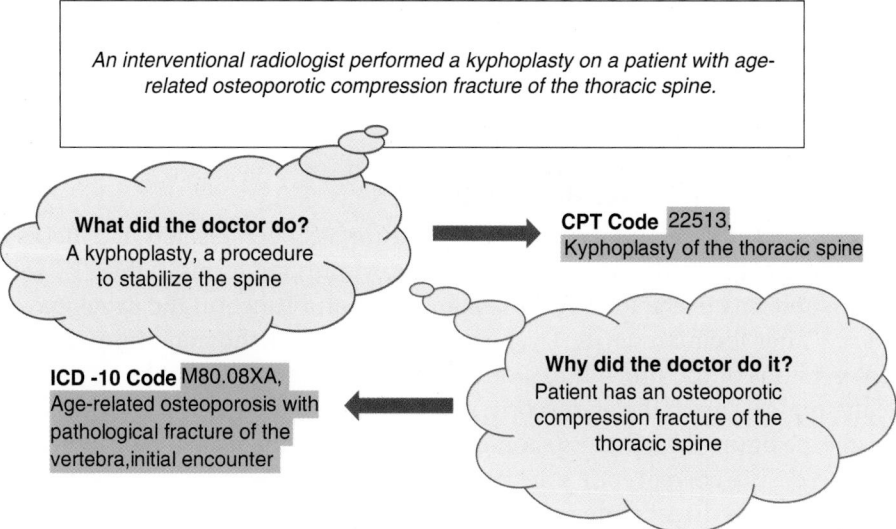

Once a coder has determined the name of the procedure, it is time to search for the main term in the CPT Index. There are four primary classes of main terms:

- *Procedure or service.* This is the action word (verb) for the procedure or service that was performed (for example, repair, excision, or endoscopy.). Chapter 11 (Surgical Services) describes these procedures in more detail.
- *Organ or anatomic site.* This is the organ or anatomic site on which the procedure was performed (for instance, femur, colon, or chest.).
- *Condition.* This is the name of the condition that was treated by the procedure (for example, abscess, Lyme disease, or spermatocele.),
- *Synonyms, eponyms, and abbreviations.* Synonyms, eponyms, and abbreviations all appear in the CPT Index as main terms. **Synonyms** are words or phrases that have the same meaning as other words or phrases. For example, *removal* and *excision* are synonyms. **Eponyms** are procedures or treatments that are named after a person. These are common in procedural coding, as procedures are

commonly named after the healthcare pioneer who invented them. An example of an eponym is *Fredet-Ramstedt procedure*, a specific type of incision into the stomach. Abbreviations are shortened versions of sometimes lengthy procedural names—for instance, EEG is the abbreviation of electroencephalography. Typically abbreviations contain a cross-reference to the full procedural name, rather than listing the CPT codes for the procedure.

Looking at figure 5.3, after asking the question: *What did the doctor do?* the coder determines that the procedure performed was a kyphoplasty, a procedure to stabilize the spine. This is the term that the coder would look up in the Index, then follow any modifying terms or cross-references, and then select a code to verify in the Tabular List.

Key to Success

If you are having trouble finding a main term in the CPT Index, try to think of as many ways as possible to look up the procedure. For example, if you cannot find the procedure name, then search for the body site or anatomic area, the type of condition being treated, and any synonyms, eponyms, or abbreviations that may apply. Sometimes the Index appears to lead you on a wild goose chase, and you may find yourself flipping back and forth through it. As you become more familiar with how procedures are listed, this process will become easier.

Modifying Terms and Cross-References

In the Index, once the main term for the procedure has been located, it is necessary to check any modifying terms and cross-references. Modifying terms in the CPT Index are much like subterms in the ICD-10-CM Main Index and function the same way. **Modifying terms** alter the main term. They are indented below the main term, and present different versions of the procedure. For example, the main term *Endoscopy* is modified by the anatomical site of the endoscopy, and then divided based on the purpose of the procedure (see figure 5.4). Coders should always review the lists of modifying terms, if available, to ensure correct code selection.

Cross-references direct coders to other main term entries that may need to be referenced. For example, in figure 5.4 the cross-reference "*See* Arthroscopy; Thoracoscopy" informs the coder that if the procedure cannot be found in the list of modifying terms that follow, then he or she should refer to the main terms *Arthroscopy* or *Thoracoscopy*.

Once the term that identifies the procedure has been located, it is necessary to refer to the code on the right-hand side of the column. Sometimes there are multiple codes listed for the procedure referenced in the Index because more than one CPT code may identify the procedure performed. Although they may represent the same procedure, each different code will include a specific detail regarding the procedure, such as the approach to the procedure, the number of elements involved in the procedure, or the exact manner in which the procedure was performed. This is yet one more reason why it is important to read code descriptions carefully. When presented with multiple code options in the Index, search for each one in the Tabular List to ensure the most appropriate code is selected.

Non-sequential codes are separated with a comma (for example, 43247, 43250, 43251), and if three or more sequential codes apply, then they are separated by a hyphen (for example, 17106 to 17108). Sometimes, several non-sequential codes apply, as well as a

Figure 5.4. Endoscopy in the CPT Index

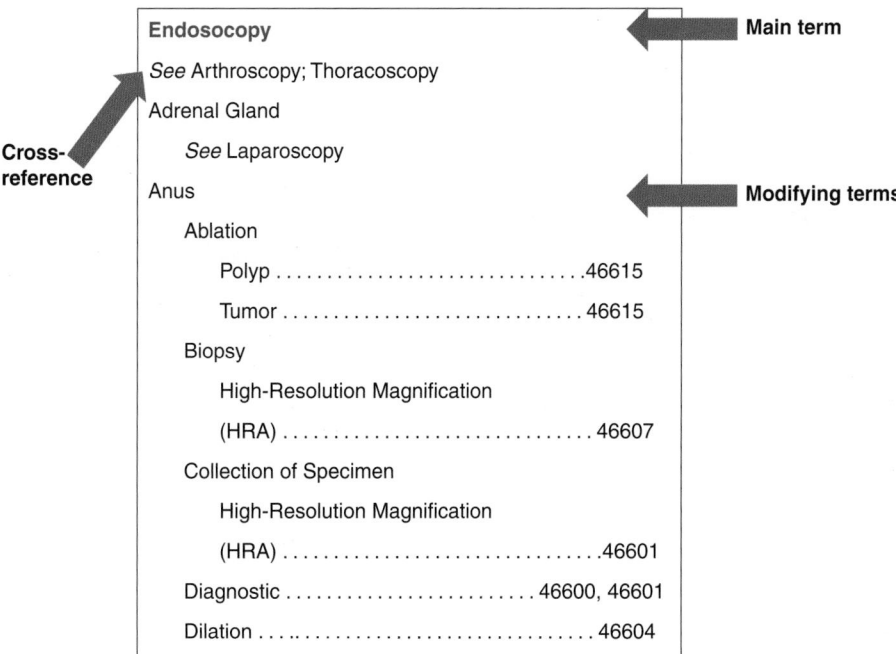

Source: AMA 2018, 876.

code range. In these cases, the codes would be separated by both commas and hyphens (for example, 36011, 36012, 36400 to 36410).

To find a procedure code in the CPT code book, coders must access the Index, locate the main term, refer to any applicable modifying terms and cross-references as necessary, and then locate the code(s) for that procedure. Once the codes are located, it is imperative to verify the codes in the Tabular List (see figure 5.5). The Tabular List of

Figure 5.5. Looking up a CPT code

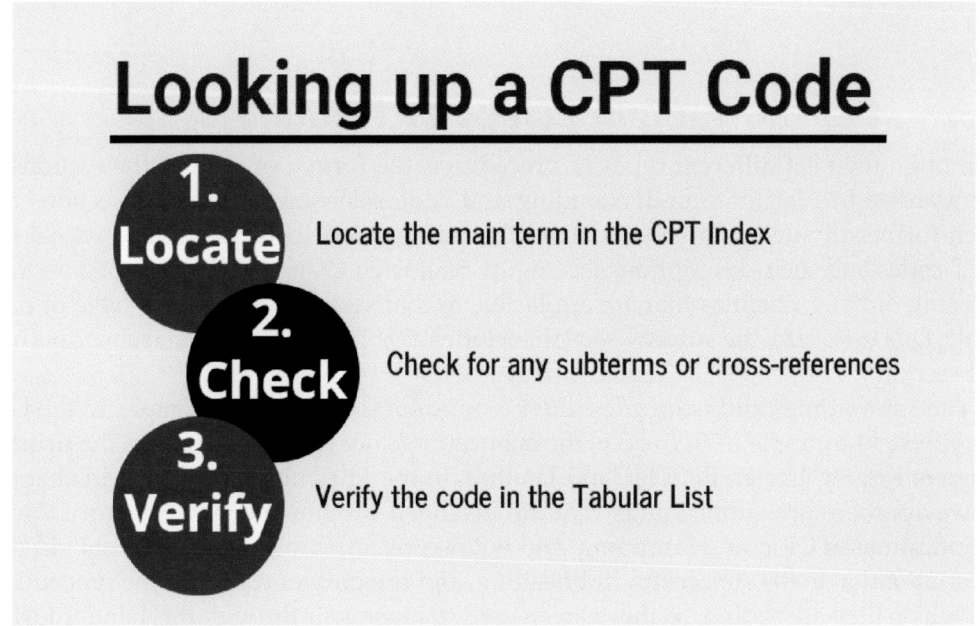

the CPT code book is the listing of Category I, II, and III codes, organized into a special format—sections, subsections, subheading, categories, and codes—for easy code identification and selection.

Complete the following practice exercises in There's a Code for That 5.3 to test your knowledge of CPT categories and appendices.

5.3

There's a Code for That

Using the CPT Index

Identify the procedural statement from the following descriptions and then look up the main term in the CPT Index and follow any cross-references and modifying terms. List the code or code ranges given by the CPT Index. The first one is already completed for you. (You do not need to verify the codes in the Tabular for this exercise, simply give the codes listed by the Index).

Example: Surgeon performed an enterotomy for the excision of a lesion.
Index entry: *44110, 44111*

1. Doctor removed 19 calculi (stones) from the gallbladder of a 35-year-old woman with cholelithiasis.

   Index entry: _____

2. Rorschach test.

   Index entry: _____

3. Salpingectomy with vaginal hysterectomy.

   Index entry: _____

4. Laparoscopic salpingectomy with vaginal hysterectomy.

   Index entry: _____

5. Surgeon amputated the gangrenous lower leg of a 75-year-old diabetic woman.

   Index entry: _____

Format of the Tabular List of CPT Codes

Although they list different types of procedures, the format of each of the sections is standardized to facilitate understanding and code selection. Category I sections are each further divided into subsections, subheadings, and then categories that list the CPT codes and their descriptions (see figure 5.6). Each Category I section begins with a listing of the guidelines that are applicable to that section, as well as a table of contents. Due to its size, the surgery section includes a table of contents for each individual subsection.

The subheadings and categories differ among subsections. For example, in the Urinary System example in figure 5.6, the subheadings are the organs within the urinary system: Kidney, Ureter, Bladder, and Urethra. In the Musculoskeletal System chapter, however, there are subheadings that are arranged around the type of procedure—Applications of Casts and Strapping, and Endoscopy/Arthroscopy. Coders should pay close attention to the subsection, subheading, and category of codes for the procedures for which they are coding, as they can be used to maneuver through the Tabular List of CPT codes to locate the correct one.

Figure 5.6. Sections, subsections, subheadings, categories, and codes

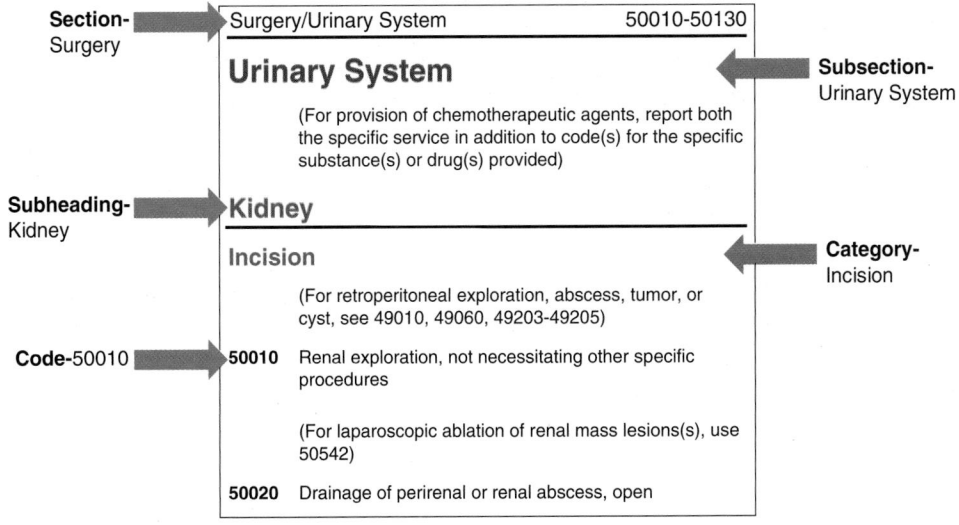

Source: AMA 2018, 339.

Key to Success

It is a good idea to locate the table of contents for each section as well as the Surgery subsections. When beginning to code from each section, review the table of contents to understand how it is divided, as well as the procedures and anatomic sites involved within it. Coders that are familiar enough with the Tabular List may find that they can locate the correct CPT codes without accessing the Index, simply by using the table of contents, subheadings, and categories within each subsection of codes.

Once the code has been identified using the Index, cross-references, and modifying terms, it must be verified in the Tabular List of CPT codes. The Tabular List contains the code descriptions, symbols, conventions, and guidelines to help coders confirm they have selected the right code, and ensure they report the code correctly. Complete the following practice exercises in There's a Code for That 5.4 to practice looking up and verifying codes in the CPT code book.

Verifying CPT codes

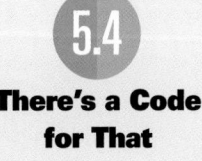

There's a Code for That

Read the procedural statement and the CPT code selected. Then verify if the CPT code selected is the correct code or not. If it is not the correct code, enter the correct code in the space provided. (The first one is done for you).

> Example: Judy selected the code 20606 for an aspiration of an ankle bursa without ultrasound guidance.
>
> Is this the correct code? *No*
>
> If not the correct code, enter it here: *20605*

1. Judy selected the code 32561 for the instillation of fibrinolytic agent for the breakup of multiloculated effusion for the third day of fibrinolytic therapy.

   Is this the correct code? _____

   If not the correct code, enter it here: _____

(Continued on next page)

5.4

Continued

2. Judy selected the code 61539 for a lobectomy of the temporal lobe with electrocorticography during the surgery.

   Is this the correct code? _____

   If not the correct code, enter it here: _____

3. Judy selected the code 33724 for the partial repair of the pulmonary vein.

   Is this the correct code? _____

   If not the correct code, enter it here: _____

4. Judy selected the code 58953 for a bilateral salpingo-oophorectomy with total omentectomy and total abdominal hysterectomy for cancer.

   Is this the correct code? _____

   If not the correct code, enter it here: _____

CPT Symbols, Conventions, and Guidelines

In the Tabular List of CPT codes there are many symbols, conventions, and guidelines that help coders navigate the codes and ensure correct code selection. Symbols are placed throughout the Tabular List, as necessary, to identify specific aspects of codes.

Symbols

Symbols are located throughout the Tabular List of the CPT code book as a visual reminder of important details that pertain to certain codes. For example, one symbol identifies codes that are exempt from modifier -51 (as discussed earlier in the chapter). This helps coders to remember that modifier -51 should not be appended to these specific codes.

Symbols are placed on the left-hand side of the code to which they apply. Not all CPT codes have applicable symbols, they only appear when necessary throughout the code listing. In the 2018 CPT code book, there are eight applicable CPT code symbols, each of which identifies a specific aspect of a particular code or codes. These symbols identify add-on codes, new and revised codes and text, modifier -51 exempt codes, codes pending FDA approval, resequenced codes, and codes that can be used to report telemedicine services.

Add-on Codes

Add-on codes are designated by the ✚ symbol. These are procedures commonly carried out in addition to the primary procedure performed. The phrases "each additional" or "(list separately in addition to primary procedure)" are generally found within the description of add-on codes to indicate they should be added onto the code for a primary procedure.

The procedures described by add-on codes include further intra-service work associated with the primary procedure (see figure 5.7). As such, add-on codes *may never be used alone*. They must always be added to the primary procedure code. Furthermore, add-on codes are exempt from modifier -51, Multiple procedures. The full list of add-on codes is included in Appendix D of the CPT code book.

Figure 5.7. Add-on code example

Source: AMA 2018, 78.

In figure 5.7, the add-on code 11201 must be appended to the code for the primary procedure, 11200. The description for code 11200 includes the removal of *up to* 15 lesions, and the add-on code identifies the removal of *each additional* 10 lesions. So, if the procedure was to remove 20 lesions, then the coder should report codes 11200 (for the first 15 lesions) and 11201 (for the additional 5 lesions), which equals 20 total lesions removed. It is permissible to report 11201 for the additional lesions because the code description is for each additional 10 lesions *or part thereof*, which means that the add-on code may be used to report the removal of less than 10 additional lesions.

Note that figure 5.7 also includes a **parenthetical note**—instructions for use of the codes, presented in parentheses throughout the Tabular List. They are intended to prevent errors and help coders report codes appropriately. These notes highlight important guidelines, like the addition of a modifier, or coding notes, such as when it may be appropriate to report codes together. They are vital in ensuring correct code selection, by helping coders certify they are reporting CPT codes correctly. For example, the parenthetical note in figure 5.7 states to use 11200 in conjunction with 11201. In this case, if the coder reports 11200 with 11201, he or she knows that is correct because the parenthetical note indicates as such.

Key to Success

Parenthetical notes are a very common component of the Tabular List, and they are easy to overlook. As you are learning coding, it may be helpful to highlight or place a star next to the parenthetical notes throughout the Tabular List, to make sure you take them into account when reporting codes throughout the CPT code book.

New and Revised Codes and Text

Each year, the CPT code book is updated to include new and revised codes and guidelines. This includes additions, deletions, and revisions of codes and guidelines. Although these are less important for beginning coders, experienced coders may find that codes used previously have been substantially altered. Therefore, the CPT code book includes three different symbols to identify new and revised codes and code guidelines or text.

New codes added to the CPT code set each year are indicated with a ● symbol to the left of the code. This symbol is to identify a completely new code that was not included in the code set the previous year.

Revised codes are identified with the ▲ symbol. These are codes that have been changed to substantially alter the procedural description. Although the code number itself has not been altered, the description of the procedure for that code has been revised. This may result in having to select a new, more appropriate code than what was used in the previous year.

New and revised text, including CPT guidelines, are identified with the symbols ▶◀ on either side of the text change. One arrow appears to the left of the text when the changes begin, and the other arrow appears to the right of the text after the change ends. In this way, the arrows append the revised or new text, making it easier for coders to identify the specific text in which changes occur or that have been added anew. The full list of additions, deletions, and revisions is included in Appendix B of the CPT code book.

Modifier -51 Exempt Codes

Some CPT codes, depending on their use and description, are modifier -51 exempt. These codes are identified with the ⊘ symbol. These codes may not be used with modifier -51 to indicate that they are multiple procedures, and have not been designated as an add-on code. For example, code 17004, Destruction (e.g., laser surgery, electrosurgery, cryosurgery, chemosurgery, surgical curettement), premalignant lesions (e.g., actinic keratoses), 15 or more lesions, is listed with the modifier -51 exempt symbol to the left of the code. This means that code 17004 may not be reported with modifier -51. The complete list of modifier -51 exempt codes is included in Appendix E of the CPT code book.

Codes Pending FDA Approval

Codes that are pending FDA approval are identified with the ⚡ symbol. This symbol is used for vaccine codes that have not been approved yet by the FDA, but are still included within the CPT code set. For example, code 90666, Influenza virus vaccine (IIV) pandemic formulation, split virus, preservative free, for intramuscular use, is still pending FDA approval but is listed within the Tabular List of the CPT code book with the lightning symbol located to the left of the code. The entire list of codes that are still pending FDA approval is included in Appendix K of the CPT code book.

Resequenced Codes

Resequenced codes are identified with the # symbol. These are codes that are not placed numerically in the Tabular List and are out of numerical sequence. The symbol is used as a navigational reference to alert coders that the code is found elsewhere. Resequencing codes allows codes to be placed within codes with related concepts and appropriate families of codes, regardless of the numerical sequencing.

Because they are out of sequence, these codes may be difficult to locate. For example, physical therapy evaluation services are reported with codes 97161 through 97164. According to the number sequence, these codes should be located after code 91750. However, since these codes have been resequenced, they are listed out of order. In these instances, the CPT book includes a statement to direct the coder where to find these codes. In this case, where code 97161 should be located, the coder will find the following: 97161, Code is out of numerical sequence. See Physical Therapy Evaluation Section. This tells the coder that the code is out of sequence and where he or she can find it. The complete list of resequenced codes is included in Appendix N of the CPT code book.

Telemedicine Codes

The ★ symbol is used to identify codes that may be reported for telemedicine services when they are appended with modifier -95. The entire list of telemedicine codes is included in Appendix P of the CPT code book.

In addition to the symbols found throughout the CPT code book, there are a few conventions and guidelines that must be discussed before diving into coding.

Conventions and Guidelines

There are a few conventions and numerous guidelines found throughout the CPT code book. The conventions are formatting and organizational practices, including the employment of standalone and indented codes. Guidelines are found in each section of the CPT code book and differ among the CPT code book sections. However, there are a few guidelines that apply to several sections across the CPT code book, and include standalone and indented codes, the time component of codes, unlisted services and special reports, and separate procedures.

Standalone and Indented Codes

To save space within the Tabular List, many codes throughout the CPT code book are indented underneath standalone codes. **Standalone codes** include the full description of the code, and do not depend on a parent code to provide more information. **Indented codes** are indented beneath a standalone code and depend on the explanation of the procedure within the standalone (or parent) code to complete the description of the indented code. Indented codes begin where the semicolon ends in the standalone code. Coders should replace the portion of the code *after* the semicolon with the description given by the indented code to complete the code description. Refer to figure 5.8 for an example of a standalone and indented code.

Figure 5.8. Standalone and indented codes

Source: AMA 2018, 77.

In figure 5.8, the standalone code is 11055, Paring or cutting of benign hyperkeratotic lesion (eg, corn or callus); single lesion. This means that code 11055 is for the cutting or paring of only *one* single lesion. Code 11056, indented below 11055, is for *2 to 4 lesions*. Because it is indented beneath the code above it, code 11056 pertains to the same procedure, *Paring or cutting of benign hyperkeratotic lesions*, but with a different number of lesions, in this case *2 to 4 lesions*. The full code description for 11056 would thus be 11056, Paring or cutting of benign hyperkeratotic lesion (e.g., corn or callus); 2 to 4 lesions. Note that the point of division between the standalone code and the indented code is the semicolon (;) in the standalone code.

There may be multiple indented codes beneath a single standalone code. As in figure 5.8, there are two indented codes: 11056 and 11057. Each one of these codes pertains to the previous parent standalone code, and they each modify the standalone code in a different way (namely, 11056 is for 2 to 4 lesions, and 11057 is for more than 4 lesions).

Time

Time is an important descriptor in many CPT codes. Some CPT codes are dependent on the amount of time taken for a procedure, from start to finish, and include that amount within the code description. Unless specific guidelines state otherwise, time is the "face-to-face" period that the healthcare professional spends directly with the patient (rather than out of the room or in his or her office working on the patient's health record or treatment). Also, unless specifically indicated in the code description, one unit of time has elapsed once the midpoint has been reached. For example, if the unit of time described within the code is for one hour, then a coder may report that unit once the halfway point has been surpassed (namely, 31 minutes). Similarly, if the unit time was two hours, then the unit could be reported at the 91-minute mark (one full hour for the first 60 minutes, and then the additional hour may be reported after the additional 31-minute mark, so 91 minutes total).

Add-on codes are frequently used with services that require concurrent procedures, or procedures that may be prolonged for a certain amount of time. If add-on codes are present, then the standalone code should be reported first and add-on codes reported according to the number of units necessary to report the full service. See figure 5.9 for an example of a time descriptor in a code, and an add-on time code.

Figure 5.9. Coding for time with standalone and add-on codes

Stand alone code: first 31 to 60 minutes

96360 Intravenous infusion, hydration; initial, 31 minutes to 1 hour

+ **96361** each additional hour (List separately in addition to code for primary procedure)

Add-on code: each additional 60 minutes

Source: AMA 2018, 678.

In figure 5.9, the first code, 96360, is for 31 to 60 minutes, and the second code, 96361, is for each additional 60 minutes. So if the intravenous infusion was performed for three hours, the appropriate codes would be 96360 (for the first hour) and then 96361 X 2 for the next two hours, equaling three hours total. Notice that the second code would be reported twice to identify two extra hours of the service performed. It is common to report certain procedures more than once. If this is the case, coders can report the services separately (that is, 96360, 96361, 96361), or by changing the number of units (that is, 96360, 96361 X 2).

Unlisted Services and Special Reports

As previously described in this chapter, there may be some services or procedures that are not found in the CPT code set. In these rare instances, a healthcare provider can report the service using an unlisted services procedure code. When an unlisted procedure code is used, the specific service should be described using a special report. A **special report** is included with the reporting of an unlisted procedure or other procedure that is rarely provided, unusual, variable, or new. Special reports should include the following:

- A complete description of the procedure, including the nature of the procedure
- Extent of the procedure performed
- Need for the procedure (that is, the medical necessity for the procedure)
- Amount of time spent on the procedure
- Effort needed to complete the procedure
- Equipment necessary to provide the service

Additional guidelines regarding special reports are found in the guidelines at the beginning of each section or subsection within the Tabular List of the CPT.

Separate Procedures

Some of the procedures or services listed throughout the CPT code book are often carried out as integral components of other procedures or services. These are designated as a **separate procedure**—a procedure that is commonly part of another, more complex procedure, but which may be performed independently or be otherwise unrelated to the procedure—within the Tabular List. Separate procedures codes should not be reported in addition to the code for the primary procedure or service of which it is considered an integral component. For example, code 20100 is designated as a separate procedure: 20100, Exploration of penetrating wound (separate procedure); neck. This means that code 20100 should *not* be reported if is it included as part of a more definitive service, such as repair to major internal structure(s) or blood vessel(s). Consider the following example.

A patient presented to the Emergency Department with a penetrating stab wound to the upper right thigh. The doctor on call explored the stab wound, including dissection, to determine that it was approximately 1.5 cm deep, noting that there was no damage to any major structures or blood vessels.

In this example, the only procedure performed was the exploration of the wound itself, without a repair done to any major structures or blood vessels. In this case, the doctor would report code 20103, Exploration of penetrating wound (separate procedure); extremity. If the doctor performed a more extensive procedure, then the code reported would be for the more extensive, primary procedure.

A patient presented to the Emergency Department with a penetrating stab wound to the abdomen. Upon exploration, the doctor on call discovered a small laceration of the liver, which he repaired using a simple suture.

In this example, the doctor did more than simply explore the wound. Upon exploration, it was determined that a more definitive procedure had to be performed (namely, a suture of the liver wound). In this case, a code for the exploration of the wound would not be reported. Rather, the coder would report the code for the definitive procedure: 47350, Management of liver hemorrhage; simple suture of liver wound or injury.

The only time that a separate procedure code should be reported is if that was the *only* procedure performed on that body site, and not part of a larger, more definitive procedure. However, a separate procedure may be reported if it was distinct from the other procedures performed at the same encounter. Combine the two previous examples:

A patient presents to the ED with a penetrating stab wound to the upper thigh as well as the abdomen. The doctor explores the thigh wound without any additional procedures, and then explores the abdomen wound, discovering and repairing a liver wound.

In this example, two codes would be reported; one for the exploration of the upper thigh wound (20103), and another for the repair of the liver (47350). The separate procedure code 20103 should be appended with modifier -59 to identify that it is a distinct procedural service.

Separate procedures have a special relationship with modifier -59. Modifier -59, Distinct procedural service, is used to identify when one procedure is considered separate from another procedure. Because coding is complex, and healthcare procedures are performed on all sites of the body, modifier -59 helps to identify when codes that would otherwise be included in other procedures (like separate procedures) are correctly reported in addition to codes for more definitive procedures. The use of modifier -59 may result in payment of a service that would otherwise be bundled into the payment for another procedure. Modifier -59 is to be used only as a last resort, when no other modifiers better identify the circumstance; this is because it is ambiguous in nature and can lead to coding errors or abuse. Therefore, CMS developed four different modifiers that can be used in lieu of modifier -59. Check payer guidelines before using these modifiers, as they may not be accepted by all payers. They are the following:

- Modifier -XE, Separate encounter, a service that is distinct because it occurred during a separate encounter
- Modifier -XP, Separate practitioner, a service that is distinct because it was performed by a different practitioner
- Modifier -XS, Separate structure, a service that is distinct because it was performed on a separate organ or structure
- Modifier -XU, Unusual non-overlapping service, the use of a service that is distinct because it does not overlap usual components of the main service

In addition to CPT codes, there is one remaining code set to discuss before beginning coding in the outpatient setting. Although not used as frequently as CPT codes, HCPCS codes are an important part of coding that allow coders to report supplies and services provided to patients in the healthcare setting, as well as to report services provided to Medicare patients. The last sections of this chapter discuss the structure, purpose, and format of HCPCS codes and the HCPCS code book.

HCPCS Code Structure

HCPCS codes and CPT codes are alike in that they are five-character codes that report services and procedures provided to patients. However, the code structure of HCPCS codes begin with a letter, rather than a number. For example, A7007, Large volume nebulizer, disposable, unfilled, used with aerosol compressor, or K0001, Standard wheelchair. Each HCPCS code begins with a letter, and similar categories of services and supplies are typically grouped together by specific letters (although this is not always the case). For example, all ambulance services begin with the letter A, and most drugs administered in the healthcare setting begin with the letter J. The letters that HCPCS codes begin with do not usually correspond to the type of service that the HCPCS code represents. For example, the administration of influenza vaccine is reported with G0008, Administration of influenza virus vaccine. A complete listing of HCPCS code categories is listed later in this chapter.

HCPCS codes are used to report supplies and services to patients in the outpatient setting. However, because the HCPCS Level II code set is created and maintained by CMS, which manages the Medicare health plan, HCPCS codes may be required to report specific services provided to Medicare patients only, such as screenings and vaccinations. The same services provided to non-Medicare patients would be reported with the appropriate CPT codes. Thus, when coding claims for reimbursement purposes, it is important to have the patient's insurance type in mind, as the billing and coding requirements will differ depending on the patient's type of insurance (for a reminder of insurance basics, review chapter 2).

The majority of HCPCS codes are used to report supplies provided to patients in the healthcare setting. When coding for healthcare encounters, this means that there is one more question that a coder should ask to ensure that he or she is coding for the encounter completely: *What supply did the doctor use to perform the procedure?* Therefore, the three questions coders should ask themselves are the following:

What did the doctor do? = Procedure code (CPT)
Why did the doctor do it? = Diagnosis code (ICD-10-CM)
What supply did the doctor use to do it? = Supply code (HCPCS)

Read the following vignette to see how asking these three questions may result in the addition of a HCPCS code.

Rudy is selecting the codes for an encounter for an IUD (intrauterine device) insertion. The patient came in for reproductive management and insertion of an IUD. She is in a monogamous relationship with her husband of five years and has two children. Her second child has just turned 6 weeks old and she has decided that she would like to get an IUD for contraception. After a brief physical examination and evaluation, the doctor decides that the IUD is appropriate for this patient and inserts the IUD into the patient's uterus. She schedules an appointment in six weeks to ensure appropriate placement of the device.

Rudy is ready to code the encounter and asks herself the first question: What did the doctor do? In this case, the doctor performed a brief evaluation and management service and then inserted the IUD into the patient's uterus. These are her procedure codes, which she will look up in the CPT code book. She then asks herself the second question: Why did the doctor do it? In this case, the doctor performed the IUD insertion for contraceptive management, as requested by the patient. It is important to note that this is not a problem-oriented visit, so the reason for the encounter is not a problem, but rather an encounter for reproductive health services. Rudy will search encounter for contraceptive management in the ICD-10-CM code book.

Now that Rudy has her first two questions answered, she must ask the third question: What supply did the doctor use to do it? In this case, the doctor supplied the patient with the actual intrauterine device, when she placed the device in the patient's uterus. Rudy will look up the intrauterine device in the HCPCS code book.

Rudy now has three types of codes to find: CPT codes for the evaluation and management and insertion of the IUD device; ICD-10-CM code for contraceptive management and insertion of IUD device; and the HCPCS code for the actual intrauterine device.

This third question may be a little bit tricky, as it refers not to the equipment or items used to treat the patient, but to any non-disposable supplies provided to the patient in the healthcare setting. In this case, the patient was given an IUD, which she will take home with her.

Key to Success

Any disposable supplies provided at the time of service—like gauze, sterile gloves, or lubricating jelly—are not coded with HCPCS codes. These expendable items are paid for by the healthcare office or facility as part of the clinical overhead expense.

As discussed in chapter 3, HCPCS code books differ depending on the book's publisher, so learning HCPCS coding relies on locating the Index and Tabular List. The coder must also follow the same process as CPT coding—locating the main term for the service or supply in the Index, checking subterms and cross-references, and then verifying the code in the Tabular List. These components are discussed in more detail in the last section of this chapter.

The HCPCS Code Book

The style, format, organization, and content of the HCPCS code book depends on the publisher of the book. However, the codes themselves are the same, no matter which organization has published the book. Because of this, it is necessary to discuss the sections of the HCPCS manual in general terms, as they may be organized in a different order. The main sections of the HCPCS code book include the Index, the Table of Drugs, list of Modifiers, Tabular List of HCPCS Level II codes, and Appendices.

Key to Success

Because HCPCS code books vary, it is a good idea to flip through your book to locate the sections discussed as follows. Although the HCPCS code book is much smaller than either of the ICD-10-CM or the CPT code books, placing tabs throughout this book for easy reference of important sections and commonly used codes is still recommended. A list of suggested tab placements is included in your student workbook.

HCPCS Index

The first section of the HCPCS code book is the Index. This index functions exactly like the indices included in the CPT and ICD-10-CM code books, with a main term listed and available subterms listed underneath the main term. Coders should reference the item, supply, or service they are looking to code in the Index first, which will refer them to a code or range of codes. Coders must then turn to the Tabular List of HCPCS codes to select the appropriate code for the supply provided or the service performed.

Looking up supplies and services in the HCPCS Index is a bit different than using the CPT or ICD-10-CM Index. Rather than searching for the condition or reason for an encounter (as in ICD-10-CM coding), or searching for a service or procedure that was performed on the patient (as in CPT coding), looking for a HCPCS code in the Index usually requires searching for the item that was supplied to the patient. When coding for a supply item, it is necessary to look up the noun or name of the item. For example, for an IUD the coder would look up *intrauterine device* or *intrauterine copper contraceptive*. Use the following when searching for codes in the HCPCS Index:

- Name of the service, test, therapy, or procedure
- Name of the item, prosthetic, orthotic, or equipment supplied
- Name of the drug or medication administered

The entries in the HCPCS code book will differ depending on the publisher of the book. Although CMS does publish an Index to each year's current HCPCS code set, individual publishers are able to rearrange, remove, and add to the Index according to how they believe the information is best presented. Thus, it may be necessary to look up items in a completely different manner than in another book. In one book it may be necessary to search for an augmentative speech generating device under *device, speech generating*, which will lead the coder to E2500, whereas in another book it may be necessary to search for the same device under *Speech generating device*, which leads the coder to the code range E2500 to E2599. Both entries lead to the same area of codes in the Tabular List, even though they were found by searching for different terms.

Key to Success

It is imperative to remain flexible when searching for any term in the Index to a coding book. As the previous example shows, you may have to search for the same supply (or condition in ICD-10-CM coding, or procedure in CPT coding) in different ways. Ultimately, it is the code selection that counts. If you find that you have searched the term in multiple ways, and it still leads to the same codes, you can be certain that you have found the right codes.

If a coder is searching for the code for a drug or medicinal substance administered in the healthcare setting—such as an antibiotic shot administered at a doctor's visit—it is necessary to search for the drug in the Table of Drugs (discussed in the next section) rather than in the Index.

Complete the following practice exercises in There's a Code for That 5.5, to practice looking up codes in the HCPCS Index.

Using the HCPCS Index

5.5

There's a Code for That

Identify the HCPCS supply or service from the following descriptions, then look up the main term in the HCPCS Index and follow any cross-references or modifying terms. List the code or code ranges given by the HCPCS Index. The first one is completed for you. (You do not need to verify the codes in the Tabular for this exercise, simply give the codes listed by the Index).

Example: Pathology of blood platelets via pheresis leukocytes reduced and irradiated.
Index entry: *P9037*

1. Body mass index (BMI).

   Index entry: _____

2. Pneumococcal vaccine administration.

   Index entry: _____

3. Dialysis supplies.

   Index entry: _____

(Continued on next page)

5.5

Continued

4. Digital hearing aid.

Index entry: _____

5. Dystrophic nail trimming.

Index entry: _____

6. Replacement microprocessor control unit for pneumatic ventricular assist device.

Index entry: _____

Table of Drugs

The Table of Drugs in the HCPCS code book is a reference tool that helps coders find the appropriate HCPCS code for drugs and medications administered in the healthcare setting. It is organized by the name of the drug or medicinal substance, dosage or unit amount given, and method of administration of the drug. The Table of Drugs is discussed in greater detail in chapter 6 (Supplies and Services).

The entries in the Table of Drugs will differ depending on the publisher of the HCPCS code book. Some tables may list drugs by their generic names, whereas others might list drugs by both generic and brand names. When coding for drugs using the Table of Drugs, it may be beneficial to refer to a Physician's Desk Reference (PDR) to help identify specific drugs and the correct routes of administration and unit dosage amounts.

HCPCS Modifiers

HCPCS modifiers are listed in a separate section from HCPCS codes. Modifiers are an important part of coding, so it is important to locate the list of modifiers in the code book table of contents for reference when coding. HCPCS modifiers may be used with either CPT or HCPCS codes, and a small selection of HCPCS modifiers are also found in Appendix A of the CPT code book. These are the most commonly used HCPCS modifiers and are included in the CPT manual for easy reference.

Tabular List of HCPCS Level II Codes

The largest section of the HCPCS code book is the Tabular List of HCPCS Level II codes. HCPCS codes range from A0021 to V5364, and are divided into multiple subsections that include

- Transport Services Including Ambulance (A0000 to A0999)

- Medical and Surgical Supplies (A4000 to A9999)

- Enteral and Parenteral Therapy (B4000 to B9999)

- CMS Outpatient Payment System (C1000 to C9999)

- Dental Procedures (D0120 to D9999)

- Durable Medical Equipment (E0100 to E8002)

- Temporary Procedures/Professional Services (G0008 to G9862)

- Behavioral Health and/or Substance Abuse Treatment Services (H0001 to H2037)

- Drugs Administered in the Medical Setting (J0100 to J8999)

- Temporary Codes Established by Different Payers (K0000 to K9999), (Q0000 to Q9999), (S0012 to S9999), (T1000 to T9999)

- Orthotics and Prosthetics (L0112 to L9900)

- Other Medical Services (M0075 to M0301)

- Laboratory Services (P0000 to P9999)

- Vision and Hearing Services (V2020 to V5364)

Coders should familiarize themselves with these sections of their HCPCS code books to help understand the services and supplies coded with this code set.

Each of the major sections includes a heading with a code range, subheadings when necessary, followed by the listing of the HCPCS codes with code descriptions, symbols, and billing notes (see figure 5.10).

Figure 5.10. HCPCS headings, subheadings, and codes

Source: AHIMA 2018, 187.

Not all headings will have subheadings, and not all codes will have symbols and billing notes. These are added throughout the Tabular List of codes on an as-needed basis. Unlike the CPT code book, the HCPCS code book does not have official guidelines listed before each major section, nor does it have guidelines in the Tabular List. Any special billing considerations, instructions, or advice is listed in the billing notes underneath the code description. Symbols also often refer to billing and coverage guidelines. It is important to note that HCPCS codes are highly variable when it comes to payment. In other words, some health carriers will pay for certain codes, while others do not. It is important to verify coverage of HCPCS services and supplies before providing them to patients.

Appendices

The last section of the HCPCS code book is the Appendices. Typically, HCPCS code books have at least one appendix at the end of the book. Sometimes, the Table of Drugs and modifiers are listed in separate appendices, along with lengthy references to Medicare billing guidelines. Other times, the appendicular information at the end of the book are references to HCPCS, billing, or coding guidelines. As always, it is important to be familiar with all sections of the HCPCS code book to be as effective and efficient as possible.

Complete the following practice exercises in There's a Code for That 5.6, to practice looking up and verifying codes in the HCPCS code book.

5.6

There's a Code for That

Verifying HCPCS codes

Read the statement for the HCPCS code selected. Then verify if the HCPCS code selected is the correct code or not. If it is not the correct code, then enter the correct code in the space provided.

1. Judy selected the code E1610 for deionizer water purification system for hemodialysis.

   Is this the correct code? _____

   If not the correct code, enter it here: _____

2. Judy selected the code L3350 for a heel wedge.

   Is this the correct code? _____

   If not the correct code, enter it here: _____

3. Judy selected the code V2500 X 2 for two PMMA spherical contact lenses.

   Is this the correct code? _____

   If not the correct code, enter it here: _____

4. Judy selected the code J3480 for the injection of potassium hydroxide preparation.

   Is this the correct code? _____

   If not the correct code, enter it here: _____

5. Judy selected the code K0006 for an extra heavy-duty wheelchair.

   Is this the correct code? _____

   If not the correct code, enter it here: _____

End of Chapter Content

Instructions: Match the symbols with the appropriate descriptions.

CPT Symbol	Meaning
1. _____ ▶◀	A. Add-on code
2. _____ ✚	B. Modifier -51 exempt
3. _____ ▲	C. Telemedicine code
4. _____ �	D. New code
5. _____ ★	E. New or revised text
6. _____ ●	F. Revised code
7. _____ ⊘	G. Resequenced code
8. _____ #	H. FDA approval pending

Instructions: Choose the best answer.

1. The CPT code answers which of the following questions?
   a. Why did the patient come in?
   b. What did the doctor do?
   c. Why did the doctor do it?
   d. What supply did the doctor use to do it?

2. The ICD-10-CM answers which of the following questions?
   a. Why did the patient come in?
   b. What did the doctor do?
   c. Why did the doctor do it?
   d. What supply did the doctor use to do it?

3. The HCPCS code answers which of the following questions?
   a. Why did the patient come in?
   b. What did the doctor do?
   c. Why did the doctor do it?
   d. What supply did the doctor use to do it?

4. Which of the following types of CPT codes is used for performance measures tracking?
   a. Category I
   b. Category II
   c. Category III
   d. Category IV

5. Which of the following types of CPT codes is composed of all numbers?
   a. Category I
   b. Category II
   c. Category III
   d. Category IV

6. How many sections of Category I codes are there?
   a. 8
   b. 6
   c. 9
   d. 3

7. Which of the following types of CPT codes ends with the letter T?
   a. Category I
   b. Category II
   c. Category III
   d. No CPT codes end with the letter T

8. If a procedure is not found in either Category I or Category III codes, how do you report the service?
   a. By using a Category II code
   b. By using an unlisted procedures code
   c. By sending a special report
   d. Do not report the service if a code does not exist

9. Which CPT appendix would you use to help identify the branches of a vascular family?
   a. Appendix K
   b. Appendix P
   c. Appendix B
   d. Appendix L

10. Which of the following types of CPT codes is indented beneath a parent code, on which it depends for the full code description?
    a. Standalone code
    b. Indented code
    c. Modifier -51 code
    d. Modifying code

11. What type of codes are used to report supplies provided to patients in the healthcare setting?
    a. CPT
    b. ICD-10
    c. Add-on codes
    d. HCPCS

12. Which of the following would be reported with a HCPCS code?
    a. Chief complaint of cough and runny nose
    b. Kyphoplasty procedure
    c. Fitting of a diaphragm
    d. Diaphragm provided to the patient

13. In which of the following ways would you search for a main term in the HCPCS Index?
    a. Name of the condition
    b. Name of the surgical procedure
    c. Name of the item or equipment supplied
    d. Name of the reason for the encounter

14. Which of the following codes is a HCPCS Level II code?
    a. 0012F
    b. 59050
    c. G0466
    d. 0042T

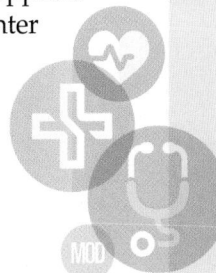

15. Find the modifiers section in the HCPCS code book. Which of the following is the modifier for Registered Dietitian?

    a. RT
    b. RD
    c. AE
    d. BA

Instructions: Answer the following questions with the appropriate code.

1. Complex repair of the scalp, 10 cm.

   CPT code(s): _____, _____

2. Debridement of eczematous skin, 20 percent of body surface.

   CPT code(s): _____, _____

3. Escharotomy, two separate incisions.

   CPT code(s): _____, _____

4. Appendectomy for ruptured appendix with generalized peritonitis, with intraoperative colonic lavage.

   CPT code(s): _____, _____

5. Hospital discharge, 30 minutes total.

   CPT code(s): _____

6. Unlisted procedure of the small intestine.

   CPT code(s): _____

7. Unlisted vascular surgical procedure.

   CPT code(s): _____

8. Barium enema colorectal cancer screening.

   HCPCS code(s): _____

9. Insertion of intrauterine device (code for the insertion and the provision of the IUD).

   CPT code(s): _____

   HCPCS code(s): _____

10. Two articulating, spring assisted underarm crutches.

    HCPCS code(s): _____

References

American Health Information Management Association. 2018. *2017 HCPCS LEVEL II, Professional Edition*. St. Louis, MO: Elsevier.

American Medical Association. 2018. *Current Procedural Terminology: 2018 Professional Edition*. Chicago: AMA.

Resources

Centers for Medicare and Medicaid Services. 2017. 2017 HCPCS Alpha-Numeric Index. https://www.cms .gov/Medicare/Coding/HCPCSReleaseCodeSets /Downloads/2017-Alpha-Numeric-Index.pdf.

Part II

Coding
In the Real World

6

CHAPTER

Supplies and Services

Learning Objectives

- Understand the basics of billing and coding; analyze and assign procedural and diagnosis codes to ambulance services.
- Understand the basics of billing and coding; analyze and assign procedural and diagnosis codes to durable medical equipment and supplies.

- Analyze the HCPCS Table of Drugs and assign HCPCS codes used to report medications given in the healthcare setting.

Key Terms

Advanced life support (ALS)
Ambulance modifier
Ambulance supplier
Basic life support (BLS)
Certificate of Medical Necessity (CMN)
Destination
Durable medical equipment (DME)

Durable medical equipment, prosthetics, orthotics, and supplies (DMEPOS)
Emergency transportation
Nonemergency transportation
Non-ambulatory
Origin
Orthotics

Physician's Desk Reference (PDR)
Prosthetics
Route of administration
Supplies
Services
Transportation indicator

In addition to medical and surgical procedures, patients commonly receive a number of miscellaneous supplies and services during healthcare encounters. Supplies are items provided to the patient in the healthcare setting, typically designed for long-term or multiple uses. Items that are used to treat the patient or help perform the procedure may also be reported with HCPCS codes. This includes medical equipment for home use (such as a pair of crutches), supplies used in patient care during an admission such as parenteral nutrition, and medications given to the patient during the encounter, such as an antibiotic injection. Services identified by HCPCS codes are miscellaneous services that may be provided to patients in the healthcare setting. Some of these services are also identified by CPT codes, such as certain vaccinations; whereas other services are only identified by codes found in the HCPCS code book, such as ambulance transportation services.

These supplies and services are coded using HCPCS Level II codes, discussed in chapter 5. While most of these codes are billed by ambulance service or durable medical equipment suppliers (both defined in the following section), some HCPCS codes (namely those for Medicare-covered services and for drugs or medications administered in the office) are commonly billed in the outpatient setting.

This chapter discusses HCPCS Level II coding within the context of a durable medical equipment office and ambulance supplier, HCPCS codes used for Medicare services in the outpatient setting, and HCPCS codes that are used to bill for drugs and medicinal substances administered in the healthcare setting.

Ambulance and Durable Medical Equipment Services

Durable medical equipment and ambulance suppliers provide a special set of healthcare services. Rather than directly providing services to a patient, such as a surgery or physical examination, durable medical equipment suppliers simply provide supplies that the patient needs in order to maintain or treat his or her health condition. Ambulance suppliers, on the other hand, are tasked with transporting a patient with a healthcare need to a provider or facility capable of treating that need. This is usually done in an emergency or urgent situation, and the emergency responders must stabilize and provide a certain level of healthcare services to the patient until he or she can receive care from a healthcare provider. Transportation is also often required in nonemergent situations, in which a patient is transported from one healthcare appointment or facility to another in order to receive a particular service not offered at the current location, such as a CT or MRI scan.

The codes used to bill for both of these services are located in the HCPCS Level II code book and are a good place to start when learning how to identify and report codes. While medical and surgical procedures may require more close attention to code description and detail, and have multiple guidelines for appropriate code selection (such as ICD-10-CM coding), HCPCS coding is a bit more simplistic. The following sections will discuss HCPCS and ICD-10-CM coding within the context of an ambulance supplier and durable medical equipment supplier's office.

Billing and coding for ambulance services requires a solid understanding of the types and uses of codes, especially HCPCS codes. All ambulance and transportation services are identified by a small selection of HCPCS codes.

Ambulance Coding Basics

There are differences between ambulance services, which are identified by HCPCS codes. The first difference is between basic life support and advanced life support services. Basic life support (BLS) is a primary level of care used for patients with life-threatening illnesses, injuries, or other severe conditions while they are transported to a facility that can provide them with complete medical care. BLS services focus on adequate blood circulation and a clear airway through the ABC's of BLS: **A**irway (protecting a clear passageway for oxygen), **B**reathing (inflating and deflation of the lungs), and **C**irculation (providing adequate blood supply). **Advanced life support** (ALS) is a higher level of care that includes life-saving protocols to further support airway, breathing, and circulation. ALS services can include manual defibrillation to restart the heart, endotracheal intubation to create an airway, placing a central venous line for venous access, or creating a surgical airway, such as a tracheotomy (opening in the trachea to establish an airway).

The next main difference in ambulance services is between emergency and nonemergency transport. Once the ambulance provider is called, **emergency transportation** responds immediately to the scene of the accident or incident to provide medical assistance and transport to a healthcare facility if necessary. For example, if an ambulance is called to respond to a car accident in which people have been injured, then that ambulance arrives as soon as possible to provide healthcare to any injured patients and then transport them to a healthcare facility for further medical care if necessary. Transportation is most commonly provided with a ground transportation vehicle, although in certain emergency situations a helicopter may be used to provide faster transport to a healthcare facility. On the other hand, **nonemergency transportation** is generally scheduled in advance and used for patient transfers from one facility to another, or to transport **non-ambulatory** patients for healthcare. Non-ambulatory means unable to walk about, so non-ambulatory patients are those that are unable to move around independently, such as a patient confined to a bed. For example, non-ambulatory patients may require transportation for activities of daily living, or transportation to and from healthcare facilities. Patient transfers are commonly performed in a nonemergency setting to transport a patient to a healthcare facility that provides more specialized healthcare.

Finally, the last major difference in ambulance services is the type of transportation—air and ground. Air ambulance services are provided by either a fixed wing (airplane) or rotary wing (helicopter) vehicle. Ground transportation vehicles are vary more and include taxi, wheelchair van, and typical on-ground ambulance carrier. If an HCPCS code does not specify that transportation is provided by either a fixed or rotary wing aircraft (air service), then the code can be used for ground transportation.

There are several additional details needed on ambulance claims, including ambulance origin and destination modifiers, transportation indicators, mileage for both ground and air transportation, and any other services or supplies that were provided to the patient during the transportation service (see figure 6.1).

Ambulance modifiers are required on ambulance claims to identify the origin and destination for each transportation. The **origin** of a transportation service is where the patient was picked up, and the **destination** is where the patient was taken. For example, the patient was taken from the scene of an accident to a hospital. In this case, the origin would be the scene of the accident, and the destination would be the hospital. Ambulance modifiers are created by combining two letters that are listed in the HCPCS code book located before the selection of ambulance codes (before A0000 to A0999). These letters are also listed in figure 6.1 for reference. The letter that corresponds to the origin is listed first, and the letter that corresponds to the destination is listed last, to build a two-letter modifier. For example, if the origin was the scene of an accident (S, Scene of accident or acute event), and the destination was a hospital (H, Hospital), then the modifier would be SH, Scene of accident or acute event to Hospital. This modifier would be appended to the end of the HCPCS code, just as in CPT coding. For example, a ground ambulance transport from the scene of an accident to a hospital would be

Figure 6.1. Ambulance billing details

 # Origin and Destination Modifiers

D = Diagnostic or therapeutic site
E = Residential, domiciliary, custodial facility
G = Hospital based ESRD facility
H = Hospital
I = Site of transfer between modes of transport
J = Freestanding ESRD facility

N = Skilled nursing facility
P = Physician's office
R = Residence
S = Scene of accident or acute event
X = Intermediate stop at physician's office on way to hospital

Transportation Indicators

Air and Ground

C1, C2, C3, C4

Ground only

C5, C6, C7

Air only

D1, D2, D3, D4

Ground transport, 20 miles

A0425 × 20

Mileage

A0425 Ground mileage, per statute mile
A0435 Fixed wing air mileage, per statute mile
A0436 Rotary wing air mileage, per statute mile

coded as such: A0429-SH, Ambulance services, basic life support, emergency transport (BLS-Emergency), Scene of accident or acute event to Hospital.

In addition to the ICD-10 diagnosis and HCPCS ambulance codes, a **transportation indicator**—a two-character code—is used to identify why the transportation service was medically necessary. These indicators provide more information regarding the circumstances as to why a patient was transported in that particular way. Transportation indicators are not usually listed in the HCPCS manual, and may or may not be necessary, depending on the patient's insurance carrier guidelines. The 11 indicators are as follows.

C1 = Transport from low-level facility to higher-level facility
C2 = Transport from one facility to another due to unavailability of service at origin facility
C3 = Response to a major incident or mechanism of injury
C4 = Excessive number of miles driven
C5 = BLS level service provided to an ALS level patient
C6 = ALS level ambulance provided for a BLS level patient
C7 = Intravenous medications required during transport
D1 = Patient condition requires long distance transport
D2 = Traffic patterns necessitating air transport
D3 = Time to get to the patient precludes ground ambulance
D4 = Pick up point not accessible by ground

For example, if a patient was stranded in a desert canyon inaccessible by vehicles and suffered a healthcare emergency, then transportation indicator D4, Pick up point not accessible by ground, would be used to identify why rotary wing (helicopter) ambulance transportation was provided. Transportation indicators C1 through C4 are used for either air or ground transportation. C5 through C7 are used for ground transportation only, and D1 through D4 are used for air transportation only.

Transportation indicators are placed in box 19 on the CMS-1500 claim form (see figure 6.2).

For each transportation service provided, the service provided should be coded with the appropriate HCPCS transportation code, and the number of miles indicated as the number of units for the service. This is done by entering the HCPCS code(s) for the transportation services in box 24.A on the CMS-1500 claim form, with the appropriate number of units identified in box 24.G. For example, if the ambulance service was 20 miles of ground transport, then the HCPCS code A0425 would be entered in box 24.A, with the number of miles identified in box 24.G (see figure 6.3). When multiple units of any HCPCS or CPT code need to be reported on a claim for services, the CPT or HCPCS code is listed, followed by the multiplication symbol (×), and then the number of units. For example, 20 miles of ground transport would be listed as A0425 × 20—A0425 identifies the ground transport and 20 identifies the number of units, in this case miles traveled (refer to figure 6.3).

Additional supplies and services are also coded for ambulance services. HCPCS codes for these supplies include oxygen and oxygen supplies, routine disposable provisions, and esophageal intubation materials.

Figure 6.2. Transportation indicators listed in box 19

Source: CMS 2017a.

Figure 6.3. Entering HCPCS codes on CMS-1500 form

Source: CMS 2017a.

Key to Success

The selection of HCPCS codes for ambulance services is relatively small, and the more familiar you become with ambulance codes in the A0021 to A0999 range, the easier it will be to ensure that you code all ambulance services correctly.

Diagnosis Coding for Ambulance Services

Emergency personnel on board the ambulance cannot diagnose a patient's condition, but this does not mean that they can send a claim for the healthcare services without a diagnosis code. Remember, as discussed in chapter 3, the diagnosis code (ICD-10-CM) on a claim indicates the medical necessity for the service. This means that there must be at least one ICD-10-CM code on the claim to prove that the ambulance service was medically necessary.

Because an emergency responder cannot determine the patient's diagnosis, he or she must record the signs, symptoms, or complaints of the patient, and code for those only. For example, if an ambulance reports to a home residence where a patient has fallen off a ladder and is complaining of severe arm pain, the code for pain in the arm would be reported on the claim. Once the patient arrives at the hospital, the healthcare providers there will determine the extent of the injury and actual diagnosis (such as a fracture).

This differs depending on the situation, however. For example, if a patient is being transferred from one healthcare facility to another for an organ transplant or surgery, then the ambulance company will have a record of the patient's actual diagnosis, which has been confirmed by a healthcare provider. In this case, the ambulance personnel may report the diagnosis that was given to them by the healthcare provider as medical necessity for the service provided.

When selecting a diagnosis code for an ambulance service, select the correct code according to one of the following three options (figure 6.4):

- Option 1: Select the appropriate code to identify the condition of the patient when they were picked up. These codes identify the patient's signs, symptoms, or other complaint.
- Option 2: Report the diagnosis code that is provided by the treating healthcare provider. This is typically only possible for patient transfers.
- Option 3: Report the ICD-10-CM code for unspecified illness:
  - R69, Illness, unspecified (ICD-10-CM)
  - R99, Ill-defined and unknown cause of mortality (ICD-10-CM)

Figure 6.4. Diagnosis coding for ambulance services

Option 1	• Select the appropriate code to identify the condition of the patient when he or she was picked up.
Option 2	• Report the diagnosis code that is provided by the treating medical provider.
Option 3	• Report the ICD-10 code for unspecified illness

The ambulance service must be fully documented to support all the codes placed on the claim. This is especially important as the detailed documentation for the ambulance service will determine whether or not the transportation service meets coverage guidelines, which will impact if the claim will be paid by the patient's insurance company. Documentation should always include the details of the trip, including the patient's medical condition and all the services provided to the patient.

Key to Success

In the following sections, selection of codes for the services provided is required. Remember the basics of code selection—examine the documentation to identify the service performed and the patient's diagnosis (when applicable); look up the main term in the Index; verify the code in the Tabular List; check any applicable guidelines, modifiers, and number of units; and assign the code!

Putting It All Together: Coding for Ambulance Services

In order to select the correct code for the service provided, it is important to carefully read the documentation of the service, then access the HCPCS code book Index and find the type of service that was provided. The HCPCS codes for ambulance services range from A0021 to A0999.

Determination of the correct codes for ambulance services relies on the following details:

- Was basic life support (BLS) or advanced life support (ALS) provided during the transport?
- Was the transport emergency or nonemergency?
- What type of transportation was used?
- What was the origin of the transport and what was the destination?
- How many miles were traveled?
- Which transportation indicator is applicable for the service?
- Was there any additional wait time, services, supplies, or personnel utilized during the service?

Study the following examples for appropriate codes for ambulance services. Then complete the practice exercises in There's a Code for That 6.1.

Example 6.1. Emergency ambulance service

Patient complaining of severe respiratory distress (shortness of breath) is transported via emergency ALS level 1 ground ambulance from her place of residence to the hospital. Total distance traveled was 8 miles.

HCPCS code: A0427-RH Ambulance service, advanced life support, emergency transport, level 1 (ALS 1-emergency); origin R-Residence; destination H-Hospital
HCPCS code: A0425 x 8 Ground mileage, per statute mile, 8 miles
ICD-10 code: R06.02 Shortness of breath

Example 6.2. Nonemergency ambulance service

A ventilator-dependent geriatric patient is transferred from a skilled nursing facility to home hospice. BLS nonemergency ground transport, 23 miles total. During transfer there was an unexpected death at the nursing facility, and the ambulance had to wait for 90 minutes before the transport could begin.

HCPCS code: A0428-NE Ambulance service, basic life support, nonemergency transport, (BLS); origin N-skilled nursing facility; destination E-residential, domiciliary, or custodial facility
HCPCS code: A0425-23 Ground mileage, per statute mile, 23 miles
ICD-10 code: Z99.11 Dependence on respirator (ventilator) status

6.1 Coding for ambulance and transportation services

There's a Code for That

Enter the correct answer for each of the following practice exercises.

1. Emergency ALS level 2 transport, rotary wing. Code just for the transportation, no mileage, without modifiers.

   HCPCS code: _____

2. Patient was transported from the scene of an accident to the hospital. What modifier would be used?

   HCPCS modifier: _____

3. Patient was picked up at the scene of an accident and transported via helicopter to a transfer pad, where he was then picked up by an on-ground ambulance and transported to a hospital. Helicopter mileage totaled 15 miles. Code only for the hospital transport, including modifier and miles traveled.

   HCPCS code: _____ - _____

   HCPCS code: _____ × _____

4. Patient with severe laceration of the right upper arm was transported from the scene of an accident via helicopter to a hospital. The total distance traveled was 13 miles. Due to heavy traffic conditions, a helicopter was dispatched to pick up the patient rather than an on-ground ambulance.

   HCPCS code: _____ - _____

   HCPCS code: _____ × _____

   Transportation indicator: _____

   ICD-10-CM code: _____

5. Nonemergency transport via wheelchair van to patient with quadriplegia and ventilator dependence. Patient was transferred from her residence to a skilled nursing facility, seven miles total distance traveled.

   HCPCS code: _____ - _____

   HCPCS code: _____ × _____

   ICD-10-CM: _____

   ICD-10-CM: _____

Durable Medical Equipment and Supplies

Durable medical equipment (DME) is a category of medical items and supplies used by patients both in and out of the healthcare setting. DME requires the following four characteristics:

- It can with stand repeated use
- It is used to serve a medical purpose
- It is not useful for a person without an illness or injury
- It can also be used in the home setting (outside of the healthcare setting)

For example, a pair of crutches supplied to a 15-year-old with a lower leg fracture are considered durable medical equipment. These crutches are: (1) used on a repetitive basis; (2) serve the purpose of helping the patient to walk; (3) are not useful for a patient without a leg injury or gait abnormality; and (4) are used everywhere that the patient goes, both in and out of the healthcare setting.

One specific type of DME are prosthetics and orthotics. **Prosthetics** are designed to replace all or part of an internal body organ (such as an artificial hip or knee replacement) or to replace an external appendage as an artificial limb (such as a lower leg prosthesis for an amputee). **Orthotics** are instruments that are used on the outside of the body to support, align, or correct deformities, or to improve the movements of joints, the spine, or the limbs (CMS 2017b). The most common types of orthotics are casts, placed on the outside of a body area to immobilize that body area and allow healing of the internal bones.

Durable medical equipment, prosthetics, orthotics, and supplies are often combined using the acronym **DMEPOS**. DMEPOS is a category of DME supplies that includes prosthetics and orthotics. Claims for DMEPOS will only be paid if the supply or equipment is considered medically necessary as determined by the healthcare provider and the patient's insurance company. For example, if a patient suffered a minor sprain to his ankle, it may not be necessary to give him a pair of crutches, but rather a supportive brace or wrap to immobilize the ankle joint. On the other hand, if a patient suffered a debilitating fracture of the femur, it may be medically necessary to supply the patient with a long leg brace and crutches until the femur bone heals.

Prior authorizations (discussed in chapter 3) may also be necessary before DME supplies are provided to the patient, when the patient's health insurance requires determination of medical necessity for the supplied item. For certain DMEPOS items, determination of medical necessity is done by using a **Certificate of Medical Necessity (CMN)** form. A CMN is an official document, completed by the physician and the DME supplier, that details the patient's diagnosis, necessity for the DME supply, and other important patient demographics and information. Usually DMEPOS items that require a CMN are over a certain dollar amount, which is why the additional attestation of medical necessity is required. For example, TRICARE insurance requires a CMN for any DME supply that has a purchase cost of $150 or more (HNFHS 2012). This form serves as proof that the DME supply was necessary to treat the patient, and will thus be covered by the patient's health insurance. Figure 6.5 displays a CMN for Positive Airway Pressure (PAP) Devices for Obstructive Sleep Apnea (CMS-10269).

The second page of the CMN contains instructions on how to complete the form. Notice that according to these directions, some sections should be completed by the physician or physician's office (Sections B and D), whereas the other sections should be

Figure 6.5. Certificate of medical necessity (CMS-10269)

DEPARTMENT OF HEALTH AND HUMAN SERVICES
CENTERS FOR MEDICARE & MEDICAID SERVICES

Form Approved
OMB No. OMB 0938-0679

CERTIFICATE OF MEDICAL NECESSITY

DME 03.03

CMS-10269: POSITIVE AIRWAY PRESSURE (PAP) DEVICES FOR OBSTRUCTIVE SLEEP APNEA

SECTION A: Certification Type/Date: INITIAL ___/___/___ RECERTIFICATION ___/___/___

PATIENT NAME, ADDRESS, TELEPHONE and HICN	SUPPLIER NAME, ADDRESS, TELEPHONE and NSC or NPI #
(_ _ _) _ _ _ - _ _ _ _ HICN _____	(_ _ _) _ _ _ - _ _ _ _ NSC or NPI # _____

PLACE OF SERVICE _____	HCPCS CODE	PT DOB ___/___/___ ; Sex ___ (M/F) ; HT.____(in.) ; WT.____(lbs.)
NAME and ADDRESS of FACILITY if applicable (See Reverse)	_____ _____ _____ _____	PHYSICIAN NAME, ADDRESS (Printed or Typed) PHYSICIAN'S NSC or NPI #: _____ PHYSICIAN'S TELEPHONE #: (_ _ _) _ _ _ - _ _ _ _

SECTION B: Information in this section may not be completed by the supplier of the items/supplies.

EST. LENGTH OF NEED (# OF MONTHS): _____ 1–99 (99=LIFETIME) | DIAGNOSIS CODES (ICD-9): _____ _____ _____ _____

ANSWERS	ANSWER QUESTIONS 1–7 FOR INITIAL EVALUATION ANSWER QUESTIONS 8–10 FOR FOLLOW-UP EVALUATION (RECERTIFICATION) (Check **Y** for Yes, **N** for No, **D** for Does Not Apply)
☐Y ☐N	1. Is the device being ordered for the treatment of obstructive sleep apnea (ICD-9 diagnosis code 327.23)? If YES, continue to Questions 2–5; If NO, Proceed to Section D
___/___/___	2. Enter date of initial face-to-face evaluation
___/___/___	3. Enter date of sleep test (If test spans multiple days, enter date of first day of test)
☐Y ☐N	4. Was the patient's sleep test conducted in a facility-based lab?
_____	5. What is the patient's Apnea-Hypopnea Index (AHI) or Respiratory Disturbance Index (RDI)?
☐Y ☐N	6. Does the patient have documented evidence of at least one of the following? Excessive daytime sleepiness, impaired cognition, mood disorders, insomnia, hypertension, ischemic heart disease or history of stroke.
☐Y ☐N ☐D	7. If a bilevel device is ordered, has a CPAP device been tried and found ineffective?
___/___/___	8. Enter date of follow-up face-to-face evaluation.
☐Y ☐N	9. Is there a report documenting that the patient used PAP ≥ 4 hours per night on at least 70% of nights in a 30 consecutive day period?
☐Y ☐N	10. Did the patient demonstrate improvement in symptoms of obstructive sleep apnea with the use of PAP?

NAME OF PERSON ANSWERING SECTION B QUESTIONS, IF OTHER THAN PHYSICIAN (Please Print):

NAME: _____ TITLE: _____ EMPLOYER: _____

SECTION C: Narrative Description of Equipment and Cost

(1) Narrative description of all items, accessories and options ordered; **(2)** Supplier's charge; and **(3)** Medicare Fee Schedule Allowance for each item, accessory, and option. *(See instructions on back)*

SECTION D: Physician Attestation and Signature/Date

I certify that I am the physician identified in Section A of this form. I have received Sections A, B and C of the Certificate of Medical Necessity (including charges for items ordered). Any statement on my letterhead attached hereto, has been reviewed and signed by me. I certify that the medical necessity information in Section B is true, accurate and complete, to the best of my knowledge, and I understand that any falsification, omission, or concealment of material fact in that section may subject me to civil or criminal liability.

PHYSICIAN'S SIGNATURE _____ DATE ___/___/___ (SIGNATURE AND DATE STAMPS ARE NOT ACCEPTABLE)

1

INSTRUCTIONS FOR COMPLETING THE CERTIFICATE OF MEDICAL NECESSITY FOR POSITIVE AIRWAY PRESSURE (PAP) DEVICES FOR OBSTRUCTIVE SLEEP APNEA (CMS-10269)

SECTION A: (May be completed by the supplier)

CERTIFICATION TYPE/DATE: If this is an initial certification for this patient, indicate this by placing date (MM/DD/YY) needed initially in the space marked "INITIAL." If this is a revised certification (to be completed when the physician changes the order, based on the patient's changing clinical needs), indicate the initial date needed in the space marked "INITIAL," and also indicate the recertification date in the space marked "REVISED." If this is a recertification, indicate the initial date needed in the space marked "INITIAL," and also indicate the recertification date in the space marked "RECERTIFICATION." Whether submitting a REVISED or a RECERTIFIED CMN, be sure to always furnish the INITIAL date as well as the REVISED or RECERTIFICATION date.

PATIENT INFORMATION: Indicate the patient's name, permanent legal address, telephone number and his/her health insurance claim number (HICN) as it appears on his/her Medicare card and on the claim form.

SUPPLIER INFORMATION: Indicate the name of your company (supplier name), address and telephone number along with the National Provider Identification (NPI) number assigned to you by the National Supplier Clearinghouse (NSC).

PLACE OF SERVICE: Indicate the place in which the item is being used, i.e., patient's home is 12, skilled nursing facility (SNF) is 31, End Stage Renal Disease (ESRD) facility is 65, etc. Refer to the DME MAC supplier manual for a complete list.

FACILITY NAME: If the place of service is a facility, indicate the name and complete address of the facility.

HCPCS CODES: List all HCPCS procedure codes for items ordered that require a CMN. Procedure codes that do not require certification should not be listed on the CMN.

PATIENT DOB, HEIGHT, WEIGHT AND SEX: Indicate patient's date of birth (MM/DD/YY) and sex (male or female); height in inches and weight in pounds, if requested.

PHYSICIAN NAME, ADDRESS: Indicate the physician's name and complete mailing address.

NPI: Accurately indicate the ordering physician's National Provider Identification number (NPI).

PHYSICIAN'S TELEPHONE NO: Indicate the telephone number where the physician can be contacted (preferably where records would be accessible pertaining to this patient) if more information is needed.

SECTION B: (May not be completed by the supplier. While this section may be completed by a non-physician clinician, or a physician employee, it must be reviewed, and the CMN signed (in Section D) by the ordering physician.)

EST. LENGTH OF NEED: Indicate the estimated length of need (the length of time the physician expects the patient to require use of the ordered item) by filling in the appropriate number of months. If the physician expects that the patient will require the item for the duration of his/her life, then enter 99.

DIAGNOSIS CODES: In the first space, list the ICD9 code that represents the primary reason for ordering this item. List any additional ICD9 codes that would further describe the medical need for the item (up to 3 codes).

QUESTION SECTION: This section is used to gather clinical information to determine medical necessity. Answer each question which applies to the items ordered, checking "Y" for yes, "N" for no, or fill in the blank if other information is requested.

NAME OF PERSON ANSWERING SECTION B QUESTIONS: If a clinical professional other than the ordering physician (e.g., home health nurse, physical therapist, dietician) or a physician employee answers the questions of Section B, he/she must print his/her name, give his/her professional title and the name of his/her employer where indicated. If the physician is answering the questions, this space may be left blank.

SECTION C: (To be completed by the supplier)

NARRATIVE DESCRIPTION OF EQUIPMENT & COST: Supplier gives **(1)** a narrative description of the item(s) ordered, as well as all options, accessories, supplies and drugs; **(2)** the supplier's charge for each item, option, accessory, supply and drug; and **(3)** the Medicare fee schedule allowance for each item/option/accessory/supply/drug, if applicable.

SECTION D: (To be completed by the physician)

PHYSICIAN ATTESTATION: The physician's signature certifies **(1)** the CMN which he/she is reviewing includes Sections A, B, C and D; **(2)** the answers in Section B are correct; and **(3)** the self-identifying information in Section A is correct.

PHYSICIAN SIGNATURE AND DATE: After completion and/or review by the physician of Sections A, B and C, the physician must sign and date the CMN in Section D, verifying the Attestation appearing in this Section. The physician's signature also certifies the items ordered are medically necessary for this patient. Signature and date stamps are not acceptable.

Source: CMS 2009.

completed by the DME supplier (Sections A and C). Any additional health records or documentation of the patient's condition may also need to be sent along with the CMN to ensure that the service will be covered. Other items that require a CMN include oxygen, pneumatic compression devices, osteogenesis stimulators, enteral and parenteral nutrition, and seat lift mechanisms, among others.

Once all the billing considerations, such as a CMN or prior authorization, have been addressed, coding for durable medical equipment is essentially as simple as identifying and reporting the correct HCPCS code(s). Perhaps one of the most problematic parts of coding from the HCPCS code book for beginning coders is locating the correct code in the book itself. Because Index entries vary by publisher and items are listed in various ways, it is sometimes difficult to locate the entry for the item being reported in the Index. It helps to be as familiar with the HCPCS code book as possible, including knowing where all sections of codes are located and placing tabs throughout the book for easy access (discussed in chapter 5).

There are numerous modifiers in the HCPCS code book that may be added to HCPCS codes for DMEPOS to provide more details about the supply or service provided, such as whether the equipment was new or used. HCPCS modifiers can identify the following:

- The type of healthcare provider
- Specifics surrounding anesthesia services
- Body areas, such as specific fingers, eyelids, or coronary arteries
- Laterality (right or left side)
- The number of wounds dressed
- That an advance beneficiary notice (ABN) or waiver of liability was given to the patient
- Specific types of treatments to patients on dialysis or with end-stage renal disease (ESRD)
- Details about the type of equipment provided

Complete the following practice exercises in There's a Code for That 6.2 to test your knowledge about HCPCS modifiers.

6.2 Identifying HCPCS modifiers

There's a Code for That

In the following exercises, code only for the HCPCS modifier as indicated.

1. Dressing for five wounds.

   HCPCS modifier: _____

2. Left foot, 4th digit.

   HCPCS modifier: _____

3. Right side.

   HCPCS modifier: _____

4. New equipment.

   HCPCS modifier: _____

5. DMEPOS item delivered via mail.

   HCPCS modifier: _____

6. Left main coronary artery.

HCPCS modifier: _____

7. Administered intravenously.

HCPCS modifier: _____

8. Upper left eyelid.

HCPCS modifier: _____

Key to Success

Because HCPCS modifiers are so varied in meaning, it is beneficial to study the list of modifiers and become as familiar with these codes as possible. Read through the HCPCS modifiers section of your HCPCS code book and note the modifier, such as RT, and then the modifier description, such as "Right side." Observe similarities and differences as you review the modifiers and note groups of modifiers that are similar in nature, such as modifiers E1 through E4 that all identify eyelids (E1, Upper left, eyelid; E2, Lower left, eyelid; E3, Upper right, eyelid; E4, Lower right, eyelid).

CPT modifiers are all numeric (they do not contain letters), whereas HCPCS modifiers all contain at least one letter (they are alphanumeric).

Diagnosis Coding for DME

When a patient is in need of DME, he or she is generally already under the care of a healthcare practitioner, and already has an established diagnosis or condition for which the DME supply is necessary. This means that when coding for DME claims, diagnostic coding (ICD-10-CM) relies on the patient's established diagnosis, which should be included on the DME supply request form from the healthcare provider. DME personnel (billers, coders, and administrative staff) are not clinical in nature and are unauthorized to diagnose patients. However, they can and may often be relied upon to abstract healthcare provider notes in order to select an ICD-10 code.

In this sense, medical necessity plays a large part in DME coding. A valid ICD-10-CM diagnosis code is always needed on the claim to indicate medical necessity for the service, and a CMN may also be needed for certain items.

Putting It All Together: Coding for Durable Medical Equipment, Prosthetics, Orthotics, and Supplies

In order to select the correct code for the supply provided, it is important to carefully read the documentation and then access the Index in the HCPCS code book and find the type of supply or equipment provided. Codes for durable medical equipment, prosthetics, orthotics, and supplies are found throughout the HCPCS code book.

Determination of the correct codes for DMEPOS relies on the following details.

- What type of supply or equipment was provided to the patient?
- Verify the details of the supply: amount per unit, size, dosage, frequency, and such.
- Are there any applicable modifiers?

Selecting the correct HCPCS code depends on coding steps similar to those of selecting CPT or ICD-10-CM codes. To find the correct HCPCS code, read through the documentation of the procedure or supply provided and then reference the Index to the HCPCS code book and also refer to any subterms or cross-references. Once a code is identified in the Index, that code should be verified in the Tabular section. Please refer to chapter 5 for a reminder of the components of the HCPCS code book. Chapter 4 includes a full discussion on identifying and selecting ICD-10-CM codes.

Example 6.3 Patient supply provided

Pediatric patient was supplied with a portable nebulizer machine to be able to provide home breathing treatments for reactive airway disease, new equipment.

HCPCS code: E0570-NU Nebulizer, with compressor
ICD-10-CM code: J45.909 Unspecified asthma, uncomplicated

Example 6.4 Patient supply provided

Patient with pre-diabetes was prescribed a home blood glucose monitor by her PCP. Supplied patient with monitor per physician's orders.

HCPCS code: E0607 Home blood glucose monitor
ICD-10-CM code: R73.03 Prediabetes

Key to Success

Remember: When locating an item in the HCPCS Index, you may find a range of codes listed rather than a single code. In this case, reference each one of the codes within that code range to ensure correct code selection.

Study the following examples for appropriate codes for DMEPOS. Then complete the practice exercises in There's a Code for That 6.3.

6.3

There's a Code for That

Coding for HCPCS supplies and services

Enter the correct answer for each of the following practice exercises.

1. Oxygen mask and two feet of tubing used in the office setting during breathing treatment provided to patient with emphysema.

   HCPCS code: _____

   HCPCS code: _____ × _____

   ICD-10-CM code: _____

2. Wheelchair-bound patient is provided with two arm pads.

   HCPCS code: _____ × _____

3. Rubber colostomy pouch, drainable, with faceplate attached.

   HCPCS code: _____

4. Patient provided with a supply of five occlusive eye patches.

HCPCS code: _____ × _____

5. Prefabricated wrist sprint.

HCPCS code: _____

Drugs Administered in the Healthcare Setting

Drugs that are administered in the healthcare setting include injections, chemotherapy drugs, inhaled solutions, and immunosuppressive drugs. They may be administered in a number of different healthcare settings. For example, a patient with a severe bacterial infection presenting to her primary care office may receive an injection of an antibiotic while in the office. On the other hand, a cancer patient presenting for chemotherapy would receive an injection of the chemotherapeutic medicinal substance while in an outpatient cancer treatment center. What differs between these drugs and over-the-counter or prescription drugs is that they are given in the healthcare setting by a healthcare professional, who then monitors the patient to ensure there will be no side effects.

HCPCS Coding for Drugs Administered in the Healthcare Setting

These drugs are coded using HCPCS codes. Although many of the HCPCS codes for drugs begin with a J, some begin with other letters, and are thus found throughout the HCPCS code book. It is important to search the Table of Drugs to identify the correct substance administered. In some instances, the drug is not listed in the Table of Drugs. In this case, turn to the HCPCS Index and search for the drug by its generic name.

HCPCS codes for Drugs Administered in the Healthcare Setting only identify the drug administered, and do not include any of the supplies that were used to administer the drug, nor the procedure code that would be billed for performing the actual administration of the drug. Additional HCPCS codes are used to report additional supplies used to administer the medication, and CPT codes are used to report the procedure performed. Furthermore, ICD-10-CM diagnosis codes are also required to indicate the medical necessity for the drug given. For example, if the patient is receiving a chemotherapy infusion drug for liver cancer, then the liver cancer would be identified with an ICD-10-CM code and included on the claim (see figure 6.6)

Figure 6.6. Coding for a chemotherapy infusion

Description	Code type	Description
Medical necessity	ICD-10-CM	C22.8, Malignant neoplasm of liver, primary, unspecified as to type
Procedure	CPT	96401, Chemotherapy administration, subcutaneous or intramuscular; non-hormonal anti-neoplastic
Supply	HCPCS	J1745, Injection, infliximab, excludes biosimilar, 10 mg

Before assigning J-codes, it is important to understand the many routes of administration. The route of administration is the way in which the drug is given to the patient. Medications may be administered in numerous ways, and the

Table of Drugs takes this into account. There are five injected routes: intra-arterial (IA), intravenous (IV), intramuscular (IM), intrathecal (IT), as well as subcutaneous (SC), inhaled (INH), oral (ORAL), various (VAR), and other routes (OTH). This allows coders to select the code for the drug based on the method of administration. Figure 6.7 provides the different routes of administration.

Figure 6.7. Routes of administration

IA = Intra-arterial (injected into an artery)
IV = Intravenous (injected into a vein)
IM = Intramuscular (injected into a muscle)
IT = Intrathecal (injected into the fluid around the spinal cord)
SC = Subcutaneous (injected into the subcutaneous layer of the skin)
INH = Inhaled (inhalation of a gas)
VAR = Various routes (enteral administrations, transdermal cream)
OTH = Other routes (rectal suppositories, otic or ophthalmic drops)
ORAL = Oral (taken by mouth)

In the HCPCS manual, the Table of Drugs (introduced in chapter 5) is a list of drugs, their dosages, and the routes of administration, cross-mapped to the corresponding J-code. Although HCPCS code books vary significantly depending on the publisher, the format of the Table of Drugs is similar to table 6.1.

Table 6.1. Table of Drugs example

Drug Name	Dosage/Unit Per	Route	Code
Nabilone	1 mg	Oral	J8650
Nalbuphine HCL	per 10 mg	IM, IV, SC	J2300
Naloxone HCL	per 1 mg	IM, IV, SC	J2310
Naltrexone, Depot Form	1 mg	IM	J2315
Nandrobolic L.A., *see* Nandrolone Decanoate			
Nandrolone Decanoate	Up to 50 mg	IM	J2320
Narcan, *see* Naloxone HCL			
Naropin, *see* Ropivacaine HCL			

This first column lists the name of the drug, by both generic and brand names. It is helpful to have access to a **Physician's Desk Reference (PDR)**, a compilation of information for prescription drugs to certify that the correct drug is selected for the service. The second column lists the dosage per one unit of the drug. For example, if the patient received 1 mg of Naloxone, then only one unit was administered. Always pay attention to the dosage or the unit per administration, as this may affect the number of units that are billed for the drug. For example, if the patient was given 2 mgs of Naltrexone, then the coder should select the code for Naltrexone, J2315, Injection, naltrexone, depot form, 1 mg, with the number of units to indicate how much was administered. The correct coding in this case would be J2315 × 2.

The third column identifies the route of administration for the drug in abbreviated form. Many drugs can be given in several different ways, and as such multiple routes of administration may be listed for a single drug.

The last column lists the HCPCS code for the drug administered. Once a HCPCS code has been identified, it is still necessary to verify the code in the Tabular List. For example, once the coder identifies the drug Naloxone HCL, coded in the Table of Drugs to J2310, he or she would then verify the code in the Tabular List by finding code J2310 within the Tabular and confirming that the code, dosage, and route of administration is correct (see figure 6.8).

Figure 6.8. Components of HCPCS drug code descriptions

Source: AHIMA 2018, 292.

Notice that some of the drugs listed in the Table of Drugs contain a cross-reference to another drug. This cross-reference directs the coder to search for the alternate drug name and then use the code listed for it. For example, in table 6.1, notice that the entry for Narcan refers the coder to *see* Naloxone HCL. The coder should then refer to this name, Naloxone HCL, and code for the drug appropriately. Some drugs are listed multiple times, with different routes of administration. In this case, select the appropriate route of administration for the drug given.

Putting It All Together: Coding for Drugs Administered in the Healthcare Setting

In order to select the correct code for the drug administered in the healthcare setting, it is important to carefully read the documentation of the service provided and then access the Table of Drugs in the HCPCS manual and locate the drug name. Then follow all cross-references, locate the correct dosage and route of administration, and find the associated HCPCS code. Be sure to verify the code in the Tabular List before making a final selection; and check the dosage of the drug that was administered to ensure that the correct number of units for the code is selected.

Determination of the correct drug code relies on the following:

- What drug was administered?
- What was the route of administration?
- What was the dosage given?

Example 6.5 Administration of medication

Patient presented to the ER in severe labor pains, asking for pain relief. This is her first pregnancy and she is dilated 2 cm. Delivery expected in excess of 4 hours. 1 mg of Stadol was administered intravenously.
HCPCS code: J0595 Injection, butorphanol tartrate, 1 mg

Example 6.6 Administration of medication

25-year-old male with gonorrhea received IM injection of Bicillin CR (100,000 units)
HCPCS code: J0558 Injection, penicillin G benzathine and penicillin G procaine, 100,000 units
ICD-10-CM code: A54.9 Gonococcal infection, unspecified

Study the following examples for appropriate codes for drugs administered in the healthcare setting. Then complete the practice exercises in There's a Code for That 6.4.

6.4

There's a Code for That

Coding for drugs administered in the healthcare setting

Enter the correct answer for each of the following practice exercises.

1. 20 mg Adalimumab administered subcutaneously.

   HCPCS code: _____

2. 35-year-old woman with bipolar I disorder was given .50 mg of Abilify.

   HCPCS code: _____ × _____

   ICD-10-CM code: _____ (Tip: Remember to look up the main term *disorder*, and then find the subterm *bipolar*.)

3. 30-year-old pregnant female with Factor V Leiden deficiency is given 10 mg Lovenox.

   HCPCS code: _____

   ICD-10-CM code: _____

4. 5-year-old patient presents to the office complaining of acute exacerbation of mild intermittent asthma. He was given 2 mgs of albuterol inhalation solution, concentrated form, via nebulizer machine.

   HCPCS code: _____ × _____

   ICD-10-CM code: _____

End of Chapter Content

Instructions: Match the terms with the appropriate descriptions.

1. _____ Intra-arterial
2. _____ Oral
3. _____ Other routes

A. Rectal suppositories, otic or ophthalmic drops
B. Inhalation of a gas
C. Injected into the fluid around the spinal cord

4. _____ Various routes

5. _____ Inhaled

6. _____ Intramuscular

7. _____ Intrathecal

8. _____ Intravenous

9. _____ Subcutaneous

D. Taken by mouth

E. Injected in to an artery

F. Injected into a muscle

G. Enteral administrations, transdermal cream

H. Injected into the subcutaneous layer of the skin

I. Injected into a vein

Instructions: Choose the best answer.

1. Which of the following types of life support would be used to provide a high level of care with life-saving protocols, such as manual defibrillation?

   a. Basic life support

   b. Advanced life support

   c. Circulation, airway, and breathing support

   d. Level 3 BLS

2. Which of the following types of transportation is scheduled in advance?

   a. Nonemergency

   b. Urgent

   c. Emergency

   d. Ground

3. Why are origin and destination modifiers appended to ambulance services?

   a. To identify why the ambulance service was medically necessary

   b. To identify the route taken by the ambulance company

   c. To justify the amount of mile driven by the ambulance

   d. To identify where the patient was picked up and where the patient was taken

4. Which of the following is the purpose of transportation indicators placed on ambulance claims?

   a. To identify the origin and destination of the transport

   b. To indicate why those particular ambulance services were medically necessary

   c. To support the ICD-10 code selected for the service

   d. To identify the type of injury or illness suffered by the patient

5. Which of the following ways may an emergency technician select a diagnosis for the ambulance services provided to a patient?

   a. Select the last code that was assigned to the patient's chart

   b. Report the code given by a family member

   c. Report the code for unspecified illness

   d. Ask the patient what his or her diagnosis is

Instructions: Answer the following questions with the appropriate code, modifier, or indicator.

1. 1 microgram (MCG) Avonex.

   HCPCS code: _____

2. Ativan, 4 mg.

   HCPCS code: _____ × _____

3. Inhaled Isuprel concentrate, 1 mg.

   HCPCS code: _____

4. 5 mg oral prednisolone.

   HCPCS code: _____

5. 5 micrograms Rebif, administered subcutaneously.

   HCPCS code: _____ × _____

6. Radioelements for brachytherapy, 15 elements.

   HCPCS code: _____ × _____

7. Plaster long-leg cast provided to 8-year-old boy with femur shaft fracture of the right leg (initial encounter).

   HCPCS code: _____

   ICD-10 code: _____

8. Nasal prosthesis.

HCPCS code: _____

9. ALS level 1 nonemergency transport provided to geriatric patient with terminal brain cancer (malignant neoplasm of brain, unspecified). Picked up from home residence and transferred to custodial facility. Total distance driven was 10 miles.

HCPCS code: _____ - _____

HCPCS code: _____ × _____

ICD-10 code: _____

10. Patient with multiple injuries was transported via rotary wing ambulance from mountain top to hospital. Emergency ALS level 2 support provided during transport, including esophageal intubation and oxygen delivered to patient during transport. 45 miles traveled.

HCPCS code: _____ - _____

HCPCS code: _____

HCPCS code: _____

HCPCS code: _____ × _____

Transportation Indicator: _____

ICD-10 code: _____

References

American Health Information Management Association. 2017. *2017 HCPCS LEVEL II, Professional Edition*. St. Louis, MO: Elsevier.

Centers for Medicare and Medicaid Services. 2017a. Details for title: CMS 1500. https://www.cms.gov/Medicare/CMS-Forms/CMS-Forms/CMS-Forms-Items/CMS1188854.html.

Centers for Medicare and Medicaid Services. 2017b. Durable Medical Equipment, Prosthetics, Orthotics, and Supplies (DMEPOS) (Rev. 3824, 08-02-17). Chapter 20 in *Medicare Claims Processing Manual*. https://www.cms.gov/Regulations-and-Guidance/Guidance/Manuals/downloads/clm104c20.pdf.

Centers for Medicare and Medicaid Services. 2009 (December). Certificate of Medical Necessity CMS-10269: Positive Airway Pressure (PAP) Devices for Obstructive Sleep Apnea. https://www.cms.gov/Medicare/CMS-Forms/CMS-Forms/Downloads/cms10269.pdf.

Health Net Federal Health Services. 2012 (September 12). Does all durable medical equipment require a certificate of medical necessity? https://www.hnfs.net/content/hnfs/home/tn/prov/provider_news/2012_prov_news_archive/cmn_dme.html.

Resources

Centers for Medicare and Medicaid Services. 2017. Ambulance (Rev. 3620, 10-07-16). Chapter 15 in *Medicare Claims Processing Manual*. https://www.cms.gov/Regulations-and-Guidance/Guidance/Manuals/downloads/clm104c15.pdf.

Centers for Medicare and Medicaid Services. 2015. Medical Conditions List and Transportation Indicators. https://www.cms.gov/Medicare/Medicare-Fee-for-Service-Payment/AmbulanceFeeSchedule/Downloads/2015-AFS-Medical-Conditions-Indicators.pdf.

CHAPTER

Behavioral Health Services

Learning Objectives

- Understand the basics of billing and coding within the specialty of behavioral health.
- Analyze the components of evaluation and management services and interpret evaluation and management coding guidelines for correct code selection.

- Examine procedural codes and guidelines for behavioral health services.
- Examine diagnosis coding and medical necessity for behavioral health services.
- Determine and apply ICD-10-CM, CPT, and HCPCS codes to behavioral health services.

Key Terms

Anxiety disorders

Attention-deficit hyperactivity disorder (ADHD)

Behavioral health services

Bipolar disorder

Contributory factors

Coordination of care

Counseling

Depression

Diagnostic and Statistical Manual of Mental Disorders (DSM-5)

Eating disorders

Electroconvulsive therapy (ECT)

Established patient

Examination

History

Inpatient

Interactive complexity

Medical decision making (MDM)

Mental health

Mental illness

Narcosynthesis for psychiatric purposes

Nature of the presenting problem

New patient

Outpatient

Partial hospitalization

Place of service (POS)

Psychotherapy

Schizophrenia

Screening, Brief Intervention and Referral to Treatment (SBIRT)

Substance abuse

Transcranial magnetic stimulation (TMS)

Vagus nerve stimulation

Behavioral health services are treatments and procedures performed by a licensed healthcare professional to address mental illnesses and substance abuse, aiming to promote well-being by preventing or intervening in mental illnesses, substance abuse, and addictive behavior. **Mental health** refers to a person's emotional, psychological, and social well-being. **Mental illness** is a condition that affects a person's thinking, feeling, or mood, and affects a person's ability to perform major life activities and functions each day. **Substance abuse** is the misuse of alcohol or drugs, which impairs a person's ability to meet daily responsibilities at home, work, or school. Behavioral health directly diagnoses, treats, and manages individuals with mental health issues or substance abuse.

Coding for behavioral health includes a basic understanding of evaluation and management (E/M) services, introduced in chapters 3 and 5, that depends on the place of service, level of service, and patient status; and it includes coding accurately for the procedures performed above and beyond the E/M service. It also depends on correctly abstracting diagnostic information to apply diagnosis codes accurately when identifying the medical necessity for the procedures performed.

Behavioral health services are performed in various settings by several different healthcare providers. This chapter discusses behavioral health coding within the context of a large behavioral health group that provides a wide range of behavioral health services including screenings and treatments provided across a number of settings.

Behavioral Health Basics

Behavioral health identifies mental health and substance abuse disorders with diagnostic screenings and tests that help identify specific behavioral disorders and manage treatment of these disorders. Unlike medical services, behavioral health services have been more restricted traditionally in terms of insurance coverage and codes that support medical necessity for the service provided. These services are now commonly covered by most health insurance policies. Approved by Congress in 2008, the Mental Health Parity and Addiction Equity Act (MHPAEA) aimed to expand behavioral health services, including mental health and substance abuse disorder benefits. The Affordable Care Act (ACA), passed in 2010, further expanded these benefits by requiring most insurance plans to cover behavioral health services, including preventive services like depression screenings for adults and behavioral screenings for children.

However, there are still discrepancies with limitations for covered services, types of providers qualified to bill for behavioral health services, the medical necessity to support services, and the actual services performed. Therefore, successful behavioral health coders must always take into consideration the patient's health insurance coverage to ensure all services are reported properly.

Behavioral health services are performed by a wide variety of providers and because state and insurance requirements vary, only certain providers can perform specific services. Additionally, the rates at which the different provider types are reimbursed differ, depending on the provider type—such as psychiatrist, social worker, or clinical psychologist. Behavioral health providers also perform their services in different settings—for example, nursing facilities, assisted living facilities, and via an interactive telemedicine interface—that must be considered on the claim.

Behavioral Health Providers

Providers that offer behavioral health services differ from those that provide medical services. Although some of them are medical doctors (MDs), others have specialty credentials that enable them to provide only behavioral health services. Behavioral health providers include

- Psychiatrist
- Clinical Psychologist (CP)
- Clinical Social Worker (CSW)
- Clinical Nurse Specialist (CN)
- Nurse Practitioner (NP)
- Physician Assistant (PA)
- Certified Nurse Midwife (CNM)
- Independently Practicing Psychologist (IPP)

It is important to understand the types of behavioral health providers because although all of the providers listed are qualified to perform behavioral health services—such as psychotherapy or counseling—their ability to bill and receive payment for their services depends on their degree, license, or credential; the state in which they practice; and the patient's insurance.

For example, a psychiatrist is a medical doctor who is legally authorized to practice in a specific state (or states), and whose behavioral health services are paid at 100 percent by Medicare. This means that Medicare pays the full amount of the allowable charge for a service provided by a psychiatrist. On the other hand, a clinical social worker (CSW) has a master's or doctoral degree in social work, and is legally authorized to perform services in the state in which they work. Medicare pays CSWs 75 percent of the allowable amount for all services. So Medicare only pays a CSW three-quarters of the amount that it would reimburse a psychiatrist. These differences in billing, including state requirements and specific insurance guidelines, vary among states and insurance plans. To learn the specifics of these requirements and guidelines, a coder or biller may have to contact each insurance company individually, as well as the state department of insurance.

Note that mid-level providers (or advanced practitioners), as discussed in chapter 1, include nurse practitioners and physician assistants who also practice in other healthcare specialties. This means that the billing variances that affect different types of behavioral health providers may also affect the billing variances for other healthcare providers. Again, it is necessary to check with payer and state regulations to determine any type of billing, coding, or payment differences between provider types.

Because the field of behavioral health is diverse, some behavioral health specialists will further subspecialize within the field. Remember, as discussed in chapter 1, a subspecialty is a specialty within a specialty. For example, a clinical psychologist may choose to subspecialize in child and adolescent psychiatry, addiction medicine, military and stress-related disorders, or marriage and family therapy.

Key to Success

It is not enough to simply select a code and report it. In addition to reporting the codes correctly, coders must keep the context of the service in mind—including who provided the service, where the service was performed, and which insurance is being billed.

Place of Service

The **place of service (POS)** is the setting or the service or where the service occurred. Behavioral health services may be performed in several different settings just as

Table 7.1. Select CPT place of service codes

Place of Service Code(s)	Place of Service Name	Place of Service Description
02	Telehealth	The location where health services and health related services are provided or received, through a telecommunication system. (Effective January 1, 2017)
03	School	A facility whose primary purpose is education. (Effective January 1, 2003)
07	Tribal 638 Free-standing Facility	A facility or location owned and operated by a federally recognized American Indian or Alaska Native tribe or tribal organization under a 638 agreement, which provides diagnostic, therapeutic (surgical and non-surgical), and rehabilitation services to tribal members who do not require hospitalization. (Effective January 1, 2003)

Source: Adapted from CMS 2016.

healthcare services may be provided in various healthcare settings, depending on the needs of the patient.

There is a special code for each POS in which a service occurred. These places of service are listed at the beginning of the CPT code book, entitled Place of Service Codes for Professional Claims. A POS code must be included on each claim, whether it is a behavioral health or any other healthcare claim for professional services, and it must correspond to the setting in which the service occurred. Table 7.1. gives some examples.

POS codes are placed in box 24.B on the CMS-1500 claim form (see figure 7.1). For example, if the service was performed in the office, then the POS code is 11, for Office. This number is placed in box 24.B on the claim form to indicate that the service was performed in the office setting.

POS codes are important in all healthcare specialties, not just in behavioral health, because healthcare services are provided in numerous settings. For behavioral health, services are commonly performed in

- Outpatient office settings (POS 11)
- Partial hospitalization programs (PHP) (POS 52)
- Community mental health centers (CMHC) (POS 53)
- Inpatient psychiatric facilities (IPF) and hospitals (POS 51)
- Long-term care and nursing facilities (POS 31 and 32)

After learning the basics of billing for behavioral health services, it is important to study and understand the actual procedures and procedure codes that are reported for behavioral health services.

Figure 7.1. Box 24.B place of service

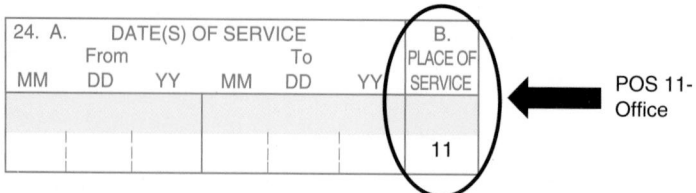

Source: CMS 2017.

Coding for Procedures in Behavioral Health

Most of the procedure codes used by behavioral health providers are evaluation and management (E/M) codes to report the medical management of patients, and psychiatry codes to report additional services such as psychotherapy and other treatments.

Key to Success

Evaluation and management codes are detailed and contain elements that must be combined to ensure correct code selection. This chapter only introduces the concepts of E/M codes and how to select them. The next chapter in this text, Primary Care, further specifies how the levels of each key component are determined. It may be helpful to refer to this chapter, and basic E/M components, when reading through chapter 8.

E/M Coding in Behavioral Health

Evaluation and management codes are used in all healthcare specialties, settings, and by all types of qualified healthcare providers. Thus, they are an extremely important part of professional outpatient coding. Any time a patient receives an evaluation by a provider (for instance, a physical examination in conjunction with counseling services), or for management of a condition (such as a medication refill request), an evaluation and management code should be reported.

Psychiatrists are medical doctors who specialize in the diagnosis and treatment of mental illnesses. Though they provide psychiatry services, they are also qualified to medically manage behavioral health patients. Many patients needing behavioral health services are given medications to treat their symptoms; others have mental health or substance abuse issues in addition to physical health issues. This requires a level of medical management for some behavioral health patients. Psychiatrists are both qualified and required to perform medical evaluation and management services for their patients, as well as any necessary mental health services, such as psychotherapy or group counseling services (discussed later in this chapter).

While mentioned briefly in previous chapters, this chapter details evaluation and management services by introducing the basic format, function, and components of E/M codes; they are also discussed further in chapter 8 (Primary Care). It is important to first present the basic components of E/M codes, and then look at the components comprehensively to determine the correct E/M code.

E/M Coding Basics

E/M codes can be reported for new or established patients, in the inpatient or outpatient setting, and even for telemedicine services. They are used to report the evaluation and management of a patient across all healthcare settings—such as outpatient office visits, inpatient hospital visits, consultations performed in both inpatient and outpatient settings, emergency departments, nursing facilities and rest homes, and home visits. E/M codes are the most commonly used codes in all professional outpatient billing as they are used to report the medical evaluation and management of a patient. Consider the following example.

A new patient presents to the office of a psychiatrist in the town where she just moved. She was under treatment for depression where she lived previously, and her new psychiatrist performs a medication history, side-effect history, and mental status examination. He then prescribes an antidepressant to the patient.

This visit would be reported with an E/M code and only an E/M code since no psychotherapy or any other services were provided.

E/M codes compose the first section of Category I codes in the CPT code book. This section is first organized by the type of service performed. There are also numerous pages of guidelines located before the codes in this section. A few of these guidelines are discussed here, with a more thorough discussion of these guidelines in chapter 8.

Key to Success

The best way to get an idea of the services reported with E/M codes is to closely look at the table of contents for the evaluation and management section of the CPT code book. Pay close attention to the main headings describing the type of services that may be reported, such as Office or Other Outpatient Services, Hospital Observation Services, and Hospital Inpatient Services. These headings designate the setting in which the service was performed as well as the type of service.

There are three key components of all E/M services—each may be documented at a different level of complexity, and may include contributory factors, all of which are combined to report the level of service that was provided to the patient. Furthermore, there are some exceptions to the general E/M format for certain behavioral health evaluation and management services. Before addressing the three key components, coders must first determine the type of E/M service by defining three factors—type of service, patient status, and place of service.

Three Factors of E/M Codes

To correctly determine the type of evaluation and management service provided, coders must first ask themselves three questions (see figure 7.2).

1. *What is the type of service?* The type of service refers to the kind of evaluation and management encounter that was given to the patient. For example, was the service an office visit, a consultation, a team conference, or a hospital discharge?

2. *What is the patient status?* There are four different types of patient status—new, established, inpatient, and outpatient. A **new patient** is one that has not received any professional services within the past three years from a healthcare provider or another healthcare provider of the same specialty and subspecialty in the same group practice. An **established patient** is one who has received professional services from the healthcare provider or another healthcare provider of the same specialty and subspecialty in the same group practice within the last three years. An **inpatient** is a patient that has been formally admitted to an inpatient hospital. In behavioral health, it is common that patients are treated in a **partial hospitalization** setting, in which they receive mental health services as an inpatient during the day, but are released to go home in the evening. Partial hospitalization services are reported as inpatient services. **Outpatients** are patients that are seen in the hospital setting, but have not been formally admitted, such as those receiving hospital observation services or emergency department services.

3. *What is the place of service?* The place of service is where the service was delivered, such as outpatient office, skilled nursing facility, or hospital setting. Note that the place of service also plays a part in the patient status of either inpatient or outpatient. For example, a patient cannot be an *inpatient* in an *office* setting (because patients are not admitted into the office setting). These questions are simply to help understand the basic components of E/M code categories and assist with code selection.

Figure 7.2. Three factors of E/M codes

Type of service	• Office visit • Consultation • Team conference • Discharge
Patient status	• Inpatient • Outpatient • New • Established
Place of service	• Outpatient office • Hospital • Skilled nursing facility • Rest home

The answers to these questions are the components of the evaluation and management service that allow the coder to locate the correct section of E/M codes for the service to report.

Read the following vignette and note how Nidia locates the E/M codes she will be using to report an E/M service.

Nidia is learning how to select the codes for the psychiatrist's evaluation and management services. She is coding for a consultation that was provided to an inpatient with substance abuse in the hospital setting. Before she can determine the level of the service, she must define the three factors of the service, which will allow her to find the correct selection of codes in the E/M section. She asks herself and answers the following questions:

    What was the type of service? A consultation
    What is the patient status? Inpatient
    What is the place of service? Hospital

With this information she can review the E/M section to find the codes needed to report this service. Looking at the table of contents in the E/M section, she can see that there is a heading for consultations, with the code ranges next to the types of consultations (see figure 7.3). She knows that she is coding for an inpatient consultation, so she looks at the entry for Inpatient Consultations, New or Established Patient (99251–99255), on page 21 in her book. She then turns to page 21 and finds a range of E/M codes, code numbers 99251 through 99255.

Figure 7.3. Consultations entry in the E/M table of contents

Source: AMA 2018, 2.

For practice finding the correct selection of evaluation and management codes, complete the There's a Code for That 7.1.

There's a Code for That

7.1 Type of service, patient status, and place of service for E/M codes

Read the following evaluation and management statements and determine the type of service, patient status, and place of service. Then use the E/M table of contents to find the correct selection of E/M codes. Note that not all of these components will be available for all E/M services. The following example is done for you.

Psychiatrist performed a consultation on a 35-year-old female inpatient in the hospital setting.

   Type of service: consultation

   Patient status: inpatient

   Place of service: hospital

   E/M codes: 99251–99255

1. Outpatient office visit for a new patient with bipolar disorder.

   Type of service: _____

   Patient status: _____

   Place of service: _____

   E/M codes: _____

2. Subsequent nursing facility care provided to a 78-year-old male admitted to a nursing facility.

   Type of service: _____

   Patient status: _____

   Place of service: _____

   E/M codes: _____

3. Behavior change intervention provided to a new patient (individual).

   Type of service: _____

   Patient status: _____

   Place of service: _____

   E/M codes: _____

4. Initial hospital inpatient service provided to a patient with schizophrenia suffering from panic attack.

   Type of service: _____

   Patient status: _____

   Place of service: _____

   E/M codes: _____

5. Emergency department visit provided to a patient in crisis.

   Type of service: _____

   Patient status: _____

   Place of service: _____

   E/M codes: _____

Three Key Components to an E/M Service

There are three key components to an E/M service, each of which represents a different part of the evaluation and management service: history, examination, and medical decision making.

- **History** is the subjective information the patient tells the provider at the encounter. There are four elements of the history key component: chief complaint (C/C), history of present illness (HPI), review of systems (ROS), and past, family, social history (PFSH). Keep in mind that this is *subjective* information. The provider typically asks pointed questions to elicit more information from the patient and help determine what he or she needs to focus on during the physical examination. For example, if the patient says she has anxiety (subjective information), then the physician will focus on the physical symptoms of anxiety (objective information) portion of the encounter.

- **Examination** is the objective information resulting from a physical examination of the patient. A healthcare provider will perform an examination of specific body areas (BAs) or organ systems (OSs), depending on the patient's needs. For example, a provider seeing a patient for anxiety may find during the physical examination that the patient has been experiencing heart palpitations. The provider will then perform an examination on the cardiovascular system as well as the neurological and psychiatric systems.

- **Medical decision making (MDM)** is the portion of the evaluation and management encounter in which the healthcare provider makes a decision about the patient's diagnosis and care or treatment plan. The MDM is comprised of the number of possible diagnoses or treatment options, the amount and/or complexity of data to be reviewed, and the risk of complications or death if the condition was to go untreated. For example, the medical decision making for a patient with anxiety includes the number of possible diagnoses, such as anxiety, heart palpitations, or any other possible complications; any labs, imaging services, or other healthcare services that should be performed or reviewed; and the risk of complications if the anxiety and heart palpitations are left untreated.

There are four different levels of work related to each one of the key components, ranging from a low to high level of work or complexity. These levels are problem focused, expanded problem focused, detailed, and comprehensive for the key component of history and examination; and straightforward, low, moderate, and high for the key component of medical decision making (note that these levels and key components are discussed later in this chapter, and in more detail in chapter 8; they are also illustrated in figures 7.4 through 7.7).

E/M codes are developed this way so that when a provider performs *more* work for a specific evaluation and management service, he or she can bill at a higher level of service and receive more payment for the service. On the other hand, if a provider performs *less* work for a specific service, then he or she will bill for a lower level of service and will be paid less for it. In this way, providers can adjust how much they bill for an evaluation and management service according to the amount of work performed for the service (see figure 7.4 for a list of the three key components and how they relate to the levels of service performed). To select the correct E/M code, the coder must determine the level of each of these three key components and then locate the corresponding E/M code.

Figure 7.4. Elements of an E/M code

Levels of Key Components

There are four levels of each of the three key components of evaluation and management codes. Each level depends on the amount of work or complexity of the service. For example, if a provider performs a comprehensive examination of all body areas and organ systems on a patient, then this is a high level of the examination component (comprehensive). On the other hand, if a provider only performs a limited examination of one body area, then this would be a low level of the examination component (problem focused). When selecting the appropriate code for an E/M service, the coder must determine the level of each of the three key components, as follows (see also figures 7.5 through 7.7).

- **History.** The levels of the history obtained from the patient range from problem focused (lowest level of history), to expanded problem-focused (next-highest level), to detailed, and finally to comprehensive (highest level of history that can be obtained from the patient). For example, if a provider completed a very low-level of history, then the lowest level of this key component would be used to select the level of history for the service—problem-focused.

- **Examination.** The levels of the examination performed by the provider range from problemfocused (lowest level of examination), to expanded problem focused, then detailed, and finally to comprehensive (highest level of difficulty of the examination component). For example, if a provider completed a very high level of examination (a complete examination of multiple body areas and organ systems), then the highest level of this key component would be used to select the level of examination for the service—comprehensive.

- **Medical decision making (MDM).** The levels of MDM performed by the provider range from straightforward (lowest level of MDM), to low, then moderate, and finally high (highest level of difficulty of MDM). For example, if a patient with a simple problem (such as a small abrasion) was seen by the provider who only needed to perform a very low level of medical decision making to treat the patient, then the lowest level of this key component would be used to select the MDM level for the service—straightforward. Figures 7.5 through 7.7 illustrate the four levels of difficulty for each of the three key components.

These levels are based on the amount of work required, information reviewed, or complexity of the data taken into account during each component of the service. For the purposes of this chapter, vignettes, examples, and exercise and review questions will state the level of each key component. For example, *detailed examination* or *low MDM*.

Figure 7.5. Levels of the history key component

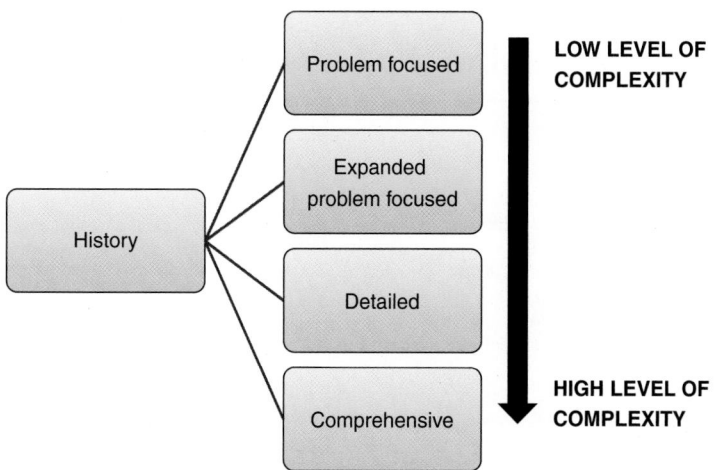

Figure 7.6. Levels of the examination key component

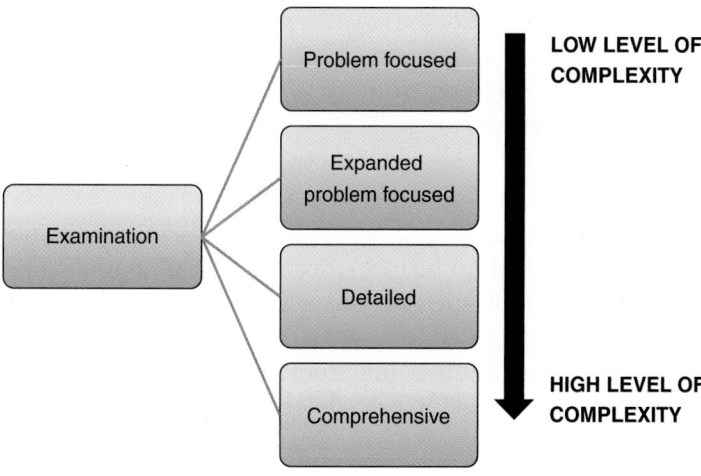

Figure 7.7. Levels of the medical decision making key component

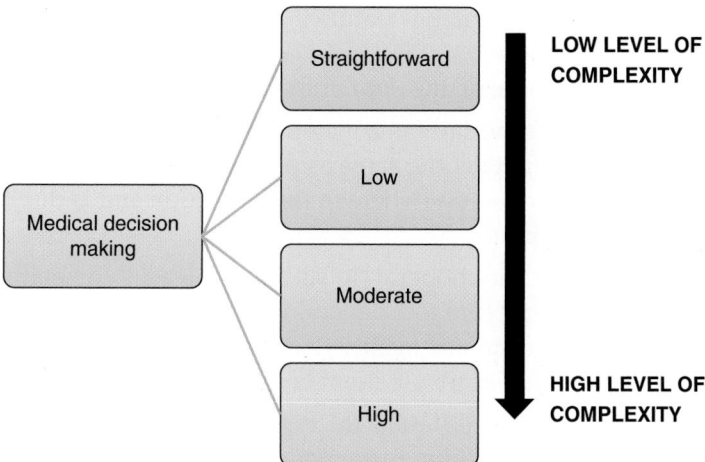

Figure 7.8. Steps to determine the level of E/M code

The following chapter, Primary Care, dives deeper into these levels, including how to select the correct level of each key component based on health record documentation. Figure 7.8 illustrates how the levels of the key components impact the level of E/M codes.

Some evaluation and management services do not depend on the levels of history, exam, and MDM, but rather on a contributory factor: counseling, coordination of care, or the nature of the presenting problem.

Contributory Factors

When the three key components are not applicable to the evaluation and management service (for example, if no standard history or physical examination is performed) and for certain E/M code categories (such as counseling codes), the levels of the three key components are not necessary for code selection. In these cases, it is necessary to consider the **contributory factors** of counseling, coordination of care, and the nature of the presenting problem, which are used to help determine the level of the E/M service.

- **Counseling** is the discussion between a healthcare provider and a patient and/or patient's family. This discussion may include
    ○ Diagnostic results, impressions, and/or recommended diagnostic studies
    ○ Prognosis (the expected outcome of the patient's medical diagnosis)
    ○ Risks and benefits of management or treatment options
    ○ Follow-up, management, or treatment instructions and compliance advice
    ○ Risk factor reduction
    ○ Education of the patient and/or family (AMA 2017)

    It is important to note, especially in behavioral health coding, that the contributory factor of counseling it *not* the same as psychotherapy counseling. Psychotherapy counseling is coded elsewhere in the CPT book and is discussed in the next section of this chapter.

- **Coordination of care** is the cooperation between at least two healthcare practitioners in providing care to a patient. Coordination of care activities might include transfer from one facility to another, or may be an agreement on treatment methodologies for a patient between a PCP and a specialist.

- **Nature of the presenting problem** is the type of condition for which the patient is receiving the evaluation and management service. A presenting problem is a disease, condition, illness, injury, symptom, sign, finding, complaint, or other reason for a healthcare encounter that prompts a patient to seek healthcare treatment. There are five levels of presenting problems:

- *Minimal.* This problem may or may not require the presence of the provider, but services are provided under the provider's supervision.
- *Self-limited or minor.* This problem either runs a definite prescribed course, is transient in nature and is not likely to permanently alter the patient's health status, or has a good prognosis with medical management.
- *Low severity.* This problem has a low risk of morbidity or mortality without treatment, and from which a full recovery is expected.
- *Moderate severity.* This problem either has a moderate risk of morbidity or mortality without treatment, or has an increased probability of prolonged functional impairment.
- *High severity.* This problem either has a high to extreme risk of morbidity or mortality without treatment, or has a high probability of severe, prolonged functional impairment. (AMA 2017)

When counseling and/or coordination of care is the determining factor of an evaluation and management service, the time spent counseling or coordinating care may be used to determine the level of the E/M service. In order to use the *time* component as the determining factor of the E/M service, more than 50 percent of the face-to-face time spent with the patient (in the outpatient setting) or floor/unit time (in a hospital or nursing facility setting) must have been spent on counseling or coordination of care. The amount of time must be clearly documented in the health record and the extent of counseling and/or coordination of care must be included.

The three key components, contributory factors, and time are all listed in E/M codes, with varying levels. The majority (although not all) E/M code descriptions are formatted so that coders can clearly select the level of each of these components and select the correct code (see figure 7.9 for the anatomy of an E/M code, which identifies all these elements within the code description). It is important to understand the format of these codes to be able to select the appropriate one.

E/M Exceptions for Behavioral Health

Some of the evaluation and management codes used in behavioral health do not fit within the typical format for E/M codes, in that they do not require identification of the levels of any of the key components or contributory factors. These E/M codes are exceptions to the rule. Medical team conferences (99366–99368), smoking and tobacco use/alcohol and/or substance abuse cessation counseling (99406–99409), telephone and online services (99441–99444), and disability evaluation services (99450) are a few of the other E/M services performed by behavioral health specialists. These codes do not include descriptions of the levels of key components, contributory factors, and patient status, even though they are included within the E/M codes section; they simply describe the service performed. For example, 99406, Smoking and tobacco cessation counseling visit; intermediate, greater than 3 minutes up to 10 minutes.

Selecting the Level of E/M Service

Evaluation and management code descriptions are carefully formatted to identify the patient status, type of service, place of service, the levels of each of the key components, contributory factors, time, and the number of key components that must be met for each specific E/M code. Study figure 7.9 to learn the anatomy of an E/M code.

Figure 7.9. Anatomy of an E/M code

Source: AMA 2018, 13.

Each E/M code begins with the description of the type and place of service (office or other outpatient visit), a description of patient status (established), and the required number of key components. The required amount of key components is the number of key components that must be met at least at the levels identified in the code description.

Sometimes, the level of *one* key component may exceed the level in the code description, whereas the levels of the other *two* key components are at the levels identified in the code description. For example, a provider might have provided a comprehensive (highest level) MDM for an encounter with a detailed history and examination, reported with 99214 (as described in figure 7.9). In this case, the coder must select the code for which all levels as required (either 2 or 3) are *at least* at the level identified in the code description. For instance, because the two lowest levels were detailed the coder cannot select a higher level than detailed. The two common denominators (detailed history and detailed examination) are the basis for code selection. Sometimes, the levels of *two* key components go beyond those identified in the code description. However, if all *three* key components must be met, the coder must select the code in which all three are at least met by the code description.

The next section of the code description is three bullet points, each identifying the required level of each key component. Then the contributory factors are listed, followed by the nature of the presenting problem(s), and the time requirement for the code. Remember that time may only be used when more than 50 percent of the time spent face-to-face (in the office or outpatient setting, or on the unit/floor in the inpatient or hospital setting) with the patient is on counseling or coordination of care.

Return to our example of Nidia, who had determined that her E/M code was within the 99251 through 99255 range for an inpatient hospital consultation.

Now that Nidia has found the code range for the service that was provided, she needs to check the documentation to determine the levels of each of the three key components so she can select the correct code within the 99251 to 99255 code range. Upon looking at the documentation, she determines that the psychiatrist provided a DETAILED HISTORY, a DETAILED EXAMINATION, and MDM OF LOW COMPLEXITY.

Nidia checks the required key components in each of the code descriptions within the code range 99251 through 99255, and notes that code 99253 also requires a detailed history, detailed examination, and MDM of low complexity. The levels of all three of the key components match, so Nidia knows this is the correct code. She assigns 99253 on the claim.

Complete the following practice exercises in There's a Code for That 7.2 to test your ability to assign codes based on the levels of the three key components.

Selecting the level of E/M services

7.2

There's a Code for That

Read the following E/M statements, determine the level of the E/M service, and assign the E/M code. Remember to check the required number of key components for each service for each category of E/M codes.

1. Office visit for a new patient with an expanded problem-focused history, an expanded problem- focused examination, and straightforward MDM.

   E/M code: _____

2. Office visit for an established patient with depression. Provider performed a comprehensive history, comprehensive examination, and MDM of moderate complexity.

   E/M code: _____

3. Problem-focused history, problem-focused examination, and straightforward MDM for an office visit for an established patient.

   E/M code: _____

4. Initial hospital care provided to a psychiatric patient. Provider performed a comprehensive history and exam, with MDM of moderate complexity.

   E/M code: _____

5. Subsequent hospital care provider to a psychiatric patient. Provider performed an expanded problem-focused history, problem-focused exam, with MDM of low complexity.

   E/M code: _____

6. Outpatient consultation provided to a patient with body dysmorphic disorder. Comprehensive history and detailed examination performed with moderate MDM.

   E/M code: _____

(Continued on next page)

7.2

Continued

7. Subsequent nursing facility care provided to a 60-year-old woman with paranoid schizophrenia. History was problem focused, examination was expanded problem focused, and MDM was low complexity.

E/M code: _____

8. Emergency department visit for an 18-year-old female presenting with suicidal ideation and anxiety. Provider performed a detailed history and examination with moderate complexity MDM.

E/M code: _____

Psychiatry Coding

Most behavioral health codes are found in the Psychiatry subsection of the Medicine section of the CPT code book, codes 90785 through 90899. These codes are for diagnostic services, psychotherapy, and other services performed on an individual, family, or group. When using the codes from this section, pay close attention to the service performed, whether or not an evaluation and management service was performed along with the service, who was involved in the service, and the length of time of the service. Codes described in this section include psychotherapy codes, other psychotherapy services or procedures, psychiatric services, and telemedicine services.

Key to Success

As with most of the subsections within the Medicine section, there are a number of guidelines within the Psychiatry section of the CPT code book. When coding from this subsection, be sure to read the guidelines and highlight, underline, make notes, or place a star next to important sections. These guidelines are the rule book for using codes from that section—make sure you utilize them!

Psychotherapy Codes

The most commonly used psychiatry codes for behavioral health providers are psychotherapy codes (90832 through 90853). **Psychotherapy** is the treatment of mental illness and behavioral disturbance in which the healthcare provider attempts to alleviate the emotional disturbances, reverse or change patterns of behavior, and encourage personality growth and development through discourse with the patient.

Depending on the needs of the patient, psychotherapy sessions can range from 30 to 60 minutes, and may or may not be performed with an evaluation and management service (which would be reported with an E/M code). Psychotherapy may be performed on an individual patient, with the patient's family (with or without the patient present), with a multi-family group, or with a non-family group. Special codes exist for psychoanalysis, psychotherapy performed on a patient in crisis, and for psychotherapy performed with interactive complexity. **Interactive complexity** is a psychotherapy service provided to a patient with specific communication factors that complicate delivery of psychiatric procedures. For example, a nonverbal adult might require the use of equipment, other physical devices, an interpreter, or a translator to help overcome communication barriers. This would be reported with the interactive complexity add-on code (for a refresher on add-on codes, see chapter 5).

An important part of coding for psychotherapy services is the use of add-on codes to report all aspects of the service performed. For example, code 90836, Psychotherapy, 45 minutes with patient when performed with an evaluation and management service, is an add-on code that should be reported in addition to the code for the primary procedure (the E/M code). If a provider performed an E/M service on a patient and then provided 45 minutes of psychotherapy, then the coder would report one code for each service: the code for the E/M service (such as 99213, Office or other outpatient visit for the evaluation and management of an established patient, which requires two out of three of the following key components: expanded problem-focused history, expanded problem-focused examination, medical decision making of low complexity), in addition to the code for the psychotherapy (90836, Psychotherapy, 45 minutes with patient when performed with an evaluation and management service). If the psychotherapy was also provided with interactive complexity, then the add-on code for interactive complexity would be coded in addition to the E/M code and the psychotherapy code.

Reporting add-on codes requires close reading, ensuring to account for all components of the patient encounter. In the previous example, the coder should report one code for the medical evaluation and management service that was performed, and then note that an additional service was performed—the 45 minutes of psychotherapy, which should also be reported with the appropriate code. Note that under the code description for 90836 is the parenthetical notation: "Use 90836 in conjunction with 99201–99255, 99304–99337, 99341–99350." This tells the coder it is appropriate to report the psychotherapy code to the code for the E/M service.

Key to Success

Add-on codes are often used in addition to other procedure codes to identify certain procedures that are performed together. If the description for the primary procedure does not include the additional services performed, then the coder should search for thee additional procedures and report any add-on codes, as necessary. For a refresher on add-on codes, see chapter 5.

Read the following example and notice how Nidia codes for the psychotherapy services performed with interactive complexity on a child.

Lisette, an 8-year-old nonverbal female with autism and bipolar disorder presents for a medication refill and monthly psychotherapy session. She is an established patient. The psychiatrist documents a medical evaluation and management encounter with an expanded problem-focused history, expanded problem-focused examination, and medical decision making of low complexity. She then completes 30 minutes of psychotherapy with the patient using interactive complexity.

Nidia chooses three codes—one for the E/M service, an add-on code for the psychotherapy, and another add-on code for the interactive complexity. She reports the following codes:

- *99213, Level 3 office visit, established patient*
- *90833, Psychotherapy, 30 minutes with patient when performed with an E/M service*
- *90785, Interactive complexity*

Once Nidia has selected her procedure codes, she then must assign the appropriate diagnosis code(s) to identify the medical necessity for the procedures.

When a non-medical clinician—such as a prescribing psychologist—performs pharmacologic management including prescription and review of medication in addition to psychotherapy services, the add-on code 90863, Pharmacologic management, should be used. This code was specifically designed for use by psychologists who are licensed to prescribe but cannot bill for an E/M code (because they are not healthcare providers). For example, if a prescribing psychologist performed a 45-minute individual psychotherapy session in addition to pharmacologic management, then the coder should report codes 90834, Psychotherapy, 45 minutes with patient, and 90863, Pharmacologic management.

Other Psychiatric Services or Procedures

In addition to psychotherapy services, there are a number of treatments and other services that can be performed for behavioral health patients. These include

- **Narcosynthesis for psychiatric purposes** (90865), or the administration of sodium amobarbitol (otherwise known as a truth serum), which hinders inhibitions so that a psychiatric interview can be conducted.
- **Transcranial magnetic stimulation (TMS)** treatment (90867 to 90869) is a non-invasive procedure that utilizes magnetic fields to stimulate areas of the brain, and is used as a treatment for depression that does not respond to medication treatment.
- **Electroconvulsive therapy (ECT)** (90870), involves the application of an electric current to a patient's brain to produce a seizure or series of seizures to alleviate mental illness; primarily depression that is nonresponsive to treatment. If the psychiatrist also administers anesthesia for the service, the anesthesia should be reported separately, in addition to the code for the ECT.
- **Vagus nerve stimulation** (95970, 95974, 95975), is the stimulation of implanted electrodes in the vagus nerve in the cranium as a treatment for depression that is resistant to medication.

Key to Success

Note that even though the codes described here are not located within the Psychiatry subsection, they are still used for behavioral health services. It is common to find codes for a certain specialty throughout the CPT code book.

The codes for these services should be reported in addition to any E/M or psychotherapy services also performed at the same session or on the same date of service. Remember that if an E/M service is performed with any additional service, modifier -25 should be appended to the E/M code to distinguish it as a significant, separately identifiable service from the psychiatry service. For a refresher on modifiers and their uses, see chapter 5.

Psychiatric Screenings

There are several psychiatric and psychological screenings, tests, and evaluations used to determine the risk of a patient having a mental illness or substance abuse issue, or whether or not the issue is already present. For example, at a six-week postnatal checkup, a mother might receive a postpartum depression screening. Even though this is a mental health screening, it is administered in the primary care setting to determine if the patient needs to be seen by a mental health practitioner. This is very common, as most mental health screenings like this are administered by a primary care practitioner, to determine if a patient is in need of behavioral health services. After a screening, if it is determined that the patient needs behavioral health services, then he or she will be transferred into the care of a behavioral health professional. Some psychiatric screenings may be covered for primary care providers only, whereas others may be covered for behavioral health providers only. This depends on the insurance billed and the patient's diagnosis.

Ultimately, whether or not the behavioral health provider gives and reports screening services depends on the individual practice. Behavioral health screening services include the following components.

- Psychiatric diagnostic evaluation, with or without medical services (90791 and 90792), which may be provided by a primary care physician.
- Behavior change interventions (99408 and 99409), such as the **Screening, Brief Intervention and Referral to Treatment (SBIRT)**, administered to patients with suspected alcohol or substance abuse. For Medicare patients, coders would use HCPCS codes G0396 and G0397 to report the administration of the same screening; and for Medicaid, coders should report HCPCS codes H0049 and H0050.
- Psychological and neuropsychological testing (96101 through 96127) services include an array of different psychological, developmental, neurobehavioral, neuropsychological, and emotional and behavioral assessments. These assessments may be provided by different practitioners, from primary care providers to therapists.
- Health and behavior assessments and interventions (96150 through 96161) are used to identify the psychological, behavioral, emotional, cognitive, and social factors vital to the prevention, treatment, or management of physical health problems. Behavioral health providers should not report these services if another, more predominant psychiatric service was performed.

Key to Success

Do not forget about the differences in billing requirements for various insurance types. An example of this is in administering drug and alcohol screenings to patients. Commercial insurance requires CPT codes 99406 through 99409, Medicare requires HCPCS codes G0396 and G0397, and Medicaid requires HCPCS codes H0049 and H0050— all for the same services! This is yet one more reason why it is important as a coder to always keep the patient's insurance in mind, as the codes may differ greatly depending on where the claim is sent and the setting in which the services are rendered.

Telemedicine Services

It is important to note that many of the behavioral health services described in the previous sections may be performed via telemedicine (as noted by the ★ symbol next to the listed codes in the CPT code book). To report a telemedicine service, the coder must report the service with the regular CPT code, appended with modifier -95, Synchronous telemedicine service. For example, if a psychiatrist performed 30 minutes of psychotherapy via a telemedicine platform for a nonmobile patient in a rural area, then he or she would report 90832, Psychotherapy, 30 minutes with patient, with modifier -95, Telemedicine service (90832-95).

MOD

Modifier -95, Synchronous telemedicine service rendered via a real-time interactive audio and video telecommunications systems must be appended to any service that is performed via a telemedicine platform. When coding for telemedicine services, check for two things: the CPT code must be a telemedicine code (it will have the ★ star symbol next to it in the CPT Tabular List and it will be listed in Appendix P), *and* it must be appended with modifier -95 to identify that the procedure was performed as a telemedicine service.

Complete the following practice exercises in There's a Code for That 7.3 to test your ability to assign psychiatric procedure codes.

7.3

There's a Code for That

Assigning psychiatric procedure codes

Read the following procedural statements and assign the appropriate psychiatric procedural codes.

1. Psychotherapy for crisis, 30 minutes.

   CPT code: _____

2. 45 minutes of individual psychophysiological therapy incorporating feedback training, with supportive psychotherapy.

   CPT code: _____

3. Psychotherapy, 30 minutes, delivered via telemedicine platform.

   CPT code: _____

4. Substance abuse screening assessment and intervention delivered to a Medicare patient, 45 minutes total service time.

   CPT code: _____

5. 60 minutes psychotherapy performed with interactive complexity.

   CPT code: _____ , _____

6. TMS, initial, delivery and management.

   CPT code: _____

Diagnosis Coding for Behavioral Health

Diagnostic coding for behavioral health services is a bit different than any other specialty. Rather than utilize the ICD-10-CM code book by itself, behavioral health providers also use the **Diagnostic and Statistical Manual of Mental Disorders**, currently in its 5th edition (DSM-5). Published by the American Psychiatric Association, the DSM-5 is the standard reference for behavioral health practitioners in the United States. For coding purposes, it is used in conjunction with the ICD-10-CM to classify mental illness and substance abuse disorders.

Coders working in the behavioral health field may use a DSM-5 code book to cross reference behavioral health diagnoses with ICD-10-CM codes, although this is not necessary. Although the DSM-5 code book does list associated ICD-10-CM codes along with descriptions of mental disorders, the ICD-10-CM code book is still the standard set of diagnosis codes that should be used for billing and reporting purposes. Ultimately, the DSM-5 is useful for coders because it can help identify the codes that should be used for diagnosed conditions; however, these codes should still be verified using the ICD-10-CM code book. Diagnosis codes for behavioral health and common behavioral health diagnoses are discussed in the following sections.

Diagnosis Codes in Behavioral Health

As in any specialty, ICD-10-CM codes identify the medical necessity for the service performed. Because insurance regulations and guidelines might be stricter regarding behavioral health services, it is important to have a clear understanding of what a patient's insurance plan will accept as medical necessity for specific behavioral health services. For example, transcranial magnetic stimulation (TMS) is typically only covered as a treatment for depression, even though research has shown that it may have a benefit for other mental health conditions such as schizophrenia (Cole 2015). So if a patient was receiving TMS treatment for schizophrenia, this would likely *not* be covered by his or her insurance plan.

The primary diagnosis for behavioral health services should reflect either the reason for the visit or the focus of the treatment. If the patient has multiple diagnoses, then as many diagnoses as necessary should be listed to accurately provide a clinical picture of the patient's mental health status. For example, if a patient is seen for a prescription refill for his attention-deficit hyperactivity disorder, and his co-occurring diagnosis of anxiety was also managed, then there would be two codes reported: F90.9, Attention-deficit hyperactivity disorder, unspecified type, and F41.9, Anxiety disorder, unspecified.

It is common for patients with substance abuse disorders to present with co-occurring mental health disorders as well as physical health issues. According to ICD-10-CM coding guidelines, coders should code all documented conditions that coexist at the time of the encounter or visit, and require or affect patient care treatment or management. Do not code conditions that previously existed and no longer exist. However, patient history codes may be necessary to identify a historical condition that impacts the patient's current care or treatment.

In ICD-10-CM, there is an additional category of codes used to represent psychosocial and environmental problems, Z55 to Z65, Persons with potential health hazards related to socioeconomic and psychosocial circumstances. These codes are used to identify additional factors that may have an impact on a patient's mental health or substance abuse issues. For example, if a patient presents with depression due to bipolar disorder, exacerbated by the fact that she was recently separated from her husband of 20 years, then the following codes would be appropriate: F31.31, Bipolar disorder, current episode depressed, mild, and Z63.5, Disruption of family by separation and divorce.

Key to Success

It might be difficult to know what you should code when reading a diagnostic statement. To make sure you have coded all possible diagnoses, a good rule of thumb is to code until you can code no longer. For example, if the diagnostic statement describes relevant patient history codes or social circumstances, check for ICD-10-CM codes to see if there are any codes that correspond to either the history or the social circumstance. This is especially important in HCC coding, which requires that each visit be coded to the full extent.

Most of the diagnosis codes used in behavioral health will be found in chapter 5 of the ICD-10-CM code book—Mental, Behavioral and Neurodevelopmental Disorders. Many of these codes are presented in a spectrum concept, including substance abuse, autism, and schizophrenia. For example, the spectrum of substance abuse goes from the earliest stages of the condition (use) to later stages (abuse and dependence). Other mental health disorders are presented in a spectrum, from a minor version of the condition to a more advanced problem.

Codes that are reported for mental health and substance abuse services often include the following types of specifications.

- Course (for example, in remission or withdrawal)
- Severity (how bad the condition is)
- Frequency (how often it occurs)
- Duration (how long the condition has persisted)
- Descriptive features (clinical features of the condition) (Reichenberg 2014)

Unspecified and other specified (NOS and NEC) versions of behavioral health diagnosis codes are also used (see chapter 4 for a description of NOS and NEC diagnosis codes). Other specified (NEC) codes should be used to identify conditions in which the symptoms of the disorder are present (and documented), but do not fully meet the code description. Unspecified (NOS) codes should be used when the provider has not fully specified the condition and the clinical criteria for the condition have not been fully documented.

The following section discusses common behavioral health conditions that are reported with ICD-10-CM codes.

Common Behavioral Health Diagnoses

Although behavioral health providers can see and treat any mental health disorder, it is common that some providers specialize in certain disorders. For example, substance abuse requires a specific type of management and course of treatment, so it is common for a provider to treat only substance abuse patients. The following lists some of the more common behavioral health diagnoses.

- **Depression** (F32 to F34) is a mental disorder that affects a person's mood, thoughts, and actions. Symptoms include weight loss or gain, feeling sad or tired, crying for no reason, lack of interest, sleeping too much or too little, thoughts of death and suicide, feeling worthless, and difficulty concentrating. Symptoms must be present every day for at least two weeks to be classified as depression. Codes for depression identify the episode, severity, and whether or not it presents with psychotic features or if it is in remission.

- Substance Use and Abuse (F10 to F19) are the only behavioral health codes that have applicable official coding guidelines (see figure 7.10). To code accurately for substance abuse or use, the substance must be identified first. There are specific categories available for alcohol, opioids, cannabis, sedatives, hypnotics and anxiolytics, cocaine, other stimulants, hallucinogens, nicotine, inhalants, and other psychoactive substances. It is then necessary to identify the severity of the condition in terms of substance use, abuse, or dependence. According to ICD-10-CM guidelines, only one code should be reported for each substance, according to the following hierarchy (see figure 7.10):
  - If abuse and use are documented for the same substance, code for abuse.

- If abuse and dependence are documented for the same substance, code for dependence.
- If use, abuse, and dependence are all documented for the same condition, code for dependence.
- If use and dependence are documented, code only for dependence.

Codes also identify the course of the substance use—for example, in withdrawal, with intoxication, and in remission. For remission status, the provider needs to document that the patient is in remission in order to be able to report the code for remission status. Note that these are complex codes that require careful reading of the code description.

- **Anxiety disorders** (F40 and F41) are mental disorders that result in constant feelings of worry, fear, and panic when faced with everyday situations. There are many types of anxiety disorders including phobias— fears of specific everyday things like going outside or being in a social environment. Codes for phobias identify the specific fear, and anxiety codes specify the type of anxiety. Note that there is one specific code for a panic attack.

- **Bipolar disorder** (F30 and F31) is a mental disorder that affects a person's mood and behavior by switching from extreme highs (mania) to extreme lows (depression). Symptoms include agitation, restlessness, sleeping less, speaking too fast, taking unnecessary risks, laughing uncontrollably inability to concentrate, depressed feelings once the manic period is over. Bipolar disorder codes specify the features of the current episode (such as manic or depressed), as well as the severity of the condition, and with or without psychotic features and if it is in remission.

Figure 7.10. OGCR I.C.5.b

---

b. Mental and behavioral disorders due to psychoactive substance use

1) In Remission

Selection of codes for "in remission" for categories F10-F19, Mental and behavioral disorders due to psychoactive substance use (categories F10-F19 with **-.11**, -.21) requires the provider's clinical judgment. The appropriate codes for "in remission" are assigned only on the basis of provider documentation (as defined in the Official Guidelines for Coding and Reporting), **unless otherwise instructed by the classification.**

Mild substance use disorders in early or sustained remission are classified to the appropriate codes for substance abuse in remission, and moderate or severe substance use disorders in early or sustained remission are classified to the appropriate codes for substance dependence in remission.

2) Psychoactive Substance Use, Abuse And Dependence

When the provider documentation refers to use, abuse and dependence of the same substance (e.g. alcohol, opioid, cannabis, etc.), only one code should be assigned to identify the pattern of use based on the following hierarchy:

- If both use and abuse are documented, assign only the code for abuse
- If both abuse and dependence are documented, assign only the code for dependence
- If use, abuse and dependence are all documented, assign only the code for dependence
- If both use and dependence are documented, assign only the code for dependence.

3) Psychoactive Substance Use *Disorders*

As with all other diagnoses, the codes for psychoactive substance use **disorders** (F10.9-, F11.9-, F12.9-, F13.9-, F14.9-, F15.9-, F16.9-) should only be assigned based on provider documentation and when they meet the definition of a reportable diagnosis (see Section III, Reporting Additional Diagnoses). The codes are to be used only when the psychoactive substance use is associated with a **physical,** mental or behavioral disorder, and such a relationship is documented by the provider.

Source: CMS 2018.

- **Eating disorders** (F50) affect the way a person eats or processes food and nutrition. There are two types of eating disorders, anorexia nervosa and bulimia. Anorexia symptoms include extreme underweight, constant thoughts about food, weight and body image, refusal to eat, fear of gaining weight, lack of menstruation, and excessive exercise. Bulimia symptoms include too much dieting and exercise, excessive use of laxatives, dehydration, lack of menstruation, poor body image, and going to the bathroom directly after eating.

- **Schizophrenia** (F20 to F29) is a mental disorder that manifests in the symptoms of delusions, hallucinations, paranoia, confused speech, isolation, outbursts of anger, and catatonic behavior that persist for at least one month. When coding for schizophrenia, it is important to note if there is any substance abuse causing the schizophrenia, or if it is related to a brain disease such as epilepsy. These may impact the schizophrenia codes reported.

- **Attention-deficit hyperactivity disorders (ADHD)** (F90) typically usually in school-age children and impact a child's school and social functioning. Symptoms include impulsivity, inattention, difficulty concentrating and following directions, difficulty completing tasks, too much energy, and restlessness. Codes for ADHD differentiate between the type (predominantly inattentive, hyperactive, combined, or other specified type). Note that although this condition is commonly seen in children, these codes can be used for patients of any age.

HCC Coding Corner

HCC

Most behavioral health codes are included in hierarchical condition categories (HCC), including depression, substance abuse, bipolar disorder, ADHD, and schizophrenia. Be careful when selecting these codes for HCC reporting purposes! Documentation for behavioral health conditions must be specific enough to support the code selected. This includes specification of the course, severity, frequency, duration, and descriptive features.

Complete the following practice exercises in There's a Code for That 7.4 to test your ability to assign behavioral health diagnosis codes.

7.4

There's a Code for That

Assigning behavioral health diagnosis codes

Read the following diagnostic statements and assign the appropriate behavioral health diagnosis codes.

1. Patient presents for major depressive disorder, mild, single episode.

   ICD-10-CM code: _____

2. 10-year-old female with history of childhood abuse presents for treatment of generalized anxiety disorder and moderate recurrent depression.

   ICD-10-CM codes: _____, _____,

   _____

3. Anorexia nervosa, binge eating/purging type.

   ICD-10-CM code: _____

4. Oppositional defiant disorder.

ICD-10-CM code: _____

5. Patient presents for treatment of opioid use. He is opioid dependent, currently in remission.

ICD-10-CM code: _____

6. Patient presents for treatment of chronic post-traumatic stress disorder due to exposure to war while in the military two years ago.

ICD-10-CM code: _____, _____

Putting It All Together: Coding for Behavioral Health Services

In order to select the correct code for the behavioral health encounter, it is important to carefully read the documentation and then access each code book to find the procedure or service provided and the corresponding diagnosis or diagnoses to support the medical necessity for the service. Procedural codes for behavioral health services are found in the CPT and HCPCS code books, and diagnosis codes are found in the ICD-10-CM code book.

Determination of the correct codes for relies on the answers to the following questions.

- What service was provided to the patient? Was an evaluation and management service provided in addition to a psychiatric service?
- Are there any applicable modifiers or add-on codes?
- What is the primary condition being treated? This will be the reason for the visit or the focus of the treatment.
- Are there any additional co-occurring mental health or physical health diagnoses?

Study the following vignette that demonstrates how to select the appropriate diagnosis and procedure codes. Then complete the following practice exercises in There's a Code for That 7.5.

Now that Nidia is finished with her training, she is responsible for coding the services provided to patients in the behavioral health clinic. She is coding both the procedural and diagnosis codes for the following encounter: A 35-year-old female established patient presented to the office for psychotherapy and medication refill for multiple personality disorder. The provider performed an evaluation and management visit with an expanded problem-focused history and MDM of low complexity, as well as 30 to 45 minutes of psychotherapy with interactive complexity using expressive art therapy.

First, she asks herself: What did the doctor do? The doctor performed an E/M encounter, psychotherapy, and art therapy (interactive complexity). She looks up the procedures codes in the CPT book and finds the following codes.

> *99213, Office or other outpatient visit for the evaluation and management of an established patient, which requires at least 2 out of 3 of the following: expanded problem-focused history, expanded problem-focused examination, medical decision making of low complexity;*
>
> *90836, Psychotherapy, 45 minutes when performed with E/M service; and*
>
> *90785, Interactive complexity.*

Now that she has her procedure codes, Nidia asks herself: Why did the doctor do it? The patient presented for treatment of multiple personality disorder. She looks up this condition in the ICD-10-CM code book and finds the following code.

> *F44.81, Dissociative identity disorder*

She then rechecks the documentation to ensure she has coded everything for the encounter and reports the chosen codes on the claim for the service.

7.5   Coding for behavioral health services

There's a Code for That

Read the following documentation from patient encounters and assign the appropriate procedure and diagnosis codes.

1. Patient presents for treatment of recurrent severe depression without psychotic symptoms, which is not responding to combination of medication and psychotherapy treatments. Today she is receiving an initial delivery and management via TMS therapy.

   CPT code: _____

   ICD-10-CM code: _____

2. Narcosynthesis evaluation of a patient with alcohol dependence with alcohol-induced bipolar disorder.

   CPT code: _____

   ICD-10-CM code: _____

3. 42-year-old new patient is brought into the office by his family for evaluation of alcohol abuse with paranoid delusions. A comprehensive history and examination were performed; MDM was high complexity. Patient was prescribed a neuroleptic and referred to an Alcoholics Anonymous program.

   CPT code: _____

   ICD-10-CM code: _____

4. Initial hospital care provided to a patient with severe psychotic features. A comprehensive history and examination are performed, with high complexity MDM. She was diagnosed with paranoid schizophrenia.

   CPT code: _____

   ICD-10-CM code: _____

5. Nurse practitioner performed 30 minutes of psychotherapy and pharmacologic management for a patient with moderate bipolar disorder without psychotic features (current episode manic), and generalized social phobia.

   CPT codes: _____, _____

   ICD-10-CM codes: _____, _____

End of Chapter Content

Instructions: Indicate whether the following statements are true or false (T or F). For false statements, rewrite the statement on the line below to make the statement true.

1. The behavioral health specialty is comprised of mental health and substance abuse services.

_____

_____

2. A child and adolescent psychiatrist is a subspecialist in the field of behavioral health.

_____

_____

3. The SBIRT is administered to patient with suspected mental illness.

_____

_____

4. Evaluation and management codes are often used in behavioral health coding.

_____

_____

5. A new patient is one who has not been seen by a healthcare provider or another healthcare provider of the same subspecialty in the same group practice within the past two years.

_____

_____

6. The three key components of an E/M service are history, evaluation, and medical decision making.

_____

_____

7. Contributory factors are the discussion between a healthcare provider and a patient or patient's family.

_____

_____

(Continued on next page)

(Continued)

8. Behavioral health procedural coding is largely comprised of E/M codes and codes within the Psychiatry subsection.

_____

_____

9. The CPT code range 90785 through 90899 includes psychiatry codes used in behavioral health coding.

_____

_____

10. The add-on code for interactive complexity is 90785.

_____

_____

Instructions: Choose the best answer.

1. Which of the following refers to a person's emotional, psychological, and social well-being?
  a. Substance abuse
  b. Mental health
  c. Mental illness
  d. Behavioral health

2. Which of the following is the misuse of alcohol or drugs, which impairs a person's ability to meet daily responsibilities?
  a. Substance abuse
  b. Mental health
  c. Mental illness
  d. Behavioral health

3. What must a behavioral health coder always consider when coding for services?
  a. The age of the patient
  b. The residency status of the patient
  c. The services requested by the patient
  d. The patient's health insurance coverage and limitations

4. What is a request from a provider of services to an insurance company to authorize a service before it is performed?
  a. Referral request
  b. Consultation
  c. Prior authorization
  d. Claim denial

5. What is placed in box 24.B of the CMS-1500 claim form?
  a. Date of service
  b. CPT code(s)
  c. ICD-10 code(s)
  d. Place of service

6. Evaluation and management code are used to report which of the following?
  a. Medical management of a patient
  b. Psychotherapy services
  c. Specialized screenings and diagnostic tests
  d. Electroconvulsive therapy

7. The type of service of an E/M code is which of the following?
  a. The patient's status as new, established, inpatient, or outpatient
  b. The type of evaluation and management encounter that was provided
  c. The setting in which the service was provided
  d. The type of provider that performed the service

8. Which patient type has been formally admitted to an inpatient hospital?
  a. Outpatient
  b. Observation
  c. Inpatient
  d. Initial

9. An established patient is one who has been seen within the last how many years?

a. Two
b. Three
c. Four
d. One

10. Which of the following is the subjective information the patient tells a provider at the encounter?

a. History
b. Examination
c. Medical decision making
d. Evaluation

11. In which portion of an E/M service does the provider make a decision regarding the patient's diagnoses and care or treatment plan?

a. History
b. Examination
c. Medical decision making
d. Evaluation

12. How many levels of each of the key components are there?

a. Four
b. Three
c. Two
d. Six

13. What are counseling, coordination of care, and nature of the presenting problem?

a. Contributory factors
b. Time components
c. Key components
d. These are not taken into account in E/M coding

14. What is the treatment of a mental illness in which the healthcare provider attempts to alleviate disturbances, reverse or change patterns of behavior, and encourage personality growth and development, through discourse with the patient?

a. Coordination of care
b. Evaluation and management service
c. Psychiatric initial evaluation
d. Psychotherapy

15. Which of the following is a non-invasive procedure that uses magnetic fields to stimulate areas of the brain?

a. Vagus nerve stimulation
b. Transcranial magnetic stimulation
c. Electroconvulsive therapy
d. Narcosynthesis

16. Which modifier should be reported with telemedicine services?

a. -51
b. -25
c. -95
d. None

17. When should other specified diagnosis codes be reported?

a. When identifying conditions in which the symptoms of the disorder are present but do not fully meet the code description
b. When the provider has not fully specified the condition and the clinical criteria have not been fully documented
c. When the condition cannot be determined to be one of two variables
d. When identifying conditions that are not fully specified in the documentation

18. The ICD-10 code book has chapter-specific guidelines on coding which of the following conditions?

a. Anxiety disorders
b. Depression
c. Substance abuse disorders
d. Attention-deficit hyperactivity disorder

Instructions: Answer the following questions with the appropriate code(s).

1. Psychotherapy provided to a patient in crisis with severe paranoid schizophrenia, 90 minutes total time.

CPT code(s): _____ , _____

ICD-10 code(s): _____

2. E/M encounter for established patient in the outpatient office setting, detailed history and examination. Psychotherapy of 45 minutes

was also performed on patient with moderate recurrent depression and acute PTSD due to her personal history of childhood neglect.

CPT code(s): _____ , _____

ICD-10 code(s): _____ ,

_____ , _____

3. ECT and necessary monitoring performed on 40-year-old female with untreatable depression (severe, recurrent, with psychotic features).

CPT code(s): _____

ICD-10 code(s): _____

4. Psychotherapy of 60 minutes provided to a male patient with recurrent depression via a telemedicine platform. His depression has been in remission for three months and is now receiving treatment for agoraphobia and panic attacks.

CPT code(s): _____

ICD-10 code(s): _____

5. Family psychotherapy performed without the patient present for a 12-year-old female with chronic PTSD due to the death of her mother approximately one year ago. She also suffers from excoriation disorder and mild intellectual disabilities.

CPT code(s): _____

ICD-10 code(s): _____ ,

_____ , _____ ,

_____

References

American Medical Association. 2018. *Current Procedural Terminology: 2018 Professional Edition*. Chicago: AMA.

American Medical Association. 2017 (January). *Current Procedural Terminology (CPT)*. Chicago: AMA.

Centers for Medicare and Medicaid Services. 2018. ICD-10-CM Official Guidelines for Coding and Reporting FY 2018. https://www.cms.gov/Medicare/Coding/ICD10/Downloads/2018-ICD-10-CM-Coding-Guidelines.pdf.

Centers for Medicare and Medicaid Services. 2017. Details for title: CMS 1500. https://www.cms.gov/Medicare/CMS-Forms/CMS-Forms/CMS-Forms-Items/CMS1188854.html.

Centers for Medicare and Medicaid Services. 2016 (November 17). Place of Service Code Set. http://www.cms.gov/Medicare/Coding/place-of-service-codes/Place_of_Service_Code_Set.html.

Cole, J. C.G. Bernacki, A. Helmer, N. Pinninti, and J.P. O'Reardon. 2015 (July–August). Efficacy of transcranial magnetic stimulation (TMS) in the treatment of schizophrenia: A review of the literature to date. *Innovations in Clinical Neuroscience* 12(7-8): 12–19. https://www.ncbi.nlm.nih.gov/pmc/articles/PMC4558786/.

Reichenberg, L.W. 2014. *DSM-5 Essentials: The Savvy Clinician's Guide to the Changes in Criteria*. Hoboken, NJ: Wiley.

Resources

Center for Medicaid and CHIP Services. 2014 (July 11). Informational Bulletin: Medication Assisted Treatment for Substance Use Disorders. https://www.medicaid.gov/Federal-Policy-Guidance/downloads/CIB-07-11-2014.pdf.

Centers for Medicare and Medicaid Services. 2016 (January). Behavioral Health Billing. https://www.cms.gov/Medicare-Medicaid-Coordination/Fraud-Prevention/Medicaid-Integrity-Education/Downloads/behavior-billing-booklet.pdf/.

Centers for Medicare and Medicaid Services. 2015 (January). Mental Health Services. https://www.cms.gov/Outreach-and-Education/Medicare-Learning-Network-MLN/MLNProducts/Downloads/Mental-Health-Services-Booklet-ICN903195.pdf.

Department of Health and Human Services. n.d. Health Insurance and Mental Health Services. https://www.mentalhealth.gov/get-help/health-insurance/index.html.

CHAPTER 8

Primary Care Services

Learning Objectives

- Understand the basics of billing and coding within the specialty of primary care.
- Examine procedural codes and guidelines for primary care services.

- Examine diagnosis coding and medical necessity for primary care services.
- Determine and apply ICD-10-CM, CPT, and HCPCS codes to primary care services.

Key Terms

Body area
Chief complaint (C/C)
Chronic obstructive pulmonary
    disease (COPD)
CLIA-waived
Diabetes mellitus
Electrocardiogram (ECG/EKG)
Foreign body
Heart failure
History of present illness (HPI)

Hypercholesterolemia
Hyperlipidemia
Hypertension
Immune globulin
Incision and drainage (I&D)
Minor surgical procedure
Organ system
Otitis
Overcoding
Past, family, social history (PFSH)

Preventive medicine services
Primary care
Primary care provider (PCP)
Review of systems (ROS)
Status asthmaticus
Undercoding
Underdose
Vaccine administration
Vaccine toxoid

Primary care healthcare providers are specialists who provide generalized, day-to-day care to patients. They act as the principal point of care and take responsibility for continuing comprehensive healthcare for patients. These providers also coordinate referrals, diagnostic testing, therapeutic treatments, and coordination of care with other providers from other specialties. There are a handful of specialties that may serve as primary care providers, including family practice, internal medicine, and pediatrics, as well as women's health or obstetrics and gynecology (OB/GYN) practitioners.

Most of the services provided by primary care practitioners are evaluation and management services, which is why E/M coding is a major component of primary care coding. Additional services are also performed, such as the administration of vaccines and in-office medical and minor surgical procedures. Patients may be seen in the primary care setting for a vast range of reasons, from signs and symptoms like sore throat and fever, to complex health issues such as diabetes mellitus, hypertension, and heart failure.

This chapter discusses the many different services that are provided within the field of primary care, with a special emphasis on evaluation and management coding (introduced in chapter 7). Additional services provided in the primary care setting are also discussed, including the administration of vaccines, in-office surgical procedures, miscellaneous medical procedures, and in-office laboratory procedures; as well as the top diagnosis codes for this specialty, including routine examinations, signs and symptoms, hypertension, diabetes, and hyperlipidemia/hypercholesterolemia.

Primary Care Basics

There are several types of healthcare specialties that qualify as primary care. Basically, whenever a doctor acts as a patient's principal point of contact, coordinates that patient's care with other providers or specialists, and takes primary responsibility for the general healthcare of a patient, he or she is acting as a **primary care provider (PCP)**. (For a reminder of the different types of healthcare specialties and the services they provide, please refer to chapter 1, Your Coding Career.)

The designation of PCP is important because many health insurance plans require a patient to select a PCP that is contracted and included within the patient's health insurance network. For some plans, the patient must make primary contact with the PCP before they are allowed to see a different provider. For example, if a patient is experiencing a digestive issue, he or she must see the PCP first and obtain a referral to a digestive disease specialist from the PCP before insurance will pay for the visit to the digestive disease specialist. In this way, the insurance company can be sure the patient needs to see the specialist (as determined by the PCP). Furthermore, the PCP can keep track of all the health issues and services that were provided to the patient.

It is important to note that not all health insurance plans require a referral to see a specialist. Some plans only require that the patient sees an in-network provider. Other plans are much more restrictive and require prior authorization to see a specialist, or may not authorize a visit to the specialist at all unless certain conditions are met. Coders must understand the relationship between a patient's insurance plan and the services that were requested and received because of these varying requirements.

Identifying a provider as a patient's PCP is also important in terms of insurance reimbursement, as the payment for health services (copayment) may be different for a PCP than for a specialist. For example, the copayment amount may differ depending on who the patient is seeing. A PCP copayment may be $30, whereas a specialist copayment is $50, and an urgent care copayment is $75. There also may be a higher amount of reimbursement, or payment for PCP services. For example, plan A may pay 90 percent of the allowable amount for PCP charges and send 10 percent to the patient deductible, whereas plan B may pay 75 percent of specialist services and send 25 percent to the patient deductible. Typically, a patient must identify a specific provider as his or her PCP, either over the phone or through the mail; some insurance plans allow patients to choose a PCP via online selection or registration.

One more consideration in terms of coding for primary care services is HCC coding (introduced in chapter 2). The data from different types of providers is used in HCC coding, but the base of data for this initiative is primary care claims. In other words, primary care provider offices are more likely to be part of accountable care organizations (ACOs)—groups of providers collectively accountable for the care they provide patients, that use performance measures to track the quality of the care provided to patients, and that receive payments linked to quality improvement initiatives (refer to chapter 2). ACO performance is evaluated on an annual basis according to specific benchmarks, one of which is the risk score assigned to the beneficiaries for that year. This risk adjustment score is based on the numerous diagnosis codes included within hierarchical condition categories as determined by the diagnosis codes selected for each patient (CMS 2016). It is important to remember that HCC coding relies on ICD-10-CM diagnosis codes, discussed in a later section in this chapter.

Procedural Coding in Primary Care

In primary care, most of the services performed are evaluation and management services because patients often present to a healthcare provider's office for the evaluation of a problem, such as an illness, and the subsequent management of it, perhaps with a medication prescription. Even when patients are not ill, there are office visits for routine examinations or preoperative exams, all of which are also reported with E/M codes. Occasionally patients undergo minor surgeries, such as cryosurgery of a wart or the incision and drainage of an abscess, so coders do have to use a few codes from the Surgery section of the CPT code book, in addition to various codes (especially vaccinations) from the Medicine section of the CPT code book.

E/M Services

Because the majority of procedures performed by PCPs are evaluation and management services, most of a PCP coder's time is spent assigning E/M codes and checking the provider's documentation to ensure it supports the level of service identified with the E/M code. E/M coding depends on the accurate identification of the numerous components of documentation that together support the levels of each key component, and ultimately the E/M code itself.

There are currently two sets of guidelines for the use of evaluation and management codes: 1995 and 1997 documentation guidelines (DGs). In 1995, due to confusion about the interpretation of E/M codes and how to select them, CMS together with AMA, developed a set of evaluation and management documentation guidelines to help direct correct code selection. However, these guidelines did not please healthcare specialists who could not receive credit for an extended examination of a single body system under the 1995 DGs (more on this later in this chapter). In 1997, the DGs were revised to include guidance for specialty providers. But the 1997 DGs were still met with opposition from the physician community. Therefore, CMS mandated that either the 1995 or 1997 DGs may be used to guide E/M code selection, as long as a provider is consistent in which one they use (AAPC 2016). Either of them may be used to determine the appropriate evaluation and management service, if a practice (or coder) does not switch between the two DGs. Furthermore, if the healthcare practice is audited, the documentation must clearly show how the specific level of E/M service was chosen based on which DGs (1995 or 1997) were used.

There are multiple elements of each of the three key components: history, examination, and medical decision making (MDM), first discussed in chapter 7. Remember, the elements of each of the key components are combined, depending on the service documented, to identify the correct level of the key component. This must be done for all three key components, which are then compared to the code descriptions for an evaluation and management service in order to find the correct code (see figure 8.1 or refer to figure 7.8).

Figure 8.1. Determine the level of E/M code

When a healthcare provider performs a complicated service, more elements are included from each of the key components, which raises the level of the E/M service and allows the provider to bill a higher amount. The level of E/M service is comprised of the levels of key components (history, exam, and MDM), so that the higher the levels of key components, the higher the level of E/M service. On the other hand, for a less complicated service less elements from each key component are included, so the level of evaluation and management service is lower and is billed at a lower amount. In this way, doctors can receive a higher amount of payment for more complicated services, and a smaller amount for less complicated services.

It is important to select the appropriate code for the services performed to avoid both undercoding and overcoding. **Undercoding** is the act of coding an E/M service at a level lower than what was performed. For example, if a doctor provided a service that could be billed with a higher level visit, such as a 99214, Office or other outpatient visit for the evaluation and management of an established patient, which requires at least 2 out of 3 of the following: *detailed* history, *detailed* examination, medical decision making of *moderate* complexity, but the coder only bills for a lower level visit, 99213, Office or other outpatient visit for the evaluation and management of an established patient, which requires at least 2 out of 3 of the following: *expanded problem-focused* history, *expanded problem-focused* examination, medical decision making of *low* complexity, then the coder is undercoding the visit. The code that should have been reported was for a higher level of service (99214) than what was actually reported (99213). This ultimately means that the doctor is not receiving payment for the service that was actually rendered.

Overcoding, on the other hand, is coding for an E/M service at a level higher than what was performed. For example, coding a level four visit, 99214, Office or other outpatient visit for the evaluation and management of an established patient, which requires at least 2 out of 3 of the following: *detailed* history, *detailed* examination, medical decision making of *moderate* complexity, when only a level three visit, 99213, Office or other outpatient visit for the evaluation and management of an established patient, which requires at least 2 out of 3 of the following: *expanded problem-focused* history, *expanded problem-focused* examination, medical decision making of *low* complexity, was performed. This is just as dangerous as it can result in a recovery audit performed by an insurance company or another company to uncover overpayments. It can result in recoupment of overpayments, in addition to more serious allegations such as billing abuse or fraud. See figure 8.2 for an illustration of undercoding versus overcoding.

Figure 8.2. Undercoding versus overcoding

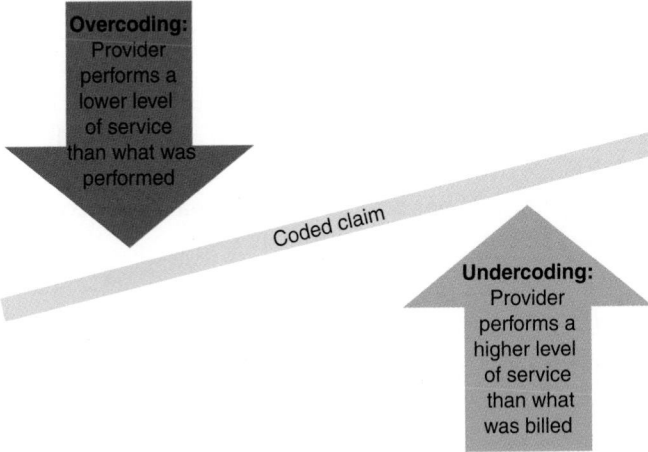

Coders must understand each of the elements included within each of the key components, so they can combine them correctly and ultimately select the appropriate E/M code. This includes understanding the individual elements involved in the three key components—the elements of history, the elements of examination, and the elements of medical decision making. Coding for PCP services also requires a solid understanding of how to code for prolonged services, preventive services, and the modifiers used with E/M codes.

Elements of History

There are four elements of the key component history: chief complaint (C/C), history of present illness (HPI), review of systems (ROS), and past, family, social history (PFSH), as shown in figure 8.3. The level of the history obtained from the patient is based on the

Figure 8.3. Elements of history

levels of each of these four elements. As discussed in chapter 7, there are four levels of history: problem focused, expanded problem focused, detailed, and comprehensive.

Remember that history is the subjective component of an evaluation and management service. It is the patient's description of the symptoms, signs, and other complaints, and does not include any components of an actual physical examination. The history component of an E/M code is only an oral account, without any physical examination or determination of the diagnosis or prescription of medications.

Chief Complaint

The **chief complaint (C/C)** is the description of the patient's symptoms, in the patient's own words. This is a concise statement that describes the problem, diagnosis (if known), condition, or other reason for the patient's encounter with the healthcare provider. It should answer the question, *Why is the patient in the office today?* For example, a chief complaint could be sore throat and fever, or needing a flu shot. The chief complaint is used to help the healthcare provider understand the reason why the patient seeks treatment. The chief complaint must be recorded for each patient encounter, but it does not impact the level of the history for the encounter.

History of Present Illness

The **history of present illness (HPI)** is a description of the development of the present illness or condition, described chronologically from the first onset of symptoms to the present encounter. The HPI is given by the patient based on questions asked by the healthcare provider. There are eight elements of HPI, each of which explains a different aspect of the current condition.

- *Location.* Where on the body the signs or symptoms are present, such as the throat.
- *Quality.* Characteristics of the signs or symptoms, such as stabbing or aching pain.
- *Severity.* The intensity of the signs or symptoms, often identified on a scale of 1 to 10.
- *Duration.* How long the problem has persisted, such as four days.
- *Timing.* When the signs or symptoms occur, such as every evening or all day long.
- *Context.* Under what circumstances do the signs or symptoms occur, such as when walking.
- *Modifying factors.* Under what circumstances do the signs or symptoms improve or worsen, such as when taking a deep breath.
- *Associated signs and symptoms.* Any other signs or symptoms related to the chief complaint, such as swelling or itching.

The healthcare provider asks pointed questions crafted around these elements to help narrow the focus of the examination. Depending on the chief complaint, the provider might require information for each of or none of these elements. The level of the HPI selected based on how many of these elements were covered in the history portion of the E/M service. There are two HPI levels—brief and extended. A brief HPI includes documentation of one to three elements, as described previously. An extended HPI includes documentation of four or more elements, or the status of three chronic conditions (CMS 1995; CMS 1997).

Read the following example of a patient history and note the eight different elements of HPI.

A 45-year-old male patient is seen complaining of abdominal pain, nausea with vomiting (three times), diarrhea (five times). He has a constant (timing) pain in the abdominal area (location), which is stabbing in nature (quality). He says that the pain is about a 7 out of 10 (severity), and it usually results in nausea and vomiting when he walks around (context). Symptoms began yesterday afternoon (duration) after eating his lunch. He recalls that the lunch smelled a little "off." He does report that lying on his left side has helped with the pain and nausea a bit (modifying factor). He is not experiencing any painful or frequent urination (associated signs and symptoms).

Review of Systems

The **review of systems (ROS)** is a series of questions aimed at obtaining more information regarding signs or symptoms the patient is experiencing. These questions are organized around the following body systems.

- *Constitutional.* General constitutional signs or symptoms, such as feeling fatigued or weak.
- *Eyes.* Signs or symptoms involving the eyes, such as discharge or visual disturbances.
- *Ears, nose, and throat.* Signs or symptoms involving the ears (such as ringing or pain), the nose (such as rhinorrhea or nose bleeds), and the throat and mouth (such as difficulty swallowing or bleeding gums).
- *Cardiovascular.* Signs or symptoms involving the cardiovascular system, such as chest pain or tightness.
- *Respiratory.* Signs or symptoms involving the respiratory system, such as shortness of breath, cough, or wheezing.
- *Gastrointestinal.* Signs or symptoms involving the gastrointestinal system, such as indigestion or diarrhea.
- *Genitourinary.* Signs or symptoms involving the genitourinary system, such as bedwetting, painful urination, or erectile dysfunction.
- *Musculoskeletal.* Signs or symptoms involving the musculoskeletal system, such as muscle cramps or joint pain or swelling.
- *Integumentary.* Signs or symptoms involving the skin (such as itching or rash) and the breasts (such as breast tenderness or lumps).
- *Neurological.* Signs or symptoms involving the neurologic system, such as dizziness, tingling, confusion, or paralysis.
- *Psychiatric.* Signs or symptoms involving the psychiatric system, such as depression or mood swings.
- *Endocrine.* Signs or symptoms involving the endocrine system, such as elevated blood sugar readings, increases in appetite or thirst, or intolerance to heat or cold.
- *Hematologic/lymphatic.* Signs or symptoms involving the hematologic and lymphatic systems, such as easily bruising and swollen glands.
- *Allergic/immunologic.* Signs or symptoms involving the allergic and immunologic systems, such as allergic reactions to certain foods or medications or frequent sneezing.

Like the answers to the HPI questions, the answers involving a review of systems help the healthcare provider determine the focus of the physical examination. There are three levels of ROS: problem pertinent, extended, and complete. A problem-pertinent ROS is the review of one system. An extended ROS is the review of two to nine systems. A complete ROS is the review of 10 or more systems (CMS 1995; CMS 1997).

Key to Success

Remember, this section of the key component of history—ROS—is still only talking with the healthcare provider. It is easy to confuse this section with an examination of each of these body systems, so it is important to keep in mind that this is only a question and answer session between the healthcare provider and patient. The answers to these questions help the provider determine what to observe in the physical examination part of the E/M service.

Past, Family, Social History

The **past, family, social history (PFSH)** is the section of the history component in which the provider asks the patient questions about his or her past healthcare history, family healthcare history, and social habits. These elements may be important in helping the healthcare provider understand the importance of certain signs or symptoms, or may raise further questions or concerns regarding the patient's health.

Figure 8.4. Relationship of the elements of history

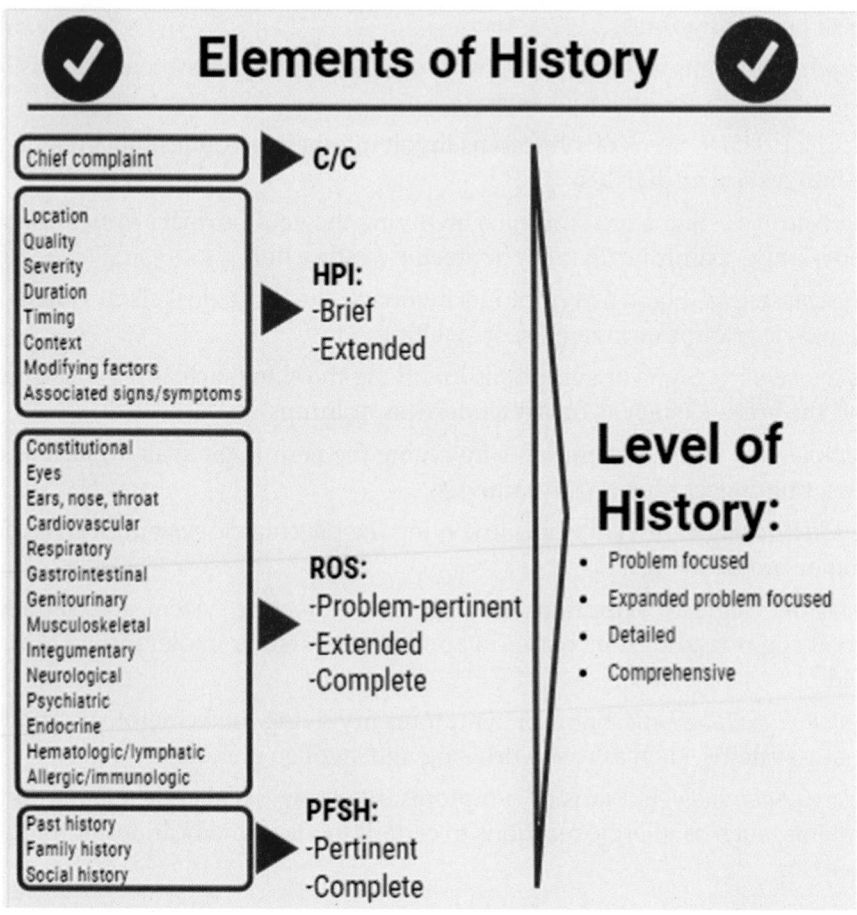

Past history includes the patient's experiences with childhood diseases, illnesses, operations, hospitalizations, treatments, and medications. Allergies can be accounted for in this section of questioning and in the review of systems, but they can only be accounted for once (either in the ROS or in the PFSH). It is important to keep in mind that these are historical conditions, meaning they are no longer active conditions.

Family history includes relevant family healthcare history, such as history of chronic conditions and malignancies, and other genetic factors like hereditary conditions.

Social history is a review of the patient's current and past social activities. This includes all relevant information regarding high-risk behaviors, such as drinking, smoking, or drug use, as well as environmental factors like the patient's work or home environment.

The amount of questions asked by the provider regarding a patient's PFSH establishes the level of PFSH obtained. There are two possible levels of past, family, social history—pertinent and complete. A pertinent PFSH is the documentation of at least one element from one of the three histories (past, family, and social). A complete PFSH depends on whether the patient is new or established. For new patients, one item from each of the three histories is required; for established patients, one item from two of the three histories is required. Refer to figure 8.4 to see how the elements of history are related to each other (CMS 1995; CMS 1997).

Putting It All Together: Determining the Level of History

The numerous factors of the elements of HPI, ROS, and PFSH are combined to determine the level of history completed for the encounter (see table 8.1). Note that the chief complaint does not factor into these calculations. It is a given that the chief complaint is considered in the documentation for each and every encounter. In table 8.1, the first column lists the level of the key component history, with the next three columns identifying the level of HPI, ROS, and PFSH, respectively, to meet that level of history. For example, a detailed history must have an extended HPI, an extended ROS, and a pertinent PFSH.

Table 8.1. Determining the level of history

Level of History	HPI	ROS	PFSH
Problem focused	Brief	N/A	N/A
Expanded problem focused	Brief	Problem pertinent	N/A
Detailed	Extended	Extended	Pertinent
Comprehensive	Extended	Complete	Complete

According to E/M documentation guidelines, to determine the level of history, three of the three elements must be met or exceeded. So the level of each of the elements of the history performed (ROS, HPI, PFSH) must meet or exceed the level performed in order to select that level (CMS 1995; CMS 1997).

For example, if a provider performed an extended HPI, extended ROS, and pertinent PFSH, then the level of history would be detailed (see table 8.2). As another

Table 8.2. Level of history: Detailed (all levels met)

Level of History	HPI	ROS	PFSH
Problem focused	Brief	N/A	N/A
Expanded problem focused	Brief	Problem pertinent	N/A
Detailed	Extended	Extended	Pertinent
Comprehensive	Extended	Complete	Complete

Table 8.3. Level of history: Expanded problem focused (lowest common denominator)

Level of History	HPI	ROS	PFSH
Problem focused	Brief	N/A	N/A
Expanded problem focused	(Brief)	Problem pertinent	N/A
Detailed	Extended	(Extended)	(Pertinent)
Comprehensive	Extended	Complete	Complete

example, if a provider performed a brief HPI, extended ROS, and pertinent PFSH, the level of history performed would be expanded problem focused (see table 8.3). In this case, three out of the three levels must be met or exceeded. Because the level of HPI did not exceed brief, the level of history performed must be selected as expanded problem focused.

The history is only one of the key components of an evaluation and management service. It is necessary to understand the elements of the remaining two key components—examination and medical decision making— to determine the level of each and ultimately the level of the E/M service performed. But first, complete the exercises in There's a Code for That 8.1.

8.1

There's a Code for That

Determine the level of history

Read the following documentation of the E/M service and determine the level of history for the encounter. You will need to determine the level of each individual element (HPI, ROS, and PFSH), and then determine the level of history provided.

1. Determine the level of HPI from the following encounter: *Established 12-year-old male presents with pain and swelling in his right knee. He plays football at his secondary school and was hit on his knee during a game three days ago by one of the other players. The pain was initially an 8 out of 10, but it quickly subsided to about a 4 out of 10. He now states that it is constantly aching is difficult to walk on, and the pain is worse in the morning. When he lies down and raises his leg with pillows, the pain does subside to a 2 or 3. He does not describe any numbness, tingling, or redness of skin.*

   How many elements of HPI are described in this passage? _____

   What is the level of HPI? _____

2. Determine the level of ROS from the same encounter: *Patient reports feeling generally fine, other than the knee pain. No allergies or immunologic problems, no rash or swelling of any areas other than the right knee, and no bruising. He does report feeling a few muscle cramps in his right thigh, especially at the end of the day after he has been on his feet all day. No tingling in the knee, just constant pain, which goes from a 2 to a 4 out of 10. Pain is generally all over the knee, he cannot tell if it is worse on the front or back, but does seem to be worse on the inner aspect of the knee.*

   How many systems were reviewed in the ROS? _____

   What is the level of ROS? _____

3. Determine the level of PFSH from the same encounter. *No known drug allergies, history of arthritis or joint problems, or immunologic problems. No relevant past injuries. No family history of osteoarthritis or joint problems. Patient is active in sports, plays football at school on a daily basis.*

Is this patient new or established? _____

How many elements of the PFSH are documented (how many elements from how many systems)? _____

What is the level of PFSH? _____

4. Using the level of HPI, ROS, and PFSH as determined, what is the level of history for this encounter? _____

Examination

The extent and subject of the examination are determined by the healthcare provider, based on his or her clinical judgment, the patient's history, and the nature of the presenting problem(s). The level of the examination performed is determined by the number of body areas and organ systems observed during the encounter. Remember that the examination is the objective component of an evaluation and management service; it is the physical study of the patient by the healthcare provider. The history is the patient *talking* with the provider, whereas the examination is the provider *doing* the examination.

Body areas are general areas of the body, rather than specific organ systems, that may be examined during an evaluation and management encounter. The CPT code book recognizes the following body areas.

- General appearance
- Head, including the face
- Neck
- Chest, including the breasts and axilla
- Abdomen
- Genitalia, groin, buttocks
- Back
- Each extremity

Organ systems are the specific groups of organs that may be examined during an evaluation and management encounter. The CPT code book recognizes the following organ systems.

- Eyes
- Ear, nose, mouth, and throat
- Cardiovascular
- Respiratory
- Gastrointestinal
- Genitourinary
- Musculoskeletal

- Skin
- Neurologic
- Psychiatric
- Hematologic/lymphatic/immunologic

The level of the examination performed depends on the number of body areas and organ systems involved in the examination. There are four levels of examination, which range from minimal to more extensive or complete.

- *Problem focused.* This is a limited examination of the affected body area or organ system.
- *Expanded problem focused.* This is a limited examination of the affected body area or organ system and other symptomatic or related organ systems.
- *Detailed.* This is an extended examination of the affected body area or organ system and other symptomatic or related organ systems.
- *Comprehensive.* This is either a general multisystem examination or a complete examination of a single organ system.

The determination of the level of examination is especially difficult because of the differences in evaluation and management guidelines. Both the 1995 and 1997 DGs require a varying number of elements in order to select a certain level of examination. For example, the 1995 guidelines require documentation of two to seven elements examined to support an expanded problem-focused exam (CMS 1995), whereas 1997 guidelines require six to eleven elements examined (CMS 1997).

The level of the examination depends on the number of body areas or organ systems that were studied (see table 8.4). For example, if one body area was examined, then the level of the exam was problem focused. If eight or more organ systems were examined, then the level of examination was comprehensive.

Table 8.4. Determining the level of examination

Level of Exam	Exam Components	Number of Body Areas/Organ Systems: 1995 Guidelines	Number of Body Areas/Organ Systems: 1997 Guidelines
Problem focused	Limited exam of affected body area/organ system	1 body area or organ system	1 to 5 body areas or organ systems
Expanded problem focused	Limited exam of affected area and other related/symptomatic organ systems	2 to 7 body areas or organ systems	6 to 11 body areas or organ systems
Detailed	Extended exam of affected area and other related/symptomatic organ systems	Extended exam of 2 to 7 body areas or organ systems	2 areas of examination from 6 organ systems
Comprehensive	General multisystem exam or complete exam of single organ system	8 or more organ systems	2 areas of examination from 9 organ systems

The final key component is medical decision making; it is the last determination needed before the level of evaluation and management service can be identified. Before reviewing this component, complete the exercise in There's a Code for That 8.2.

Determine the level of examination

Read the following documentation of the E/M service and determine the level of examination for the encounter.

1. Determine the level of exam from the following encounter (note that this is the same patient from There's a Code for That 8.1):

   - *EENT: not examined*
   - *Cardiovascular: within normal limits*
   - *Respiratory: within normal limits*
   - *Lymphatic: no lymphadenopathy noted*
   - *Musculoskeletal: pain upon palpitation of right patella, complete range of motion, swelling of knee joint (right), left knee within normal limits*
   - *Genitourinary: not examined*
   - *Gastrointestinal: not examined*
   - *Integumentary: no visible bruising or redness, scratches, or superficial injuries*

   How many different body areas or organ systems were examined?

   _____

   What is the level of examination? _____

Medical Decision Making

As discussed in chapter 7, there are three considerations in determining the level of medical decision making for an E/M service—number of diagnoses and management options, amount and/or complexity of data to be reviewed, and risk of complications and/or morbidity or mortality (AMA 2017). The levels of work for each of these three elements are identified to determine the level of medical decision making. If the key component history is *talking*, and the key component examination is *doing*, then the key component medical decision making is *thinking* (see figure 8.5). The MDM component of an E/M service is the pivotal component in an encounter, and appropriate documentation can guarantee or prevent the accurate selection of the E/M service level. It is important to ensure that the MDM is documented fully.

Figure 8.5. Three key components

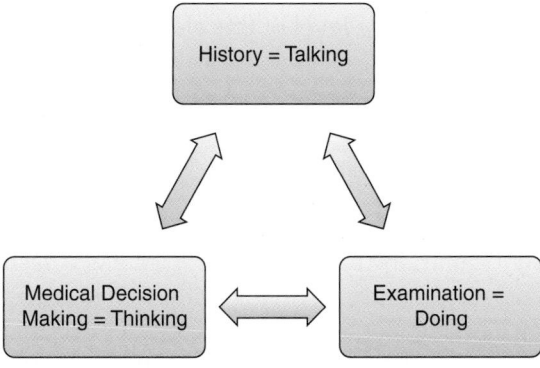

MDM consists of assembling findings from the patient's history and examination, determining a diagnosis (if possible), and weighing the pros and cons of certain treatments, while taking into account the risk of the condition and any additional tests that should be ordered or reviewed. In other words, MDM is the healthcare provider doing what they have been trained to do—use his or her medical expertise to make a decision regarding the patient's condition.

Number of Diagnoses and Management Options

The number of diagnoses and management options is the element of MDM that considers other possible diagnoses or treatment options for the patient, based on the relative difficulty in determining the patient's diagnosis, as well as the status of the problem (such as if it is worsening or stable).

E/M auditing tools are commonly used to help coders determine the exact level of the three key components, including the level of medical decision making. These audit tools are pre-formatted forms with specific sections for each key component (history, examination, and MDM), and include separate areas to indicate if each element of each key component has been documented or performed (see figure 8.6). These forms usually break down each element into points that can be tallied according to the amount of each element documented in the health record from a specific visit, and then calculated to determine the exact level of each key component.

E/M auditing forms are varied and differ from payer to payer. Some are based on 1995 DGs, whereas others are based on 1997 DGs; and many auditing forms allow the coder to use either 1995 or 1997 DGs. The points system used in the forms may vary from payer to payer, so it is important to check with the insurance payer before using a specific form.

There are four levels of complexity for this element of medical decision making: minimal, limited, multiple, and extensive. Using a point system aligned with E/M documentation guidelines (either 1995 or 1997, or both), coders can determine which level to choose based on the documentation (see table 8.5). On most audit forms, a minor problem that would likely resolve if the patient had not come in for treatment, may be worth one point. A patient usually has more than one of these minor problems, but only a maximum of two points may be counted no matter the amount of minor problems. Established, stable, or improving conditions would each be worth one point. Established, worsening conditions would be two points. A health problem that is new to the provider, but that does not require any additional workup, is three points (this can only be counted once, even if there is more than one new problem present). A health problem that is new to the provider and requires additional workup would be four points.

The points are added to create a total score for the number of diagnoses and management options, which determines the level of this element, as follows (Novitas 2017).

- Minimal: One point
- Limited: Two points
- Multiple: Three points
- Extensive: Four points

For example, if a patient came saw a provider for a localized rash that did not require any further workup and was already resolving without treatment, this problem would be assigned one point. The level assigned for the number of diagnoses and management options would be *minimal*. On the other hand, if the same patient came in with a severe rash that was worsening by spreading to other areas of the body, and this

Figure 8.6. Example E/M auditing form

History

Refer to data section (table below) in order to quantify. After referring to data, circle the entry farthest to the *RIGHT* in the table, which best describes the HPI, ROS and PFSH. If one column contains three circles, draw a line down that column to the bottom row to identify the type of history. If no column contains three circles, the column containing a circle farthest to the *LEFT*, identifies the type of history.

After completing this table which classifies the history, circle the type of history within the appropriate grid in Section 5.

HPI: Status of chronic conditions: ❏ 1 condition ❏ 2 conditions ❏ 3 conditions **OR**		❏ Status of 1-2 chronic conditions		❏ Status of 3 chronic conditions	
HPI (history of present illness) elements: ❏ Location ❏ Severity ❏ Timing ❏ Modifying factors ❏ Quality ❏ Duration ❏ Context ❏ Associated signs and symptoms		❏ Brief (1-3)		❏ Extended (4 or more)	
ROS (review of systems): ❏ Constitutional ❏ Ears,nose, ❏ GI ❏ Integumentary ❏ Endo (wt loss, etc) mouth, throat ❏ GU (skin, breast) ❏ Hem/lymph ❏ Eyes ❏ Card/vasc ❏ Musculo ❏ Neuro ❏ All/immuno ❏ Resp ❏ Psych ❏ All others negative	❏ None	❏ Pertinent to problem (1 system)	❏ Extended (2-9 systems)	❏ *Complete	
PFSH (past medical, family, social history) areas: ❏ Past history (the patient's past experiences with illnesses, operation, injuries and treatments) ❏ Family history (a review of medical events in the patient's family, including diseases which may be hereditary or place the patient at risk) ❏ Social history (an age appropriate review of past and current activities)		❏ None	❏ Pertinent (1 history area)	❏ **Complete (2 or 3 history areas)	
	PROBLEM FOCUSED	**EXP.PROB. FOCUSED**	**DETAILED**	**COMPRE-HENSIVE**	

Examination

Refer to data section (table below) in order to quantify. After referring to data, identify the type of examination. Circle the type of examination within the appropriate grid in Section 5.

Limited to affected body area or organ system (one body area or system related to problem)	**PROBLEM FOCUSED EXAM**
Affected body area or organ system and other symptomatic or related organ system(s) (additional systems up to total of 7)	**EXPANDED PROBLEM FOCUSED EXAM**
Extended exam of affected area(s) and other symptomatic or related organ system(s) (additional systems up to total of 7 or more depth than above)	**DETAILED EXAM**
General multi-system exam (8 or more systems) or complete exam of a single organ system (complete single exam not defined in these instructions)	**COMPREHENSIVE EXAM**

Body areas: ❏ Head, including face ❏ Chest, including breasts and axillae ❏ Abdomen ❏ Neck ❏ Back, including spine ❏ Genitalia, groin, buttocks ❏ Each extremity **Organ systems:** ❏ Constitutional ❏ Ears,nose, ❏ Resp ❏ Musculo ❏ Psych (e.g., vitals, gen app) mouth, throat ❏ GI ❏ Skin ❏ Hem/lymph/imm ❏ Eyes ❏ Cardiovascular ❏ GU ❏ Neuro	❏ 1 body area or system	❏ Up to 7 systems	❏ Up to 7 systems	❏ 8 or more systems
	PROBLEM FOCUSED	**EXP.PROB. FOCUSED**	**DETAILED**	**COMPRE-HENSIVE**

Figure 8.6. *(Continued)*

Medical Decision Making

Number of Diagnoses or Treatment Options

Identify each problem or treatment option mentioned in the record. Enter the number in each of the categories in Column B in the table below. (There are maximum number in two categories.)

Number of Diagnoses or Treatment Options

A	B	X	C	=	D
Problem(s) Status	**Number**		**Points**		**Result**
Self-limited or minor (stable, improved or worsening)	*Max = 2*		1		
Est. problem (to examiner); stable, improved			1		
Est. problem (to examiner); worsening			2		
New problem (to examiner); no additional workup planned	*Max = 1*		3		
New prob. (to examiner); add. workup planned			4		
			TOTAL		

Multiply the number in columns B & C and put the product in column D. Enter a total for column D.

Bring total to **line A** in Final Result for Complexity (table below)

Amount and/or Complexity of Data Reviewed

For each category of reviewed data identified, circle the number in the points column. Total the points.

Amount and/or Complexity of Data Reviewed	
Reviewed Data	**Points**
Review and/or order of clinical lab tests	1
Review and/or order of tests in the radiology section of CPT	1
Review and/or order of tests in the medicine section of CPT	1
Discussion of test results with performing physician	1
Decision to obtain old records and/or obtain history from someone other than patient	1
Review and summarization of old records and/or obtaining history from someone other than patient and/or discussion of case with another health care provider	2
Independent visualization of image, tracing or specimen itself (not simply review of report)	2
TOTAL	

Bring total to **line C** in Final Result for Complexity (table below)

Risk of Complications and/or Morbidity or Mortality

Use the risk table below as a guide to assign risk factors. It is understood that the table below does not contain all specific instances of medical care; the table is intended to be used as a guide. Circle the most appropriate factor(s) in each category. The overall measure of risk is the highest level circled. Enter the level of risk identified in Final Result for Complexity (table below).

Level of Risk	Presenting Problem(s)	Diagnostic Procedure(s) Ordered	Management Options Selected
Minimal	• One self-limited or minor problem, e.g., cold, insect bite, tinea corporis	• Laboratory tests requiring venipuncture • Chest x-rays • EKG/EEG • Urinalysis • Ultrasound, e.g., echo • KOH prep	• Rest • Gargles • Elastic bandages • Superficial dressings
Low	• Two or more self-limited or minor problems • One stable chronic illness, e.g., well controlled hypertension or non-insulin dependent diabetes, cataract, BPH • Acute uncomplicated illness or injury, e.g., cystitis, allergic rhinitis, simple sprain	• Physiologic tests not under stress, e.g.,pulmonary function tests • Non-cardiovascular imaging studies with contrast, e.g., barium enema • Superficial needle biopsies • Clincal laboratory tests requiring arterial puncture • Skin biopsies	• Over-the-counter drugs • Minor surgery with no identified risk factors • Physical therapy • Occupational therapy • IV fluids without additives
Moderate	• One or more chronic illnesses with mild exacerbation, progression, or side effects of treatment • Two or more stable chronic illnesses • Undiagnosed new problem with uncertain prognosis, e.g., lump in breast • Acute illness with systemic symptoms, e.g., pyelonephritis, pneumonitis, colitis • Acute complicated injury, e.g., head injury with brief loss of consciousness	• Physiologic tests under stress, e.g., cardiac stress test, fetal contraction stress test • Diagnostic endoscopies with no identified risk factors • Deep needle or incisional biopsy • Cardiovascular imaging studies with contrast and no identified risk factors, e.g., arteriogram cardiac cath • Obtain fluid from body cavity, e.g., lumbar puncture, thoracentesis, culdocentesis	• Minor surgery with identified risk factors • Elective major surgery (open, percutaneous or endoscopic) with no identified risk factors • Prescription drug management • Therapeutic nuclear medicine • IV fluids with addititives • Closed treatment of fracture or dislocation without manipulation
High	• One or more chronic illnesses with severe exacerbation, progression, or side effects of treatment • Acute or chronic illnesses or injuries that may pose a threat to life or bodily function, e.g., multiple trauma, acute MI, pulmonary embolus, severe respiratory distress, progressive severe rheumatoid arthritis, psychiatric illness with potential threat to self or others, peritonitis, acute renal failure • An abrupt change in neurologic status, e.g., seizure, TIA, weakness or sensory loss	• Cardiovascular imaging studies with contrast with identified risk factors • Cardiac electrophysiological tests • Diagnostic endoscopies with identified risk factors • Discography	• Elective major surgery (open, percutaneous or endoscopic with identified risk factors) • Emergency major surgery (open, percutaneous or endoscopic) • Parenteral controlled substances • Drug therapy requiring intensive monitoring for toxicity • Decision not to resuscitate or to de-escalate care because of poor prognosis

Final Result for Complexity

Draw a line down any column with 2 or 3 circles to identify the type of decision making in that column. Otherwise, draw a line down the column with the 2nd circle from the left. After completing this table, which classifies complexity, circle the type of decision making within the appropriate grid in Section 5.

A	Number diagnoses or treatment options	≤ 1 Minimal	2 Limited	3 Multiple	≥ 4 Extensive
B	Highest Risk	Minimal	Low	Moderate	High
C	Amount and complexity of data	≤ 1 Minimal or low	2 Limited	3 Multiple	≥ 4 Extensive
	Type of decision making	STRAIGHT-FORWARD	LOW COMPLEX.	MODERATE COMPLEX.	HIGH COMPLEX.

(left margin, vertical) **MEDICAL DECISION MAKING**

Table 8.5. Example of the number of diagnoses and management options

Number of Diagnoses and Management Options	Points
Minor problem (self-resolving)	1 each for a maximum of 2
Established (stable or improving)	1 each
Established (worsening)	2 each
New problem (no additional workup)	3
New problem (with additional workup)	4
Total	

Source: Adapted from Novitas 2017.

problem was new to the treating provider who ordered additional workup by testing the patient for allergies, this would be assigned four points (a new problem with additional workup). The level assigned for the number of diagnoses and management options for this problem would be *extensive*.

The number of diagnoses and management options is only the first part of the calculation to determine the level of medical decision making for an evaluation and management service. The next component is the amount and/or complexity of data to be reviewed.

Amount and/or Complexity of Data

The amount and/or complexity of data to be reviewed is a measure of the need to order or review tests, or the need to gather and review additional data regarding the patient's condition. The work involved in this element includes planning, scheduling, and performing, as well as reviewing lab tests, radiologic services, and other diagnostic services. It also includes the review of past healthcare history and requesting and reviewing old health records.

There are also four levels of complexity for this element of medical decision making: minimal or none, limited, moderate, and extensive. A points system aligned with E/M documentation guidelines (either 1995 or 1997, or both), can be used to determine the level of work involved for this element of medical decision making (see table 8.6). Review of clinical labs, medical tests, and radiological tests would be assigned one point. No matter how many different tests were reviewed, only one point should be assigned

Table 8.6. Example of the amount and/or complexity of data

Amount and/or Complexity of Data	Points
Lab ordered or reviewed	1 maximum
Radiologic exam ordered or reviewed	1 maximum
Medicine section test ordered or reviewed	1 each
Discussion of results with performing provider	1
Decision to obtain old records or history	1
Reviewing and summarizing old records, history, or discussion with other health provider	2
Independent interpretation of test results	2
Total	

Source: Adapted from Novitas 2017.

for lab or radiologic tests. As many points as necessary may be assigned for tests from the Medicine section of the CPT code book. The following are examples of how points may be assigned for calculating the amount and/or complexity of data.

- Discussing the results of a test with another healthcare provider = one point.
- Deciding to obtain old records or additional healthcare history from a person other than the patient = one point.
- Reviewing and summarizing data from old records or additional history gathered from a person other than the patient = two points.
- Independent or secondary interpretation of a lab specimen or diagnostic examination results = two points (keep in mind that this is not ordering the test or reviewing another provider's interpretation, but providing a new, independent interpretation of the test results). (Novitas 2017)

The points are added to create a total score for the amount and/or complexity of data to be reviewed, which determines the level of this element, as follows (Novitas 2017):

- Minimal or none: Zero to one point
- Limited: Two points
- Moderate: Three points
- Extensive: Four points

For example, if a patient came in complaining of a sore throat and the provider chose to perform a strep throat swab in the office (a clinical lab test), then this would be assigned one point (for lab ordered and reviewed). The level for this element would be *minimal*. But if the same patient presented with trouble swallowing and a swallow study was performed (a medicine section test—one point), and the doctor made the decision to order old health records from the patient's previous doctor (one point), as well as discuss the results from a previous swallow study with another healthcare provider (one point), then three total points would be assigned for this element. The level for this element of medical decision making would be *moderate*.

The last component in the calculation of the level of medical decision making is the risk of complications and/or morbidity or mortality posed by the patient's condition.

Risk of Complications and/or Morbidity or Mortality

The last element that must be considered in medical decision making is the risk of complications and/or morbidity or mortality from the patient's condition. In other words, how dangerous is the patient's condition? The risk is based on the healthcare provider's determination of the probability that the patient will become seriously ill or diseased, experience complications from the condition, or die. There are a few components considered in this calculation of risk, including the nature of the presenting problem, urgency of the visit, any comorbid (coexisting) conditions, and the need for surgery.

There are four levels of complexity for this element of medical decision making: minimal, low, moderate, and high. Unlike the other two elements, a points system is not used to determine the level of this element of medical decision making. According to both 1995 and 1997 DGs, the levels of this element are determined according to the nature of the presenting problem, diagnostic procedures ordered, and management options selected.

- Minimal: One self-limited or minor problem
- Low:
  - Two or more self-limited or minor problems, *or*
  - One stable chronic illness, *or*
  - Acute uncomplicated illness or injury
- Moderate:
  - One or more chronic illnesses with mild exacerbation, progression, or side effects, *or*
  - Two or more chronic stable illnesses, *or*
  - Undiagnosed new problem with uncertain prognosis, *or*
  - Acute illness with systemic symptoms, *or*
  - Acute complicated injury
- High:
  - One or more chronic illnesses with severe exacerbation, progression, or side effects, *or*
  - Acute or chronic illness/injury that poses a threat to life or bodily function, *or*
  - An abrupt change in neurologic status (CMS 1995; CMS 1997)

Once all levels of the three elements of medical decision making are determined, it is necessary to combine them to determine the level of the medical decision making for the encounter.

Putting It All Together: Determining the Level of Medical Decision Making

To determine the level of the medical decision making for the encounter, it is necessary to identify the number of diagnoses or management options, the amount and/or complexity of data to be reviewed, and the risk of complications and/or morbidity or mortality. There are four levels of MDM: straightforward, low complexity, moderate complexity, and high complexity (see table 8.7). To qualify for a certain level of MDM, two out of the three levels must be met or exceeded.

For example, if a patient came in for an evaluation and management encounter and the number of diagnoses or treatment options involved was minimal, the data reviewed was limited, and the risk involved was low, then the level of MDM would be *low* because two out of the three levels were met or exceeded (see table 8.8). If, however,

Table 8.7. Determine the level of medical decision making

Level of MDM	Number of Diagnosis or Management Options	Amount and/or Complexity of Data	Risk Involved
Straightforward	Minimal	Minimal or none	Minimal
Low	Limited	Limited	Low
Moderate	Multiple	Moderate	Moderate
High	Extensive	Extensive	High

Table 8.8. Level of MDM: Low (two levels met or exceeded)

Level of MDM	Number of Diagnosis or Management Options	Amount and/or Complexity of Data	Risk Involved
Straightforward	Minimal	Minimal or none	Minimal
Low	Limited	Limited	Low
Moderate	Multiple	Moderate	Moderate
High	Extensive	Extensive	High

Table 8.9. Level of MDM: Moderate (two levels met or exceeded)

Level of MDM	Number of Diagnosis or Management Options	Amount and/or Complexity of Data	Risk Involved
Straightforward	Minimal	Minimal or none	Minimal
Low	Limited	Limited	Low
Moderate	Multiple	Moderate	Moderate
High	Extensive	Extensive	High

the number of diagnoses was extensive, the amount of data to be reviewed was moderate, and the risk involved was low, then the level of MDM for the encounter would be *moderate* (see table 8.9). Complete the exercises in determining the level of medical decision making in There's a Code for That 8.3.

8.3

There's a Code for That

Determine the level of medical decision making

Read the following documentation of the E/M service for the patient from There's a Code for That 8.1 and 8.2 and determine the level of MDM for the encounter. You will need to determine both the level of each individual element (HPI, ROS, and PFSH) and then the level of history provided.

1. Calculate the points for the number of diagnoses and management options for this encounter, using the following table: *This is a new problem to the provider today, condition seems stable but will require additional work up to determine diagnosis.*

Number of Diagnoses and Management Options	Points
Minor problem (self-resolving)	1 each for a maximum of 2
Established (stable or improving)	1 each
Established (worsening)	2 each
New problem (no additional workup)	3
New problem (with additional workup)	4
Total	

How many points are scored for the number of diagnoses? _____

What is the level of this element of MDM? _____

2. Calculate the points for the amount and/or complexity of data to be reviewed for this encounter, using the following table: *Ordered complete x-ray of right knee, will review radiologist report and follow-up as needed.*

Amount and/or Complexity of Data	Points
Lab ordered or reviewed	1 maximum
Radiologic exam ordered or reviewed	1 maximum
Medicine section test ordered or reviewed	1 each
Discussion of results with performing provider	1
Decision to obtain old records or history	1

Reviewing and summarizing old records, history, or discussion with other health provider	2
Independent interpretation of test results	2
Total	

How many points are scored for the amount and/or complexity of data?

_____

What is the level of this element of MDM? _____

3. Calculate the points for the risk of complications and/or morbidity or mortality for this encounter, using the following table: *Working diagnosis of knee joint pain secondary to injury.*

Level of MDM	Presenting Problem(s)
Minimal	• One self-limited of minor problem
Low	• Two or more self-limited or minor problems • One stable chronic illness • Acute uncomplicated illness or injury
Moderate	• One or more chronic illnesses with mild exacerbation, progression, or side effects • Two or more stable chronic illnesses • Undiagnosed new problem with uncertain prognosis • Acute illness with systemic complications • Acute uncomplicated injury
High	• One or more chronic illnesses with severe exacerbation, progression, or side effects • Acute or chronic illness/injury that poses a threat to life or bodily function • An abrupt change in neurologic status

Source: Adapted from CMS 1995; CMS 1997.

What is the level of this element of MDM? _____

4. Using the level of number of diagnoses, amount and/or complexity of data, and risk, what is the level of MDM for this encounter? _____

_____

Determine the Level of the E/M Service

Once the levels of the three key components have been determined, it is possible to establish the level of the E/M service. As a review from chapter 7, there are three key components to an E/M service—history, examination, and medical decision making. There are four levels of complexity for each of these key components, as follows.

- History: problem focused, expanded problem focused, detailed, comprehensive
- Examination: problem focused, expanded problem focused, detailed, comprehensive
- Medical decision making: straightforward, low, moderate, high

Once the levels of each of the three key components are identified, they must be matched to the description of an E/M code, according to how many of the key components are necessary. Look at the description for the following code and notice which of the key components are needed for code selection:

99213, Office or other outpatient visit for the evaluation and management of an established patient, which requires at least 2 of the 3 key components:

- An expanded problem focused history
- An expanded problem focused examination
- Medical decision making of low complexity

This code requires that at least two of the three key components be at or above the level identified in the code description. Some E/M codes require that all three levels of the key components match, such as E/M codes for new patients, initial inpatient or hospital observation care, consultations, and emergency department visits. When this is the case, the levels of all three key components must be at or above the levels identified in the code description.

Use the information from There's a Code for That 8.1, 8.2, and 8.3 to determine the E/M code in There's a Code for That 8.4.

8.4

There's a Code for That

Determine the level of E/M code

Using the level of history from There's a Code for That 8.1, the level of exam from There's a Code for That 8.2, and the level of MDM from There's a Code for That 8.3, what is the E/M code for this encounter? _____

Prolonged Services

In certain circumstances, a healthcare provider may spend an inordinate amount of time with a patient, either face-to-face or without direct patient contact, to manage or treat the patient's condition. These are considered **prolonged services**. These codes are useful for those rare instances when a patient is extremely sick or extra time is required to treat or manage the patient's condition, or to counsel the patient regarding his or her health status. Codes for prolonged services (99354 through 99416) are used when the healthcare practitioner provides an E/M service that is longer or more difficult than what could be represented by the highest level of E/M code. The prolonged service code is reported in addition to the code for the primary evaluation and management procedure (for example, 99211 through 99215).

There are three types of prolonged service codes:

- Prolonged services with direct patient contact (99354 to 99357).
  - Office or other outpatient setting (99354 and 99355)
  - Inpatient or observation setting (99356 and 99357)

- Prolonged services without direct patient contact (99358 and 99359)
- Prolonged clinical staff services with physician or other qualified health care professional supervision (99415 and 99416)

All prolonged service codes are time-based codes—the only factor considered during selection of these codes is the extra amount of service time that was provided to the patient. Most prolonged service codes are also add-on codes that must be added to the primary code for the evaluation and management service, such as an outpatient office visit code. For example, code 99354, Prolonged evaluation and management or psychotherapy service(s) (beyond the typical service time of the primary procedure) in the office or outpatient setting requiring direct patient contact beyond the usual service; first hour, identifies one extra hour of direct face-to-face time provided to the patient in the outpatient office setting. Each type of prolonged service has additional add-on codes, which should be used to identify additional time over the first hour of prolonged service time. For the outpatient office setting, this code is 99355, Prolonged evaluation and management or psychotherapy service(s) (beyond the typical service time of the primary procedure) in the office or outpatient setting requiring direct patient contact beyond the usual service; each additional 30 minutes.

Coding for prolonged services requires a careful calculation of the extra time spent with the patient. Each E/M code identifies a specific amount of time, on which the level of the code should be based (if using time as the determining factor for code selection)—the time spent with the patient that is calculated as part of the initial E/M service. For example, see the description for code 99215 in figure 8.7.

Code 99215 includes 40 minutes of face-to-face time spent with the patient. So if the healthcare provider spent 90 minutes in the office face-to-face with the patient, then it would necessitate reporting a prolonged service code because 90 minutes exceeds the 40 minutes reported by code 99215. Note that in order to bill for a prolonged service, the time limit listed in the primary code (like the 40 minutes in code 99215) must be *over* 30 minutes. The prolonged service codes should not be reported for anything less than an additional 30 minutes. In the outpatient setting, anything over the first additional 30 minutes, over the 40 minutes identified in the code for the primary procedure, should be reported with a prolonged services codes.

Figure 8.7. Code description for 99215

| 99215 | **Office or other outpatient visit** for the evaluation and |

management of an established patient, which requires

at least 2 of these 3 key components:

- **A comprehensive history**

- **A comprehensive examination**

- **Medical decision making of high complexity**

Counseling and/or coordination of care with other

physicians, other qualified healthcare professional, or

agencies are provided consistent with the nature of the

problem(s) and the patient's and/or family's needs.

Usually, the presenting problem(s) are of moderate to

high severity. Typically, **40 minutes are spent face-to-** 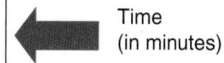 Time (in minutes)

face with the patient and/or family.

For example, if the patient was treated in the outpatient office setting for 90 minutes, then the codes selected would be as follows: 99215, Office or other outpatient visit for the evaluation and management of an established patient, which requires at least 2 of these 3 key components: comprehensive history, comprehensive examination, and medical decision making of high complexity, as well as 99354, Prolonged evaluation and management or psychotherapy service(s) (beyond the typical service time of the primary procedure) in the office or outpatient setting requiring direct patient contact beyond the usual service; first hour. 99215 identifies the first 40 minutes, and 99354 identifies the remaining 50 minutes of time. Note that even though only 50 minutes of extra time were spent with the patient, this amount is greater than 30 minutes, so the code can still be reported.

Key to Success

Assigning the correct codes for prolonged services requires careful identification of the total time spent, and then careful selection of the appropriate prolonged services code(s) to account for the correct amount of time. Remember to use your CPT code book as a guide to help you find the correct CPT codes. The CPT Professional Edition includes helpful tables that identify the amount of time spent on the E/M service, as well as how to report the prolonged service codes appropriately.

If the prolonged service is *more* than one hour over the time identified in the primary service, then an add-on code should be reported to identify the additional time. The add-on code should be reported as many times as necessary to identify the full amount of time spent with the patient. For example, if the provider spent 120 minutes (2 hours) in the office face-to-face with the patient, then the codes reported would be as follows: 99215, (Level 5 established patient office visit), 99354 (prolonged service, first hour), and then 99355, Prolonged evaluation and management or psychotherapy service(s) (beyond the typical service time of the primary procedure) in the office or outpatient setting requiring direct patient contact beyond the usual service; each additional 30 minutes.

Preventive Services

In addition to evaluation and management encounters that involve the three key components of history, examination, and medical decision making, there is another important type of E/M service common in primary care—preventive medicine services.

Also known as routine general healthcare examinations, checkups, or well-child exams, **preventive medicine services** are comprehensive health evaluations that involve a physical examination and include an age and gender appropriate history, counseling and anticipatory guidance and health risk factor reduction interventions, and the ordering of laboratory and diagnostic procedures. Preventive examinations are typically performed on an annual basis, unless the patient is under the age of three (in which case he or she would receive additional preventive exams throughout the year).

The E/M codes used to report preventive services are significantly more simplistic. When coding for a preventive service, coders only need to know two things: (1) if the patient was considered new or established and (2) the age of the patient. For example, code 99384, Initial comprehensive preventive medicine service, adolescent (age 12 through 17) is for a new patient from 12 to 17 years old.

Preventive services become a bit more complicated when they are performed on the same day as an additional E/M service. It is common that during a preventive exam, the healthcare provider might encounter an additional problem or abnormality. If the problem or abnormality does not require any additional work, then no additional E/M service codes should be reported. However, if additional work is required to evaluate, treat, or otherwise manage the abnormality, then it may be necessary to include an additional E/M service code.

If a problem or abnormality encountered during a preventive examination is extensive enough to require additional work to perform the key components of a problem-oriented E/M service, then the appropriate office visit code should be reported along with the preventive medicine code. Modifier -25 should be appended to the office visit code to identify that it was a significant, separately identifiable service, provided by the same provider on the same date of service (refer to chapter 5 for a reminder of the uses and functions of modifiers).

This scenario is quite common in primary care coding, especially pediatrics and family practice. Consider the following example.

A one-year-old child presents for a routine preventive examination and vaccinations and while in the office the parent tells the doctor that the baby has been tugging at her ear lately, has been a bit fussy, and was running a fever the night before. In addition to the comprehensive preventive examination, including the growth and the development of the child, the pediatrician also performs a problem-oriented visit—obtaining a brief history of the present illness; examining the child's ears, eyes, nose and throat; and determining that the child has otitis media and prescribes an antibiotic.

In this scenario, the pediatrician would code for the well-child examination using code 99392, Preventive medicine service, early childhood (age 1 through 4 years), as well as 99213, Level 3 office visit, to report the additional E/M service. The additional E/M code, 99213, would be appended with modifier -25, to indicate that it was a significant, separately identifiable service.

> Modifier -25, Significant, separately identifiable evaluation and management service by the same physician or other qualified health care professional on the same day of the procedure or other service, is perhaps one of the most important modifiers in all of procedural coding. Without adding modifier -25, the additional service would be bundled into the primary service (in this case the preventive examination) by the payer. When this happens, the payer only pays for the primary service and does not pay for any of the additional service that was performed. By not effectively using modifier -25, coders may be preventing reimbursement for thousands of dollars to which the healthcare provider is rightfully entitled.
>
> **MOD**

Other than modifier -25, there are a handful of other modifiers that are used with evaluation and management services. They describe different scenarios and provide additional information regarding the primary E/M service.

Modifiers Used with E/M Services

There are several CPT modifiers that are specifically designed for use with E/M services only. They describe modified circumstances, such as modifier -95, Telemedicine service, and can make a significant difference in reimbursement, such as modifier -25,

Significant, separately identifiable service. Additional CPT modifiers that may be used with E/M codes include

- Modifier -24, Unrelated E/M service by the same physician or other qualified health care professional during a postoperative period. This modifier is used to indicate that an E/M service was performed during a postoperative period for a reason unrelated to the original procedure. This is an important modifier for reimbursement purposes. For example, a 60-year-old male received a pacemaker 20 days ago. Because this is a major procedure, it has a 90-day global period, which means that any routine follow-ups or diagnostic services performed in relation to the pacemaker are bundled into the code for the primary procedure (the code for pacemaker insertion). So if the same patient comes in to the same physician during the postoperative period for a visit unrelated to the pacemaker—such as hypertension—then the coder should append modifier -24 to the E/M code. This will indicate to the payer that the E/M service was *not* related to the pacemaker insertion and it should be paid separately.

- Modifier -32, Mandated services. This modifier should be appended to a code for a procedure that has been mandated by an official organization, such as a physical examination as required by a third-party payer, government, legislative, or regulatory requirement. Although it can be used with other procedures (when mandated by an official body), it can also be used with E/M service codes.

- Modifier -57, Decision for surgery. This modifier should be appended on an evaluation and management procedure that resulted in the initial decision to perform a surgery. For example, if a patient comes into the office complaining of intense right lower quadrant abdominal pain, and it is determined that there is an immediate need for surgery to remove a burst appendix, then the E/M code for the ED service would be appended with modifier -57 to indicate that the E/M service resulted in the decision to perform the surgery.

Now, complete the practice exercises for coding for E/M services in There's a Code for That 8.5.

8.5

There's a Code for That

E/M services

Read the following documentation of the E/M service and code for the encounter.

1. Routine physical examination for newborn infant, never seen in this practice before.

   CPT code: _____

2. Annual wellness exam for 45-year-old female established patient.

   CPT code: _____

3. Routine well-child exam of established 2-year-old female. During well check it was found that she had acute serous OM of the right ear. Additional E/M performed with problem-focused history and exam, with MDM of low complexity.

   CPT codes: _____, _____ - _____

4. 60-year-old patient seen for a preventive routine physical examination, as mandated by his life insurance policy.

CPT code: _____ - _____

5. A 15-year-old female was seen in the office and a decision for surgery was made. What modifier would be appended to the E/M service code?

Modifier: _____

Vaccinations

After E/M services, the most common procedures performed by primary care specialists are vaccinations. Often performed alongside an E/M service, vaccinations may be administered on a set schedule, as is the case with infants and small children who receive vaccines per a timetable set by the state in which they live. Vaccines also may be given to patients on an annual basis, such as the flu shot, or on an as-needed basis per health recommendations, such as the Tdap (tetanus, diphtheria, and pertussis) vaccine that is recommended for pregnant women and once every 10 years for adults.

It is important to keep in mind that not all injections given in a healthcare office are vaccines. Some are injections of antibiotics or therapeutic substances. These injections are coded differently than vaccinations. **Immune globulins** (codes 90281 through 90399) are serum globulins extracted from human blood, or recombinant immune globulin products created in a laboratory through genetic modification of human and/or animal proteins. These substances are injected as a post-exposure prophylaxis, meaning that they are given after the patient has been exposed to the disease. For example, the rabies immune globulin (90375, 90376) is given after a patient has been exposed to the rabies virus via an animal bite, scratch, or lick. Although the codes for these injections are listed before the codes for vaccine administrations, vaccine administration codes are not used to report the injection of immune globulins. Rather, the code for the injections of a therapeutic substance should be used. Pay careful attention to the guidelines before each section of codes to help identify which codes to use.

When coding for vaccines, to the coder should understand the two components needed to report a vaccine administration correctly—the administration of the vaccine and the vaccine serum itself. The way the vaccine was administered will also impact the administration codes used. To report a vaccine administration accurately, it is necessary to report two codes, at a minimum. At least one code is required for the administration of the vaccination, and another code is required for the vaccine serum itself (see figure 8.8).

Figure 8.8. Vaccine coding components

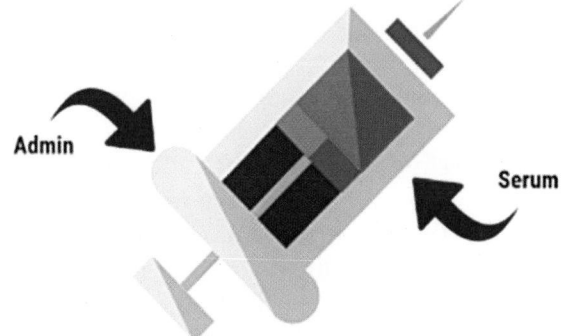

Administration

Vaccine administration is the act of giving the patient the vaccine, such as by injecting the needle into the muscle or spraying the vaccine into the nose or mouth. When coding for the administration of a vaccine, it is important to know the following:

- What was the route of administration: Was it an oral/nasal vaccine, or was it injected?
- The age of the patient: Was the patient under the age of 18 years?
- Was counseling provided to the patient?
- Are there multiple components to the vaccine serum?
- How many vaccines were given and what were they?

There are six different vaccine administration codes and to the coder must know the answers to these questions before he or she can determine which administration codes to report. Vaccine administration codes fall into three categories:

- 90460 and 90461 report adminstrations that were provided with counseling to pediatric patients.
- 90471 and 90472 report administration of injected vaccines.
- 90473 and 90474 report administration of oral or nasal vaccines.

The most basic vaccine administration codes are 90471, Immunization administration (includes percutaneous, intradermal, subcutaneous, or intramuscular); 1 vaccine, and 90472, each additional vaccine. These codes are for the administration of a vaccine via injection (that is, needle), no matter what type of injection is used (for example, intramuscular, intradermal, subcutaneous, and such). Furthermore, the words "single or combination vaccine/toxoid" are found in parentheses after each code, and indicate that no matter the vaccine serum if it was given via an injection, then code 90471 should be used to identify the first injection. If a patient received more than one injection, then 90471 is used for the first injection, and the add-on code 90472 is used for each additional injection (see figure 8.9).

Figure 8.9. Example of vaccine injections using 90471 and 90472

A patient received three total vaccines that were administered intradermally.

90471 (for the first vaccine)	OR 90471 (for the first vaccine)
90472 (for the second vaccine)	90472 × 2 (for the next two vaccines)
90472 (for the third vaccine)	

Many third-party payers have specific requirements regarding how they will process vaccine codes. For example, some require the coder to list each individual vaccine administration individually, whereas a different insurance plan may allow coders to report multiple units (illustrated by using the × symbol) and combine administration codes. Still other payers may require the codes to be ordered in a specific manner. What is imperative is that each vaccine serum is reported alongside the appropriate administration codes.

The next vaccine administration codes are 90473, Immunization administration by intranasal or oral route; 1 vaccine, and 90474, each additional vaccine. Again note that after each code description in parentheses are the words "single or combination vaccine/toxoid," and remember the only thing that matters with these codes is if the vaccine was delivered orally or intra-nasally. If a patient received more than one oral or nasal vaccine, then the administration of the first vaccine would be reported with 90473 and 90474 would be reported for each additional vaccine (see figure 8.10).

Figure 8.10. Example of vaccine administrations using 90473 and 90474

> *A patient received two vaccines. One was administered nasally and the other was administered orally.*

90473 (for the first vaccine)
90474 (for the second vaccine)

This gets trickier when the vaccines administered are both injected and oral vaccines. It is very common, especially in pediatric patients, that multiple vaccines are given at a single encounter. Often this includes both injected and oral or nasal vaccines and in this case codes 90471 and 90473 (for the first administration) may *never* be used together. One or the other must take precedence. Instead of using both 90471 for the first injected vaccine and 90473 for the first oral/nasal vaccine, either 90471 or 90473 would be used depending on which vaccine was first, and then 90472 and 90474 would be used for the additional vaccines (see figure 8.11).

Figure 8.11. Example of vaccine administrations using a combination of injections and oral/nasal vaccines

> *A patient received three injected vaccinations, one oral vaccine, and one nasal vaccine.*

90471 (for the first injected vaccine given)
90472 (for the second injected vaccine)
90472 (for the third injected vaccine)   90471 (for the first injected vaccine given)
90474 (for the oral vaccine)   OR   90472 × 2 (for the next two injected vaccines)
90474 (for the nasal vaccine)   90474 × 2 (for the oral and nasal vaccines)

The last two vaccine administration codes necessitate the most attention to detail. These are the only two vaccine administration codes that require counseling by the physician or other qualified healthcare practitioner. They may also only be used with pediatric patients (up to the age of 18). Administration codes 90460, Immunization administration through 18 years of age via any route of administration, with counseling by physician or other qualified health care professional; first or only component of each vaccine or toxoid administered, and 90461, Immunization administration through 18 years of age via any route of administration, with counseling by physician or other qualified health care professional; each additional vaccine or toxoid component administered, take into account the counseling provided to patients, and were developed in response to the heavy amount of counseling that some healthcare providers must give their patients regarding the safety and efficacy of vaccines. These administration codes were specially developed to capture this extra counseling, for *each component* of *each vaccine* given.

Components are the individual toxoid elements that are present within a vaccine. There are several combination vaccines—such as the MMR vaccine that combines toxoids for measles (M), mumps (M), and rubella (R). This is an example of a three-component vaccine; for the administration of an MMR vaccine, there are three components. 90460 would be used to report the first component, and 90461 (× 2) would be used to report the second and third components (see figure 8.12).

Figure 8.12. Example of component coding using 90460 and 90461

> *A pediatric patient received the MMR injection with counseling.*

90460 (for the first component)   90460 (for the first component)
90461 (for the second component)   OR   90461 × 2 (for the next two components)
90461 (for the third component)

If a patient received multiple vaccines, each with several components, then code 90460 (and any additional component administration codes) would be used for each vaccine. For example, if a patient received three vaccines—MMR (three components), DTaP (three components), and flu mist vaccines—then code 90460 would be used *three* times, one for each of the first components. 90461 would be used four times, to report the additional two components for the MMR and DTaP vaccines (see figure 8.13).

Figure 8.13. Example of component coding using 90460 and 90461 with multiple vaccines

A pediatric patient received an MMR and DTaP injection, and flu mist nasal vaccine with counseling.

90460 (for the first component of MMR)	90460 (for the first component of MMR)
90461 (for the second component of MMR)	90461 × 2 (for the next two components of MMR)
90461 (for the third component of MMR)	90460 (for the first component of DTaP)
90460 (for the first component of DTaP) OR	90461 × 2 (for the next two components of DTaP)
90461 (for the second component of DTaP)	90460 (for the one component of flu mist)
90461 (for the third component of DTaP)	
90460 (for the one component of flu mist)	

Key to Success

Note that with administration codes 90460 and 90461, the route of administration does not matter. Codes for vaccine administration provided to a pediatric patient with counseling do not differ depending on whether the vaccine was given orally, nasally, or injected (see figure 8.14).

Vaccination coding is not complete without also reporting the serum that was administered. Vaccine serum, or toxoid, codes identify the substance that was injected into the patient.

Figure 8.14. Vaccine administration codes

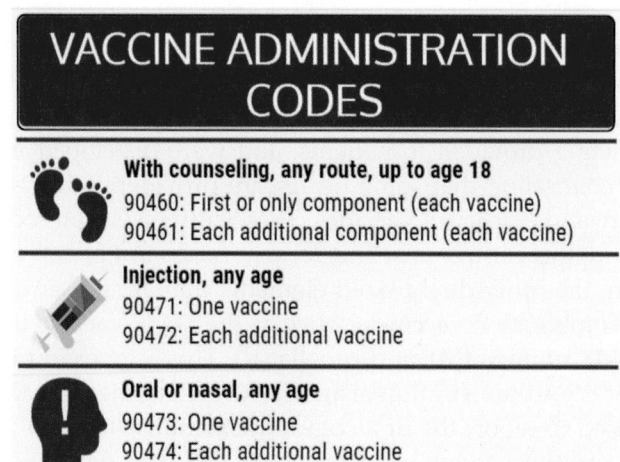

Vaccine Serums/Toxoids

The **vaccine toxoid** is the actual substance that is injected or given to a patient and that creates an immune response from the patient. There are a number of vaccine toxoid codes, each of which identify the specific substance that was injected into the patient at the encounter. One code should be selected to identify each vaccine administered. When coding vaccine toxoids, it is important to pay attention to the following:

- *The specific toxoid administered.* Codes may describe the formulation of the vaccine, such as 90649, Human papillomavirus vaccine, types 6, 11, 16, 18, quadrivalent (4vHPV) versus 90650, Human papillomavirus vaccine, types 16, 18, bivalent (2vHPV).

- *The age group for the vaccine.* Codes may differ depending on age of the patient, such as 90634, Hepatitis A vaccine pediatric/adolescent dosage, versus 90636, Hepatitis A and hepatitis B vaccine, adult dosage.

- *The dosing schedule of the vaccine.* Codes sometimes differ, depending on the dosing schedule for which they are formulated, such as 90647, Haemophilus influenza type b vaccine, 3 dose schedule, versus 90648, Haemophilus influenza type b vaccine, 4 dose schedule.

- *The route of administration.* Codes will differ based on the route of administration, such as 90658, Influenza virus vaccine, trivalent, for intramuscular use, versus 90660, Influenza virus vaccine, trivalent, for intranasal use.

- *The components of the vaccine.* As previously discussed, combination vaccines include components for multiple diseases. Pay careful attention to the components included, as there are many similar combinations.

Putting It All Together: Coding for Vaccinations

Procedural coding for vaccines requires *at least* two codes: one for the administration of the vaccine and one for the serum administered. In the real world, it is important to also pay attention to the third-party payer involved in the claim, as the patient's insurance may require vaccination codes in a certain order or reported with additional information in order to cover the vaccines. Certain insurances may also only cover specific vaccines, so it is also important to verify that each vaccine is covered under the patient's insurance policy. For example, Medicare may restrict the number or type of vaccinations covered for Medicare beneficiaries. Furthermore, Medicare requires different vaccine administration codes for three vaccines:

- G0008, Administration of influenza virus vaccine
- G0009, Administration of pneumococcal virus vaccine
- G0010, Administration of hepatitis B vaccine

If a Medicare patient presents for either an influenza, pneumococcal, or hepatitis B vaccine, then one of these three vaccine administration codes should be used, rather than the administration codes identified previously (90460 through 90474). The serum code is still reported with the administration, so if a Medicare patient received an influenza vaccine, then it would be coded as follows: G0008, Administration of influenza virus vaccine, and 90658, Influenza virus vaccine, trivalent (IIV3), split virus, 0.5 mL dosage, for intramuscular use. Practice selecting the appropriate vaccine or E/M codes in the exercises in There's a Code for That 8.6.

Vaccine coding

8.6

There's a Code for That

Read the following documentation and select the appropriate vaccine and/or E/M codes.

1. Patient with commercial insurance was given seasonal influenza vaccine (trivalent, split virus), 0.25mL, via injection.

   CPT codes: _____, _____

(Continued on next page)

8.6

Continued

2. Vaccine administration provided to a 5-year-old patient with counseling. Vaccines administered were DTaP and varicella.

CPT codes (DTaP admin): _____, _____ × _____

CPT code (DTaP): _____

CPT code (varicella admin): _____

CPT code (varicella): _____

3. Patient was given HPV vaccine via IM injection (4vHPV) in the office, patient also received meningococcal conjugate vaccine (MCV4).

CPT codes (HPV admin and serum): _____, _____

CPT codes (meningococcal admin and serum): _____, _____

4. Routine physical examination for 18-month-old female with Medicaid. Hepatitis B, IPV, rotavirus (RV5), and influenza (LAIV3) vaccines all given in the office.

CPT code (E/M service): _____

CPT codes (hep B admin and serum): _____, _____

CPT codes (IPV admin and serum): _____, _____

CPT codes (rotavirus admin and serum): _____, _____

CPT codes (influenza admin and serum): _____, _____

In-Office Procedures

In addition to evaluation and management encounters and vaccinations, primary care specialists perform several minor in-office procedures, miscellaneous medical procedures, and certain lab tests. Some of these in-office procedures are specialized in nature—such as avulsion of an ingrown toenail performed by a podiatrist, or removal or insertion of an IUD device performed by a gynecologist. Ultimately, the procedures performed by a primary care specialist will depend on his or her area of specialty, the needs of the patient, and available resources. It is also important to remember the impact of modifiers on procedures performed at the same time as an evaluation and management service, as these will greatly impact payment for the services provided.

Minor Surgical Procedures

Minor surgical procedures may be found throughout the CPT code book, and may be performed across several different healthcare specialties. Unlike major invasive surgeries, minor surgical procedures are minimally invasive, in that they only break the skin or mucous membranes and connective tissues. Minor surgical procedures do not require any general anesthesia or respiratory assistance during the procedure. However, they might involve local anesthesia, such as application of a numbing cream to the skin. Some of these in-office medical procedures include

- *Wart cryosurgery.* An integumentary system procedure, cryosurgical removal of warts is a common in-office medical procedure. It involved using a can of medical grade liquid nitrogen to freeze off the nonmalignant lesion and is reported with code 17110, Destruction (e.g., laser surgery, electrosurgery, cryosurgery, chemosurgery, surgical curettement), of benign lesions other than skin tags or cutaneous vascular proliferative lesions; up to 14 lesions.

- *Lysis of penile adhesions.* Common in circumcised male infants, penile adhesions occur when the skin of the glans of the penis adheres to the skin of the shaft of the penis. This must be separated via lysis before it grows together and requires surgical intervention. It is reported with 54162, Lysis or excision of penile post-circumcision adhesions.

- *Repair of lacerations and suture removal.* Although it is more common for patients to receive sutures in an emergency department or urgent care clinic, some primary care providers may perform simple laceration repairs in-office. Codes for simple repair of the integumentary system (12001 through 12021), depend on the site of the repair and the total length of the repair. For example, if the doctor sutures three lacerations on the cheek, the lengths of which add up to 3 cm total, then code 12013, Simple repair of superficial wounds of face, ears, eyelids, nose, lips, and/or mucous membranes; 2.6 cm to 5.0 cm, would be reported. If areas other than the face, ears, eyelids, nose, lips and/or mucous membranes (as listed in this code description) were repaired, then these anatomical sites would be grouped into a different CPT code, as necessary. To code for the simple repair of superficial wounds, both the anatomical sites and the size of the repair are grouped into the same code. Removal of sutures is more common in the primary care office. Most patients who receive sutures in an emergency department or urgent care clinic return to the office of their primary care doctor for removal of the sutures. There is no code that captures the work involved in removing sutures that were placed by another provider. This is because the removal of simple sutures is included in the code for the placement of the sutures; the two procedures are bundled into the same code. Instead, an E/M code that is appropriate to the level of work involved would be reported for the removal of sutures.

- *Biopsy.* Whether or not a primary care specialist performs a biopsy will depend on the needs of the patient and available resources. Typically, more invasive or specialized biopsies, such as the biopsy of a breast lump via fine needle aspiration, are performed by a specialized provider. Simple biopsies, such as the biopsy of a mole or nevus, may be performed by a primary care specialist. This procedure includes the simple shaving or excision of a portion of the lesion to send to pathology for a biopsy, and would be reported with codes 11100, Biopsy of skin, subcutaneous tissue and/or mucous membrane (including simple closure), unless otherwise listed; *single lesion*, and 11101, Biopsy of skin, subcutaneous tissue and/or mucous membrane (including simple closure), unless otherwise listed; *each separate/additional lesion.*

- *Incision and drainage (I&D) of abscess.* An **incision and drainage** is a surgical treatment performed for soft tissue abscesses, for which medical treatment alone is insufficient. In this procedure, the abscess is incised with a sharp blade and drained of material. It is sometimes packed with gauze or other medicinal agents to reduce the infection. Codes for I&D of abscess are 10060, Incision and drainage of abscess (e.g., carbuncle, suppurative hidradenitis, cutaneous or subcutaneous abscess, cyst, furuncle, or paronychia); simple or single, and 10061, Incision and drainage of abscess (e.g., carbuncle, suppurative hidradenitis, cutaneous or subcutaneous abscess, cyst, furuncle, or paronychia): complicated or multiple. When coding for an incision and drainage, it is important to identify the type of cyst or lesion on which the procedure was performed, as there are additional codes for the I&D of acne lesions, pilonidal cysts, and for the removal of foreign bodies.

- *Removal of foreign bodies.* A foreign body is any unnatural object that is present in the human body. Removal of foreign bodies can be as varied as the removal of a splinter from under the skin, to the removal of a bean stuck in a child's nose or ear. Depending on the site and type of the foreign body, this procedure may be performed in the primary care office or in the hospital setting. For example, the removal of a foreign body from the nose may not be possible in the outpatient setting, if the child is uncooperative or if the foreign body is stuck too far in the nasal cavity to remove with forceps. If this is the case, then the child would be sent to the hospital for general anesthesia or for a more invasive procedure. When coding for foreign body removal, go to the entry for *Removal* in the CPT Index, locate the subterm *Foreign body*, and verify the code selection in the Tabular List.

Medical Procedures

Besides minor surgical procedures, multiple miscellaneous procedures from the Medicine section of the CPT code book are commonly used to report the different procedures and services provided to patients. These procedures range from therapeutic injections, to hearing and visual screening screenings, developmental evaluations, and codes used to report services provided outside normal office hours. The procedures performed will again depend on the type of primary care practitioner, the patients he or she serves, and available resources. They include the following.

- **Electrocardiogram** (ECG or EKG). ECGs are common procedures that record the heart's electrical activity as a line tracing on paper and can be used to evaluate heart rhythm and function. The code for a routine ECG is 93000, Electrocardiogram, routine ECG with at least 12 leads; with interpretation and report. However, this is not the only ECG code available. Note that the code description read "with interpretation and report." This means that the provider's office both performed the ECG test (which includes placing leads on the patient's chest and performing the procedure), as well as providing a report of the ECG findings. Code 93000 should only be reported if both of these conditions were met. Code 93005, Electrocardiogram, routine ECG with at least 12 leads; tracing only, without interpretation and report should be reported when the office performed the ECG procedure but the healthcare provider did not read and provide a report of the tracing findings. Code 93010, Electrocardiogram, routine ECG with at least 12 leads; interpretation and report only, should be reported when the healthcare provider reviews and provided a report of the ECG tracing, but a different office provides the actual ECG tracing. Keep in mind that there are additional ECG codes within the Cardiography section of the CPT code book. Be sure to read the code descriptions carefully.

Key to Success

The differences in the codes for electrocardiograms describe the technical versus the professional components of the service. The technical component of the service is the performance of the test. The professional component of the service is the healthcare provider's interpretation of the findings of the test. These two components also make up numerous radiology codes as well as some cardiovascular codes, so it is important to keep them in mind as you learn more about the codes in the CPT code book.

- *Therapeutic injections.* Unlike vaccinations, therapeutic injections are given to patients for some sort of therapeutic treatment. For example, a very sick patient may require an injection of an antibiotic in the office to begin antibiotic treatment immediately, or a patient with an intractable migraine may be given a shot of medication to help with the pain immediately. Like vaccine coding, these injections require at least two codes—one for the administration of the injection and one for the substance injected. Code 96372, Therapeutic, prophylactic, or diagnostic injection (specify substance or drug), subcutaneous or intramuscular, should be used to report the intramuscular injection of a therapeutic substance as described previously. The substance injected is reported with the appropriate HCPCS code to identify the medication administered by the injection. These therapeutic substances are reported with the appropriate HCPCS code, found in the Table of Drugs, as discussed in chapter 5.

- *Screenings.* Primary care practitioners, as the first line of care for patients, perform a number of different screenings. These include vision, hearing, psychological, and developmental screenings, among others. These screenings are often performed together with a preventive medicine service to check for any patient abnormalities. If any abnormalities are present, then the primary care practitioner will likely refer the patient to a healthcare specialist, or he or she may order further diagnostic tests. To find the codes for the specific screening service performed, refer to the CPT Index and search under the specific name of the test, or the body area or organ system, and reference the screening performed.

- *Respiratory services.* Respiratory services are common in the primary care office. These include spirometer tests, breathing treatments, and pulmonary function tests, and are reported with codes from the Pulmonary subsection, 94010 to 904799.

Laboratory Procedures

The last type of procedures that are often performed in the primary care setting are in-office laboratory procedures. Whether laboratory procedures are performed in the office and which procedures are performed depends on office specifics. For example, some offices may not perform any laboratory procedures, whereas others might have a CLIA-waived status that allows them to perform certain in-office laboratory procedures, such as blood counts and bacterial cultures. CLIA stands for the Clinical Laboratory Improvement Amendments of 1988, which regulates facilities that perform laboratory tests on human specimens. CLIA-waived laboratory tests are simple and have low risk for erroneous results, although they are not error-proof. Some of the laboratory tests that are performed in-office include:

- Urinalysis procedures are commonly done to identify a specific substance in the urine, such as glucose, or to indicate if a urinary tract infection is present. They are reported with codes from the Urinalysis subsection of the CPT code book, 81000 through 81099. Usually done with a reactive strip, urine pregnancy tests are administered when a patient may be pregnant and are coded with 81025, Urine pregnancy test, by visual color comparison methods.

- Throat and nasal swabs are performed to obtain a sample of the mucous membrane lining from the back of the throat or nasal passages. Two frequently performed throat swabs are for streptococcus, 87880, Streptococcus, group A, and mononucleosis, 86308, Heterophile antibodies, screening. Influenza tests are performed via a nasopharyngeal swab and are reported with 87804, Influenza.

- Blood counts identify the specific amounts of certain cells within a blood sample. For example, a red blood cell count will determine the amount of red blood cells that are present in a blood sample. The code used to report the blood count depends on what type of count it was, such as complete blood count (CBC), white blood cell count (WBC), or red blood cell count (RBC), and other factors that identify the type of hematology procedure performed. They are located in the Hematology and Coagulation subsection of the CPT code book, 85004 through 85049.

MOD

It may be necessary to append modifier -QW, CLIA-waived test, at the end of the CLIA-waived laboratory tests performed in your office. It identifies that the procedure was a CLIA-waived test that was performed in your office, rather than sent to a laboratory. This depends on carrier discretion, so some payers might require this and others may not.

Key to Success

Codes for laboratory services might be difficult to locate in the CPT code book. If you are stuck, it is helpful to look up the infectious agent or screening in as many ways as possible and to check all cross-references. Start by searching for the infectious agent by name, or by locating the type of screening, and go from there. It may take some time, but the more familiar you become with laboratory codes, the easier it will be to find what you are looking for.

Modifiers for In-Office Procedures

It is common that an in-office procedure and an evaluation and management procedure are both performed at the same encounter on the same patient. When this happens, it is appropriate to report one code for the evaluation and management service as well as the code for the in-office procedure, as long as the E/M service is a significant, separately identifiable service from the in-office procedure. When this is the case, it is important to remember to append the correct modifiers to the procedure codes. Whether or not to add a modifier depends on the insurance payer, as well as the specifics of the encounter. According to CPT guidelines, if an E/M code is billed with any type of additional procedure modifier -25, Significant, separately identifiable evaluation and management service by the same physician or other qualified healthcare professional on the same day of the procedure or other service, must be appended to the E/M code to identify the E/M service as separately identifiable from the additional procedure. This identifies the E/M as a unique and different service from the other procedure that was performed, so that the insurance payer will pay for each service separately (both the E/M service as well as the additional procedure). Documentation should clearly identify that an E/M service was performed in addition to the procedure, and that the two services were distinct from each other. Additional important modifiers in the primary care setting include

- Modifier -59, Distinct procedural service. This modifier is used to identify procedures or services, other than E/M services, that are not normally reported together but are appropriate under the circumstances. For example, an E/M service performed with an in-office procedure, such as wart cryosurgery. These two procedures are not commonly reported together, so the cryosurgery code would be appended with modifier -59. Modifier -59 should be used when the documentation supports a different session, different procedure or surgery, different site or organ system, separate excision or incision, separate lesion, or separate injury, not ordinarily encountered on the same day or at the same encounter. Refer to chapter 5 for additional information on modifier -59.

- Modifier -76, Repeat procedure or service by same physician or other qualified health care professional. This modifier is useful when a particular procedure must be repeated. For example, if a patient receives a nebulizer breathing treatment in the office to treat asthma with status asthmaticus, and then the provider must administer another nebulizer breathing treatment because the first one was not effective enough, then modifier -76 would be used to indicate the procedure had to be repeated. The procedure code would be billed with two units (depending on how many times the procedure was performed), and appended with modifier -76.

Now, practice selecting the appropriate procedure or E/M codes in the exercises in There's a Code for That 8.7.

Primary care procedures

8.7

There's a Code for That

Read the following documentation and select the appropriate procedure and/or E/M codes.

1. Newborn seen in the office for suspected urinary tract infection. Doctor performed a detailed history and examination, and moderate complexity medical decision making for the E/M encounter for this new patient. A straight urinary catheter was inserted to obtain urine sample, and qualitative urinalysis performed.

   CPT code (E/M service): _____ - _____

   CPT code (urinalysis): _____

   CPT code (catheterization): _____

2. Wart cryosurgery performed on three painful warts on 28-year-old female patient.

   CPT code: _____

3. Routine preventive well-child exam performed on established 4-year-old patient. Screening test for visual acuity also performed.

   CPT codes: _____ , _____

Diagnosis Coding in Primary Care

Because primary care specialists are the first point of contact for patients, these providers see healthcare conditions across the entire spectrum of the ICD-10-CM code book. A primary care coder should therefore be familiar with how to select codes from all chapters of the ICD-10-CM code book. Furthermore, because PCPs are often the first healthcare provider that a patient sees when he or she begins to experience problems, they are more likely to see patients with signs, symptoms, and conditions that may not be definitive in nature. For example, a patient with fatigue and thinning hair may need more workup before the provider can diagnose the patient with a specific disease or condition. For the time being, it is necessary to report the patient symptoms, which are typically unspecified in nature. For these reasons, PCPs are more likely to report unspecified (NOS) codes. Therefore coders should strive to select the most specific code possible, based on the provider's documentation of the patient's healthcare conditions.

Remember, if a provider has documented that a condition is "suspected," "possible," "rule-out," or in any way questions that the patient may not actually have the condition, then the diagnosis code for the suspected condition should not be reported. If there is no definitive diagnosis recorded in the patient's health record, then it is necessary to code for the signs and symptoms only.

When coding for primary care services, there are a few chapters within the ICD-10-CM code book with which coders should be more familiar, as well as a few conditions of which they should be especially aware. These are chapter 18: Symptoms, Signs and Abnormal Clinical and Laboratory Findings, Not Elsewhere Classified; and Z-codes, located in chapter 21: Factors Influencing Health Status and Contact with Health Services. The end of this section will also discuss some of the top conditions for this specialty, as well as certain conditions that are important in HCC coding.

Signs and Symptoms

Chapter 18: Symptoms, Signs and Abnormal Clinical and Laboratory Findings, Not Elsewhere Classified, contains code for signs and symptoms that are reported when a more definitive diagnosis cannot be confirmed. This chapter includes symptoms, signs, abnormal results of clinical or other investigative procedures, and ill-defined conditions regarding which no diagnosis classifiable elsewhere is recorded. According to the OCGR for chapter 18 (see also figure 8.15):

- Codes that describe symptoms and signs are acceptable when a definitive diagnosis has not been established by the provider.
- Codes for signs and symptoms may be reported in addition to a related definitive diagnosis when the sign or symptom is not routinely associated with that

Figure 8.15. OGCR I.C.18.a, I.C.18.b, I.C.18.c

---

18. Chapter 18: Symptoms, Signs, and Abnormal Clinical and Laboratory Findings, Not Elsewhere Classified (R00-R99)

Chapter 18 includes symptoms, signs, abnormal results of clinical or other investigative procedures, and ill-defined conditions regarding which no diagnosis classifiable elsewhere is recorded. Signs and symptoms that point to a specific diagnosis have been assigned to a category in other chapters of the classification.

a. Use of symptom codes

Codes that describe symptoms and signs are acceptable for reporting purposes when a related definitive diagnosis has not been established (confirmed) by the provider.

b. Use of a symptom code with a definitive diagnosis code

Codes for signs and symptoms may be reported in addition to a related definitive diagnosis when the sign or symptom is not routinely associated with that diagnosis, such as the various signs and symptoms associated with complex syndromes. The definitive diagnosis code should be sequenced before the symptom code.

Signs or symptoms that are associated routinely with a disease process should not be assigned as additional codes, unless otherwise instructed by the classification.

c. Combination codes that include symptoms

ICD-10-CM contains a number of combination codes that identify both the definitive diagnosis and common symptoms of that diagnosis. When using one of these combination codes, an additional code should not be assigned for the symptom.

Source: CMS 2018.

diagnosis. The definitive diagnosis should be sequenced before the symptom or sign code.

- Codes for signs and symptoms that are commonly associated with a disease process should not be assigned as additional codes, unless otherwise instructed by ICD-10-CM notations.
- If a combination code exists that includes the definitive diagnosis along with the sign or symptom, it is not necessary to assign an additional code for the symptom.

In short, do not code for signs and symptoms that are routinely associated with a disease process. For example, if the definitive diagnosis is a fractured wrist, then it is not necessary to include a code for wrist pain. On the other hand, if a sign or symptom is not commonly associated with the disease process, it is acceptable to report a sign or symptom code to better describe the condition. For example, a patient experiencing fainting spells in addition to being diagnosed with an ear infection.

Note that not all signs and symptoms are located within chapter 18. Some specific signs and symptoms are located within the chapters for their respective organ system or body area. Some of the more common sign and symptoms reported in primary care are

- **Abdominal pain (R10).** Abdominal pain codes are specific as to the type and location of the pain. Types include acute abdomen (severe generalized abdominal pain), localized pain, abdominal tenderness, rebound abdominal tenderness, colic, and generalized abdominal pain. The sites for abdominal pain are quite specific, and include left or right upper or lower quadrants, periumbilic, or epigastric sites (see figure 8.16) for an illustration of abdominopelvic regions and quadrants that may be identified by ICD-10-CM codes for abdominal pain.
- **Fever (R50).** There are five possible fever codes: drug induced, post-procedural, post-vaccination, post-transfusion, or unspecified. If the type of fever is not identified as one of the former types, the NOS code should be selected: R50.9, Fever, unspecified.

Figure 8.16. Abdominopelvic regions and quadrants

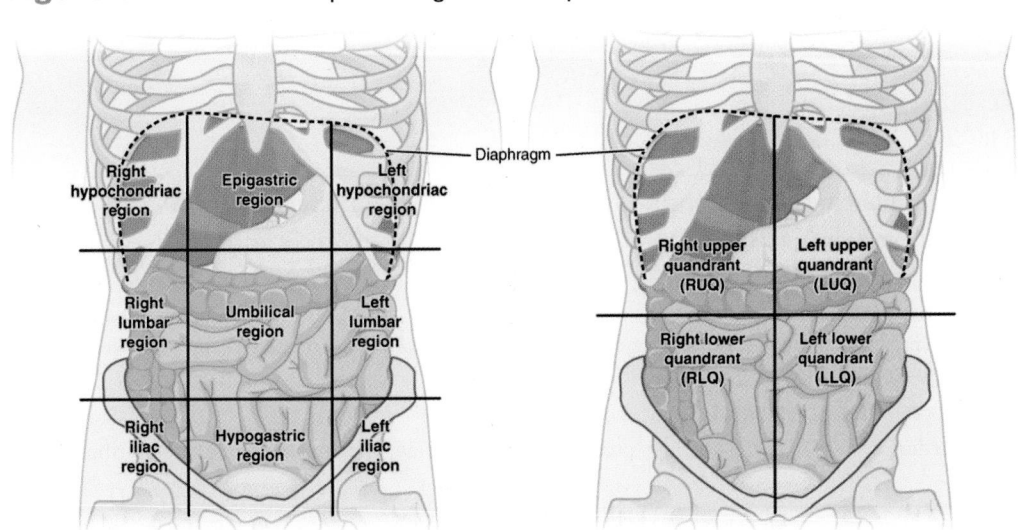

(a) Abdominopelvic regions   (b) Abdominopelvic quadrants

Source: OpenStax 2013.

- **Chest pain (R07).** Chest pain codes are divided on the site and type of the chest pain, including pain in throat, chest pain on breathing, precordial pain, pleurodynia, intercostal pain, other specified, or unspecified chest pain. If the chest pain is not identified as one of the former types, then the NOS code should be selected: R07.9, Chest pain, unspecified.

- **Abnormal glucose (R73).** Abnormal glucose codes should be reported when a lab finding has resulted in an atypical reading of the glucose level in the blood. Codes for abnormal glucose in the signs and symptoms chapter do not include low glucose levels (E16.2, Hypoglycemia), rather only raised or prediabetic levels (hyperglycemia). The codes include impaired fasting glucose, impaired oral glucose tolerance, prediabetes, other specified type of abnormal glucose, or hyperglycemia, unspecified.

Z-Codes

Chapter 21: Factors Influencing Health Status and Contact with Health Services includes numerous codes used in the primary care setting. These codes are different than codes in the other ICD-10-CM chapters, as they identify reasons for encounters other than when a patient is ill such as an encounter for a preventive exam, and specifics that add more information to the encounter, such as relevant family healthcare history or a past medical event. The official guidelines for the use of codes from this chapter are extensive, so it is important to read and understand these guidelines before selecting codes from this chapter. The following guidelines should be noted (see also figure 8.17):

- Z codes may be used in any healthcare setting, and they may be used as either a first-listed or secondary diagnosis code. Certain Z-codes are designated only as first-listed diagnosis codes.

- Z codes are not procedure codes. They may seem very similar to procedure codes, but do not confuse the two. Z-codes are used to identify the reason for a patient encounter. If the encounter is for a preventive examination, then the reason for the encounter is preventive examination (see category Z00.0, Encounter for general adult medical examination). Keep in mind that both an ICD-10-CM code and a CPT code must be used together to report a healthcare encounter completely.

Figure 8.17. OGCR I.C.21.a, I.C.21.b

---

21. **Chapter 21: Factors Influencing Health Status and Contact with Health Services (Z00-Z99)**

NOTE The chapter specific guidelines provide additional information about the use of Z codes for specified encounters.

a. **Use of Z codes in any healthcare setting**

Z codes are for use in any healthcare setting. Z codes may be used as either a first-listed (principal diagnosis code in the inpatient setting) or secondary code, depending on the circumstances of the encounter. Certain Z codes may only be used as first-listed or principal diagnosis.

b. **Z Codes indicate a reason for an encounter**

Z codes are not procedure codes. A corresponding procedure code must accompany a Z code to describe any procedure performed.

Source: CMS 2018.

- There are 16 categories of Z-codes, and not all of them are listed here. It is helpful to read through the OGCR and the description of categories within the chapter to understand the guidelines for each.

Some of the more common Z-codes that are reported in primary care include

- *Persons encountering health services for examinations (Z00 to Z13).* This category includes preventive examinations. For preventive examination codes, it is important to select the appropriate code according to the age of the patient (adult, newborn under 8 days old, newborn 8 to 28 days old, child over 28 days old), and whether or not any abnormal findings were encountered. An abnormal finding includes anything that is considered an additional finding by the healthcare provider. This could range from a problem in growth or development, to an illness or chronic healthcare condition. This category also includes codes for special examinations, such as vision and hearing screening, gynecological exams, screening exams for malignant neoplasms, and preoperative examinations. See figure 8.18 for the OGCR related to preventive examination services.

- *Patient status codes.* Status codes indicate that a patient is either a carrier of a disease or has the sequelae or residual of a past disease or condition. These codes identify patient status such as the presence of a prosthetic or mechanical device from a past healthcare treatment, the fact that a patient has a healthcare condition, or a condition that is likely to impact his or her health, acquired absences, and the presence of artificial openings (such as a gastrostomy). See figure 8.19 for the OGCR related to patient status codes.

Figure 8.18. OGCR I.C.21.c.13

---

13) Routine and administrative examinations

The Z codes allow for the description of encounters for routine examinations, such as, a general check-up, or, examinations for administrative purposes, such as, a pre-employment physical. The codes are not to be used if the examination is for diagnosis of a suspected condition or for treatment purposes. In such cases the diagnosis code is used. During a routine exam, should a diagnosis or condition be discovered, it should be coded as an additional code. Pre-existing and chronic conditions and history codes may also be included as additional codes as long as the examination is for administrative purposes and not focused on any particular condition.

Some of the codes for routine health examinations distinguish between "with" and "without" abnormal findings. Code assignment depends on the information that is known at the time the encounter is being coded. For example, if no abnormal findings were found during the examination, but the encounter is being coded before test results are back, it is acceptable to assign the code for "without abnormal findings." When assigning a code for "with abnormal findings," additional code(s) should be assigned to identify the specific abnormal finding(s).

Pre-operative examination and pre-procedural laboratory examination Z codes are for use only in those situations when a patient is being cleared for a procedure or surgery and no treatment is given.

The Z codes/categories for routine and administrative examinations:

Z00	Encounter for general examination without complaint, suspected or reported diagnosis
Z01	Encounter for other special examination without complaint, suspected or reported diagnosis
Z02	Encounter for administrative examination
	Except: Z02.9, Encounter for administrative examinations, unspecified
Z32.0-	Encounter for pregnancy test

Source: CMS 2018.

Figure 8.19. OGCR I.C.21.c.3

---

3) Status

Status codes indicate that a patient is either a carrier of a disease or has the sequelae or residual of a past disease or condition. This includes such things as the presence of prosthetic or mechanical devices resulting from past treatment. A status code is informative, because the status may affect the course of treatment and its outcome. A status code is distinct from a history code. The history code indicates that the patient no longer has the condition.

A status code should not be used with a diagnosis code from one of the body system chapters, if the diagnosis code includes the information provided by the status code. For example, code Z94.1, Heart transplant status, should not be used with a code from subcategory T86.2, Complications of heart transplant. The status code does not provide additional information. The complication code indicates that the patient is a heart transplant patient.

For encounters for weaning from a mechanical ventilator, assign a code from subcategory J96.1, Chronic respiratory failure, followed by code Z99.11, Dependence on respirator [ventilator] status.

The status Z codes/categories are:

Z14   Genetic carrier

        Genetic carrier status indicates that a person carries a gene, associated with a particular disease, which may be passed to offspring who may develop that disease. The person does not have the disease and is not at risk of developing the disease.

Z15   Genetic susceptibility to disease

        Genetic susceptibility indicates that a person has a gene that increases the risk of that person developing the disease.

        Codes from category Z15 should not be used as principal or first-listed codes. If the patient has the condition to which he/she is susceptible, and that condition is the reason for the encounter, the code for the current condition should be sequenced first. If the patient is being seen for follow-up after completed treatment for this condition, and the condition no longer exists, a follow-up code should be sequenced first, followed by the appropriate personal history and genetic susceptibility codes. If the purpose of the encounter is genetic counseling associated with procreative management, code Z31.5, Encounter for genetic counseling, should be assigned as the first-listed code, followed by a code from category Z15. Additional codes should be assigned for any applicable family or personal history.

Z16   Resistance to antimicrobial drugs

        This code indicates that a patient has a condition that is resistant to antimicrobial drug treatment. Sequence the infection code first.

Z17   Estrogen receptor status

Z18   Retained foreign body fragments

Z19   Hormone sensitivity malignancy status

Z21   Asymptomatic HIV infection status

        This code indicates that a patient has tested positive for HIV but has manifested no signs or symptoms of the disease.

Z22   Carrier of infectious disease

        Carrier status indicates that a person harbors the specific organisms of a disease without manifest symptoms and is capable of transmitting the infection.

Z28.3   Underimmunization status

Z33.1   Pregnant state, incidental

        This code is a secondary code only for use when the pregnancy is in no way complicating the reason for visit. Otherwise, a code from the obstetric chapter is required.

Z66   Do not resuscitate

        This code may be used when it is documented by the provider that a patient is on do not resuscitate status at any time during the stay.

Z67   Blood type

Z68   Body mass index (BMI)

        As with all other secondary diagnosis codes, the BMI codes should only be assigned when they meet the definition of a reportable diagnosis (see Section III, Reporting Additional Diagnoses).

Z74.01	Bed confinement status
Z76.82	Awaiting organ transplant status
Z78	Other specified health status

Code Z78.1, Physical restraint status, may be used when it is documented by the provider that a patient has been put in restraints during the current encounter. Please note that this code should not be reported when it is documented by the provider that a patient is temporarily restrained during a procedure.

Z79	Long-term (current) drug therapy

Codes from this category indicate a patient's continuous use of a prescribed drug (including such things as aspirin therapy) for the long-term treatment of a condition or for prophylactic use. It is not for use for patients who have addictions to drugs. This subcategory is not for use of medications for detoxification or maintenance programs to prevent withdrawal symptoms in patients with drug dependence (e.g., methadone maintenance for opiate dependence). Assign the appropriate code for the drug dependence instead.

Assign a code from Z79 if the patient is receiving a medication for an extended period as a prophylactic measure (such as for the prevention of deep vein thrombosis) or as treatment of a chronic condition (such as arthritis) or a disease requiring a lengthy course of treatment (such as cancer). Do not assign a code from category Z79 for medication being administered for a brief period of time to treat an acute illness or injury (such as a course of antibiotics to treat acute bronchitis).

Z88	Allergy status to drugs, medicaments and biological substances

Except: Z88.9, Allergy status to unspecified drugs, medicaments and biological substances status

Z89	Acquired absence of limb
Z90	Acquired absence of organs, not elsewhere classified
Z91.0-	Allergy status, other than to drugs and biological substances
Z92.82	Status post administration of tPA (rtPA) in a different facility within the last 24 hours prior to admission to a current facility

Assign code Z92.82, Status post administration of tPA (rtPA) in a different facility within the last 24 hours prior to admission to current facility, as a secondary diagnosis when a patient is received by transfer into a facility and documentation indicates they were administered tissue plasminogen activator (tPA) within the last 24 hours prior to admission to the current facility.

This guideline applies even if the patient is still receiving the tPA at the time they are received into the current facility.

The appropriate code for the condition for which the tPA was administered (such as cerebrovascular disease or myocardial infarction) should be assigned first.

Code Z92.82 is only applicable to the receiving facility record and not to the transferring facility record.

Z93	Artificial opening status
Z94	Transplanted organ and tissue status
Z95	Presence of cardiac and vascular implants and grafts
Z96	Presence of other functional implants
Z97	Presence of other devices
Z98	Other postprocedural states

Assign code Z98.85, Transplanted organ removal status, to indicate that a transplanted organ has been previously removed. This code should not be assigned for the encounter in which the transplanted organ is removed. The complication necessitating removal of the transplant organ should be assigned for that encounter.

See section I.C19. for information on the coding of organ transplant complications.

Z99	Dependence on enabling machines and devices, not elsewhere classified

NOTE   Categories Z89-Z90 and Z93-Z99 are for use only if there are no complications or malfunctions of the organ or tissue replaced, the amputation site or the equipment on which the patient is dependent.

HCC Coding Corner

HCC

Patient status codes are often important in HCC coding and risk adjustment, as they identify past healthcare conditions and treatments that may still have an impact on the patient's overall health. For example, nearly all codes within category Z94, Transplanted organ and tissue status, qualify as HCC codes. The fact that a patient has a past organ transplant is likely to impact his or her current and future healthcare needs, even though it might not be an issue at the present time.

- *Encounter for inoculation or vaccination.* In strict contrast to the complexity of CPT coding for vaccine administrations, identifying the medical necessity for ICD-10-CM codes is much easier. Code Z23, Encounter for immunization, is to be used to identify the medical necessity for all vaccines or inoculations.
- *Personal and family healthcare history.* There are two types of history codes—personal and family history. Personal history codes explain a patient's past healthcare condition that no longer exists and for which he or she is no longer receiving treatment, but that has the potential for recurrence and therefore may require continued monitoring. For example, an organ transplant or absence of an organ is an important part of personal history that has the potential to

Figure 8.20. OGCR I.C.21.c.4

4) History (of)

There are two types of history Z codes, personal and family. Personal history codes explain a patient's past medical condition that no longer exists and is not receiving any treatment, but that has the potential for recurrence, and therefore may require continued monitoring.

Family history codes are for use when a patient has a family member(s) who has had a particular disease that causes the patient to be at higher risk of also contracting the disease.

Personal history codes may be used in conjunction with follow- up codes and family history codes may be used in conjunction with screening codes to explain the need for a test or procedure. History codes are also acceptable on any medical record regardless of the reason for visit. A history of an illness, even if no longer present, is important information that may alter the type of treatment ordered.

The history Z code categories are:

Z80	Family history of primary malignant neoplasm
Z81	Family history of mental and behavioral disorders
Z82	Family history of certain disabilities and chronic diseases (leading to disablement)
Z83	Family history of other specific disorders
Z84	Family history of other conditions
Z85	Personal history of malignant neoplasm
Z86	Personal history of certain other diseases
Z87	Personal history of other diseases and conditions
Z91.4-	Personal history of psychological trauma, not elsewhere classified
Z91.5	Personal history of self-harm
Z91.81	**History of falling**
Z91.82	**Personal history of military deployment**
Z92	Personal history of medical treatment
	Except: Z92.0, Personal history of contraception Except: Z92.82, Status post administration of tPA (rtPA) in a different facility within the last 24 hours prior to admission to a current facility

Source: CMS 2018.

impact healthcare needs. Another example of pertinent personal history would be a personal history of cancer, which could also impact the patient's current or future healthcare needs. Family history codes are used when a patient has a family member or members who have had a particular disease that poses a risk to the patient—if he or she may also contract the disease, or if the family history impacts the well-being of the patient. History codes are often used together with other ICD-10-CM codes that identify a reason for an encounter. History codes should never be sequenced as the first-listed code. See figure 8.20 for the OGCR related to personal and family history codes.

Key to Success

When looking up a history code, go to the entry for *History* in the Index. There are two major divisions under this entry: *family* and *personal*. It is easy to get mixed up between these two sections when searching for a code in the history entry. It is a best to draw a line after the family history section, and before the personal history section, in order to keep these two sections separate.

- **Counseling.** Primary care practitioners commonly perform different counseling services. As the primary point of contact for healthcare and health services, PCPs must sometimes counsel their patients regarding their health. This counseling includes encounters for contraceptive management (Z30) and counseling for victims of abuse (Z69)

- **Body mass index (BMI).** BMI codes (category Z68) are based on two different scales—adult and pediatric. Pediatric BMI codes identify the weight percentile, either less than 5th percentile, 5th percentile to less than 85th percentile, 85th to 95th percentile, and greater than or equal to 95th percentile for age. Adult BMI codes, on the other hand, identify the specific BMI number, ranging from 19 or less to 70 or greater. Note that BMI codes should never be used as the first-listed diagnosis code, it is only acceptable as a secondary code.

For practice assigning primary care diagnoses, complete the exercises in There's a Code for That 8.8.

Primary care diagnoses

8.8

Read the following documentation and select the appropriate diagnosis code(s).

There's a Code for That

1. Patient presents with fever, headache, and sore throat. Rapid flu test performed in office is positive for influenza A.

   ICD-10-CM code: _____

2. Patient presents with fever, headache, and sore throat. All labs performed in the office are negative.

   ICD-10-CM codes: _____, _____, _____

3. 40-year-old male presents with lower right quadrant abdominal pain, nausea, and vomiting. STAT CT scan ordered and admitted to hospital.

   ICD-10-CM codes: _____, _____

(Continued on next page)

Continued

4. 3-day-old female presents for initial routine well-child examination.

   ICD-10-CM code: _____

5. 40-year-old female presents for routine annual checkup without abnormal findings. She had breast cancer three years ago, status post right-sided mastectomy, and is currently still in remission. She is also given a flu shot in the office.

   ICD-10-CM codes: _____, _____, _____,
   _____

Top Primary Care Conditions

Primary care practitioners see countless conditions ranging from otitis media, to diabetes, to hypertension. The specific conditions seen and treated depend on the specialty of the provider and available resources. For example, a pediatrician is likely to see more ear infections and fewer cases of high blood pressure. An internal medicine doctor is more likely to treat diabetes, hyperlipidemia, and chronic obstructive pulmonary disease.

Available resources also affect the most commonly seen conditions for PCPs. For example, in a rural area the town doctor may see all conditions, as there are few to no specialists that can treat specialized conditions. On the other hand, a PCP in a large city with many specialists close at hand is less likely to treat and manage conditions such as congestive heart failure or neoplastic diseases; instead these patients would be referred to healthcare specialists.

Coders in the primary care setting also need to keep in mind HCC codes, especially if their office belongs to an ACO, as many of these top conditions are included within HCC coding and risk adjustment. Keep an eye out for the **HCC** symbol as you read through this section. This symbol identifies codes that are important in risk adjustment. When coding for these conditions, it is imperative to select codes to the highest level of specificity, based on clear and complete provider documentation.

The following sections discuss the top conditions in primary care coding.

Asthma

Asthma (J45) codes are based on severity— mild, moderate, or severe—and its recurrence, in terms of intermittent or persistent. Each type of asthma is further specified as uncomplicated, with acute exacerbation, or with status asthmaticus. Report the uncomplicated code unless the healthcare provider documents that the patient presents with exacerbation (such as wheezing or shortness of breath), or status asthmaticus. Status asthmaticus is an extreme form of asthma exacerbation that does not respond to treatment and can result in hypoxia and ultimately respiratory failure.

Chronic Obstructive Pulmonary Disease

Chronic obstructive pulmonary disease, or COPD, is a lung disease characterized by chronically poor airflow. Symptoms include shortness of breath, chronic cough, and sputum production. Coding for COPD is a bit complicated, as it often presents with additional conditions like chronic or acute bronchitis, emphysema, or another respiratory condition.

To look up COPD in the Index in the ICD-10-CM code book, search first for the term *Disease*, then reference the subterm *pulmonary* or *lung*, then find the subterm *chronic obstructive*. This will lead you to the section of codes in the Index for COPD. Select the code that most closely matches your diagnosis description and verify the code in the Tabular List.

There are three codes for COPD:

- J44.0, COPD with acute lower respiratory infection
- J44.1, COPD with (acute) exacerbation
- J44.9, COPD, unspecified

Coding for COPD gets complicated when a patient presents with COPD and acute lower respiratory infection and acute exacerbation. For example: *A patient with acute bronchitis presents with acute exacerbation of his COPD.* This case would require three codes: one to identify the COPD with acute lower respiratory tract infection (J44.0, COPD with acute lower respiratory infection), one code to identify the COPD as exacerbated (J44.1, COPD with (acute) exacerbation), and one code to identify the acute bronchitis (J20.9, Acute bronchitis, unspecified). This may seem a bit like overcoding, but the two COPD codes are necessary—one to identify the exacerbation and one to identify the additional lower respiratory infection. Figure 8.21 presents the guidelines for COPD coding.

Figure 8.21. OGCR I.C.10.a.1

---

10. Chapter 10: Diseases of the Respiratory System (J00-J99)

    a. Chronic Obstructive Pulmonary Disease [COPD] and Asthma

        1) Acute exacerbation of chronic obstructive bronchitis and asthma

            The codes in categories J44 and J45 distinguish between uncomplicated cases and those in acute exacerbation. An acute exacerbation is a worsening or a decompensation of a chronic condition. An acute exacerbation is not equivalent to an infection superimposed on a chronic condition, though an exacerbation may be triggered by an infection.

Source: CMS 2018.

Diabetes

Diabetes mellitus is a condition in which the body does not control the amount of glucose (sugar) in the blood, and the kidneys excrete large amounts of urine. It occurs when the body does not make enough insulin or cannot control the amount of insulin secreted.

Codes for diabetes mellitus are found in chapter 4: Endocrine, Nutritional, and Metabolic Disease, in categories E08 through E13. There are five categories of diabetes.

- E08, Diabetes mellitus due to underlying condition. This category should be used when the diabetes is a result of an underlying condition, such as Cushing's syndrome or pancreatitis. When using codes from this category it is important to also identify the underlying condition with an additional code(s), and sequence the diabetes code *after* the code for the underlying condition.

- E09, Drug or chemical induced diabetes mellitus. This category should be used when the diabetes is a result of a drug or chemical. An additional code should be used to identify the toxic effect. If the drug or chemical was not taken or administered correctly, and it resulted in the diabetes, code the toxic effect as a poisoning, and sequence the poisoning code *before* the diabetes code. If the drug or chemical was taken therapeutically and correctly prescribed and administered, code the toxic effect as an adverse effect, and sequence the adverse effect code *after* the diabetes code.

- E10, Type 1 diabetes mellitus. Type I diabetes is also referred to as juvenile or early-onset, and it is insulin-dependent. Patients with type I diabetes must take insulin for the rest of their lives. It usually develops before the age of 40, most cases beginning in early adulthood or during adolescence.

- E11, Type 2 diabetes mellitus. Type 2 diabetes develops later in life and is a result of the body not producing enough insulin for proper function, or when the body creates insulin resistance by not responding to insulin. Type 2 diabetes may be controlled by weight loss, exercise, following a healthy diet, and monitoring blood glucose levels. Some type 2 diabetics must take insulin daily, whereas others may not.

- E13, Other specified diabetes mellitus. This category should be used for diabetes that does not fit within any other category. This includes diabetes due to genetic defects of beta-cell function, genetic defects in insulin action, post-pancreatectomy diabetes, or postprocedural diabetes.

Once the type of diabetes has been determined, one code should be reported for each complication experienced by the patient. If there are no diabetic complications, report the diabetes code from the correct category without complications (namely, E11.9, Type 2 diabetes mellitus without complications). Except for the uncomplicated code (given), diabetes codes are all combination codes that describe the type of diabetes as well as the complication. Complications that present with diabetes include:

- Hyperosmolarity
- Ophthalmic complications. Ophthalmic complication codes are very complex. Codes identify the specific type of complication, as well as the laterality of the eye involved. If both eyes are involved, assign the bilateral code.
- Neurological complications
- Circulatory complications
- Other specified complications. Be careful with diabetes with skin ulcer codes, as they require an additional code to identify the site of the ulcer.
- Unspecified complications

Assign one code for each complication. This may seem like overcoding, but one code must be selected for each complication included in the documentation. If the provider reports that the diabetes is "uncontrolled," "poorly controlled," or "out of control," assign an additional code to identify this complication, as with hyperglycemia (that is, E11.65, Type 2 diabetes mellitus with hyperglycemia).

When assigning codes for diabetes, follow these steps (see also figures 8.22 and 8.23):

1. Determine the type of diabetes (categories E08 through E13). If the patient is pregnant, assign a code from category O24, Diabetes mellitus in pregnancy, childbirth, and the puerperium. Note that category O24 includes codes for both pre-existing diabetes in pregnancy and gestational diabetes. Codes for pre-existing diabetes should be used for patients who already had diabetes prior to becoming pregnant. Codes for gestational diabetes should be used for patients who developed diabetes during pregnancy.

2. Select one code for each complication. Assign an additional code for diabetes with hyperglycemia if the condition is identified as uncontrolled.

3. Assign a code for any long-term use of insulin or oral hypoglycemics: Z79.4, Long-term (current) use of insulin, or Z79.84, Long-term (current) use of

oral hypoglycemic drugs. Note that neither of these codes should be used with category E10 codes (type 1 diabetes). Because type 1 diabetics must use insulin, it is implied that they are on long-term use of insulin so it is not necessary to use these codes. Do not assign either of these codes if insulin is only temporarily given to lower blood sugar. Also note that these codes should be assigned *after* the code(s) for diabetes or diabetic complications.

4. Identify all additional codes and sequence them according to ICD-10-CM guidelines. Additional codes may be required to identify any underlying conditions, toxic effects, stage of chronic kidney disease, the site of a skin ulcer, or other complication or manifestation of the disease.

Figure 8.22. Diabetes coding

Figure 8.23. OGCR I.C.4.a

---

4. Chapter 4: Endocrine, Nutritional and Metabolic Diseases (E00-E89)

a. Diabetes mellitus

The diabetes mellitus codes are combination codes that include the type of diabetes mellitus, the body system affected, and the complications affecting that body system. As many codes within a particular category as are necessary to describe all of the complications of the disease may be used. They should be sequenced based on the reason for a particular encounter. Assign as many codes from categories E08 – E13 as needed to identify all of the associated conditions that the patient has.

1) Type of diabetes

The age of a patient is not the sole determining factor, though most type 1 diabetics develop the condition before reaching puberty. For this reason type 1 diabetes mellitus is also referred to as juvenile diabetes.

2) Type of diabetes mellitus not documented

If the type of diabetes mellitus is not documented in the medical record the default is E11.-, Type 2 diabetes mellitus.

3) Diabetes mellitus and the use of insulin and oral hypoglycemics

If the documentation in a medical record does not indicate the type of diabetes but does indicate that the patient uses insulin, code E11, Type 2 diabetes mellitus, should be assigned. **An additional code should be assigned from category Z79 to identify the long-term (current) use of insulin or oral hypoglycemic drugs. If the patient is treated with both oral medications and insulin, only the code for long-term (current) use of insulin should be assigned. Code Z79.4 should not be assigned if insulin is given temporarily to bring a type 2 patient's blood sugar under control during an encounter.**

4) Diabetes mellitus in pregnancy and gestational diabetes

See Section I.C.15. Diabetes mellitus in pregnancy.

See Section I.C.15. Gestational (pregnancy induced) diabetes

(Continued on next page)

Figure 8.23. *(Continued)*

---

5) Complications due to insulin pump malfunction

   (a) Underdose of insulin due to insulin pump failure

   An underdose of insulin due to an insulin pump failure should be assigned to a code from subcategory T85.6, Mechanical complication of other specified internal and external prosthetic devices, implants and grafts, that specifies the type of pump malfunction, as the principal or first-listed code, followed by code T38.3x6-, Underdosing of insulin and oral hypoglycemic [antidiabetic] drugs. Additional codes for the type of diabetes mellitus and any associated complications due to the underdosing should also be assigned.

   (b) Overdose of insulin due to insulin pump failure

   The principal or first-listed code for an encounter due to an insulin pump malfunction resulting in an overdose of insulin, should also be T85.6-, Mechanical complication of other specified internal and external prosthetic devices, implants and grafts, followed by code T38.3x1-, Poisoning by insulin and oral hypoglycemic [antidiabetic] drugs, accidental (unintentional).

6) Secondary diabetes mellitus

   Codes under categories E08, Diabetes mellitus due to underlying condition, E09, Drug or chemical induced diabetes mellitus, and E13, Other specified diabetes mellitus, identify complications/manifestations associated with secondary diabetes mellitus. Secondary diabetes is always caused by another condition or event (e.g., cystic fibrosis, malignant neoplasm of pancreas, pancreatectomy, adverse effect of drug, or poisoning).

   (a) Secondary diabetes mellitus and the use of insulin or *oral* hypoglycemic drugs

   For patients with secondary diabetes mellitus who routinely use insulin or oral hypoglycemic drugs, an additional code from category Z79 should be assigned to identify the long-term (current) use of insulin or oral hypoglycemic drugs. If the patient is treated with both oral medications and insulin, only the code for long-term (current) use of insulin should be assigned. Code Z79.4 should not be assigned if insulin is given temporarily to bring a secondary diabetic patient's blood sugar under control during an encounter.

   (b) Assigning and sequencing secondary diabetes codes and its causes

   The sequencing of the secondary diabetes codes in relationship to codes for the cause of the diabetes is based on the Tabular List instructions for categories E08, E09 and E13.

   (i) Secondary diabetes mellitus due to pancreatectomy

   For postpancreatectomy diabetes mellitus (lack of insulin due to the surgical removal of all or part of the pancreas), assign code E89.1, Postprocedural hypoinsulinemia. Assign a code from category E13 and a code from subcategory Z90.41-, Acquired absence of pancreas, as additional codes.

   (ii) Secondary diabetes due to drugs

   Secondary diabetes may be caused by an adverse effect of correctly administered medications, poisoning or sequela of poisoning.

   See section I.C.19.e for coding of adverse effects and poisoning, and section I.C.20 for external cause code reporting.

Source: CMS 2018.

Heart Failure

Heart failure, also called congestive heart failure or CHF, is a condition in which the heart cannot pump enough blood to meet the body's needs. Heart failure can only affect one or the other side of the heart, and it can be acute, chronic, or acute on chronic. Codes for heart failure (I50) will depend on the site of the failure and its acuity.

Hyperlipidemia/Hypercholesterolemia

Hyperlipidemia is a condition in which there are high levels of lipids, or fats, in the blood. **Hypercholesterolemia** is a condition in which there are high levels of cholesterol in the blood. Codes for both conditions are included within the same category: E78, Disorders of lipoprotein metabolism and other lipidemias.

Hypertension

Hypertension, or high blood pressure, is a common condition in adults. There are five categories of hypertension, as follows.

- I10, Essential (primary) hypertension. This is high blood pressure without any related heart disease or chronic kidney disease, which is not a result of an underlying condition.

- I11, Hypertensive heart disease. This category of hypertension should be used when heart disease is a result of hypertension, or if the provider documents "hypertensive heart disease." If the provider documents a different cause of the heart disease, use one code for the heart disease and code I10, Essential (primary) hypertension. Codes differ depending on if the patient presents with or without heart failure. If the patient has heart failure, use an additional code to identify the heart failure (I50, Heart failure).

- I12, Hypertensive chronic kidney disease. This category should be used when a patient has both hypertension and chronic kidney disease (CKD). However, if the provider documents a cause other than hypertension, use code I10, Essential (primary) hypertension, along with the code identifying the CKD. Codes differ based on the stage of chronic kidney disease, either stage 5 CKD or end-stage renal disease (ESRD), or stage 1 through 4 or unspecified CKD. Either way, an additional code to identify the stage of CKD should be included sequenced after the code for the hypertension, as follows:
  - N18.1, Chronic kidney disease, stage 1
  - N18.2, Chronic kidney disease, stage 2 (mild)
  - N18.3, Chronic kidney disease, stage (moderate)
  - N18.4, Chronic kidney disease, stage (severe)
  - N18.5, Chronic kidney disease, stage
  - N18.6, End-stage renal disease (ESRD)

- I13, Hypertensive heart and chronic kidney disease. This category is to be used when the patient has both hypertensive heart disease as well as hypertensive chronic kidney disease. As in the previous categories, codes differ based on the stage of CKD as well as whether the heart disease presents with or without heart failure. Assign an additional code to identify the stage of CKD, as well as to identify the heart failure (if present).

- I15, Secondary hypertension. Secondary hypertension is due to an underlying condition. Assign one code for the hypertension and one code for the underlying disease. Sequencing of the two codes will depend on which condition is the primary reason for the encounter.

There are additional types of hypertension codes, such as I16, Hypertensive crisis, which is an acute severe increase in blood pressure; and codes for hypertension within certain organs, such as pulmonary hypertension, hypertension in the vessels of the eye and the brain, and hypertension complicating pregnancy, childbirth, and the puerperium.

Also called "white coat syndrome," transient hypertension is a temporary elevated high blood pressure reading, without the diagnosis of hypertension. It is assigned code R03.0, Elevated blood pressure reading without diagnosis of hypertension, and should be used until a diagnosis of hypertension is established. See figure 8.24 for the OGCR pertaining to hypertension.

Figure 8.24. OGCR I.C.9.a

---

9. Chapter 9: Diseases of the Circulatory System (I00-I99)

a. Hypertension

The classification presumes a causal relationship between hypertension and heart involvement and between hypertension and kidney involvement, as the two conditions are linked by the term "with" in the Alphabetic Index. These conditions should be coded as related even in the absence of provider documentation explicitly linking them, unless the documentation clearly states the conditions are unrelated.

For hypertension and conditions not specifically linked by relational terms such as "with," "associated with" or "due to" in the classification, provider documentation must link the conditions in order to code them as related.

Source: CMS 2018.

Otitis

Otitis, otherwise known as an ear infection, can occur in the outer ear canal as *otitis externa* (H60, Otitis externa), or in the middle ear, *otitis media* (H65, Nonsuppurative otitis media, H66, Suppurative and unspecified otitis media, H67, Otitis media in diseases classified elsewhere). It is a common condition in pediatric patients. Codes for otitis depend on the type of ear infection and the laterality (either right, left, or bilateral). When coding for otitis, it is important to also code for any known exposure to or use of tobacco or tobacco products, as this results in the selection of an additional code. This includes environmental exposure to tobacco, such as second-hand smoke. Some otitis media codes are combination codes that include associated ruptured tympanic membrane (ear drum), whereas others are not. If an associated ruptured tympanic membrane is present, and it is not included in the code description, then assign an additional code to identify the rupture.

As previously mentioned, primary care practitioners see patients with diagnoses from across the spectrum of available ICD-10-CM codes. When coding for primary care services, it is important to pay attention to the many different signs and symptoms, and when they should be reported rather than, or in addition to, a definitive diagnosis. HCC coding also requires that documentation be complete, clear, and as specific as possible so coders can report all appropriate codes necessary for risk adjustment coding.

Underdosing

Unlike an overdose, in which a patient takes too much of a certain substance, or an adverse effect, when a patient takes something correctly prescribed but suffers some sort of problem due to the substance taken, an **underdose** occurs when a patient does not take the properly prescribed amount of a medication. When a patient presents to the PCP's office and is suffering an ill-effect because he or she is not taking medication as prescribed, it should be coded as an underdose.

When coding for an underdose, the primary code should identify the problem bing experienced by the patient as a result of the underdose, followed by the underdose code. For example, if a type 2 diabetic patient is suffering from high blood sugar episodes because she keeps forgetting to take her medication regularly (and hence underdosing), then the codes would be as follows: E11.65, Type 2 diabetes mellitus with hyperglycemia, and then T38.3X6A, Underdosing of insulin and oral hypoglycemic [antidiabetic] drugs, initial encounter. The additional code Z91.130, Patient's unintentional underdosing of medication regimen due to age-related debility, would also be assigned to identify the patient's noncompliance with her medication regimen (in this case unintentional because she keeps forgetting). See figure 8.25 for the OGCR related to underdosing.

Figure 8.25. OGCR I.C.19.e.5.c.

> **(c) Underdosing**
>
> Underdosing refers to taking less of a medication than is prescribed by a provider or a manufacturer's instruction. For underdosing, assign the code from categories T36-T50 (fifth or sixth character "6").
>
> Codes for underdosing should never be assigned as principal or first-listed codes. If a patient has a relapse or exacerbation of the medical condition for which the drug is prescribed because of the reduction in dose, then the medical condition itself should be coded.
>
> Noncompliance (Z91.12-, Z91.13-) or complication of care (Y63.6-Y63.9) codes are to be used with an underdosing code to indicate intent, if known.

Source: CMS 2018.

When assigning an underdosing code, at least two codes are required: one for the negative effect of the underdosing, and one to identify the underdosing itself. To find the underdosing code, it is necessary to go to the Table of Drugs in the ICD-10-CM code book, and refer to the drug that the patient was supposed to be taking. The sixth column in the Table of Drugs lists the underdosing codes. It is still necessary to verify the code in the Tabular List and identify the episode of care for the encounter. For a refresher on using the Table of Drugs and assigning encounters for services, refer to chapter 4. For more practice on assigning top primary care diagnosis codes, complete the exercises in There's a Code for That 8.9.

Coding for top primary care diagnoses

8.9

There's a Code for That

Read the following documentation and select the appropriate diagnosis code(s).

1. Diabetes, unspecified.

   ICD-10-CM code: _____

2. Patient presents with type 2 diabetes mellitus with mild bilateral nonproliferative diabetic retinopathy without macular edema, and diabetic cataract in the right eye. She is on long-term use of oral hypoglycemic drugs.

   ICD-10-CM codes: _____, _____, _____

3. Diabetes secondary to Cushing's disease. Patient seen today for treatment of her Cushing's.

   ICD-10-CM codes: _____, _____

4. Patient presents for follow-up on her recently diagnosed type 2 diabetes. Her healthcare conditions are also significant for essential hypertension, hyperlipidemia, and obesity due to excess calories. Her current BMI is 34.

   ICD-10-CM codes: _____, _____, _____,
   _____, _____

5. 10-year-old male with juvenile diabetes presents for management of his condition. He is currently well-controlled with his current insulin regimen.

   ICD-10-CM code: _____

6. Hypertensive heart disease with acute systolic heart failure.

   ICD-10-CM codes: _____, _____

(Continued on next page)

8.9

Continued

7. Patient is seen for management of his hypertensive CKD (stage 3). He also has DMII with peripheral neuropathy and CHF (congestive heart failure), which is not related to the hypertension.

   ICD-10-CM codes: _____, _____,

   _____, _____

8. COPD and acute bronchitis.

   ICD-10-CM codes: _____, _____

9. Pediatric patient presents with moderate persistent asthma with acute exacerbation. He is exposed to secondary smoke in the home.

   ICD-10-CM codes: _____, _____

Putting It All Together: Coding for Primary Care Services

To select the correct codes for a primary care encounter, it is important to carefully read the documentation, then access each code book to find the procedure or service provided as well as the corresponding diagnosis or diagnoses to support the medical necessity for the service. Procedural codes for PCP services are found in the CPT and HCPCS code books, and diagnosis codes are found in the ICD-10-CM code book.

Determination of the correct codes relies on the answers to the following questions.

- What services were provided to the patient?
  - Was an E/M service provided?
  - Were any in-office medical procedures provided?
  - Were any in-office surgical procedures performed?
  - Were any in-office labs completed?
- Are there any applicable modifiers or add-on codes?
- What is the primary condition being treated? The primary reason for the encounter should be the first-listed diagnosis.
- Are there any additional signs, symptoms, conditions, or Z-codes that should be reported?

Study the following vignette and note how to select the appropriate diagnosis and procedure codes. Then complete the following practice exercises in There's a Code for That 8.10.

One year ago, Audrey graduated from a health information management program. She learned the basics of evaluation and management coding and is preparing to take her coding certification exam in six months. Currently, she is working as a coder in a large primary care group practice and has learned a lot about primary care in general. Audrey is getting better at selecting the correct level of E/M code, even though the process is still a bit confusing for her. She is currently working on the following encounter.

History: 67-year-old female presents for medication follow-up. She is currently taking 10 mg gabapentin every four hours to control symptoms of peripheral neuropathy. She is not taking any other medications, and is not allergic to any medications. Her neuropathy began seven years ago, when she noticed tingling and stabbing pains in her fingers and toes. Some days she notes that her entire arms begin to tingle and feel achy all over. She reports that she must take her prescribed dosage every four hours as directed or her symptoms reappear. Today, she has a slight burn on her right hand, which happened as she was baking a cake. She reports that her hands are difficult to control at times.

Exam: Patient looks well, awake and well-oriented to surroundings. Eye, cardio, respiratory, and gastro all within normal limits. Skin is notably dry in patches. Complete range of motion of both arms and legs, neuro exam of toes reveals slight pain to the touch and lack of response to stimuli in three of the left toes. Hand grip strength is generally strong, but lower on the right hand than the left.

MDM: Based on patient's reports, peripheral neuropathy seems to be controllable with current dosage of gabapentin. Continue meds as prescribed and follow up in six months.

First, Audrey asks herself: *What did the doctor do?* The doctor performed an E/M encounter. There were no additional medical or surgical procedures or lab tests. She now begins to audit the E/M encounter to determine the correct code. The first component that she audits is the history component, and Audrey scores it as follows:

> 67-year-old female presents for medication follow-up *(chief complaint).* She is currently taking 10 mg gabapentin every four hours to control symptoms of peripheral neuropathy *(PFSH: past medical-current medications).* She is not taking any other medications, and is not allergic to any medications *(PFSH-past medical-no allergies).* Her neuropathy began seven years ago *(HPI: duration),* when she noticed tingling and stabbing *(HPI: quality)* pains in her fingers and toes *(HPI: location).* Some days she notes that her entire arms begin to tingle and feel achy all over *(ROS: neurologic).* She reports that she must take her prescribed dosage every four hours as directed or her symptoms reappear *(HPI: modifying factors).* Today, she has a first degree burn on her right hand, which happened as she was baking a cake *(HPI: associated signs and symptoms).* She reports that her hands are difficult to control at times *(ROS: neurologic).*

Audrey has scored the following for the history component for this encounter:

- HPI-5 elements, level of HPI is *extended*
- ROS-1 element, level of ROS is *problem-pertinent*
- PFSH-2 from past medical, level of *pertinent*

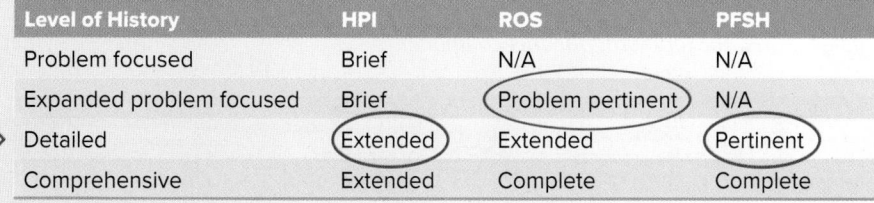

Level of History	HPI	ROS	PFSH
Problem focused	Brief	N/A	N/A
Expanded problem focused	Brief	Problem pertinent	N/A
Detailed	Extended	Extended	Pertinent
Comprehensive	Extended	Complete	Complete

She determines that the *level of history* for the encounter is *detailed.*

Now, Audrey scores the examination component of the encounter, as follows:

Patient looks well, awake and well-oriented to surroundings (general appearance). *Eye, cardio, respiratory, and gastro all within normal limits* (eye, cardiovascular, and gastrointestinal organ systems). *Skin is notably dry in patches* (integumentary organ system). *Complete range of motion of both arms and legs, neuro exam of toes reveals slight pain to the touch and lack of response to stimuli in three of the left toes* (neurological organ system). *Hand grip strength is generally strong, but lower on the right hand than the left* (neurological organ system).

Audrey has scored the following for this component:

- *Limited exam of affected area and other related/symptomatic organ systems*

Level of Exam	Exam Components	Number of Body Areas/Organ Systems: 1995 guidelines	Number of Body Areas/Organ Systems: 1997 guidelines
Problem focused	Limited exam of affected body area/organ system	1 body area or organ system	1 to 5 body areas or organ systems
Expanded problem focused	Limited exam of affected area and other related/symptomatic organ systems	2 to 7 body areas or organ systems	6 to 11 body areas or organ systems
Detailed	Extended exam of affected area and other related/symptomatic organ systems	Extended exam of 2 to 7 body areas or organ systems	2 areas of examination from 6 organ systems
Comprehensive	General multisystem exam or complete exam of single organ system	8 or more organ systems	2 areas of examination from 9 organ systems

She determines that the level of examination *for the encounter is* expanded problem focused.

Now Audrey scores the final component of the encounter, medical decision making:

Based on patient's reports, peripheral neuropathy seems to be controllable with current dosage of gabapentin. Continue meds as prescribed and follow up in six months.

- *Number of diagnoses: Established problem—stable (peripheral neuropathy, controllable, continue meds as prescribed), 1 point. Level is* minimal.
- *Amount of data to be reviewed: None. Level is* none (minimal).
- *Risk of complications, morbidity, or mortality: One stable chronic condition. Level is* minimal.

Audrey has scored the following for this component:

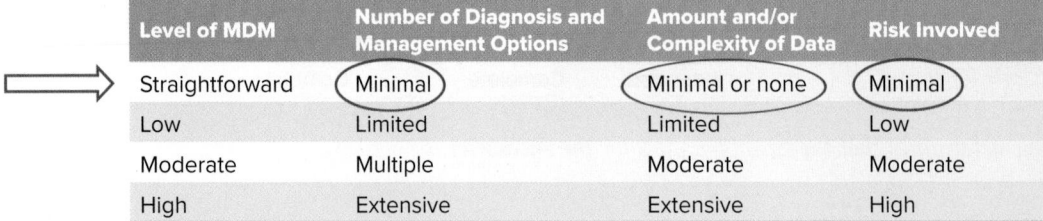

Level of MDM	Number of Diagnosis and Management Options	Amount and/or Complexity of Data	Risk Involved
Straightforward	Minimal	Minimal or none	Minimal
Low	Limited	Limited	Low
Moderate	Multiple	Moderate	Moderate
High	Extensive	Extensive	High

She determines that the level of MDM *for the encounter is* straightforward.

Now that Audrey has all three levels of the key components, she determines the type of service, place of service, and patients status in order to find the correct section of codes in the E/M section of the CPT code book. This is an outpatient office visit for an established patient, so Audrey goes to codes 99211 through 99215 in the CPT code book, and selects the code that matches the following (remember that for established patients, only two out of the three levels of the key components are required to match):

- *Detailed history*
- *Expanded problem-focused examination*
- *Straightforward medical decision making*

Audrey's code is: 99213, Office or other outpatient visit for the evaluation and management of an established patient, which requires at least 2 out of 3 of the following: expanded problem-focused history, expanded problem-focused examination, medical decision making of low complexity

Now that she has her procedure code, Audrey asks herself: Why did the doctor do it? The patient presented for a follow-up on her established diagnosis of peripheral neuropathy. She also has a first degree burn on her right hand. She looks up these conditions in the ICD-10-CM code book and finds the following codes:

Neuropathy, peripheral (use the default code as there are no more specifics on the type of neuropathy): G62.9, Polyneuropathy, unspecified

Burn, hand, right, first degree, initial encounter: T23.101A, Burn of first degree of right hand, unspecified site, initial encounter

She then rechecks the documentation to ensure she has coded everything for the encounter, and reports the chosen codes on the claim for the service.

Coding for primary care services

8.10

There's a Code for That

Read the following documentation from patient encounters and assign the appropriate procedure and diagnosis codes.

1. 18-month-old established female presents with acute suppurative OM of the right ear with rupture of tympanic membrane. Physician performed a E/M service with detailed history, expanded problem-focused exam, and MDM of low complexity. During the exam, a large accumulation of impacted cerumen was noted in the left ear, which was removed with instrumentation by the physician.

   CPT codes: _____ - _____, _____

   ICD-10-CM codes: _____, _____

(Continued on next page)

8.10

Continued

2. 72-year-old female presents for treatment of treatment-resistant urinary tract infection. She came in two days ago and urine culture was taken, which tested positive for MRSA. Provider performed a problem-focused history and examination, with moderate complexity medical decision making.

CPT codes: _____

ICD-10-CM codes: _____ , _____

3. 45-year-old female presents to the office of her internist with anemia in CKD, stage 3. Internist performs a detailed history, detailed examination, and MDM of moderate complexity. CBC (automated and automated differential WBC count) performed in office indicates that anemia is improving.

CPT codes: _____ , _____

ICD-10-CM codes: _____ , _____

4. 67-year-old established male patient is seen in the clinic with DM2 and mild nonproliferative diabetic retinopathy with macular edema, as well as a diabetic cataract on his right eye. His DM is controlled daily with insulin. Physician performed a detailed history and with comprehensive examination and medical decision making of high complexity. Due to worsening of visual problem, physician also performed a bilateral visual acuity screen and referred the patient to an ophthalmologist.

CPT codes: _____ , _____

ICD-10-CM codes: _____ , _____ , _____

5. 45-year-old male presents for routine physical examination. Patient is a healthy middle-aged male, no abnormal findings. Flu shot (IIV3) also administered in the office.

CPT codes: _____ , _____ , _____

ICD-10-CM codes: _____ , _____

HCC

End of Chapter Content

Instructions: Indicate whether the following statements are true or false (T or F). For false statements, rewrite the statement on the line below to make the statement true.

1. Primary care practitioners specialize in the care of neoplasms.

_____

_____

2. A women's health practitioner may be considered a primary care practitioner.

_____

_____

3. PCP stands for primary care patient.

_____

_____

4. HCC coding is not important for accountable care organizations.

_____

_____

5. Most of the procedures performed by primary care providers are E/M encounters.

_____

_____

6. HPI stands for history of the patient's illness.

_____

_____

7. There are four different elements that make up the key component of history.

_____

_____

8. The key components of history and examination are both made up of the same elements.

_____

_____

9. Modifier -25 may not be appended to evaluation and management services.

_____

_____

10. Biopsy is an example of a minor surgical procedure that would be performed in the office.

_____

_____

Instructions: Choose the best answer.

1. In some health insurance plans, patients are required to select which of the following?
   a. A patient care coordinator
   b. A primary care provider
   c. Designated procedure codes
   d. Mental health services

2. Which of the following is the best description of an ACO?
   a. A group of patients who engage in risk management reduction
   b. A billing and coding group that specializes in auditing claims
   c. A group of healthcare providers that collectively utilizes performance measures
   d. A group of insurance companies that engages in risk adjustment education

3. Which of the following types of CPT is most commonly billed in primary care coding?
   a. Evaluation and management codes
   b. Vaccination codes
   c. In-office surgical procedure codes
   d. Medicine codes

4. The elements of the key component history are: chief complaint; history of present illness; past, family, social history; and which of the following?
   a. Body areas
   b. Organ systems
   c. Risk
   d. Review of systems

5. What is the act of coding an E/M service at a level lower than what was performed?
   a. Undercoding
   b. Overcoding
   c. Fraud
   d. Abuse

6. Which of the following describes an organ system?
   a. A specific organ system that may be examined during an E/M encounter
   b. A general area of the body that may be examined during an E/M encounter
   c. A specific area of the body that is reviewed in the review of systems
   d. A general organ system that is reviews in the review of systems

7. In E/M coding, which key component asks the question: How dangerous or risky is the patient's healthcare condition?
   a. History
   b. Examination
   c. Medical decision making
   d. None of the above

8. In coding for vaccines, the two codes that must be reported are the administration and which of the following?
   a. Administration
   b. Serum
   c. Immune globulin
   d. Therapeutic substance

9. Which of the following best describes an encounter that includes a comprehensive health evaluation and anticipatory guidance?
   a. Evaluation and management encounters
   b. Preventive services
   c. Chronic care management
   d. Vaccination administration

10. When two E/M services are performed on the same day, which modifier is necessary to report?
   a. Modifier -32
   b. Modifier -95
   c. Modifier -24
   d. Modifier -25

11. Which of the following vaccine administration codes would be used for an injection provided to a pediatric patient with counseling?
   a. 90471
   b. 90473
   c. 97632
   d. 90460

12. Which of the following vaccine administration codes would be used for a nasal administration of a flu vaccine?
   a. 90471
   b. 90473
   c. 97632
   d. 90460

13. Offices may perform laboratory procedures in the office if they are which of the following?

    a. Provider approved
    b. Sent to the patient deductible
    c. Pre-authorized by the insurance plan
    d. CLIA-waived

14. Which of the following modifiers should be appended to a procedure that was repeated on the same date of service?

    a. Modifier -59
    b. Modifier -QW
    c. Modifier -76
    d. Modifier -XU

15. In ICD-10-CM coding, Z-codes are used to report which of the following reasons for encounter?

    a. Signs and symptoms
    b. Preventive examinations
    c. Patient history
    d. Patient status

16. For hypertension with CKD, one code should be selected for the hypertension, and another code for the:

    a. Heart failure
    b. Diabetes
    c. Stage of CKD
    d. End-stage renal disease

Instructions: Answer the following questions with the appropriate code(s).

1. 56-year-old female with DMII presents with recently diagnosed mild open-angle bilateral glaucoma and right eye cataract. Her diabetes is poorly controlled with daily insulin use. (Remember to use an additional code for hyperglycemia because the DM is identified as poorly controlled). Provider performed a detailed history, comprehensive examination, and high complexity MDM. Referred to endocrinologist.

   CPT code(s): _____

   ICD-10-CM code(s): _____,
   _____, _____, _____,
   _____, _____

2. 56-year-old new male patient is seen for stage 4 CKD with congestive heart failure due to hypertension. Provider performed a detailed history and exam with MDM of moderate complexity.

   CPT code(s): _____

   ICD-10-CM code(s): _____,
   _____, _____

3. 21-year-old female is seen with severe persistent asthma with acute exacerbation. Pulse oximetry taken in the office revealed oxygen level of 88 percent. Pressurized nebulizer breathing treatment immediately administered using albuterol sulfate inhalation solution. Post-neb oxygen level was a steady 95 percent. Provider performed a problem-focused history, detailed examination, and high complexity MDM.

   CPT code(s): _____,
   _____, _____

   ICD-10-CM code(s): _____

References

American Academy of Professional Coders. 2016. *Study Guide: CEMC Evaluation and Management.* Salt Lake City, UT: AAPC.

American Medical Association. 2017 (January). *Current Procedural Terminology (CPT).* Chicago: AMA.

Centers for Medicare and Medicaid Services. 2018. ICD-10-CM Official Guidelines for Coding and Reporting FY 2018. https://www.cms.gov/Medicare/Coding/ICD10/Downloads/2018-ICD-10-CM-Coding-Guidelines.pdf.

Centers for Medicare and Medicaid Services. 2016 (March). Accountable Care Organizations: What Providers Need to Know. https://www.cms.gov/Medicare/Medicare-Fee-for-Service-Payment/sharedsavingsprogram/Downloads/ACO_Providers_Factsheet_ICN907406.pdf.

Centers for Medicare and Medicaid Services. 1997. 1997 Documentation Guidelines for Evaluation and Management Services. https://www.cms.gov/Outreach-and-Education/Medicare-Learning-Network-MLN/MLNEdWebGuide/Downloads/97Docguidelines.pdf.

Centers for Medicare and Medicaid Services. 1995. 1995 Documentation Guidelines for Evaluation and Management Services. https://www.cms.gov/Outreach-and-Education/Medicare-Learning-Network-MLN/MLNEdWebGuide/Downloads/95Docguidelines.pdf.

Novitas Solutions. 2017. E/M Documentation Auditor's Instructions. https://www.novitas-solutions.com /webcenter/content/conn/UCM_Repository/uuid /dDocName:00004966.

OpenStax. "Regions and Quadrants of the Peritoneal Cavity." 2013. Digital Image. Accessed December, 2017. https://cnx.org/contents/F-TuqKAF@3/Anatomical -Terminology#fig-ch01_06_05.

Resources

American Health Information Management Association. 2016. *ICD-10-CM Code Book: 2017*. Chicago: AHIMA.

Beck, D. and D. Margolin. 2007. Physician Coding and Reimbursement. https://www.ncbi.nlm.nih.gov/pmc /articles/PMC3096340/.

Centers for Disease Control and Prevention. 2017. Clinical Laboratory Improvement Amendments (CLIA). https:// wwwn.cdc.gov/clia/resources/waivedtests/.

Menahem, S., A. Nazarenko, and P. Shvartzman. 2014 (March 25). Minor surgical procedures and musculoskeletal injections by primary care physicians - an Israeli experience. *Israel Journal Health Policy Research* 3:12. https://www.ncbi.nlm.nih.gov/pmc/articles /PMC3987677/.

Practice Management Institute. 2012. *E/M Coding Workshop*. San Antonio: Assistex, Inc.

CHAPTER 9

Eye and Vision Services

Learning Objectives

- Understand the basics of billing and coding within the specialties of optometry and ophthalmology.
- Examine procedural codes and guidelines for eye and vision services.
- Examine diagnosis coding and medical necessity for eye and vision services.
- Identify and apply ICD-10-CM, CPT, and HCPCS codes to optometry and ophthalmology cases.

Key Terms

Acquired condition
Congenital condition
Comprehensive ophthalmological services
Cortical cataract
Enucleation
Evisceration
Exenteration
Extracapsular cataract extraction (ECCE)
Glaucoma
Goniolens

Intermediate ophthalmological services
Intracapsular cataract extraction (ICCE)
Intraocular pressure
Lifestyle impairments
Macular degeneration
Nuclear cataract
Ocular adnexa
Ophthalmologist
Ophthalmology
Optometrist

Optometry
Phacoemulsification
Refraction
Refractive surgery
Retinal detachment
Slit lamp
Strabismus
Subcapsular cataract
Trabeculectomy
Vision insurance

Eye and vision services are performed by two different, yet interrelated healthcare specialists—optometrists and ophthalmologists. Optometrists examine the eyes for visual defects, such as myopia (nearsightedness), and prescribe lenses to correct the defect (either glasses or contact lenses). Ophthalmologists specialize in pathology and diseases of the eyeball, and perform surgeries to correct eye problems.

Often, to determine visual acuity, optometrists see patients with defects in vision and perform vision screenings and refractions. A refraction is a test performed to determine if a patient has any abnormalities with his or her vision, and is used to identify the appropriate prescription for eyeglasses or contact lenses. However, optometrists sometimes see patients with medical problems of the eye, such as a corneal ulcer, and provide medical treatment. Therefore, optometrists sometimes see patients with vision diagnoses, and other times they see patients with medical diagnoses. This results in complications when billing and coding for eye services, as some healthcare insurance plans will pay for vision procedures, while others will only pay for medical procedures.

This chapter discusses the basics of coding for optometry and ophthalmology services, for both visual and medical conditions. This includes the differences between the two specialties, in addition to the different procedures and diagnoses used in coding for eye and vision services. Eye services also employ a special set of ophthalmology evaluation and management codes that may be used as an alternative to medical evaluation and management codes—making eye and vision services an interesting offshoot from general coding.

Optometry and Ophthalmology Basics

There are two major divisions within eye and vision services—optometry and ophthalmology—each of which provides a specific type of service. An optometrist is a specialist in optometry, and practitioners in this field perform examinations of the ophthalmological system, in addition to medical treatment and management of eye conditions. For example, an optometrist would perform an evaluation and management of a patient's ophthalmological system, and a refraction to determine any visual defects. Then the optometrist would provide a prescription for corrective lenses to correct any visual defect.

On the other hand, an ophthalmologist is a specialist in ophthalmology and practitioners in this field specialize in the anatomy, physiology, and pathology of diseases of the eyeball; they also perform medical and surgical procedures on the eye. For example, an ophthalmologist would be the healthcare provider to repair a retinal detachment or perform an intraoperative lens procedure.

It is important to understand the distinction between the two types of providers to understand which codes are reported in each of these specialties. Billing and coding for eye and vision services is also particularly unique because of the difference between vision insurance and healthcare insurance, as identified by the diagnosis code submitted to identify the medical necessity for the service (see figure 9.1).

The eye is one of the most complex anatomical structures in the human body, so it is essential to review eye anatomy and physiology.

Billing and Coding Basics

The difference between optometrists and ophthalmologists is more than just a side note. Because the two specialties are inherently different, there are major differences in billing and coding for their respective services. The first important thing to note is the difference between insurance plans. Depending on the type of service and the patient's

Figure 9.1. Optometry versus ophthalmology

diagnosis, it is necessary to send the claim for services to either a vision insurance plan or a healthcare insurance plan. Furthermore, documentation requirements to support medical necessity for services are more extensive and a simple statement of patient diagnosis may not be enough to support certain services.

Type of Patient Insurance

Like behavioral health services, certain vision services are not covered under healthcare insurance. Rather, these services are paid under a separate vision insurance policy. **Vision insurance** is similar to health insurance, but it only covers services related to visual acuity assessments, refractions, and corrective lenses. Services covered by vision insurance typically include

- Routine (ophthalmological) wellness examinations
- Contact lens fitting
- Hardware, such as frames and lenses

Vision insurance plans vary widely. For example, some plans will cover contact lens fitting, while others may not. Many also place limits on the frequency of services, such as one wellness examination per year. There are also limits on the amount of payment for services—such as insurance will pay $150 for a pair of glasses with lenses, but any amount over the $150 the patient would pay out of pocket.

Healthcare insurance covers services that are necessary due to a medical diagnosis. Even though services are performed on the eye, they are covered by healthcare insurance if the patient has a medical condition that affects the eye, such as hypertension. Services covered by healthcare insurance for eye procedures include

- Office visits
- Diagnostic tests
- Surgical procedures
- Office procedures due to a medical diagnosis

Unlike vision insurance, healthcare insurance has few limitations on the amount or frequency of visits. Instead of once per year, patients may receive medical eye services as often as medically necessary. Because it does not cover vision services, healthcare insurance does not pay for lenses, frames, or contact lenses.

In short: Vision insurance pays for eyesight care, and medical insurance pays for eye care.

Vision and healthcare insurance are not always separate. It is possible to have a plan with combined coverage, so a patient may have one plan that covers both medical and vision procedures. Other insurance plans—such as Medicaid and Medicare—include coverage for certain vision services through the healthcare plan. For example, most Medicaid plans permit one eye screening per year and allow a certain amount of coverage for lenses (eyesight care), and cover injuries or medical conditions of the eyes, like corneal lacerations or glaucoma (eye care).

When coding, the differences between insurance plans and types of insurance cannot be understated. Because the majority of outpatient coding is used for payment, it is helpful to know the special requirements of the insurance plan being billed. Codes reported for eye and vision services differ, depending on which insurance plain is being billed. So when coding for eye and vision services, either for an optometrist or an ophthalmologist, first identify the insurance plan for the patient and determine which services may be reported and how.

Key to Success

The rest of this chapter discusses the numerous codes used for different insurance plans and for various services. Do not get preoccupied with these billing differences as you are learning ICD-10-CM and CPT coding. It is more important to focus on learning how to code accurately by correctly reporting the procedure performed and the condition treated. Differences in billing will become more significant when you are a more experienced coder.

Healthcare versus Vision Diagnoses

It is important to differentiate between vision diagnoses and medical diagnoses of the eye. When coding for vision services (billed through vision insurance), use only vision diagnosis codes from the ICD-10-CM code book, such as codes for amblyopia or presbyopia, that affect eyesight and require corrective lenses. However, when coding for medical eye services (billed through healthcare insurance) the necessary ICD-10-CM diagnosis code can be used to identify the condition affecting the eyes, such as foreign body on the eye or diabetic retinopathy, both of which are medical problems impacting the eyes.

Specific diagnostic coding information for common conditions is discussed later in this chapter, but at this point it is important to briefly discuss instances when more than a simple diagnosis code is needed.

Medical Necessity for Eye Services

Before discussing the specific diagnosis codes used in eye and vision services, medical necessity for eye procedures should be addressed, as the requirements to support medical necessity for some procedures are more extensive than simply stating the procedure code.

Medical necessity to support procedures that treat such conditions as cataracts, capsular opacification, and blepharoptosis, must identify lifestyle impairments suffered by the patient due to the condition. Lifestyle impairments are descriptions of how the patient's eye condition has negatively impacted his or her lifestyle, including

- How decreased vision affects daily living activities
- Eyelids that rest on the eyelashes

- Restriction of peripheral vision
- Continued complaints of glare, or lack of distance or near vision
- Patient must raise eyelashes to see better

These functional impairments and ones like them must be documented before the surgery to correct the condition. If additional surgeries are needed, then the new lifestyle impairments must be sufficient to support the medical necessity for the new service. To ensure that the patient's diagnosis qualifies as a lifestyle impairment, and that the service provided will be considered medically necessary, it may be necessary to contact the patient's insurance payer to confirm that the service will be covered. Some insurance policies may require a prior authorization for certain services before they may be provided.

As a coder in an optometry or ophthalmology practice, coding may entail more than simply selecting and reporting a code. Certain services may need to be reported with health records, or with pre-certification or preauthorization documents that support the need for the procedure.

Anatomy and Physiology of the Eye and Ocular Adnexa

The eye and ocular adnexa are some of the most complex structures in the human body. It is necessary to be familiar with the anatomy and physiology of the eye, to ensure correct code selection. The Eye and Ocular Adnexa section in the CPT code book is organized anatomically, starting with the eye and then moving to the adnexa and accessory structures. Review figure 9.2 and identify the following:

- Eyeball
- Anterior segment (consists of the cornea, anterior chamber, anterior sclera, iris, ciliary body, and lens).
- Posterior segment (consists of the vitreous, retina, choroid, and posterior sclera)

Figure 9.2. Anatomy of the eye

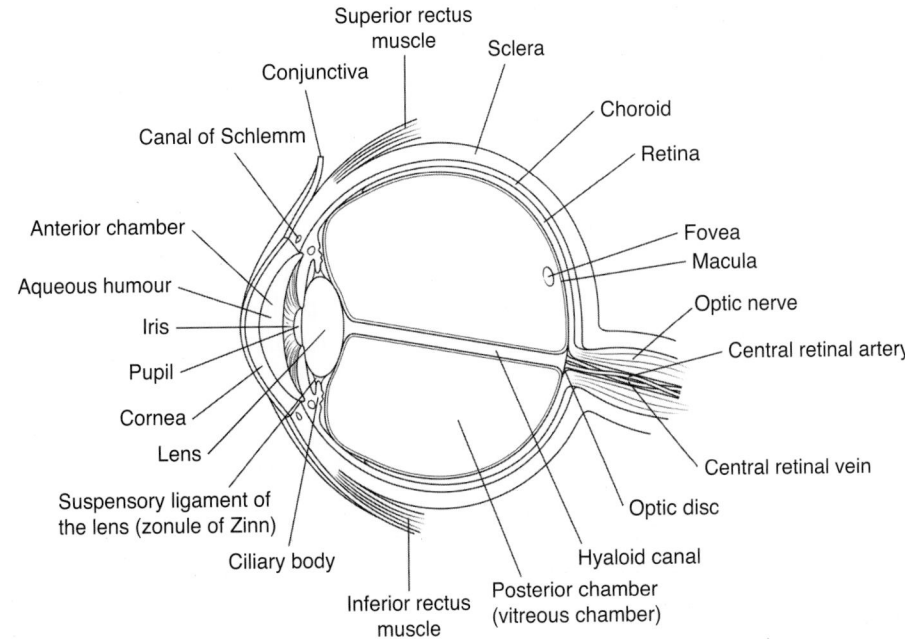

Source: ©AHIMA.

Figure 9.3. Extrinsic eye muscles

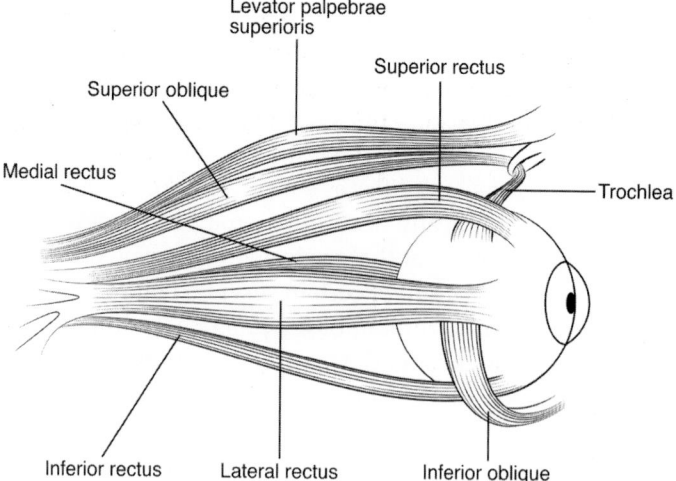

Source: ©AHIMA.

Figure 9.4. Lacrimal apparatus

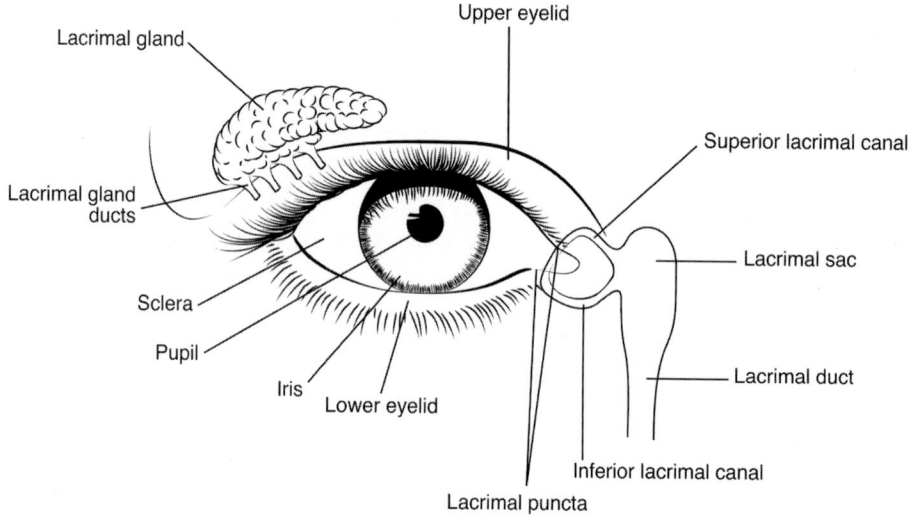

Source: ©AHIMA.

Ocular adnexa are the accessory structures of the eye including the extraocular muscles, eyelids, lacrimal system, orbit, and optic nerve and pathways. Surgical procedures on these structures are also found in the Eye and Ocular Adnexa subsection of the CPT code book (with the exception of the optic nerve and pathways, found in the Nervous System subsection of the CPT code book). Review figures 9.2 through 9.4 and identify the following:

- Extraorbital muscles
- Orbit
- Eyelids
- Conjunctiva
- Lacrimal System

Key to Success

The medical terms for eye and ocular structures may be unfamiliar to most coders, especially those new to the field. As you read this chapter (and other chapters with distinct terminology), be sure to use a high quality medical dictionary. Learning the terminology now will ensure that you have what it takes to complete a certification exam or begin working as a coder in this field.

Procedural Coding in Optometry and Ophthalmology

Procedural coding for optometry and ophthalmology services is based on a unique set of procedure codes. Although eye service providers may bill E/M codes, there are several other sections within the CPT code book that are specifically devoted to the eye. The majority of eye and vision service codes are located in three different areas of the CPT code book: the E/M section, the Eye and Ocular Adnexa subsection in the Surgery section, and the Ophthalmology subsection of the Medicine section. Additional codes from the Radiology section (ultrasounds of the eye and orbital contents) and Category III (new and emerging eye technology) codes may also be used for eye and vision services.

Key to Success

The specialty of eye and vision services will determine which codes you use most often. For example, optometry coding relies more on evaluation and management of eye conditions and healthcare services, and so coding for an optometrist will require spending most of your time in the E/M and Medicine sections of the CPT code book. On the other hand, ophthalmology coding relies heavily on the surgical procedure performed by the ophthalmologist, so coding within this specialty means that you will spend more time in the Surgery section of the CPT code book. It is necessary to remain flexible in whichever specialty you work, and code for the service that was performed rather than coding only from one section of the book.

Coding for eye and vision services is perhaps best understood by dividing the two specialties—optometry coding and ophthalmology coding. However it is first necessary to discuss the E/M codes that may be used by either specialty, including when to use ophthalmology E/M codes rather than medical E/M codes, and vice-versa. Finally, this section discusses the handful of modifiers that are often used in optometry and ophthalmology services.

Ophthalmology E/M Services

Coding for eye and vision encounters is flexible, because there is a special selection of evaluation and management codes that are only used for ophthalmological services. Eye specialists can use evaluation and management codes (Office or Other Outpatient Services, 99201 through 99215), from the E/M section of the CPT code book, or ophthalmological service E/M codes (Ophthalmology, 91010 through 92499) from the Medicine section of the CPT code book.

There are four ophthalmological service E/M codes that are divided depending on patient status (new or established) and level of the service (intermediate or comprehensive). These codes are used when a provider performs an evaluation of the ophthalmological system including history, general observation, external and ophthalmoscopic examinations, gross visual field, and sensorimotor examination. These are integrated services and medical decision making cannot be separated from the examining techniques used. Unlike medical E/M codes, ophthalmological services do not include a history related to all aspects of the patient's health, such as a review of all body areas or organ systems, nor do they include a physical examination or more than just the ophthalmological system. They only focus on the eye and accessory structures. The four ophthalmology E/M codes are as follows.

- 92002, Ophthalmological services: E/M with initiation of diagnostic and treatment program; *intermediate, new patient*
- 92004, Ophthalmological services: E/M with initiation of diagnostic and treatment program; *comprehensive, new patient*
- 92012, Ophthalmological services: E/M with initiation or continuation of diagnostic and treatment program; *intermediate, established patient*
- 92014, Ophthalmological services: E/M with initiation of diagnostic and treatment program; *comprehensive, established patient*

There are two levels of complexity for ophthalmological services—intermediate and comprehensive (see table 9.1). **Intermediate ophthalmological services** include an evaluation of a new or existing condition complicated with a new diagnosis. **Comprehensive ophthalmological services** include a general evaluation of the complete ophthalmological system. An ophthalmologist may also decide to use a medical E/M code (discussed as follows), instead of one of the four ophthalmology E/M codes. Note also that these ophthalmological services (92002 through 92014) codes are to be used in conjunction with codes to report any other services performed on the same date.

Table 9.1. Ophthalmological services E/M codes

Ophthalmologic Services	Intermediate	Comprehensive
New	92002	92004
Established	92012	92014

Notice that the last two digits in the ophthalmologic services codes are the same as if they were medical evaluation and management codes. A low-level intermediate E/M encounter for a new patient is coded with 99202, Office or other outpatient visit for the evaluation and management of a new patient, which requires these three key components: an expanded problem-focused history; an expanded problem-focused examination; straightforward medical decision making; and the low-level ophthalmologic services encounter for a new patient is coded with 92002, Ophthalmological services: E/M with initiation of diagnostic and treatment program; intermediate, new patient. Correspondingly, the higher-level E/M code is 99214, Office or other outpatient visit for the evaluation and management of an established patient, which requires at least 2 of these 3 key components: a detailed history; a detailed examination; medical decision making of moderate complexity; and the comprehensive level ophthalmological services codes is 92014, Ophthalmological services: E/M with initiation of diagnostic and treatment program; comprehensive, established patient. However, ophthalmological

Figure 9.5. E/M and ophthalmological services examples

Case #1: Evaluation and Management Code	Case #2: Ophthalmological Services Code
A 68-year-old new patient presented to the office of an ophthalmologist for an eye checkup. He states that his glasses might be "slightly off." After further questioning, he states that his vision has been slightly blurry for the past three months, at all distances. Ophthalmologist performed a comprehensive eye examination with refraction and diagnosed the patient with a senile nuclear cataract and glaucoma suspect. Additional testing in the office included pachymetry, and retinal photos. Will follow up in one week for intraocular pressure and optical coherence tomography.	*68-year-old established patient presents to the ophthalmology office for his follow-up from one week ago. Ophthalmologist performed an intermediate examination and diagnosed the patient with primary open-angle glaucoma. Optical coherence tomography and extended visual field examination was performed in the office. Prescribed Xalatan and will follow up in two weeks.*
Procedure codes:	**Procedure codes:**
99204, Level 4 E/M encounter, new patient 92015, Determination of refractive state 76514, Diagnostic ophthalmic ultrasound; corneal pachymetry 92250, Fundus photography with interpretation and report	92012, Ophthalmological services; intermediate, established patient 92133, Scanning computerized ophthalmic diagnostic imaging, posterior segment, with interpretation and report; optic nerve 92083, Visual field examination, with interpretation and report; extended examination
Diagnosis codes:	**Diagnosis codes:**
H25.10, Age-related nuclear cataract, unspecified eye H40.009, Preglaucoma, unspecified, unspecified eye	H40.1190, Primary open-angle glaucoma, unspecified eye, stage unspecified
Justification of code use:	**Justification of code use:**
In this case, the patient came in for just a checkup but the provider completed a comprehensive evaluation and found two significant medical problems: cataracts and glaucoma suspect.	In this case, the patient came in for an evaluation of an existing condition complicated by a new diagnostic problem, with initiation of diagnostic and treatment program.

services should not be coded when the provider performs an evaluation of the patient's ophthalmological system for a medical diagnosis.

Evaluation and management codes (99201 through 99215) may be used in lieu of the ophthalmological services codes when the provider performs an encounter for a medical diagnosis, which involves more than the patient's ophthalmological system. For example, if an optometrist performs a routine visual examination of a patient with diabetic retinopathy, she would use an E/M code (99201 through 99215), rather than an ophthalmological services code (92002 through 92014).

Both sets of E/M codes are used by either optometrists or ophthalmologists, depending on the circumstances of the encounter. Review figure 9.5 to see examples of each type of encounter.

Besides evaluation and management services, there are several additional procedures performed on the eyes and accessory structures. It is helpful to discuss these services separately, depending on if they are optometry or ophthalmology services, as well as briefly cover some of the modifiers that are used in coding optometry and ophthalmology procedures.

Optometry Procedures

Optometry services are focused on the health and wellness of the eye and the ability to see. Optometry procedures are surgically non-invasive—and do not include surgical treatments of the eyes—and consist mostly of eye examinations, the provision of glasses and corrective lenses, screenings and diagnostic tests for eye conditions, and miscellaneous ophthalmological services.

Figure 9.6. Examples of refraction coding

Case #1: Commercial Insurance	Case #2: Medicaid
Intermediate eye examination performed on 10-year-old established female patient, including refraction.	Intermediate eye examination performed on 10-year-old established female patient, including refraction.
Procedure codes:	**Procedure code:**
92012, Ophthalmological services; intermediate, established patient 92015, Determination of refractive state	S0621, Routine ophthalmological examination including refraction, established patient

Eye Exams and Refractions

Eye examinations are coded with either medical E/M codes or with ophthalmological services E/M codes, as described in the previous section. It is important to note that eye examination codes do not include refraction. A refraction test is a common component of a typical eye examination performed by an optometrist for a prescription for corrective lenses that which may be coded separately from the eye examination itself using code 92015, Determination of refractive state. After a refraction is performed, it may be determined that the patient needs glasses or corrective lenses.

However, using this refraction code depends on the patient's insurance policy. If the patient has Medicaid, there are two HCPCS codes that include the refraction in addition to the eye examination: S0620, Routine ophthalmological examination *including refraction*, new patient, and S0621, Routine ophthalmological examination *including refraction*, established patient. Notice that in the example presented in figure 9.6 the encounter description is the same, yet the procedure codes billed differ based on the patient's insurance company.

Glasses and Corrective Lenses

Many optometry offices also provide glasses and corrective lenses to their patients, which are coded using the appropriate HCPCS or CPT code.

HCPCS codes for vision services, V0000 through V2999 are used to bill various supplies used for vision services, such as corrective lenses. The act of refracting the patient's vision or performing any actual procedures on the patient's vision are reported with CPT codes and are discussed as follows. These HCPCS codes are used to report the corrective lenses or other vision products that are supplied to the patient. They include

- Frames
- Spectacle lenses (single vision, bifocal, trifocal, and variable asphericity)
- Contact lenses
- Low vision aids
- Prosthetic eyes
- Intraocular lenses
- Miscellaneous vision services

As previously mentioned, CPT codes are used to report the procedures specific to fitting contact lenses, either for correcting a patient's vision or for managing a health condition. They include the following:

- 92071, Fitting of contact lens for treatment of ocular surface disease. This code is used when a contact lens is prescribed to provide dressing to the eye. For example, a contact lens may be fitted over a corneal abrasion to act as a bandage and allow healing.

- 92072, Fitting of contact lens for management of keratoconus, initial fitting. Keratoconus is a condition in which the cornea of the eye protrudes in a cone shape. Contact lenses for keratoconus help to reshape the cornea and restore vision.

- Contact lens services. These services include the prescription and fitting of contact lenses and the instructions and training of the wearer. Incidental revision of the lens during the trial period is also included in these services (for example, fitting a different set of lenses within the trial period if the initial pair were uncomfortable or did not fit well). These services are coded with 92310, Prescription of optical and physical contact characteristics of and fitting of contact lens, with medical supervision of adaptation; corneal lens, both eyes, except for aphakia, through 92317, Prescription of optical and physical characteristics of contact lens, with medical supervision of adaptation and direction of fitting by independent technician; corneoscleral lens, and depend on the type of lens, the condition being treated, and the individual that is completing the fitting component of the contact lens service. In addition to the contact lens fitting, the appropriate HCPCS V-code (as listed previously) should also be used to identify the lenses supplied to the patient.

For example, when a patient goes into the office for the fitting of contact lenses, the actual fitting and prescription of the lens is reported with the appropriate CPT code. The lens itself is reported with the appropriate HCPCS code.

Screenings and Miscellaneous Eye Services

Similar to medical specialties, optometrists perform a number of different screenings used to either test for a specific condition (such as glaucoma), or to test for visual acuity. There are also several different ophthalmological services performed by optometrists.

- G0117 and G0118, Glaucoma screening for high risk patient, is used for Medicare patients who meet the criteria for a glaucoma screening.

- 92020, Gonioscopy, is an examination of the front part of the eye (the anterior chamber), between the cornea and the iris. This examination is used to determine a buildup of pressure, which could indicate glaucoma.

- 92100, Serial tonometry, is yet another way to screen for glaucoma. This consists of multiple measurements of intraocular pressure over an extended period of time on the same day. Note that a tonometry measurement is included in an ophthalmological examination, and that this procedure is designated as a separate procedure. It should only be reported if it is the only procedure performed on the date of service.

- 76514, Ophthalmic ultrasound, diagnostic; corneal pachymetry, unilateral or bilateral (determination of corneal thickness) is performed for various reasons, including screening for keratoconus and glaucoma.

Additional codes for miscellaneous ophthalmological services, visual acuity assessments, and ophthalmoscopy codes are also listed throughout the ophthalmology subsection of the CPT code book. Minor surgical procedures are also performed by optometrists. Keep in mind that these procedures are not invasive surgeries, like those performed by ophthalmologists.

Figure 9.7. Slit lamp examination of the eye

Source: US Air Force, Seltmann 2012.

Minor Surgical Procedures

Minor surgical procedures performed by optometrists are minimally invasive, and usually are done to treat a minor or uncomplicated problem. They include the following:

- 65205 through 65222, Removal of foreign body, external eye. These codes report the removal of a foreign body from the external eye, including the cornea or conjunctiva. Foreign bodies that are deeper than the external eye may require patient anesthesia and a more complex removal. These codes depend on the depth of the foreign body, the area from which the foreign body was removed, and whether or not a slit lamp was used. A **slit lamp** is a high-intensity light that can be focused into a thin sheet to shine into the eye. Slit lamps are commonly used during eye examinations to find abnormalities in the anterior of the eye (see figure 9.7).

- 65435, Removal of corneal epithelium; with or without chemocauterization (abrasion, curettage). Also called corneal epithelial debridement, this procedure treats irregularities of the epithelium (skin) of the cornea.

- 67820, Correction of trichiasis; epilation, by forceps only. Trichiasis in a condition in which the eyelashes are ingrown or misdirected, and must be manually removed using forceps and a biomicroscope.

- 68761, Closure of the lacrimal punctum; by plug, each. In this procedure, the provider inserts a small plug into the lacrimal punctum, which reduces drainage from the eye. It is often performed as a treatment for dry eye syndrome.

Practice coding optometry procedures by completing the exercises in There's a Code for That 9.1.

9.1

There's a Code for That

Optometry procedures

Read the following documentation of the optometry service and code for the encounter.

1. Comprehensive ophthalmological examination with refraction performed on an established patient with senile nuclear sclerosis and hypermetropia.

   CPT codes: _____, _____

2. Optometrist performed a comprehensive ophthalmological examination on a new patient with open angle glaucoma and type 1 diabetes mellitus. Additional procedures included a bilateral corneal pachymetry, scanning computerized ophthalmic diagnostic imaging (SCODI) of the anterior segment, and extended bilateral visual field examination using Humphrey visual field analyzer.

   CPT codes: _____, _____, _____,

   _____

3. Routine ophthalmological examination with refraction performed on an established Medicaid patient. Optometrist furnished patient with spectacle frames with lenses. Lens #1 (right): single vision, plano to 1.75. Lens #2 (left): single vision, plano to 1.90. Both with anti-reflective coating. (Hint: Since this is a Medicaid patient, use the appropriate HCPCS code for the service. Supplies are also coded with HCPCS codes. Modifiers should identify the right and left sides).

   HCPCS codes: _____, _____, _____ -

   _____, _____ - _____, _____

4. Patient with pain in the left eye was found upon examination (new patient, level 3 encounter) to have a foreign body in the cornea. Optometrist removed FB from the cornea with slit lamp assistance. Hint: Upon examination, the provider made the decision to perform the FB removal surgery.

   CPT codes: _____ - _____, _____

Ophthalmology Procedures

Ophthalmologists may perform both medical and ophthalmological E/M services, but their specialty is focused on surgical interventions to treat eye conditions. Procedures consist of several specialized eye surgeries, but the most common are refractive surgeries, trabeculectomies, cataract surgeries, orbital surgeries, and strabismus surgery.

Key to Success

At the beginning of the Eye and Ocular Adnexa subsection within the Surgery section of the CPT code book, note the statement placed before the listing of CPT codes: *Do not report code 69990 in addition to codes 65091–68850.* Codes 65091 through 68850 are all Eye and Ocular Adnexa surgery codes. Code 69990, Operating microscope, should be reported when a surgical microscope is employed during microsurgery. However, the use of a surgical microscope is integral to ophthalmological procedures, and so it may not be reported separately when coding from this subsection of the CPT code book.

Refractive Surgeries

Refractive surgeries are performed to reshape the cornea of the eye and improve eye sight. They may be either elective or functional. Elective refractive surgery would be done solely to improve idiopathic myopia, hyperopia, and astigmatism. Functional refractive surgery would be done to correct a defect in vision due to a medical diagnosis, such as a traumatic injury. The surgery is performed by using a laser to re-shape the cornea, and only takes a few minutes.

There are a number of different codes for refractive surgeries, which differ depending on the reason for the surgery and the type of surgery performed.

- Laser-assisted refractive surgeries are procedures in which a laser is used to incise the eye and reshape the cornea. The two most common are
  - S0800, Laser in situ keratomileusis (LASIK). Although it is not covered by Medicare, a handful of commercial insurance payers may pay for LASIK surgery to correct vision conditions.
  - S0810, Photorefractive keratectomy (PRK), is the second most common refractive laser surgery (after LASIK).
- If astigmatism is a result of ocular trauma or has been surgically induced, refractive surgery may be performed to reshape the cornea and restore vision. These procedures are coded with 65772, Corneal relaxing incision for correction of surgically induced astigmatism, and 65775, Corneal wedge resection for correction of surgically induced astigmatism.
- If none of the previous codes are applicable because of differences in the manner in which the procedure was performed, it would be appropriate to use 66999, Unlisted procedure, anterior segment of the eye, for either LASIK or PRK.

Trabeculectomy

A **trabeculectomy** is performed as a treatment for glaucoma, by lowering the **intraocular pressure** (the pressure inside the eyeball). It consists of the ophthalmologist using a laser to open a drainage canal in the eye to allow for the outflow of aqueous humor by removing a part of the trabecular meshwork of the eye. The resulting outflow of aqueous humor drains into a bleb on the upper portion of the eye, covered by the eyelid. By draining the pressure of the aqueous humor, a trabeculectomy may slow the damage caused by glaucoma but cannot restore any vision lost from glaucoma (see figure 9.8). Procedure codes for trabeculectomies include the following:

- 66170, Fistularization of sclera for glaucoma; trabeculectomy ab externo, and 66172, Fistularization of sclera for glaucoma; trabeculectomy ab externo with scarring from previous ocular surgery or trauma. These codes are the basic trabeculectomy codes for the treatment of glaucoma.
- 65850, Trabeculotomy ab externo, and 65855, Trabeculoplasty by laser surgery are performed for congenital glaucoma. These procedures are less invasive than trabeculectomies, and are less likely to cause cataracts.

Figure 9.8. Trabeculectomy

Source: International Glaucoma Association 2017.

- 65820, Goniotomy. Also performed as a treatment for congenital glaucoma, this procedure uses a device called a **goniolens** (an ophthalmic endoscope) to see the anterior chamber of the eye and make an incision into the trabecular meshwork, reducing intraocular pressure. Note that if the goniolens is used, the add on code 66990, Use of ophthalmic endoscope, should also be reported.

Key to Success

Be careful when reading and selecting surgical procedure codes, as differences in procedure names are usually only a few letters. For example, a trabecul*ectomy* is a completely different procedure than a trabecul*otomy*. Reading either of these terms too quickly makes it easy to miss the small differences in spelling, and may ultimately result in selecting the wrong code.

Cataract Surgery

Cataracts are a common cause of vision loss and affect, to some degree, over half of all adults over the age of 65 (Johns Hopkins University 2017). A cataract occurs when the lens, which lies behind the iris and pupil of the eye, becomes clouded, impeding vision.

There are three main types of cataracts.

- **Nuclear cataracts** form in the nucleus of the lens and are often associated with aging. They may also be referred to as senile cataracts.
- **Subcapsular cataracts** form at the back of the lens and are more common in individuals with diabetes mellitus or patients on high doses of steroids.
- **Cortical cataracts** begin on the peripheral edges of the lens and work their way inward toward the center. (AAO 2017)

Cataract surgery consists of replacing the clouded lens with an artificial lens to restore vision. It is a commonly performed surgery that takes about 30 minutes to complete. **Phacoemulsification** is a technique used during extracapsular cataract excision that uses ultrasound vibrations to break up the cloudy lens and extract it through a small hollow tube. There are two types of cataract extractions:

- **Extracapsular cataract extraction (ECCE).** In this procedure the lens is either broken up via phacoemulsification or it is surgically removed in one piece, leaving the lens capsule intact. ECCEs are reported with codes
    - 66982, Extracapsular cataract removal with insertion of intraocular lens prosthesis, manual or mechanical technique, complex, requiring devices or techniques not generally used in routine cataract surgery, and
    - 66984, Extracapsular cataract removal with insertion or intraocular lens prosthesis, manual or mechanical technique.
- **Intracapsular cataract extraction (ICCE).** This procedure removes both the lens and the lens capsule, and is performed only in rare cases. ICCE is reported with code
    - 66983, Intracapsular cataract extraction with insertion of intraocular lens prosthesis.

Orbital Surgery

Orbital surgeries are performed to treat defects resulting in acquired absence of the eye, eye tumors, or for removal of the eye for medical reasons.

Codes for the removal of ocular contents are based on the extent of the removal:

- **Evisceration** of the ocular contents is the removal of the contents of the globe of the eye, while leaving the remaining structures intact. This procedure is coded with:
  - 65091, Evisceration of ocular contents; *without implant*, or
  - 65093, Evisceration of ocular contents, *with implant*.
- **Enucleation** is removing the eyeball while leaving the orbital structures intact, including the extraocular muscles. Codes for enucleation are divided depending on whether an implant was placed after the removal of the eye, and whether the extraocular muscles were attached to the implant (if placed). They are:
  - 65101, Enucleation of eye, *without implant*,
  - 65103, Enucleation of eye; *with implant, muscles not attached to implant*, and
  - 65105 Enucleation of eye; *with implant, muscles attached to implant*.
- **Exenteration** of the orbit includes the removal of the eye and ocular adnexa. These codes are based on the extent of the removal. They are:
  - 65110, Exenteration of orbit, removal of orbital contents; only,
  - 65112, Exenteration of orbit, removal of orbital contents; with therapeutic removal of bone, and
  - 65114, Exenteration of orbit, removal of orbital contents; with muscle or myocutaneous flap.

Strabismus Surgery

Strabismus is a misalignment of the eye muscles that can be surgically corrected by repositioning and strengthening the muscles of the eye. Codes for strabismus surgery (67311 through 67340) are based on the type or muscle (horizontal, vertical, or superior oblique), and the number of extraocular muscles involved in the procedure.

Modifiers Used in Eye and Vision Services

There are a handful of important modifiers that a coder may need to append to eye and vision service codes. They identify the laterality of the procedure (either right or left), as well as the specific eyelid being worked on (when applicable). Additional modifiers may identify specific stages of the operative period, or the decision for surgery.

- Modifier -LT, Left side and modifier -RT, right side. Theses modifiers are used with paired organs to identify the side of the body on which the procedure was performed. For example, if the patient had strabismus surgery on the right eye, then the modifier -RT should be appended to the strabismus surgery code.
- Eyelid modifiers are used to identify the specific eyelid on which the procedure is being performed. It is not necessary to also use the -RT or -LT modifiers with these, as the laterality is already built into the modifier.
  - Modifier -E1, Upper left, eyelid
  - Modifier -E2, Lower left, eyelid
  - Modifier -E3, Upper right, eyelid
  - Modifier -E4, Lower right, eyelid
- Modifier -54, Surgical care only. This modifier is used when the surgeon performed only the surgery on the patient, and did not provide either the pre-or postoperative care. For example, if the ophthalmologist performed an extracapsular cataract extraction (ECCE), and then transferred the care of the patient to an optometrist, he would bill the code for the ECCE (66984) with modifier -54

If you are not sure whether or not to include the laterality or eyelid modifiers, append the modifiers to the appropriate procedure codes, just in case. It is better to have a modifier and not need it, than to need a modifier and not have it. Usually if an informational modifier is reported and the insurance plan does not require the modifier, they will simply ignore it. However, if the insurance *does* require the modifier and it was not reported, they may deny the charge.

MOD

to indicate that he only performed the surgery on the patient: 66984-54, Extracapsular cataract removal with insertion or intraocular lens prosthesis, manual or mechanical technique, *surgical care only*. The payment for the surgery will be reduced accordingly.

- Modifier -55, Postoperative management only. This modifier should be appended when one healthcare provider performed the surgical procedure, and a different healthcare provider performed the postoperative care. It should be appended to the code for the primary procedure, when reported by the provider who only managed the postoperative care. For example, an optometrist postoperatively manages a patient that just received an ECCE. He would report the code for the ECCE with modifier -55: 66984-55, Extracapsular cataract removal with insertion or intraocular lens prosthesis, manual or mechanical technique, *postoperative management only*. Even though the optometrist did not perform the cataract removal, it is coded as if he did, but with modifier -55 to identify that it was only the postoperative care. Modifier -55 will result in a minimal payment for the service, according to the work that was performed; for example, about 20 percent of the regular payment amount.

- Modifier -57, Decision for surgery. This modifier is important in optometry coding, as it can indicate that a decision for surgery was made during an evaluation and management encounter. For example, if it was determined during the encounter that a patient with glaucoma needed surgical intervention to treat the condition, then modifier -57 would be appended to the E/M code.

- Modifier -58, Staged or related procedure or service by the same physician or other qualified health care professional during the postoperative period. This modifier should be used when a procedure is performed in stages, and it should be appended to the second or subsequent code for the additional stage of surgery. For example, a surgeon performed a blepharoplasty (plastic repair of the eyelid), which was reported with code 67971, Reconstruction of eyelid, full thickness by transfer of transconjunctival flap from opposing eyelid; *up to two-thirds of eyelid, 1 stage or first stage*. It was determined that this surgical repair would not be sufficient, and the patient returned to the operating room on a different day after the initial surgery, and a second stage of the repair was done. The second stage repair should be reported as 67975, Reconstruction of eyelid, full thickness by transfer of transconjunctival flap from opposing eyelid; *second stage*, appended with modifier -58, as such: 67975-58.

Complete the exercises in There's a Code for That 9.2 to practice coding ophthalmology procedures.

9.2

There's a Code for That

Ophthalmology procedures

Read the following documentation of the ophthalmology service and code for the encounter.

1. Photocoagulation of localized retinal lesion of the right eye.

   CPT code: _____

2. Laser-assisted in situ keratomileusis.

   HCPCS code: _____

3. Goniotomy performed on two-year-old female with congenital glaucoma with ophthalmological endoscopic assistance.

   CPT code: _____, _____

4. ECCE with insertion of IOL prosthesis.

   CPT code: _____

5. Excision of two chalazion on right upper eyelid.

   CPT code: _____

Diagnostic Coding in Optometry and Ophthalmology

Diagnostic codes used in optometry and ophthalmology include a vast range of conditions affecting the eye and ocular adnexa, as well as comorbid conditions (as discussed in chapter 2) like hypertension or diabetes mellitus, which may complicate or even cause eye diseases. Diagnosis codes used in eye and vision services can be separated into two main types: screenings or examinations, and eye conditions.

Key to Success

The diagnosis code used should be selected carefully, taking into account the patient's insurance—whether it is vision or healthcare insurance. Remember that healthcare insurance will not pay for an examination or treatment of a vision condition or general eye wellness examination. Rather, healthcare insurance will only pay for eye services performed for an actual diagnosis.

Eye Screenings and Examinations

Routine wellness examinations are performed on the ophthalmological system by optometrists and ophthalmologists, just as they are performed on the entire physical body by primary care practitioners. Optometrists perform annual wellness examinations to check for disease processes and to care for the vision of patients with vision needs. If, after examination, an optometrist discovers indicators for a disease, he or she will determine if there is a need for a further diagnostic test for the suspected condition. The diagnosis codes used to identify the medical necessity for these services depend on the type of service performed and if any abnormalities or disease conditions were encountered.

- Z01.00, Encounter for examination of eyes and vision, without abnormal findings, and Encounter Z01.01, for examination of eyes and vision, with abnormal findings, should be used when a patient presents for a routine eye wellness examination. If no abnormal findings are encountered, then code Z01.00 should be reported. If any abnormal findings are encountered, then code Z01.01 should be reported, with secondary codes to identify the abnormality. This includes any abnormal condition, even a vision problem. For example, if a patient is seen for a routine eye check and it is discovered that she has irregular astigmatism of the right eye, then the coder should report Z01.01, Encounter for examination of eyes and vision, with abnormal findings, along with H52.211, Irregular astigmatism, right eye.

- Z13.5, Encounter for screening of eye and ear disorders, should be reported when a patient presents for a diagnostic test for an eye condition and there was no diagnosis confirmed as a result of the test. For example, if a patient comes in for a diagnostic screening for macular degeneration, and the diagnosis of macular degeneration is confirmed at that visit, then only the code for macular degeneration should be reported. On the other hand, if the diagnosis of macular degeneration was *not* confirmed, then the code for the diagnostic screening should be reported. If specific signs and symptoms that prompted the test are present, the coder should report the codes for the signs and symptoms. The screening code should only be reported if the diagnostic test was ordered without any signs, symptoms, illness, or injury recorded.

- Z96.1, Presence of intraocular lens, should be reported for any patient who has an intraocular lens prosthesis (pseudophakia).

Diagnostic Eye Coding

Besides eye screenings and examinations, optometrists and ophthalmologists commonly see a number of different medical diagnoses of the eye. Furthermore, there are a few specific guidelines when it comes to coding for eye conditions including laterality, diabetic complications, and congenital conditions.

Laterality and Eyelids

Because the eyes are paired organs, many of the diagnosis cods for eye conditions specify the laterality of the condition. Remember that in CPT coding, specific modifiers (-LT, Left side; -RT, Right side; and -50, Bilateral procedure) identify the laterality of the procedure. Laterality also exists in ICD-10-CM coding for eye conditions. However, in ICD-10-CM coding, laterality is identified by selecting the correct code for the laterality documented, rather than adding a modifier to identify the laterality, as in CPT coding. It is important to be particularly careful when coding for eye conditions and the procedures performed on them, to ensure that the laterality identified in the ICD-10-CM code matches the laterality identified by the CPT modifier (if applicable).

The laterality of the eye conditions may be specified as right, left, or bilateral. If there is no laterality specified in the documentation, then the unspecified laterality code should be reported. For conditions affecting the eyelids, diagnosis codes may specify the exact eyelid affected by the condition. They include the right upper, right lower, left upper, and left lower eyelids. As with the laterality, if the specific eyelid is not documented, then select the code for the unspecified eyelid. For example, the codes for stye (H00.01-, Hordeolum externum) identify both the eyelid involved (upper or lower) as well as the laterality of the condition (right or left). A stye on the upper right eyelid would be coded as H00.011, Hordeolum externum right upper eyelid. However, if the provider's documentation did not specify which side (laterality) or eyelid on which the stye was located, then the unspecified version of the code would be reported (H00.019, Hordeolum externum unspecified eye, unspecified eyelid).

Key to Success

When selecting diagnosis codes for eye conditions, be sure that the laterality (or eyelid) of the diagnosis code matches the laterality (or eyelid) identified by the CPT modifier. For example, if the procedure code modifier is -RT for a right-sided procedure, then the diagnosis code should identify that the condition affected the right eye. If the laterality or the eyelids do not match, then it may cause problems with claim processing.

Diabetic Eye Complications

Chronic high blood sugar, like that which happens with diabetes mellitus, can have negative effects on the eyes. So it is common for eye conditions to present along with diabetes. When this happens, it is necessary to code for both the eye condition and the diabetes, by type. The following diabetes codes are combination codes that identify both the type of diabetes and the ophthalmological complication.

- E08.3-, Diabetes mellitus due to underlying condition with ophthalmic complications
- E09.3-, Drug or chemical-induced diabetes mellitus with ophthalmic complications
- E10.3-, Type 1 diabetes mellitus with ophthalmic complications
- E11.3-, Type 2 diabetes mellitus with ophthalmic complications
- E12.3-, Other specified diabetes mellitus with ophthalmic complications

If no combination code exists that identifies both the diabetes and the complication, then it is necessary to code for the two conditions separately.

Use the steps that follow to look up diabetes with ophthalmic complications and code for them correctly. Remember that one code should be used to identify each diabetic complication, so if the patient has multiple ophthalmologic conditions, then one code should be reported to identify each individual complication.

1. Identify the type of diabetes—diabetes due to underlying condition, drug or chemical-induced diabetes, type 1, type 2, or other specified diabetes.
2. Identify each ophthalmic complication—diabetic retinopathy, diabetic cataract, diabetic macular edema, or other diabetic ophthalmic complication. Diabetic retinopathy codes are very specific, and identify the type of retinopathy (proliferative or nonproliferative), the severity (mild, moderate, or severe), and whether it presents with or without macular edema.
3. If no combination code exists that identifies both the diabetes and the complication, then select the code for *other diabetic complication,* such as E11.39, Type 2 diabetes mellitus with other diabetic ophthalmic complication, and add an additional ICD-10-CM code to identify the specific complication.

Congenital versus Acquired Conditions

A **congenital condition** is one that was present at or before birth. An **acquired condition**, on the other hand, is one that develops over the course of a person's life.

Congenital conditions affect every part of the human body not just the eyes, so the difference between congenital and acquired conditions should be kept in mind for coding for conditions throughout the ICD-10-CM code book.

Congenital codes are all coded from chapter 17: Congenital Malformations, Deformations, and Chromosomal Abnormalities of the ICD-10-CM code book. Acquired conditions of the eyes are coded from chapter 7: Diseases of the Eye and Adnexa of the ICD-10-CM code book. If a condition is stated as *congenital*, then it should be coded from chapter 17. To look up a congenital anomaly in the ICD-10-CM code book, search for the condition in the Main Index and then select the congenital version of the condition. For example, when searching for congenital aphakia (absence of the lens of the eye), look up the term *aphakia* in the ICD-10-CM Main Index, and then reference the subterm *congenital*, which leads you to code Q12.3. Verify the code in the Tabular List: Q12.3, Congenital aphakia.

Eye Conditions

Coding for eye conditions usually requires knowledge of the laterality of the condition, as well as specifics of the severity of the condition. Generally speaking, coders should report one code for each eye condition, per eye, unless the condition presents bilaterally and a bilateral code exists. Top diagnoses for eye conditions include glaucoma, injuries, cataracts, macular degeneration, vision problems, and retinal detachments, all of which can be found in the Main Index of the ICD-10-CM code book and verified in the Tabular List.

Glaucoma

Glaucoma (H40 to H42) is a buildup of intraocular pressure that causes damage to the eye's optic nerve over time, and may eventually lead to irreversible vision loss. Treatments for glaucoma include medication and surgical intervention (trabeculectomy). There are many types of glaucoma, which may be caused by injury to the eye, inflammatory conditions, severe eye infections, or a blockage of blood vessels in the eye. They are as follows:

- Open-angle glaucoma, also called wide-angle glaucoma, in which the trabecular meshwork of the eye does not properly allow for the outflow of aqueous humor.
- Angle-closure glaucoma, also called chronic angle-closure or narrow-angle glaucoma, in which drainage of aqueous humor from the eye due to the angle between the iris and cornea being too narrow.
- Congenital glaucoma (Q15.0, Congenital glaucoma), is when a child is born with glaucoma due to a congenital defect in the eye's drainage structure.
- Secondary glaucomas occur because of an underlying medical condition, such as poorly controlled diabetes or hypertension.

Glaucoma ICD-10-CM codes are perhaps the most specific eye condition codes, so a coder must be careful with code selection and pay attention to the OGCR for this condition. As many codes as possible should be assigned to identify the type of glaucoma, the affected eye, and the stage of the glaucoma. When a patient has bilateral glaucoma, and both eyes are documented as having the same type and stage of glaucoma, then the bilateral code option should be selected. If the glaucoma is bilateral, but the stage or type is different, then assign one glaucoma code for each eye, rather than the bilateral code option. If the stage of the glaucoma cannot be determined, then use the code option for *indeterminate* stage. This is different from *unspecified* stage, which should be

Figure 9.9. OGCR I.C.7.a

---

7. Chapter 7: Diseases of the Eye and Adnexa (H00-H59)

a. Glaucoma

1) Assigning Glaucoma Codes

Assign as many codes from category H40, Glaucoma, as needed to identify the type of glaucoma, the affected eye, and the glaucoma stage.

2) Bilateral glaucoma with same type and stage

When a patient has bilateral glaucoma and both eyes are documented as being the same type and stage, and there is a code for bilateral glaucoma, report only the code for the type of glaucoma, bilateral, with the seventh character for the stage.

When a patient has bilateral glaucoma and both eyes are documented as being the same type and stage, and the classification does not provide a code for bilateral glaucoma (i.e. subcategories H40.10, H40.11 and H40.20) report only one code for the type of glaucoma with the appropriate seventh character for the stage.

3) Bilateral glaucoma stage with different types or stages

When a patient has bilateral glaucoma and each eye is documented as having a different type or stage, and the classification distinguishes laterality, assign the appropriatecode for each eye rather than the code for bilateral glaucoma.

When a patient has bilateral glaucoma and each eye is documented as having a different type, and the classification does not distinguish laterality (i.e. subcategories H40.10, H40.11 and H40.20), assign one code for each type of glaucoma with the appropriate seventh character for the stage.

When a patient has bilateral glaucoma and each eye is documented as having the same type, but different stage, and the classification does not distinguish laterality (i.e. subcategories H40.10, H40.11 and H40.20), assign a code for the type of glaucoma for each eye with the seventh character for the specific glaucoma stage documented for each eye.

4) Patient admitted with glaucoma and stage evolves during the admission

If a patient is admitted with glaucoma and the stage progresses during the admission, assign the code for highest stage documented.

5) Indeterminate stage glaucoma

Assignment of the seventh character "4" for "indeterminate stage" should be based on the clinical documentation. The seventh character "4" is used for glaucomas whose stage cannot be clinically determined. This seventh character should not be confused with the seventh character "0", unspecified, which should be assigned when there is no documentation regarding the stage of the glaucoma.

Source: CMS 2018.

used when the documentation does not specify the stage of glaucoma. Refer to figure 9.9 for the OGCR related to coding for glaucoma.

Key to Success

Be careful when selecting codes for glaucoma, as many of them require a seventh-character extension to identify the stage of the condition. If the glaucoma is due to an underlying condition, underlying eye disorder, or an adverse effect, additional codes are needed to identify the causative conditions.

Eye Injuries

Eye injuries are coded from chapter 19: Injury, Poisoning, and Certain Other Consequences of External Causes, from category S05, Injury of eye and orbit. Remember that all injury codes require a seventh-character extension to identify the encounter (A-initial, D-subsequent, S-Sequela). To code for an injury of the eye, check the documentation for the specific type of eye injury (contusion, laceration, penetrating wound), and the laterality of the condition. Bilateral eye injury codes do not exist, so if there are both right and left sided injuries, assign one code per ocular injury.

Cataracts

Diagnosis cods for cataracts (H25 to H28) specify the type and laterality of the condition. Types include age-related (also called senile), infantile or juvenile, traumatic (resulting from a traumatic injury), complicated (by neovascularization, other eye disorder, or glaucoma), drug-induced, or secondary cataract. If the same cataract presents bilaterally, then assign the bilateral code option. If the condition presents bilaterally but the type of cataract is different, assign one code for each side. Furthermore, additional codes may be needed to identify the underlying disease or eye condition, or the causative substance in drug-induced cataracts.

Macular Degeneration

Macular degeneration (H35.3-) is a deterioration of the central portion of the retina, called the macula. In its early stages macular degeneration does not affect eyesight, but as the disease progresses patients may experience blurry or wavy vision, and in its most severe stages it can lead to complete loss of the central area of vision. Be diligent when reporting codes for macular degeneration, as some require seven characters, while others require only six. Codes for nonexudative (or dry) and exudative (or wet) age-related macular degeneration (AMD) require seven characters. The seventh character identifies the stage of the AMD.

Vision Impairments

Because optometrists treat vision and refractive disorders, there are several diagnoses for vision impairments that are commonly coded (H52 and H53). These include myopia (nearsightedness), astigmatism, presbyopia (farsightedness), and other visual disturbances such as scotomas (blind spots) and color blindness.

Retinal Detachment

A retinal detachment (H33) occurs when the retina, a layer of tissue at the back of the eye, detaches from the eye tissues. It causes irreversible and immediate vision impairment and requires urgent treatment. Diagnosis codes for retinal detachments identify the laterality of the condition as well as the type of tear: retinal break, single break, multiple breaks, giant retinal tear, retinal dialysis, or total retinal detachment.

Coding for eye and vision diagnoses requires an eye for detail, as many codes require identification of the laterality and severity of the condition; and most ICD-10-CM codes are six to seven characters long, making them some of the more complex diagnosis codes in ICD-10-CM coding. For practice assigning optometry and ophthalmology diagnosis codes, complete the exercises in There's a Code for That 9.3.

Diagnostic coding for optometry and ophthalmology

9.3

There's a Code for That

Read the following documentation and assign the appropriate diagnosis code(s) for the encounter.

1. Patient presents for a routine eye exam with no abnormal findings.

ICD-10-CM code: _____

(Continued on next page)

9.3

Continued

2. Patient presents for a routine eye examination. During the exam, it is noted that the patient has developed regular astigmatism of the right eye since the last visit. Spectacle glasses were provided as well as lenses with anti-reflective coating.

ICD-10-CM codes: _____, _____

3. Patient is a known diabetic (type 2), diagnosed with proliferative diabetic retinopathy with macular edema of the right eye and proliferative diabetic retinopathy without macular edema of the left eye.

ICD-10-CM codes: _____, _____

4. Congenital cataract in a 1-year-old female patient.

ICD-10-CM code: _____

5. Patient has primary open-angle glaucoma of the right and left eyes, mild stage.

ICD-10-CM code: _____

6. 28-year-old male hockey player presents for evaluation of his partially resolved cataract of the left eye, which is a late effect of blunt force trauma to the eye from a hockey stick. (Hint: Remember that a late effect is a sequela of a previous injury).

ICD-10-CM codes: _____, _____

7. Age-related macular degeneration.

ICD-10-CM code: _____

Putting It All Together: Coding for Eye and Vision Services

To select the correct codes for an eye and vision service encounter, a coder must carefully read the documentation, then access each code book to find the procedure or service provided and the corresponding diagnosis or diagnoses to support the medical necessity for the service. Procedural codes for optometry and ophthalmology services are found in the CPT and HCPCS code books, and diagnosis codes are found in the ICD-10-CM code book.

Determination of accurate codes relies on the answers to the following questions.

- What services were provided to the patient?
    - Was an E/M service provided? Was it a E/M service or an ophthalmological E/M service?
    - Were any additional procedures performed?
    - Was a surgery performed?
- Are there any applicable modifiers or add-on codes?
- Is there a definitive diagnosis for the encounter? If yes, this should be the first-listed diagnosis code. If no, then use the appropriate eye screening code. If signs or symptoms are present, code for the signs and symptoms.

- Are there any additional signs, symptoms, conditions, or z-codes for screenings, examinations, or patient history that should be reported?

Study the following vignette that demonstrates how to select the appropriate diagnosis and procedure codes. Then complete the following practice exercises in There's a Code for That 9.4.

Terrence is coding an encounter for a 42-year-old female that was seen yesterday at her optometrist's office. The woman has been suffering from bilateral dry-eye syndrome for many years and has elected for punctal occlusion. After a level 4 medical examination of this established patient, the optometrist closed the left and right lacrimal punctum via plug occlusion.

First, Terrence asks himself: What did the doctor do? The doctor performed a level 4 medical examination for an established patient, and then inserted four plugs into the patient's lacrimal ducts (right upper, right lower, left upper, and left lower lacrimal ducts). He assigns code 99214 for the E/M service, and determines that the code for the lacrimal occlusion is 68761. Because the doctor plugged all four of the lacrimal ducts, he assigns the code four times with the appropriate modifier to identify the location of the procedure:

> *99214, Office or other outpatient visit for the evaluation and management of an established patient, which requires at least 2 of these 3 key components: a detailed history, a detailed examination, medical decision making of moderate complexity*
>
> *68761-E1, Closure of the lacrimal punctum; by plug, each (upper left eyelid)*
>
> *68761-E2, Closure of the lacrimal punctum; by plug, each (lower left eyelid)*
>
> *68761-E3, Closure of the lacrimal punctum; by plug, each (upper right eyelid)*
>
> *68761-E4, Closure of the lacrimal punctum; by plug, each (lower right eyelid)*

Now that he has his procedure codes, Terrence asks himself: Why did the doctor do it? In this case, the patient has bilateral dry-eye syndrome. He looks up the condition in the ICD-10-CM code book and finds the following code:

> *H04.123, Dry eye syndrome of bilateral lacrimal glands*

He then rechecks the documentation to make sure he has coded everything for the encounter, and reports the chosen codes on the claim for the service.

Diagnostic and procedural coding for eye and vision services

9.4

There's a Code for That

Read the following documentation and assign the appropriate CPT, HCPCS, and ICD-10-CM code(s) for the encounter.

1. Extended ophthalmoscopy with retinal drawing, with interpretation and report. Patient has been experiencing visual discomfort and visual halos, and has vitreous floaters of the left eye.

   CPT codes: _____

   ICD-10-CM codes: _____, _____, _____

(Continued on next page)

9.4

Continued

2. Ophthalmologist performed a strabismus surgery of the left eye on two horizontal muscles (medial rectus muscle), and one vertical muscle (superior rectus muscle), employing posterior fixation technique, without muscle recession. Patient is 22-year-old female with monocular esotropia of the left eye.

CPT codes: _____ - _____, _____ - _____,

_____ - _____

ICD-10-CM codes: _____

3. Repair of retinal detachment via photocoagulation on a 62-year-old with retinal detachment with single break of the right eye.

CPT codes: _____ - _____

ICD-10-CM codes: _____

HCC

End of Chapter Content

Instructions: Indicate whether the following statements are true or false (T or F). For false statements, rewrite the statement on the line below to make the statement true.

1. Optometrists treat vision and ophthalmologists surgically treat eye conditions.

_____

_____

2. Vision insurance pays for your eyes, and healthcare insurance pays for your glasses.

_____

_____

3. There are five ophthalmological E/M encounter codes.

_____

_____

4. Optometrists and ophthalmologists may code for encounters with either E/M codes or ophthalmological E/M codes.

_____

_____

5. Ophthalmology procedures are typically noninvasive.

_____

_____

6. A trabeculectomy is a procedure to treat cataracts.

_____

_____

7. Eyelid modifiers should be used on diagnosis codes to identify the laterality of the eyelid.

_____

_____

8. Congenital eye conditions are present at birth.

_____

_____

Instructions: Choose the best answer.

1. Which of the following types of insurance would pay for an optometrist to perform a routine eye examination?

  a. Healthcare insurance

  b. Vision insurance

  c. Dental insurance

  d. Insurance will not pay for this service

2. Which of the following is a good example of a lifestyle impairment that would prove medical necessity for an ophthalmological service?

  a. Inability to get a job due to poor life management skills

  b. Patient must lose weight to function better

  c. Restriction of peripheral vision

  d. The statement of the diagnosis

3. Which of the following is included as a component of the ocular adnexa?

  a. Cornea

  b. Anterior chamber

  c. Vitreous

  d. Conjunctiva

4. If an optometrist performed an examination of the ophthalmological system for presbyopia, which of the following E/M codes might she report?

  a. 99213

  b. 92002

  c. 99214

  d. 92015

5. Which of the following would be an appropriate code for the fitting of a contact lens for a corneal abrasion injury?

  a. 92071

  b. 92310

  c. 92072

  d. 92311

6. LASIK is one type of which type of surgery?

  a. Phacoemulsification

  b. Cataract surgery

  c. Refractive surgery

  d. Goniotomy

7. If a patient has two types of glaucoma, one in each eye, how should it be reported?

  a. With one code to identify both of the conditions

  b. With a bilateral code

  c. With one code for each condition to identify them individually

  d. With two codes for the same type of glaucoma, with a right and left modifier

8. Which of the following conditions is a buildup of intraocular pressure?

  a. Cataracts

  b. Macular degeneration

  c. Retinal detachment

  d. Glaucoma

Instructions: Answer the following questions with the appropriate code(s).

1. 30-year-old female patient presented to the office with a central corneal ulcer of the right eye. Level 4 E/M performed for this new patient, with fitting of contact lens. Gas permeable scleral contact lens provided to the patient in office.

   CPT code(s): _____

   ICD-10-CM code(s): _____

2. Evisceration of left eye with implant due to malignant neoplasm of left eye.

   CPT code(s): _____

   ICD-10-CM code(s): _____

3. 67-year-old male presents for routine eye examination, intermediate ophthalmological E/M encounter performed with no new treatment plan established. Patient's history is relevant for cataract surgery two years ago, and he has an intraocular lens in the left eye. He also has presbyopia and irregular astigmatism.

   CPT code(s): _____

   ICD-10-CM code(s): _____

References

American Academy of Ophthalmology. 2017 (October 4). Cataract. http://eyewiki.org/Cataract.

Centers for Medicare and Medicaid Services. 2018. ICD-10-CM Official Guidelines for Coding and Reporting FY 2018. https://www.cms.gov/Medicare/Coding/ICD10/Downloads/2018-ICD-10-CM-Coding-Guidelines.pdf.

International Glaucoma Association. 2017. https://www.glaucoma-association.com/about-glaucoma/treatments/surgery/trabeculectomy.

John's Hopkins University. n.d. Cataracts FAQ. http://www.hopkinsmedicine.org/wilmer/conditions/cataracts_faq.html.

US Air Force, Seltmann, D. "Luke AFB eye exam.jpg." Digital Image. Wikimedia Commons. April, 2012. Accessed December 2017. https://commons.wikimedia.org/wiki/Category:Slit_lamp#/media/File:Luke_AFB_eye_exam.jpg.

Resources

American Academy of Ophthalmology. 2017 (October 30). Enucleation. http://eyewiki.org/Enucleation.

American Medical Association. 2013. *Advanced Anatomy and Physiology for ICD-10-CM/PCS.* Salt Lake City, UT: Contexo Media.

Asbell, R.L. 2004 (February 1). Coding for corneal surgery requires distinction between cosmetic and functional. *Ocular Surgery News U.S. Edition.* http://www.healio.com/ophthalmology/news/print/ocular-surgery-news/%7B17138fd4-b050-4108-a2b5-5639286885ac%7D/coding-for-corneal-surgery-requires-distinction-between-cosmetic-and-functional.

Blue Cross Blue Shield of Rhode Island. 2013 (September 5). Payment Policy | Ophthalmology Examinations and Refractions: Correct Coding and Benefits Adjudication. https://www.bcbsri.com/sites/default/files/polices/Opthalmology_Examinations.pdf.

Cibis, G.W. 2017 (March 13). Primary Congenital Glaucoma Treatment & Management. https://emedicine.medscape.com/article/1206081-treatment#d9.

Centers for Medicare and Medicaid Services. 2017 (January). Medicare Vision Services. https://www.cms.gov/Outreach-and-Education/Medicare-Learning-Network-MLN/MLNProducts/downloads/VisionServices_FactSheet_ICN907165.pdf.

The Coding Institute. 2017 (February). Use Expert Examples to Avoid These Common Eye Coding Errors. *Ophthalmology and Optometry Coding Alert* 20(2): 9–16. https://codinginstitute-upload.s3.amazonaws.com/product_images/afc0ba_opc.jpg.

Vijaya, L., P. Manish, G. Ronnie, and B. Shantha. 2011 (January). Management of Complications in Glaucoma Surgery. *Indian Journal of Ophthalmology* 59(Suppl1): S131–S140. https://www.ncbi.nlm.nih.gov/pmc/articles/PMC3038515/.

CHAPTER 10

Urgent Care and Emergency Department Services

Learning Objectives

- Understand the basics of billing and coding in urgent care and emergency department services.
- Examine procedural codes and guidelines for urgent care and emergency department services.

- Examine diagnosis coding and medical necessity for urgent care and emergency department services.
- Determine and apply ICD-10-CM, CPT, and HCPCS codes to urgent care and emergency department services.

Key Terms

Appendicitis
Burn codes
Cardiopulmonary resuscitation (CPR)
Closed procedure
Corrosion codes
Dislocation reduction
Emergency services
Emergent
Endotracheal intubation
Foreign body (FB)
Hemothorax

Incision and drainage (I&D)
Lumbar puncture
Lund-Browder classification
Moderate (conscious) sedation
Motor vehicle accident (MVA)
Myocardial infarction
Nasal packing
Open procedure
Oximetry
Penetrating wound
Pleural effusion
Pneumothorax

Professional component
Rule of nines
Sepsis
Septic shock
Systemic inflammatory response syndrome (SIRS)
Technical component
Thoracostomy
Tracheostomy
Tracheotomy
Urgent care

Urgent care and emergency department services are provided on an as-needed basis to patients with urgent and emergent (life-threatening) medical issues. Although they sound similar, urgent care and emergency department services should not be confused, as they each provide a different level of service to patients depending on their health-care needs.

This chapter discusses the basics of coding for both urgent care and emergency department services, which include a wide range of procedure and diagnosis codes. It also discusses the differences between the two healthcare settings—including services provided, E/M codes used, and the types of healthcare providers that practice in each setting. Coding for urgent care and emergency department services requires the ability to differentiate between signs and symptoms versus a definitive diagnosis, the ability to effectively utilize many portions of both the CPT and ICD-10-CM code books, and an understanding of the difference between urgent and emergent services and conditions.

Urgent Care and Emergency Department Basics

Coding for urgent care and emergency department (ED) services requires a solid understanding of both the CPT and ICD-10-CM code books; and how to read, interpret, and apply the coding guidelines, while keeping in mind the billing and coding differences between the two settings. It also entails an understanding of how the billing details of the facility may impact coding for services performed in each setting, respectively. Although both types of facilities treat patients who have immediate medical needs, the level of urgency differs between the two settings. Furthermore, because of the differences in the available resources and urgency of the healthcare services, pricing structure and reimbursement also differ greatly.

Please note that some EDs may report ICD-10-PCS codes, depending on how the facility is organized. This chapter only discusses ICD-10-CM, CPT, and HCPCS codes in the setting of the ED or urgent care clinic.

Urgent Care Services

Urgent care services are provided to patients who need healthcare for non–life-threatening situations, illnesses, or injuries. Most urgent care practices are open after-hours and on weekends, and have on-site x-ray and laboratory access.

Urgent care services are provided to patients who need services urgently—but the patient is not in danger of losing life or limb—such as when a patient's regular doctor is not available and he or she cannot wait for an appointment. For example, a pediatric patient rapidly develops a fever and rash on a Friday evening, but the child's regular doctor's office is closed for the weekend. The parent of the child can take him to an urgent care clinic for an examination, any necessary lab tests, and a medication prescription.

Urgent care clinics take patients on a walk-in basis, without scheduling an appointment beforehand. Though the patient has the benefit seeing a healthcare provider without an appointment, it also means that patients are generally seen on a first-come, first-seen basis, and he or she may need to wait a long time. Urgent care centers are typically non-hospital based, and open seven days a week for usually 13 or more hours each day, which means that healthcare services are almost always available.

Because urgent care clinics are not primary care practices and only provide care to patients on an as-needed basis, claims for urgent care services must be submitted with a specific place-of-service (POS) code (refer to chapter 7 for a refresher on place of service codes). Urgent care centers are designated as outpatient offices, but are not considered primary care offices, as their purpose is to treat outpatients seeking immediate healthcare. So when billing for services provided at an urgent care clinic, it is necessary to use place-of-service code 20, Urgent Care Facility, on the CMS-1500 form when sending claims to third-party payers. According to the CPT code book, POS code 20 should be used for any "location, distinct from a hospital emergency room, an office, or a clinic, whose purpose is to diagnose and treat illness or injury for unscheduled, ambulatory patients seeking immediate medical attention" (AMA 2017). The POS code is listed in box 24.B of the CMS-1500 claim form (see figure 10.1).

Figure 10.1. CMS-1500 box 24.B: Place-of-service code 20-Urgent Care Facility

24. A.	DATE(S) OF SERVICE					B. PLACE OF SERVICE	C. EMG
	From			To			
MM	DD	YY	MM	DD	YY		
						20	

Source: CMS 2017.

Because the basic structure of the clinic is an outpatient facility that provides healthcare encounters at a level of care lower than an emergency room (for instance, operations and complex medical procedures are not possible at urgent care centers), then it is necessary to use outpatient office E/M codes when billing for urgent care encounters. Coders should report codes 99201 through 99215 (Office or Other Outpatient Services) for E/M encounters provided to patients in the urgent care setting.

Emergency Department Services

Emergency services are provided to patients in a life-threatening situation, when loss of life or limb is imminent. These patients are in immediate need of an x-ray, surgical procedure, or interventional procedure for trauma or other life-threatening situations. An example of an emergency is a patient with a severe laceration of the arm from a chainsaw injury who is at risk of losing either his life or his limb (see figure 10.2).

Figure 10.2. Urgent versus emergent

Urgent <————> Emergent

Services needed urgently   Loss of life or limb is imminent

Emergency services are provided in a designated emergency department (ED) or emergency room (ER), which is a hospital-based facility, open 24 hours a day. Like urgent care clinics, patients do not need an appointment to be seen at an emergency department, but patients are not seen on a first-come, first-seen basis. Emergency department services are allocated so that patients with the most severe injuries or illnesses are seen before patients with less severe or life-threatening situations. For example, if a patient with a high fever signs into the ED before the patient with the arm laceration, the ED will take the arm laceration patient for treatment before the patient with the fever. This arm injury is more life-threatening than the fever. This may result in patients waiting much longer for treatment at an emergency department than they would at an urgent care clinic, depending on the reason for the visit.

Billing and coding for ED services requires an understanding of the different POS and E/M codes used to bill for services performed there. There is also a separate box on the CMS-1500 form to identify emergent services.

Place of Service and Fees for Emergency Department Services

Emergency departments are a designated portion of a hospital that is open to patients 24 hours a day and used to diagnose and treat illnesses, injuries, and other life-threatening conditions. As a designated space apart from the hospital, it has its own POS code. When billing for services that were performed in the ED, it is necessary to use POS code 23, Emergency Room-Hospital, as the place of service. POS code 23 should be use for "a portion of a hospital where emergency diagnosis and treatment of illness or injury is provided" (AMA 2017). The POS code is listed in box 24.B of the CMS-1500 claim form (see figure 10.3).

Figure 10.3. CMS-1500 box 24.B: Place-of-service code 23-Emergency Room-Hospital

24. A. DATE(S) OF SERVICE						B. PLACE OF SERVICE	C. EMG
From			To				
MM	DD	YY	MM	DD	YY		
						23	

Source: CMS 2017.

Because of the additional available resources in the emergency department setting, ED services have their own section of E/M codes listed in the CPT code book—99281 through 99288. These codes should be used rather than outpatient E/M codes when E/M encounters are performed in the ED setting.

Key to Success

When coding for services, the POS code must match the service that was performed. For example, if you report an emergency department E/M code, but the POS code does not indicate that the place of service was the emergency department, then the insurance company will not pay for the claim. POS codes are easy to overlook, but they are a fundamental component of coding for services.

Box 24.C, Emergency

On the CMS-1500 claim form, there is an additional area that must be completed when coding for emergency services. Box 24.C, Emergency, should be filled out with a "Y" to identify that the service was provided on an emergent basis (see figure 10.4). If the service is not an emergency, then the box can be left blank.

This is an important designation to make, as emergency services are usually excluded from prior authorization requirements for medical procedures. For example, if a patient emergently presented to the ER with a severe head injury and a CT scan was performed to rule out a subdural hematoma, then this service should be indicated as an emergency in box 24.C of the CMS-1500 claim form. On the other hand, if a patient

Figure 10.4. CMS-1500 box 24.C: Emergency

Source: CMS 2017.

came into the outpatient office with a severe headache and the doctor wanted to order a CT scan, then a prior authorization or quality review would likely be needed before the service would be authorized by the insurance, because the headache is not an emergency. This is yet another example of the close connection between the intricacies of healthcare coding and billing for reimbursement.

The procedures performed in either the urgent care or ED settings vary, and coders will utilize all areas of the CPT code book and the HCPCS code book, including E/M services, labs, some surgeries, radiological procedures, and medical procedures. ICD-10-CM coding is just as varied; patient conditions range from anxiety attacks to severe traumatic injuries.

Procedural Coding for Urgent Care and ED Services

Urgent care services are provided to patients who need care right away. Emergency services are provided to patients in a life-threatening situation. Because sometimes the line between an urgent situation and a life-threatening situation is difficult to discern, urgent care clinics and emergency departments provide some of the same services.

However, there are some important differences. First, the E/M codes used in either setting are completely different. Urgent care clinics use E/M codes 99201 through 99215, whereas EDs use E/M codes 99281 through 99288. Urgent care services are also less invasive, as surgical procedures performed in the urgent care setting are typically minor. Both urgent care clinics and EDs perform medical evaluations and services, x-rays, and labs, but emergency departments perform more surgically complex procedures that require a specialized level of medical training. This ED must also keep more resources on-hand, such as a sterile operating room, advanced imaging equipment, and the ability to perform more complex laboratory tests.

Procedures Performed in the Urgent Care Setting

Procedures performed in the urgent care setting range from simple evaluation and management encounters to more complex healthcare encounters, which may involve laboratory tests, x-rays or other imaging procedures, and additional medical procedures like breathing treatments or injections. Urgent care clinic resources are more limited than ED resources, and staff are not trained to treat all emergency situations. Therefore, sometimes an urgent care clinic will call for an ambulance to transport a patient to the hospital, although this is rare. Urgent care centers perform E/M encounters as well as additional procedures.

The E/M codes used in the urgent care setting are the same as those used in outpatient facility billing and the primary care setting, as discussed in chapter 8. They range from 99201 to 99215. As a reminder, codes 99201 through 99205 are for new patients, and 99211 through 99215 are for established patients. Urgent care centers may see new or established patients, so it is important to remember how to differentiate the two. Refer to chapter 7 for the basics on how to select a new versus an established patient.

For a review of the key components of E/M codes and how to select the level of E/M code based on the provider documentation, refer to chapter 7 (Behavioral Health Services) and chapter 8 (Primary Care Services) of this text.

Besides healthcare evaluation and management services, urgent care clinics perform countless procedures, all aimed at diagnosis and initial treatment of medical conditions. Most of the procedures performed are either diagnostic or therapeutic. There are also revenue codes that identify the urgent care encounter as a special service and can pay an extra amount for the service.

Diagnostic Procedures

Diagnostic procedures performed in urgent care include lab tests and blood analysis, x-rays, oximetry, and electrocardiograms (ECGs). These tests are designed to evaluate the severity of the patient's condition or to determine the patient's definitive diagnosis.

Laboratory Tests

Laboratory tests are designed to determine patient diagnosis, mostly for infectious diseases such as strep throat, influenza, bacterial and fungal infections, and sexually transmitted infections (gonorrhea, chlamydia, herpes). Common blood tests performed are complete blood counts (CBC), lipid panels, basic metabolic panels (BMET) and comprehensive metabolic panels (CMP), hepatic function panels, thyroid stimulation hormone tests, and tests for heterophile antibodies. Note that this is not an all-inclusive list of all lab tests performed at urgent care centers. Laboratory procedures are coded from the Laboratory and Pathology section of the CPT code book. To look up a laboratory procedure, it helps to first look under the entry *Pathology and Laboratory* in the Index, and then find the subterm(s) for the substance being tested for, such as angiotensin converting enzymes (ACE). Another way to look up a lab procedure is to search for the type of lab test performed, such as *Blood Cell Count*, and then find the subterm(s) for the type of blood count performed.

X-rays and Imaging Procedures

X-rays and imaging procedures are found in the Radiology section of the CPT code book. When coding for x-rays, go to *X-ray* in the Index, and search for the subterm that identifies the body area being studied in the x-ray. For example, a patient coming into the urgent care clinic with a wrist injury would likely receive an x-ray of the wrist to rule out a fracture. To look up this x-ray, go to *X-ray* in the Index, and find the subterm *wrist*. This leads you to code range 73100 to 73110. Now, go to that range of codes in the Radiology section of the CPT code book. There are two wrist x-ray codes available (note that code 73115, Radiological examination, wrist, arthrography, radiological supervision and interpretation, is an arthrography code, which uses contrast material into the joint to diagnosis joint problems).

- 73100, Radiologic examination, wrist; *2 views*
- 73110, Radiologic examination, wrist; *complete, minimum of 3 views*

The two codes for x-ray of the wrist differ based on the number of views. The number of views is the number of images taken at different angles during the x-ray. For example, the x-ray technician may take two views—one anterior view x-ray of the wrist and one lateral view x-ray of the wrist. X-ray CPT codes differ based on the number of views taken during the x-ray. If the x-ray code is described as *complete*, then it will identify the minimum number of views required for a complete x-ray. Anything over that amount of views is included within that code. For example, if the x-ray tech took four views of the wrist, then the code selected would be 73110, Radiologic examination, wrist; *complete, minimum of 3 views.*

Oximetry

Oximetry is a noninvasive test that measures a patient's oxygen saturation level. A sensor is placed over a portion of the body with thin skin with vascular structures underneath such as the fingertip, earlobe, or, in the case of infants, foot. This procedure is performed to determine if the patient is in any type of respiratory distress, by identifying if the level of oxygen in the blood is decreased. Normal pulse oximetry levels are between 95 and 100, and anything under 92 to 90 is considered low (Hackethal 2017). If the has a low blood oxygen level, then a breathing treatment or additional interventions may be started, depending on how low the reading is. The codes for oximetry differ, depending on the number of readings taken.

- 94760, Noninvasive ear or pulse oximetry for oxygen saturation; *single determination*
- 94761, Noninvasive ear or pulse oximetry for oxygen saturation; *multiple determinations (e.g., during exercise)*
- 94762, Noninvasive ear or pulse oximetry for oxygen saturation; *by continuous overnight monitoring (separate procedure)*

Electrocardiogram (ECG or EKG).

As discussed in chapter 8 (Primary Care) an electrocardiogram measures the electrical impulses of the heart and can be used to identify arrhythmias and other heart issues. Codes for ECGs are 93000 to 93042, and differ depending on the type of ECG taken and the work involved in the test. The most common codes are the following:

- 93000, Electrocardiogram, routine ECG with at least 12 leads; *with interpretation and report*
- 93005, Electrocardiogram, routine ECG with at least 12 leads; *tracing only, without interpretation and report*
- 93010, Electrocardiogram, routine ECG with at least 12 leads; *interpretation and report only*

Note that the codes differ based on interpretation and report, and tracing. There are two components to an ECG: the work involved in taking the test (that includes placing the leads and performing the test), and the interpretation of test results and written report of the findings. Tracing is the work involved in taking the test, also called the **technical component** of the test. The interpretation and report are the **professional components** of the test that consists of the healthcare provider interpreting the results from the test, determining a diagnosis or next steps in treatment or diagnosis, and providing a written report of his or her findings. Because most urgent care centers own the testing equipment and perform the test (technical component), and employ the healthcare provider who reads and interprets the report (professional component), urgent care centers typically bill for the codes that include both of these components (93000, Electrocardiogram, routine ECG with at least 12 leads; *with interpretation and report*). If the facility performs only one portion of the service (technical or professional), then they would bill *only* for the service performed.

Therapeutic Procedures

Therapeutic procedures are performed to treat either a confirmed diagnosis or a patient's signs or symptoms in the urgent care clinic. Most of the time, treatments are minimal or initial enough to ensure that the patient is not in any immediate medical danger. The patient is then referred to his or her primary care physician or healthcare specialist for follow-up and definitive treatment, and in rare cases the patient may be advised to go to the hospital via ambulance. These therapeutic procedures include injections, vaccinations, breathing treatments, injury treatments, and wound repair.

Injections

Injections are given to treat medical conditions therapeutically with a medicinal substance. Injections should not be confused with vaccinations, and are *not* coded with vaccination administration codes. Rather, use code 96372, Therapeutic, prophylactic, or diagnostic injection (specify substance or drug); subcutaneous or intramuscular. The substance injected should be identified with an HCPCS code. For example, if a patient with a severe bacterial infection presents to the urgent care clinic, the healthcare provider may choose to inject an antibiotic in the office rather than wait for a prescription to be filled and oral antibiotics taken. This would be coded with 96372, and the HCPCS code for the antibacterial substance injected into the patient (such as J0696, Injection, ceftriaxone sodium, per 250 mg).

Vaccinations

Vaccinations are also given in the urgent care setting, such as a tetanus vaccine administered to a patient with an injury from a rusty nail, or the seasonal flu vaccine. Refer to chapter 8 (Primary Care) for the basics of vaccine coding. The only difference between coding for vaccines in the urgent care setting rather than the primary care setting would be the change of the POS code, to identify the place of service when the vaccination was administered.

Breathing Treatments

Breathing treatments are given to patients in respiratory distress or if they have a low blood oxygen level due to an asthma exacerbation, respiratory infection, or other respiratory condition like pneumonia or chronic obstructive pulmonary disease (COPD). Breathing treatments use pressurized air mixed with a steroid solution that is inhaled by the patient. This procedure helps open airway passages to allow the patient to breathe more easily. To find the codes for breathing treatments, search in the Index under the term *Inhalation Treatment*, and select the subterm for the type of breathing treatment administered.

Treatment for Injuries

Injury treatments provided in the urgent care setting depend on the type of injury suffered by the patient. Urgent care centers are not trained nor equipped to operate on patients, perform casting procedures, or repair complex injuries (these would be performed in the emergency department setting). Furthermore, urgent care centers do not have healthcare providers that are trained in all medical procedures, such as setting fractures or reducing dislocations. Because of these limitations, most of the injury treatments performed are aimed at stabilizing the injury and reducing pain or discomfort, so that the patient may receive more definitive treatment from his or her PCP or a specialty provider. For example, an injury treatment for a fracture would include the application of a temporary splint to immobilize the fracture until the patient could be seen by an orthopedist (bone doctor). Any splint, brace, or other immobilizing device would be reported with the appropriate HCPCS codes to identify the device, and the application or provision of the device would be included in the E/M code for the visit. An immobilizing device is called an orthotic device, otherwise known as an orthosis, an externally applied device designed for a particular body area to protect and support injuries, reduce pain, and assist in the healing process (discussed in chapter 6). To look up orthotic devices in the HCPCS code book, search under the term *Orthotic additions*, or by the body area (wrist, ankle, hand).

If more than one injury is treated, then the one procedure that required the most work is reported first, with less work-intensive procedures listed after the more work-intensive procedures. This should also correspond with the injury diagnosis codes, as they should also be listed before the codes for less severe injuries (this is discussed in greater depth in the following diagnosis coding section).

Wound Repair

Wound repair codes (12001 to 13160) are found in the Integumentary section of the CPT code book. Complex, penetrating, or otherwise life-threatening wounds would be seen in the emergency setting. Wounds treated in urgent care consist of lacerations, cuts, abrasions, and superficial injuries; and wound repair would consist primarily of repairs of the skin such as suturing, stapling, or cleaning and bandaging wounds on the skin. Would repair codes are divided into three types—simple, intermediate, and complex repairs, and code selection depends on the site and size of the wound. If the wound is repaired using adhesive strips as the only repair material, then the wound repair is included in the E/M code and not coded separately.

- Simple wound closure codes (12001 to 12021) are used when the wound is superficial or involves subcutaneous tissues but does not involve any deeper structures. This type of repair requires only one layer of closure.

- Intermediate wound repair codes (12031 to 12057) are used for wounds that require layered closure of one or more of the deeper layers of subcutaneous tissue and superficial fascia, in addition to closure of the skin (see figure 10.5). Closure of wounds that are heavy in particulate matter or otherwise require extensive cleaning are also categorized as intermediate.

- Complex wound repair codes (13100 to 13153) are used for wounds that require more than layered closure, such as scar revision, debridement due to traumatic lacerations or avulsions, extensive undermining, stents, or retention sutures. Because of the complex nature of this type of repair, it is less commonly performed at urgent care centers than the two former types of wound repair.

Figure 10.5. Intermediate wound repair (layered skin closure)

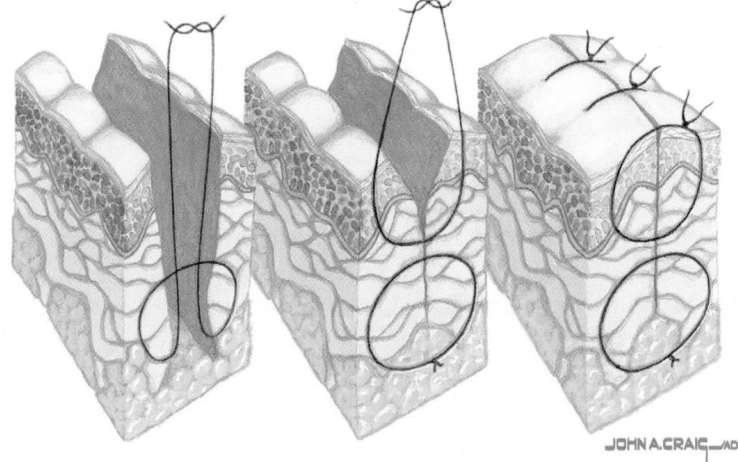

JOHN A. CRAIG—AD

When coding wound repair, pay attention to three important components of wound repair codes:

1. *The site of the wound repair.* Each wound repair code identifies a group of anatomical regions, all of which may be included in the same repair code. For example, code 13120, Repair, complex, scalp, arms, and/or legs; 1.1 cm to 2.5 cm, groups repairs of the skin on scalp, arms, or legs.

2. *The size (in centimeters) of the repair.* Each wound repair code identifies the total size of the repair, for that specific anatomical site. For example, code 13120, Repair, complex, scalp, arms, and/or legs; 1.1 cm to 2.5 cm identifies a total repair of 1.1 to 2.5 centimeters total for those specific body areas.

3. *The complexity of the repair.* Each repair code identifies the complexity of the repair procedure, in terms of simple, intermediate, or complex. For example, code 13120, Repair, complex, scalp, arms, and/or legs; 1.1 cm to 2.5 cm identifies a complex repair of the skin on the specified anatomical sites.

Combine the lengths of the wounds from each body site by complexity. For example, if there is a 1.0 cm simple repair of the right cheek, a 0.5 cm simple repair of the left cheek, and a 0.75 cm repair of the forehead, then these repairs would be added together—because they are the same complexity (simple) and the same body site: (face)—to total a simple repair of the face of 2.25 cm. The code selected in this example would be 12011, Simple repair of superficial wounds of face, ears, eyelids, nose, lips and/or mucous membranes; 2.5 cm or less. The coder should add the lengths of wound in the same complexity and the same body area (see figure 10.6).

Figure 10.6. Wound repair

Wounds of different complexities or body area should be coded separately. For example, if the wound repair was a 1.0 cm simple repair of the right cheek and a 0.75 cm intermediate repair of the left cheek, then the two codes selected would be 12011, Simple repair of superficial wounds of face, ears, eyelids, nose, lips and/or mucous membranes; 2.5 cm or less, and 12051, Repair, intermediate, wounds of face, ears, eyelids, nose, lips and/or mucous membranes; 2.5 cm or less.

Just as in coding for injury treatments, sequence the more complex wound repair code followed by the least complex wound repair code(s).

Note that according to CPT guidelines, when more than one classification of wounds is repaired (in terms of anatomical site, size, and complexity), then the most complicated repair should be listed first, followed by the least complicated repairs. Additional repair codes should be appended with modifier -59, Distinct procedural service, to identify that the repair procedures were distinct from each other. If any nerves, blood vessels, or tendons were repaired as part of a complex repair service, then these procedures should be coded separately and appended with modifier -59 to indicate that these procedures were distinct from the primary service.

MOD

Key to Success

All wound repair codes are reported in centimeters. The conversion factor from inches to centimeters is 1 inch to 2.54 centimeters. So if the documentation reads 1 inch, then this should be converted to 2.54 centimeters. To perform the conversion, multiply the number of inches by 2.54, and the result is the number of centimeters. For example, if the wound repair was 1.5 inches, then multiply the number of inches (1.5) by 2.54, and the result is the number of centimeters, or 3.81 centimeters.

Additional Urgent Care Codes

There are additional codes that can be added to certain services provided in the urgent care setting to increase the amount of revenue for that service. The revenue codes used in urgent care are as follows.

- S9088, Services provided in an urgent care center. This code should be added to all services provided at the urgent care center, except for Medicaid and Medicare (that do not accept the code). This code allows urgent care clinics to get an extra amount of revenue to help offset the extra expenses of providing urgent care services.

- 99051, Service(s) provided in the office during regularly scheduled evening, weekend, or holiday office hours, in addition to basic service. This code should only be used for services that are provided during evening hours (typically after 5 p.m.), on the weekend (Saturday or Sunday), or on a holiday, regularly scheduled by the urgent care clinic. This code should be added to the basic service provided, but only for those services that occur at the off-times as indicated by the code description. Like the previous code, it is designed to obtain additional revenue to offset costs by regularly staying open during off-hours.

- S9083, Global fee urgent care centers, should only be used when there is a specific agreement between the urgent care center and the insurance company. To see if this fee is necessary, the healthcare practice would have to verify by calling the insurance company to see if it is required. This is a global fee, and if using this code, then the urgent care does not charge for any specific services provided during the patient encounter; rather, they are reimbursed a set fee for the global urgent care charge.

The procedures performed in the urgent care setting are less invasive, less costly, and less dangerous. However, procedures performed in the ED setting are by nature more invasive, more costly, and more dangerous due to the life-threatening nature of the patient's medical condition. For practice assigning procedure codes for urgent care services, complete the exercises in There's a Code for That 10.1.

Urgent care procedures

There's a Code for That

Read the following documentation and select the appropriate procedure and/or E/M codes.

1. 8-year-old female new patient seen after having sustained a wrist injury from a fall on the playground at school. She appears in acute distress. Complete x-ray of the wrist confirms Colles' fracture of the left wrist. Wrist was immobilized using compression bandages and referral was given for patient to see ortho next week. Expended problem-focused history and examination, with moderate medical decision making (MDM).

   CPT code (E/M service): _____

   CPT code (x-ray): _____

   CPT code (revenue code): _____

2. 12-year-old established Medicaid patient seen for fever and sore throat during evening hours. Mother reports that the entire family has been sick for the last week, and now her daughter has reported feeling ill. Streptococcal (group A) swab performed in the office is negative. CBC (automated with automated WBC count) shows low WBC count. Prescribed amoxicillin and follow up with PCP if not improved within a week. Detailed history and examination with moderate complexity MDM.

   CPT code (E/M service): _____

   CPT code (labs): _____, _____

   CPT code (revenue code): _____

3. Patient seen for multiple wound repairs after having walked through a plate glass window. Following wounds were repaired: simple repair of 7 cm laceration on right upper thigh, 3 cm laceration of right hip, and 2 cm on abdomen. Intermediate double layer repair done on a 3 cm laceration of the right forearm, 2 cm laceration on right shoulder, and 2.75 cm laceration on forehead. (Remember, when sequencing codes for injuries, sequence the repair for the worst injury first, followed by the least complex repairs.)

   CPT codes: _____, _____ - _____,

   _____ - _____

   CPT code (revenue code): _____

4. 25-year-old sexually active established male patient presents during weekend hours, suspecting that he has a UTI. Gonorrhea immunoassay tests positive. Azithromycin prescribed. Detailed history performed with moderate complexity MDM.

   CPT codes: _____, _____

   CPT code (revenue codes): _____, _____

Procedures Performed in the ED Setting

Procedures performed in the emergency department setting are by nature more complex and risky, due to the life-threatening medical conditions of the patients. However, some patients who present to the ED for treatment are not experiencing true life- or limb-threatening situations. These patients will still be treated, but their services will be more similar to those performed in an urgent care setting. Note that one difference between urgent care and ED procedures is in the treatment of fractures. Where an urgent care center may provide a temporary cast and refer to an orthopedist for definitive treatment, an ED may provide the definitive treatment for the fracture. Fracture diagnosis and treatment is discussed in detail in two later chapters in this text—chapter 13 (Radiology) and chapter 15 (Orthopedics).

Evaluation and management encounters in the ED setting are assigned to a special code range of E/M services: emergency department services (99281 to 99288). Additional procedures performed in the ED include life-saving surgical procedures and other less invasive procedures.

E/M Encounters in the Emergency Department

Emergency department E/M encounters are coded from the Emergency Department Services section of the CPT code book, with codes 99281 through 99288. While there are many similarities between these codes and outpatient office E/M codes, there are a couple of notable differences.

First, all of the key components of the E/M service are the same—history, examination, and medical decision making; the levels and elements of each key component; and the nature of the presenting problem included in the code description. However, the component of time is *not* a consideration in emergency department E/M coding. Because of the variable intensity of the nature of ED services, and that most providers see many patients at multiple times throughout their services, it is difficult to determine the total time spent on any emergency department service, so it is not included in the code descriptions.

Key to Success

Time is a factor in many E/M codes, including outpatient office and inpatient evaluation and management services. However, time is *not* a component of code selection for E/M services rendered in the emergency department setting. Coders should not use time as a deciding factor for the level of emergency department E/M service and instead rely on the complexity of the service performed.

There is also no differentiation between new or established patients in the ED setting as there is no additional classification of codes for new patients versus established patients. When coding for emergency department E/M services, coders should rely on the documentation of the level of history, examination, and medical decision making, while considering the nature of the presenting problem. Note that these E/M codes require all three key components to match the level described in the code description in order to select the code.

Surgical Procedures

Surgical procedures performed in the emergency department are performed either to treat the patient's illness or injury (such as the reduction of a dislocated shoulder or incision and drainage of an abscess), to help diagnose the patient (for example, a lumbar puncture), or to help stabilize the patient before he or she is taken to the operating room or is admitted to the hospital for another procedure (such as endotracheal intubation, or chest tube placement). An inherent component of many of these procedures is conscious sedation, administered by the ED provider to help reduce the sensation of pain during the procedure. Additional procedures performed in the ED setting include foreign body removals and penetrating wound explorations.

Emergency Intubation and Tracheostomy

An emergency intubation is performed to open the airway to prevent asphyxiation. There are two types of intubations—endotracheal and tracheostomy.

An **endotracheal intubation** (also called intubation) is performed to maintain an open airway, or to allow the administration of certain drugs, such as anesthesia. On critically ill patients, an emergent intubation is performed to help ventilate the lungs and prevent asphyxiation and airway obstruction. The procedure is performed by carefully inserting a laryngoscope through the mouth and into the larynx to help view the procedure, and the endotracheal tube is placed directly in the trachea. The laryngoscope is then removed and the endotracheal tube is left in place (see figure 10.7).

Figure 10.7. Endotracheal intubation

To code for an emergency endotracheal intubation, report code 31500, Intubation, endotracheal, emergency procedure.

An emergency tracheostomy is performed for the same reasons as an emergency endotracheal intubation—to open the airway to prevent asphyxiation or to allow ventilation of the lungs. However, this procedure is performed when the mouth or upper airway is either compromised due to trauma or obstruction of the upper airway. In this procedure, a **tracheotomy** is performed, which cuts through the trachea to allow for the insertion of a tracheostomy tube, or trach tube (Ahmadinejad 2011). The trach tube is then left in place to allow for ventilation (see figure 10.8). The **tracheostomy** is the connection that is established by the insertion of the tube.

Figure 10.8. Tracheostomy

Key to Success

Note the differences at the end of the words trache*otomy* and trache*ostomy*. A tracheotomy procedure is an incision that allows access into the body cavity, whereas a tracheostomy is a connection established after the tube is inserted (as it connects the inside of the body cavity to the outside for drainage). Understanding the differences between these two suffixes (*-otomy* and *-ostomy*) is imperative in understanding the procedure performed and, in some instances, which code to report for the procedure performed. *-Otomy* means to make an incision, and *-ostomy* means to make an opening from inside the body cavity to the outside.

There are two emergency tracheostomy codes that depend on the type of incision used to perform the procedure. A transtracheal incision cuts horizontally through the tracheal cartilage, while the cricothyroid membrane incision cuts though vertically through the cricothyroid membrane at the upper end of the trachea.

The codes for tracheostomy are: 31603, Tracheostomy, emergency procedure; transtracheal, and 31605, Tracheostomy, emergency procedure; cricothyroid membrane. Note that these are both identified as emergency procedures. Tracheostomies are also performed in nonemergent situations, when patients require long-term ventilation. For example, patients with severe brain injuries often need ventilation through a tracheostomy tube due to the presence of a large amount of secretions in the lungs and the inadequacy of natural breathing (Ahmadinegad 2011). When a tracheostomy is planned, the coder should report 31600, Tracheostomy, planned, or 31601, Tracheostomy, younger than 2 years.

Moderate (Conscious) Sedation

Moderate (conscious) sedation is used during ED procedures to anesthetize patients during a medical or surgical procedure. Moderate sedation is a drug-induced depression of consciousness that still allows the patient to respond to commands and tactile stimulation. During moderate sedation, no additional interventions are required to maintain cardiovascular or respiratory function.

Moderate sedation codes (99151 through 99157) are based on the provider who performed the service, age of the patient, and time spent under sedation. There are three components of moderate sedation:

- *Preservice work.* This includes assessment of the patient's history including experiences with sedation, drug allergies, a physical examination, a pre-sedation assessment, informed consent, and initial IV access and the administration of fluids (among other components).
- *Intraservice work.* This begins with the administration of the sedating agent(s) and ends when the procedure is complete and the administering physician ends personal face-to-face time with the patient. Intraservice work requires continuous face-to-face attendance of the physician and monitoring of the patient's response to the sedating agent.
- *Postservice work.* This component includes any additional face-to-face time, after the continuous face-to-face time during the procedure has ended. Such as monitoring the patient until he or she can safely be transferred from the anesthesia or treatment area and readied for discharge. It is not included in the intraservice work time.

To select the correct code for a moderate sedation procedure, it is necessary to identify the intraservice work time involved in the procedure, as the code selection is based on the intraservice time only. Although the preservice and postservice work is included within the service, it is not reported nor calculated into the moderate sedation time, as it is considered integral to the moderate sedation procedure. For example, if the total sedation time was 1 hour with 15 minutes of preservice work, 15 minutes of intraservice work, and 30 minutes of postservice work, then the coder should report 99152, Moderate sedation services provided by the same physician or other qualified health care professional performing the diagnostic or therapeutic service that the sedation supports, requiring the presence of an independent trained observer to assist in the monitoring of the patient's level of consciousness and physiological status; initial 15 minutes of intraservice time, patient age 5 years or older. Code 99152 reports 15 minutes of the intraservice work, which is the only item reported, even though the entire procedure took 1 hour.

Additional time over 15 minutes is reported with the appropriate add-on code to identify additional intraservice time in 15-minute increments. For example, if the intraservice work during the sedation required 45 minutes of time, then the codes reported would be 99152 (for the first 15 minutes), and 99153, Moderate sedation services provided by the same physician or other qualified health care professional performing the diagnostic or therapeutic service that the sedation supports, requiring the presence of an independent trained observer to assist in the monitoring of the patient's level of consciousness and physiological status; one for each additional 15 minutes of intraservice time (× 2 for the additional 30 minutes). In this example, if 45 minutes of time was spent on the service, then it would be coded with 99152, 99153, and 99153 (or 99152 and 99153 × 2).

Incision and Drainage

Incision and drainage (I&D) is a procedure performed on an abscess or cyst that requires drainage. It consists of cutting into the skin above the cyst or abscess to allow for drainage of the pustular material. Emergency physicians may need to perform an I&D to drain a postoperative wound or skin infection. Codes selected for the incision and drainage (10040 to 10180) depend on the reason for the procedure including acne surgery, abscess, pilonidal cyst, removal of a foreign body, hematoma, seroma, or other fluid collection, or postoperative wound infection. Codes are further divided based on whether the procedure was simple/single or complicated/multiple. For example, if an emergency physician performed an I&D on a single uncomplicated MRSA cyst on the buttock of a 25-year-old patient, the code reported would be 10060, Incision and drainage of abscess (e.g., carbuncle, suppurative hidradenitis, cutaneous or subcutaneous abscess, cyst, furuncle, or paronychia); simple or single.

Foreign Body Removal

Sometimes related to an incision and drainage are foreign body removals. A **foreign body (FB)** is any unnatural object that is present inside the body or organ structure. Foreign bodies include ingested (for example, a swallowed marble or coin) or inhaled (such as an aspirated pill) materials introduced through trauma (like a bullet from a gunshot wound), or injury (for instance, retained pieces of asphalt from a road rash incident or a splinter), or purposefully inserted into a natural opening (such as a bead in a child's nose).

Accordingly, codes for foreign body removal range from invasive surgery to remove deeply imbedded FBs, to removal of FBs requiring nothing more than forceps or a pair of tweezers. Foreign body removals may be performed on natural body openings such as the ears, nose, eyes, or on the external structure of the body like the skin. More complex foreign body removals may be performed on the internal structures of the body, such as airways or gastrointestinal tract. Code selection depends on the area from which the foreign body was removed, as well as the manner of the removal.

To find the code for a FB removal, search under the term *Removal* in the CPT Index, and then refer to the subterm *Foreign Body* and locate the site of the foreign body and available codes, then verify the code in the Tabular List. Codes listed in the Tabular may differ based on the complexity of the procedure or the technique used to remove the FB. For example, if an ED physician removed a bead from the nose of the patient via lateral rhinotomy (an incision into the side of the nose), then the code reported would be 30320, Removal of foreign body, intranasal; by lateral rhinotomy.

Penetrating Wound Exploration

A **penetrating wound** is one that results from a trauma that pierces the skin and goes into the body's deeper structures, such as a stab or gunshot wound. Due to the life-threatening nature of this type of injury, patients with a penetrating wound are often brought to the ED for evaluation and treatment. This requires exploration of the penetrating wound to evaluate the damage caused by the wound. If severe damage is found, the patient may be transferred to the operating room for emergency surgery. If no significant damage is done, the ED physician may decide to repair the wound in the ED.

There are four codes for wound exploration: 20100, Exploration of penetrating wound (separate procedure); neck, 20101, Exploration of penetrating wound (separate procedure); chest, 20102, Exploration of penetrating wound (separate procedure); abdomen/flank/back, and 20103, Exploration of penetrating wound (separate procedure); extremity, that depend on the area being explored—the neck, chest, abdomen/flank/back, or an extremity. These codes identify the surgical exploration, enlargement, and extension of the wound, debridement, removal of foreign body, and minimal ligation of blood vessels. If a major repair is done, then the wound exploration code is not reported, as this would be included in the code for the major procedure (such as a major blood vessel repair).

Lumbar Puncture

A lumbar puncture, also called a spinal tap, is a diagnostic procedure used to evaluate cerebrospinal fluid that surrounds the brain and spinal cord. Lumbar punctures are performed in the ED setting to diagnose conditions such as meningitis or subarachnoid hemorrhage, both of which can be life-threatening diseases. During the procedure, a needle is inserted into the spinal canal in the lumbar area, and a hollow tube is threaded into the space to obtain a sample of the cerebrospinal fluid (see figure 10.9).

Figure 10.9. Lumbar puncture

Lying Position · Sitting Position

Source: Blausen.com staff 2013.

There is one code for lumbar puncture when it is performed for diagnostic purposes: 62270, Spinal puncture, lumbar, diagnostic.

Needle and Tube Thoracostomy

A thoracostomy is an opening created in the thoracic cavity, otherwise known as a chest tube. It acts as a drain for the thoracic cavity to drain blood, fluid, or air from around the lungs, heart, or esophagus. A thoracostomy can be performed either by a needle or a tube. In a needle thoracostomy, a hollow needle is directly inserted into an intercostal space (between the ribs) to allow for drainage. A tube thoracostomy consists of a trocar being placed between the ribs, through which a hollow tube is inserted into the chest and secured in place to allow for continuous drainage (USNLM 2017). A trocar is a surgical instrument that contains a long, pointed tube through which other instrumentation can be passed. Thoracostomies are performed in the ED to emergently treat patients suffering from **pneumothorax** (collapsed lung), **hemothorax** (blood in the pleural cavity), or **pleural effusion** (fluid buildup in the chest).

Codes for thoracostomies depend on the type of procedure performed (either by needle or tube), and the reason for the procedure.

- 32035, Thoracostomy; *with rib resection for empyema*, and 32036, Thoracostomy; *with open flap drainage for empyema*. These thoracostomies are performed specifically for empyema, a type of pleural effusion.

- 32551, Tube thoracostomy, includes connection to drainage system (e.g., water seal), when performed, open (separate procedure). This code should be reported for any thoracostomy performed as a separate procedure for drainage of the pleural space (besides that done for empyema).

- 32554-32557, Thoracentesis, needle or catheter, aspiration of the pleural space. This range of codes identifies needle aspirations of the pleural cavity, performed with or without imaging guidance.

Additional Procedures

Additional procedures performed in the emergency department are noninvasive in nature and require external manipulation or therapy to an organ or body part. Remember that emergency departments still provide all the services that are also provided by an urgent care clinic including labs, x-rays and imaging services, and treatment of injuries. The next sections discuss ED procedures such as reduction of dislocations, cardiopulmonary resuscitation, and control of nasal hemorrhage.

Dislocation Reduction

Dislocation reduction is the act of relocating a joint to its original location, in the case of joint dislocation or subluxation (partial dislocation). Depending on the joint and the patient, reductions may be performed under moderate sedation. If the joint is unable to be reduced into the socket successfully, then the patient would be admitted to the hospital so that the reduction could be performed surgically.

Codes for dislocation reduction depend on the site of the dislocation or subluxation, and whether the reduction was performed open or closed. An **open procedure** is one in which the skin is incised (or cut into) to perform the procedure. A **closed procedure** is one in which the skin is not opened to perform the procedure. Closed reductions are performed without opening the skin; the healthcare provider manipulates the joint back into place externally. Open reductions are performed surgically, by cutting into the skin and surgically putting the joint back into place.

To search for a dislocation reduction code, search for the term *Dislocation* in the Index, then locate the subterm for the body site of the dislocation, and find the code for either open or closed reduction. Verify the code in the Tabular List.

Cardiopulmonary Resuscitation

Cardiopulmonary resuscitation, otherwise known as CPR, is a medical procedure that involves the healthcare provider repeatedly compressing a patient's chest in an attempt to circulate the blood and restore breathing to a patient who has suffered cardiac arrest (a stopping of the heart).

There is one code for CPR: 92950, Cardiopulmonary resuscitation (e.g., in cardiac arrest).

Control of Nasal Hemorrhage

Nasal packing is performed for uncontrollable hemorrhage from the nose (epistaxis or bloody nose). Nasal packing codes are located in the Respiratory subsection of the CPT code book and depend on the type of packing performed (30901 to 30906). Anterior nasal hemorrhage control consists of either cauterization of the blood vessels, or nasal packing materials (such as cotton balls, gauze, or nasal tampons) that are placed in the front of the nose to control the bleeding. Posterior control is the cautery of blood vessels or the packing of the posterior nasal cavity to control the hemorrhage (see figure 10.10).

Figure 10.10. Control of nasal hemorrhage

For practice assigning procedure codes to emergency department services, complete the exercises in There's a Code for That 10.2.

Emergency department procedures

10.2

There's a Code for That

Read the following documentation and select the appropriate procedure and/or E/M codes.

1. 4-year-old male patient seen in the ED with a FB in his nose. Mother reports that she was cooking breakfast when her son walked up to her with tears in his eyes and pointing to his nose. Small plastic brick toy was visible at the time, when she tried to remove the toy with tweezers the toy became lodged further into the nasal cavity. Toy is now barely visible upon rhinoscopic inspection. Under conscious sedation, foreign body was removed from the nose via lateral rhinotomy without complications. Total intraservice time was 10 minutes. Expanded problem- focused history and examination with moderate complexity MDM.

   CPT code (E/M service): _____ - _____

   CPT code (FB removal): _____

   CPT code (conscious sedation): _____

2. Patient with severe anaphylactic reaction presented to the ER in respiratory distress. Endotracheal intubation performed.

   CPT code (intubation and injection): _____

3. Limited cautery of uncontrollable epistaxis.

   CPT code: _____

4. 45-year-old male presents with multiple stab wounds in upper left shoulder and forearm from a bar fight. Penetrating wound exploration performed with extension of dissection and surgical exploration. No major damage was noted and wounds were repaired. (Note: because there were no major repairs performed, code only for the wound exploration).

   CPT code: _____

5. 7-year-old female presents with severe headache and stiff neck. Mother reports that the symptoms came on suddenly and worsened over the course of the day. CSF obtained through lumbar puncture, tested positive for bacterial meningitis. Comprehensive history and examination with MDM of high complexity.

   CPT code (E/M service): _____ - _____

   CPT code (lumbar puncture): _____

Diagnostic Coding for Urgent Care and ED Services

The diagnosis code selected for the urgent care or emergency department service should identify the medical necessity for the service provided. Because patients may have a wide range of different conditions, signs, symptoms, or diagnoses, it is necessary to employ the entire ICD-10-CM code book while coding.

Key to Success

This section discusses coding for urgent care and emergency department services separately, although these conditions may be seen in either setting depending on the circumstances.

Diagnostic Coding for Urgent Care Services

Coding for urgent care services requires a solid understanding of the differences between signs and symptoms and a definitive diagnosis, and when to code for both, as well as the ability to code for infectious diseases. Injuries are also commonly seen in the urgent care center, the codes for which require detailed analysis of the healthcare documentation to extract all necessary details and select the required external cause codes.

Signs and Symptoms

Often when a patient seeks services at an urgent care clinic it is due to a sudden-onset sign or symptom that happens when the patient's primary care provider is not available. Remember when coding for signs and symptoms, if a definitive diagnosis is determined then do not code for the related signs and symptoms. On the other hand, if a definitive diagnosis cannot be determined, then code only for the signs and symptoms. The only time it is necessary to code for both the signs and symptoms and a definitive diagnosis is when the signs and symptoms are not related.

When a patient presents to the clinic with signs and symptoms, diagnostic testing is usually performed to confirm the diagnosis. For example, if a patient presents with painful urination, and a urinalysis performed confirms a urinary tract infection (UTI), then the patient's definitive diagnosis is a UTI. The confirmed diagnosis of the UTI is the only diagnosis code that is needed to support the medical necessity for the urinalysis procedure, and the painful urination code does not need to be reported.

If a definitive diagnosis has been determined, but additional, *unrelated* signs or symptoms are also present, code for both the definitive diagnosis and the unrelated signs and symptoms. For instance, if a patient is diagnosed with a UTI but also has dizziness unrelated to the UTI diagnosis, then the coder would report the UTI as well as the symptom of dizziness. Refer to figure 10.11 for a flowchart to help decide when it is appropriate to code for the signs and symptoms versus a definitive diagnosis.

Infectious Diseases

Often when a diagnostic test for a sign or symptoms results in a definitive condition, the diagnosis code is for an infectious disease. Infectious diseases are coded from chapter 1: Certain Infectious and Parasitic Diseases, of the ICD-10-CM code book. Other conditions, while due to an infectious disease, may be coded from different chapters of the ICD-10-CM code book, such as respiratory conditions and ear infections.

Common infectious diseases seen in the urgent care setting are also commonly seen in the primary care setting, such as mononucleosis, streptococcal pharyngitis (strep throat), otitis media (ear infection), influenza, and conjunctivitis (pink eye). When coding for any type of infectious disease, if the specific pathogen is known (etiology), it should be identified with a code to identify the organism. Refer to chapter 4 for a discussion of etiology and manifestations including relevant OGCR.

The only exception to this is if a combination code exists that identifies the etiology and manifestation of the disease in one code. Combination codes include both

Figure 10.11. Signs and symptoms versus definitive diagnosis

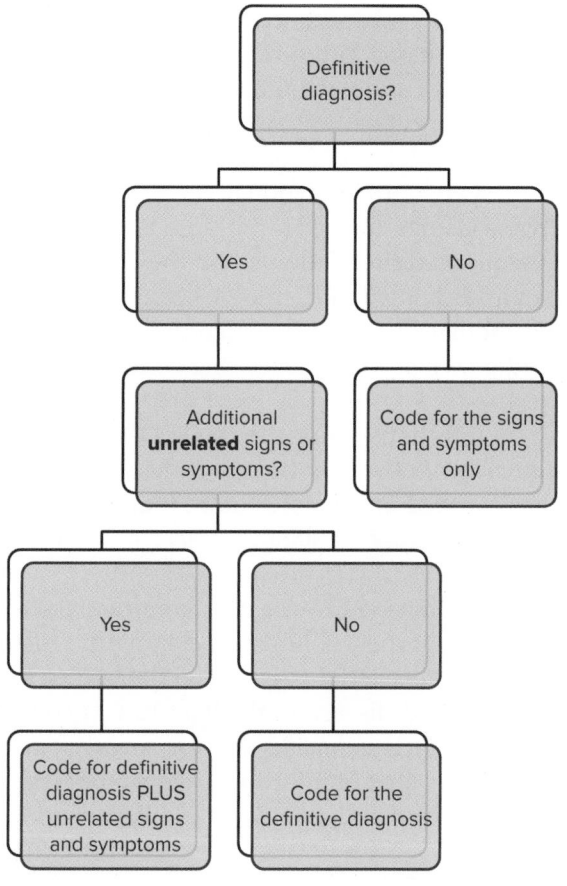

the etiology (cause of the disease) and the manifestation (signs or symptoms of the disease) all into one code. For example, if a patient presents to the urgent care clinic complaining of fever with cough, chills, nausea, and headache, and it is confirmed that the patient has influenza, then the code for unspecified influenza should be used, J11.1, Influenza due to unidentified influenza virus with other respiratory manifestations. In this case, the one code (J11.1) identifies both the etiology (influenza, the infectious organism), as well as the manifestations of the disease (other respiratory manifestations).

However, if the specific influenza viral strain (etiology) is identified by the clinic, then it should be reported with the appropriate combination code to identify both the viral infection (influenza with other manifestation), and the specific infectious disease (etiology). For example, if the patient came into the office with a viral pneumonia and it was identified that the patient had influenza with pneumonia due to the novel influenza A virus, then the appropriate code would be J09.X1, Influenza due to identified novel influenza A virus with pneumonia.

When there is no combination code to identify both the infectious organism (when known) and the etiology, then the two conditions must be coded separately. For instance, if a patient is diagnosed with a lung abscess due to *Klebsiella pneumoniae* without pneumonia, then the coder should report one for the lung abscess, J85.2, Abscess of lung without pneumonia, and B96.1, Klebsiella pneuomoniae [K. pneumoniae] as the cause of disease classified elsewhere.

When identifying the etiology and manifestation of a disease with separate codes, select the "B" code for the infectious disease, *as the cause of disease classified elsewhere.*

This indicates that the infectious organism caused the manifestation identified by the other code. B codes are ICD-10-CM codes, located in chapter 1: Certain Infectious and Parasitic Diseases, and located in the section Bacterial and viral infectious agents (B95 to B97). Beneath the category name in the ICD-10-CM code book, there is a note that these categories are for use as a supplementary or additional code, and used to identify the infectious agent (etiology) of a disease classified elsewhere in the ICD-10-CM manual. This is an important category of codes to understand, as these codes are only to be used in conjunction with a primary code to identify the manifestation.

Sequencing of the two codes should be as indicated in the ICD-10-CM code book: the manifestation code is sequenced first, followed by the code to identify the etiology of the disease. Remember, as discussed in chapter 4, sequencing of these codes is guided by the notations in the Tabular List, including "code first" and "use additional code." These notations tell coders when to sequence one code before another and in which situations.

When searching for an infectious disease in the ICD-10-CM code book, look up the main term *Infection, infected, infective*, and then find the subterm for the specific pathogen. If the pathogen has resulted in a manifestation that is coded elsewhere, be sure to select the subterm *as cause of disease classified elsewhere*, and then verify the code in the Tabular List.

Sexually transmitted infections (STIs) are also commonly seen in the urgent care setting. These include genital herpes, gonorrhea, chlamydia, trichomoniasis, syphilis, human papillomavirus (HPV), bacterial vaginosis, HIV/AIDS, and viral hepatitis. To search for a sexually transmitted disease in the ICD-10-CM code book, search for the name of the type of infectio, (such as *syphilis* or *trichomoniasis*) and then search for the subterm to identify the specific type of infection; excepts for HIV and AIDS, which are discussed in chapter 14: Independent Laboratory and Pathology Services,

Injuries and External Causes

Injuries are often seen in the urgent care setting, especially since wait times are relatively short and most urgent care clinics have imaging services on-site, like x-rays. Thus, a patient with a possible fracture can be seen for a quick determination of the extent of the injury, receive initial treatment, and receive a referral for further treatment, if necessary. Also, some injuries like skin lacerations can be immediately repaired in the urgent care setting. Injuries commonly seen in the urgent care setting include muscle and joint sprains and strains, cuts and lacerations, minor burns, and fall injuries.

When a patient has multiple injuries, the coder should report one code for each injury, with the most severe injury sequenced first, followed by the less severe injuries. When coding for multiple injuries, remember:

Worst Comes First

External causes of injury codes are also common in ED encounters, each of which require a solid understanding of the episode of service for the encounter.

External Causes of Injury

When coding for injuries, the healthcare provider needs to document the actual injury, rather than a sign or symptom. For example, if a patient presents with wrist pain, an inconclusive x-ray is taken, and the healthcare provider documents suspected wrist fracture, then the coder should report wrist pain (or another appropriate, documented sign or symptom), and *not* a code for a wrist fracture, as this diagnosis was not confirmed. Remember coders cannot report a diagnosis that is *suspected, unconfirmed, rule-out,* or *questionable* in the outpatient setting (refer to chapter 4, OGCR IV.H).

When coding for any type of injury, it is necessary to include up to four codes for the external causes of the injury. As discussed in chapter 4, external cause codes are always sequenced after the codes for the primary medical condition (such as the injury suffered). External cause codes provide additional information surrounding the circumstances of the injury or illness, but do not clearly identify the medical necessity for the service, so they have no impact on reimbursement. There are four possible external cause code categories.

- The injury mechanism is the manner in which the injury happened, such as kicked by a horse, W55.12XA, Struck by horse, initial encounter.
- The activity in which the patient was engaged when the injury happened, such as riding a horse, Y93.52, Activity, horseback riding.
- The place of occurrence is where the injury occurred, such as in a rodeo arena, Y92.39, Other specified sports and athletic area as the place of occurrence of the external cause.
- The status of the patient at the time of the activity, such as sport done for pay, Y99.0 Civilian activity done for income or pay.

Key to Success

The need to code for external causes depends on the state in which the healthcare services are provided. Some states do not require external cause codes, while other states do mandate them. In some areas, it may be necessary to report external cause codes to certain payers who require them, whereas other payers will not process and may deny claims with external cause codes. It is imperative to understand the specific requirements for the encounter for which you are coding and report those codes accordingly. This text assumes that external causes are necessary to report, so as you read and come across an external cause described in the documentation, then you should assign the appropriate code(s). Remember, external cause codes are always listed *after* the codes for the patient's medical condition(s).

Identify the Encounter
When coding for injuries, a coder must identify the encounter for the injury (refer to chapter 4). Remember that the seventh character A-initial represents any encounter for which the patient is in *active treatment.* D-subsequent is when the patient is in the healing phase, and S-sequela is for a late effect, or sequela, of that condition. As most patients seen in the urgent care setting are experiencing acute conditions, the majority of the encounters will be A-initial. If, however, a patient received stitches two weeks ago in the urgent care clinic and returns today for the removal of the stitches, then the encounter would be D-subsequent.

For all initial encounters (ending with an *A*), it is necessary to identify all four external cause codes (if possible). For all encounters other than initial encounters to the coder only needs to report the external cause code for the injury mechanism, with either a D-subsequent or S-sequela, seventh character, depending on the circumstances. See figure 10.12 for the OGCR related to coding for external causes of morbidity.

Figure 10.12. OGCR I.20

---

20. Chapter 20: External Causes of Morbidity (V00-Y99)

The external causes of morbidity codes should never be sequenced as the first-listed or principal diagnosis.

External cause codes are intended to provide data for injury research and evaluation of injury prevention strategies. These codes capture how the injury or health condition happened (cause), the intent (unintentional or accidental; or intentional, such as suicide or assault), the place where the event occurred the activity of the patient at the time of the event, and the person's status (e.g., civilian, military).

There is no national requirement for mandatory ICD-10-CM external cause code reporting. Unless a provider is subject to a state-based external cause code reporting mandate or these codes are required by a particular payer, reporting of ICD-10-CM codes in Chapter 20, External Causes of Morbidity, is not required. In the absence of a mandatory reporting requirement, providers are encouraged to voluntarily report external cause codes, as they provide valuable data for injury research and evaluation of injury prevention strategies.

a. General External Cause Coding Guidelines

1) Used with any code in the range of A00.0-T88.9, Z00-Z99

An external cause code may be used with any code in the range of A00.0-T88.9, Z00-Z99, classification that **represents** a health condition due to an external cause. Though they are most applicable to injuries, they are also valid for use with such things as infections or diseases due to an external source, and other health conditions, such as a heart attack that occurs during strenuous physical activity.

2) External cause code used for length of treatment

Assign the external cause code, with the appropriate 7th character (initial encounter, subsequent encounter or sequela) for each encounter for which the injury or condition is being treated. Most categories in chapter 20 have a 7th character requirement for each applicable code.

Most categories in this chapter have three 7th character values: A, initial encounter, D, subsequent encounter and S, sequela. While the patient may be seen by a new or different provider over the course of treatment for an injury or condition, assignment of the 7th character for external cause should match the 7th character of the code assigned for the associated injury or condition for the encounter.

3) Use the full range of external cause codes

Use the full range of external cause codes to completely describe the cause, the intent, the place of occurrence, and if applicable, the activity of the patient at the time of the event, and the patient's status, for all injuries, and other health conditions due to an external cause.

4) Assign as many external cause codes as necessary

Assign as many external cause codes as necessary to fully explain each cause. If only one external code can be recorded, assign the code most related to the principal diagnosis.

5) The selection of the appropriate external cause code

The selection of the appropriate external cause code is guided by the Alphabetic Index of External Causes and by Inclusion and Exclusion notes in the Tabular List.

6) External cause code can never be a principal diagnosis

An external cause code can never be a principal (first-listed) diagnosis.

7) Combination external cause codes

Certain of the external cause codes are combination codes that identify sequential events that result in an injury, such as a fall which results in striking against an object. The injury may be due to either event or both. The combination external cause code used should correspond to the sequence of events regardless of which caused the most serious injury.

8) No external cause code needed in certain circumstances

No external cause code from Chapter 20 is needed if the external cause and intent are included in a code from another chapter (e.g. T36.0X1- Poisoning by penicillins, accidental (unintentional)).

b. Place of Occurrence Guideline

Codes from category Y92, Place of occurrence of the external cause, are secondary codes for use after other external cause codes to identify the location of the patient at the time of injury or other condition.

Generally, a place of occurrent code is assigned only once, at the initial encounter for treatment. However, in the rare instance that a new injury occurs during hospitalization, an additional place of occurrence code may be assigned. No 7th characters are used for Y92.

Do not use place of occurrence code Y92.9 if the place is not stated or is not applicable.

c. Activity Code

Assign a code from category Y93, Activity code, to describe the activity of the patient at the time the injury or other health condition occurred.

An activity code is used only once, at the initial encounter for treatment. Only one code from Y93 should be recorded on a medical record.

The activity codes are not applicable to poisonings, adverse effects, misadventures or sequela.

Do not assign Y93.9, Unspecified activity, if the activity is not stated.

A code from category Y93 is appropriate for use with external cause and intent codes if identifying the activity provides additional information about the event.

d. Place of Occurrence, Activity, and Status Codes Used with other External Cause Code

When applicable, place of occurrence, activity, and external cause status codes are sequenced after the main external cause code(s). Regardless of the number of external cause codes assigned, there should be only one place of occurrence code, one activity code, and one external cause status code assigned to an encounter. However, in the rare instance that a new injury occurs during hospitalization, an additional place of occurrence code may be assigned.

e. If the Reporting Format Limits the Number of External Cause Codes

If the reporting format limits the number of external cause codes that can be used in reporting clinical data, report the code for the cause/intent most related to the principal diagnosis. If the format permits capture of additional external cause codes, the cause/intent, including medical misadventures, of the additional events should be reported rather than the codes for place, activity, or external status.

f. Multiple External Cause Coding Guidelines

More than one external cause code is required to fully describe the external cause of an illness or injury. The assignment of external cause codes should be sequenced in the following priority:

If two or more events cause separate injuries, an external cause code should be assigned for each cause. The first-listed external cause code will be selected in the following order:

External codes for child and adult abuse take priority over all other external cause codes.

See Section I.C.19., Child and Adult abuse guidelines.

External cause codes for terrorism events take priority over all other external cause codes except child and adult abuse.

External cause codes for cataclysmic events take priority over all other external cause codes except child and adult abuse and terrorism.

External cause codes for transport accidents take priority over all other external cause codes except cataclysmic events, child and adult abuse and terrorism.

Activity and external cause status codes are assigned following all causal (intent) external cause codes.

The first-listed external cause code should correspond to the cause of the most serious diagnosis due to an assault, accident, or self-harm, following the order of hierarchy listed above.

g. Child and Adult Abuse Guideline

Adult and child abuse, neglect and maltreatment are classified as assault. Any of the assault codes may be used to indicate the external cause of any injury resulting from the confirmed abuse.

For confirmed cases of abuse, neglect and maltreatment, when the perpetrator is known, a code from Y07, Perpetrator of maltreatment and neglect, should accompany any other assault codes.

See Section I.C.19. Adult and child abuse, neglect and other maltreatment

h. Unknown or Undetermined Intent Guideline

If the intent (accident, self-harm, assault) of the cause of an injury or other condition is unknown or unspecified, code the intent as accidental intent. All transport accident categories assume accidental intent.

1) Use of undetermined intent

External cause codes for events of undetermined intent are only for use if the documentation in the record specifies that the intent cannot be determined.

i. Sequelae (Late Effects) of External Cause Guidelines

1) Sequelae external cause codes

Sequela are reported using the external cause code with the 7th character "S" for sequela. These codes should be used with any report of a late effect or sequela resulting from a previous injury.

See Section I.B.10 Sequela (Late Effects)

2) Sequela external cause code with a related current injury

A sequela external cause code should never be used with a related current nature of injury code.

(Continued on next page)

Figure 10.12. *(Continued)*

3) Use of sequela external cause codes for subsequent visits

Use a late effect external cause code for subsequent visits when a late effect of the initial injury is being treated. Do not use a late effect external cause code for subsequent visits for follow- up care (e.g., to assess healing, to receive rehabilitative therapy) of the injury when no late effect of the injury has been documented.

j. Terrorism Guidelines

1) Cause of injury identified by the Federal Government (FBI) as terrorism

When the cause of an injury is identified by the Federal Government (FBI) as terrorism, the first-listed external cause code should be a code from category Y38, Terrorism. The definition of terrorism employed by the FBI is found at the inclusion note at the beginning of category Y38. Use additional code for place of occurrence (Y92.-). More than one Y38 code may be assigned if the injury is the result of more than one mechanism of terrorism.

2) Cause of an injury is suspected to be the result of terrorism

When the cause of an injury is suspected to be the result of terrorism a code from category Y38 should not be assigned. Suspected cases should be classified as assault.

3) Code Y38.9, Terrorism, secondary effects

Assign code Y38.9, Terrorism, secondary effects, for conditions occurring subsequent to the terrorist event. This code should not be assigned for conditions that are due to the initial terrorist act.

It is acceptable to assign code Y38.9 with another code from Y38 if there is an injury due to the initial terrorist event and an injury that is a subsequent result of the terrorist event.

k. External cause status

A code from category Y99, External cause status, should be assigned whenever any other external cause code is assigned for an encounter, including an Activity code, except for the events noted below. Assign a code from category Y99, External cause status, to indicate the work status of the person at the time the event occurred. The status code indicates whether the event occurred during military activity, whether a non-military person was at work, whether an individual including a student or volunteer was involved in a non-work activity at the time of the causal event.

A code from Y99, External cause status, should be assigned, when applicable, with other external cause codes, such as transport accidents and falls. The external cause status codes are not applicable to poisonings, adverse effects, misadventures or late effects. Do not assign a code from category Y99 if no other external cause codes (cause, activity) are applicable for the encounter.

An external cause status code is used only once, at the initial encounter for treatment. Only one code from Y99 should be recorded on a medical record.

Do not assign code Y99.9, Unspecified external cause status, if the status is not stated.

Source: CMS 2018.

For practice assigning diagnosis codes to urgent care services, complete the exercises in There's a Code for That 10.3.

Urgent care diagnoses

There's a Code for That

Read the following documentation and select the appropriate diagnosis code(s).

1. Patient with left knee pain presents to urgent care clinic after a wrestling injury. All x-rays performed were negative, suspect ligamentous injury. Refer to ortho for follow-up and further imaging.

   ICD-10-CM code: _____, _____

2. Patient seen for multiple lacerations after having walked through a plate glass window. Following wounds were noted: simple wounds of right upper thigh, right hip, and abdomen. Intermediate wounds on right forearm, right shoulder, and forehead. *Do not code for the external causes.*

   ICD-10-CM codes: _____, _____, _____,
   _____, _____, _____

3. 32-year-old female established patient seen for lymphadenopathy, sore throat, and hyperpyrexia. Lab tests performed included group A strep, influenza, and mono spot. Mono spot was positive for infectious mononucleosis.

   ICD-10-CM code: _____

4. X-ray performed on patient with severe cough, chest pain, and fever shows pneumonia infiltrates. Lab culture of sputum test positive for streptococcal pneumoniae.

   ICD-10-CM code: _____

5. Patient suffered impact injury during soccer practice at a local athletic field. She was practicing in her off-hours for a recreational soccer league. She was running toward another player when they collided and fell to the ground, after which two other players toppled over and fell on top of the patient. She is now complaining of chest pain and difficulty breathing. X-ray negative for any fracture or internal injuries. Impression: Contusion of right ribs.

   ICD-10-CM code (injury): _____

   ICD-10-CM codes (external causes): _____, _____,
   _____, _____

Diagnostic Coding for ED Services

Diagnoses for conditions seen in the emergency department setting typically revolve around life-threatening illnesses and injuries. These include cardiovascular conditions, skin infections, appendicitis, motor vehicle accidents, burns, sepsis, septicemia, and systemic inflammatory response syndrome (SIRS). Patients present to the ED for treatment with various conditions, some of which are true life-threatening emergencies, while others are simple problems that do not require any treatment. Coding diagnoses for ED services relies on the coder's ability to utilize the entire ICD-10-CM code book and read and interpret ICD-10-CM coding guidelines.

Cardiovascular Problems and Myocardial Infarctions

Chest pain, cardiac dysrhythmias, congestive heart failure, and myocardial infarctions are all conditions that may be seen in the ED setting.

Chest pain may be a symptom of an injury, such as a broken rib or soreness from a cough; or it may be more serious, such as an impending myocardial infarction (MI) or lower respiratory infection. This is why it is a condition that is commonly evaluated in the emergency department. Codes for chest pain identify the type of chest pain. If the chest pain is determined to be a symptom of a more definitive condition, such as myocardial infarction, then code for the MI and not the symptom of chest pain.

Other cardiovascular problems in the ED may include cardiac dysrhythmias and congestive heart failure, vascular diseases, and deep vein thromboses and pulmonary embolisms.

A myocardial infarction (MI), otherwise known as a heart attack, is the death of a portion of the heart muscle due to lack of oxygen supply. Heart attacks vary in the site and type of the infarction, and codes depend on whether the MI is a STEMI (ST elevation myocardial infarction) or NSTEMI (non-STEMI), as well as if the MI is initial or subsequent.

HCC

An initial MI (category I21) is the either the first MI, or an MI that occurs more than 28 days (4 weeks) after an initial MI. For example, if the patient had a heart attack two years ago and presents to the ED today with a new heart attack, then it would be coded with an I21 code to identify it as an initial MI.

A subsequent MI (category I22) is a heart attack that occurs within 28 days (4 weeks) of an initial MI. For example, if the patient that came in two weeks ago with a heart attack presents today with a different MI (an infarction of a different site), then the MI for this encounter would be coded as a subsequent MI (I22). An additional code would be assigned to identify the initial MI. If the previous MI is older than 28 days, then code I25.2, Old myocardial infarction, should be used to identify the previous MI. The old MI code may be used for any old MI, even if it occurred 10 years ago or more.

Review the following flowchart (figure 10.13) to help identify when an MI would be identified as either initial or subsequent, and the sequencing of each. See also figure 10.14 for the OGCR related to coding myocardial infarctions.

Figure 10.13. Acute versus subsequent MI flowchart

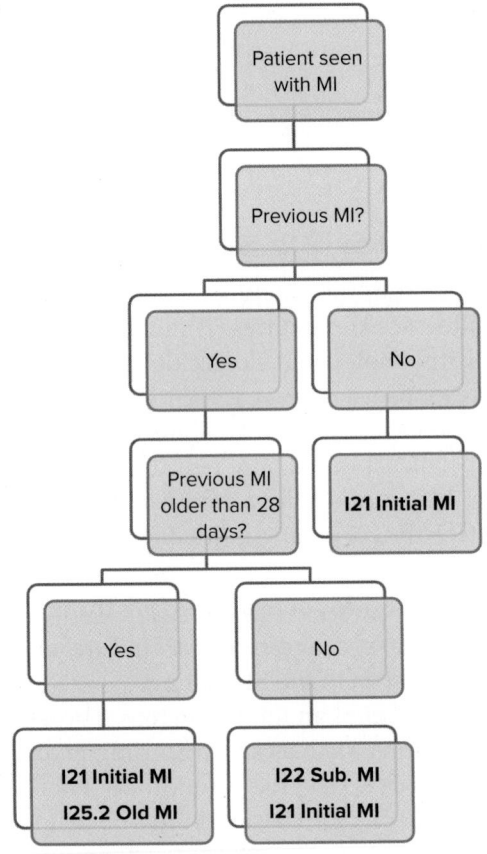

HCC Coding Corner

Note that all myocardial infarction codes are HCC codes, which means careful coding of these conditions is required and documentation should be complete and follow all HCC guidelines. The old MI code, I25.2, Old myocardial infarction, is an important code in HCC coding in any setting because even if the patient was not seen for a current heart attack or cardiovascular problem, the code should still be added to the claim to identify relevant patient medical history.

Figure 10.14. OGCR I.C.9.e

---

e. Acute myocardial infarction (AMI)

1) ST elevation myocardial infarction (STEMI) and non ST elevation myocardial infarction (NSTEMI)

The ICD-10-CM codes for **type 1** acute myocardial infarction (AMI) identify the site, such as anterolateral wall or true posterior wall. Subcategories I21.0-I21.2 and code I21.3 are used for **type 1** ST elevation myocardial infarction (STEMI). Code I21.4, Non-ST elevation (NSTEMI) myocardial infarction, is used for **type 1** non ST elevation myocardial infarction (NSTEMI) and nontransmural MIs.

If **a type 1** NSTEMI evolves to STEMI, assign the STEMI code. If **a type 1** STEMI converts to NSTEMI due to thrombolytic therapy, it is still coded as STEMI.

For encounters occurring while the myocardial infarction is equal to, or less than, four weeks old, including transfers to another acute setting or a postacute setting, and the myocardial infarction meets the definition for "other diagnoses" (see Section III, Reporting Additional Diagnoses), codes from category I21 may continue to be reported. For encounters after the 4 week time frame and the patient is still receiving care related to the myocardial infarction, the appropriate aftercare code should be assigned, rather than a code from category I21. For old or healed myocardial infarctions not requiring further care, code I25.2, Old myocardial infarction, may be assigned.

2) Acute myocardial infarction, unspecified

Code **I21.9, Acute myocardial infarction, unspecified**, is the default for unspecified acute myocardial infarction **or unspecified type**. If only **type 1** STEMI or transmural MI without the site is documented, assign code I21.3, **ST elevation (STEMI) myocardial infarction of unspecified site.**

3) AMI documented as nontransmural or subendocardial but site provided

If an AMI is documented as nontransmural or subendocardial, but the site is provided, it is still coded as a subendocardial AMI.

See Section I.C.21.3 for information on coding status post administration of tPA in a different facility within the last 24 hours.

4) Subsequent acute myocardial infarction

A code from category I22, Subsequent ST elevation (STEMI) and non ST elevation (NSTEMI) myocardial infarction, is to be used when a patient who has suffered **a type 1 or unspecified** AMI has a new AMI within the 4 week time frame of the initial AMI. A code from category I22 must be used in conjunction with a code from category I21. The sequencing of the I22 and I21 codes depends on the circumstances of the encounter.

Do not assign code I22 for subsequent myocardial infarctions other than type 1 or unspecified. For subsequent type 2 AMI assign only code I21.A1. For subsequent type 4 or type 5 AMI, assign only code I21.A9.

5) Other Types of Myocardial Infarction

The ICD-10-CM provides codes for different types of myocardial infarction. Type 1 myocardial infarctions are assigned to codes I21.0-I21.4.

Type 2 myocardial infarctions, and myocardial infarction due to demand ischemia or secondary to ischemic balance, is assigned to code I21.A1, Myocardial infarction type 2 with a code for the underlying cause. Do not assign code I24.8, Other forms of acute ischemic heart disease for the demand ischemia. Sequencing of type 2 AMI or the underlying cause is dependent on the circumstances of admission. When a type 2 AMI code is described as NSTEMI or STEMI, only assign code I21.A1. Codes I21.0-I21.4 should only be assigned for type 1 AMIs.

Acute myocardial infarctions type 3, 4a, 4b, 4c and 5 are assigned to code I21.A9, Other myocardial infarction type.

The "Code also" and "Code first" notes should be followed related to complications, and for coding of postprocedural myocardial infarctions during or following cardiac surgery.

Source: CMS 2018.

Sepsis, Septicemia, and SIRS

Sepsis, also referred to as septicemia or bacteremia, is a complication of an infection outside of the bloodstream, such as a tooth abscess or skin infection. Once a patient is deemed septic, the infectious organism has invaded the bloodstream and carried throughout the blood to other sites of the body. This may result in acute organ dysfunction, and the patient is deemed to have severe sepsis that can result in septic shock and ultimately death.

Codes for sepsis identify the condition as either sepsis or severe sepsis. Severe sepsis is when the sepsis has caused any acute organ dysfunction or organ failure. The specific type of organ failure must also be identified in the documentation with a separate ICD-10-CM code. **Septic shock** is a severe drop in blood pressure caused by sepsis that can lead to organ failure or death. If the sepsis is documented as occurring with septic shock, the coder should report the code for the septic shock.

Coding for sepsis requires multiple codes, depending on the condition.

- *Sepsis only.* To code for sepsis (or septicemia) without severe sepsis (no organ dysfunction), assign a code to identify the infectious organism, from category A40 and A41.

- *Severe sepsis (with organ dysfunction).* To code for severe sepsis, a minimum of three codes is required. One to identify the sepsis (septicemia code from category A40 and A41), one to identify the infection as severe sepsis, with or without septic shock (R65.2-), and a third code to identify the specific associated organ dysfunction (such as acute kidney failure N17.- or acute respiratory failure J96.0-).

- **Systemic inflammatory response syndrome (SIRS)** is a noninfectious process, such as heatstroke or a traumatic injury. Although this condition is not due to an infectious process, it is coded similarly, from the same category as severe sepsis (R65). Coding for SIRS requires at least two codes—one for the underlying trauma or condition, and one to identify the SIRS, either with or without acute organ dysfunction (R65.10, Systemic inflammatory response syndrome (SIRS) of non-infectious origin without acute organ dysfunction, or R65.11, Systemic inflammatory response syndrome (SIRS) of non-infectious origin with acute organ dysfunction). An additional code should be reported to identify the acute organ dysfunction, if applicable, such as K72.0, Acute and subacute hepatic failure.

Sequencing of the codes involved in sepsis, severe sepsis, and SIRS depends on the coder's ability to identify and interpret coding guidelines in the ICD-10-CM code book (see figure 10.15). For sepsis, the code for septicemia should be sequenced before the code for severe sepsis, and the code for the acute organ dysfunction should follow the severe sepsis code. For SIRS, the code for the underlying condition or injury should be sequenced first, followed by the SIRS code, and finally the code for the acute organ dysfunction (if applicable).

Appendicitis

Coding for appendicitis is markedly less difficult than coding for sepsis and SIRS, but because it is a common condition seen in the ED, it bears mention here. Right lower quadrant (RLQ) abdominal pain is a possible indicator of appendicitis that commonly results in an imaging procedure performed in the ED, such as an ultrasound or CT scan of the abdomen.

Appendicitis is inflammation of the appendix that can be a life-threatening condition if it ruptures, which can cause a systemic infection. Codes for appendicitis (K35 through K37) identify the condition as either acute, chronic/recurrent, or unspecified. Acute appendicitis codes are divided depending on if any localized or generalized peritonitis is present, due to a rupture of the inflamed appendix, such as K35.3, Acute appendicitis with localized peritonitis.

Figure 10.15. OGCR I.C.1.d

---

d. Sepsis, Severe Sepsis, and Septic Shock

1) Coding of Sepsis and Severe Sepsis

(a) Sepsis

For a diagnosis of sepsis, assign the appropriate code for the underlying systemic infection. If the type of infection or causal organism is not further specified, assign code A41.9, Sepsis, unspecified organism.

A code from subcategory R65.2, Severe sepsis, should not be assigned unless severe sepsis or an associated acute organ dysfunction is documented.

(i) Negative or inconclusive blood cultures and sepsis

Negative or inconclusive blood cultures do not preclude a diagnosis of sepsis in patients with clinical evidence of the condition, however, the provider should be queried.

(ii) Urosepsis

The term urosepsis is a nonspecific term. It is not to be considered synonymous with sepsis. It has no default code in the Alphabetic Index. Should a provider use this term, he/she must be queried for clarification.

(iii) Sepsis with organ dysfunction

If a patient has sepsis and associated acute organ dysfunction or multiple organ dysfunction (MOD), follow the instructions for coding severe sepsis.

(iv) Acute organ dysfunction that is not clearly associated with the sepsis

If a patient has sepsis and an acute organ dysfunction, but the medical record documentation indicates that the acute organ dysfunction is related to a medical condition other than the sepsis, do not assign a code from subcategory R65.2, Severe sepsis. An acute organ dysfunction must be associated with the sepsis in order to assign the severe sepsis code. If the documentation is not clear as to whether an acute organ dysfunction is related to the sepsis or another medical condition, query the provider.

Source: CMS 2018.

Motor Vehicle Accidents

A **motor vehicle accident (MVA)** is an accident that involves any type of motor vehicle. Some MVAs occur with only one vehicle, others may involve a vehicle and a pedestrian or bicycle, or they may involve multiple vehicles of different types. When a patient is injured in a motor vehicle accident, he or she is typically transported to the ED via ambulance. Injuries sustained in car accidents can range from nonexistent to the most severe, resulting in death.

Coding for an MVA requires one code for the actual injury sustained by the patient, such as a fracture, laceration, or whiplash injury. Additional codes that identify the circumstances surrounding the MVA should be included. Codes for MVAs are found in the following ICD-10-CM categories.

- Pedestrian injured in transport accident (V00 to V09)
- Pedal cycle rider injured in transport accident (V10 to V19)
- Motorcycle rider injured in transport accident (V20 to V29)
- Occupant of three-wheeled motor vehicle injured in transport accident (V30 to V39)
- Car occupant injured in transport accident (V40 to V49)
- Occupant of pick-up truck or van injured in transport accident (V50 to V59)
- Occupant of heavy transport vehicle injured in transport accident (V60 to V69)
- Bus occupant injured in transport accident (V70 to V79)
- Other land transport accidents (V80 to V89)

MVA codes are detailed codes that identify the person injured, how the injury happened, any other vehicles or objects involved in the accident, the person driving the transport vehicle, and the encounter (initial, subsequent, sequela). For example, if a patient suffered a whiplash injury while he was driving a car, when he accidentally hit the car in front of him in traffic because he was distracted by his cell phone, the ICD-10-CM code reported would be V43.52XA, Car driver injured in collision with other type car in traffic accident, initial encounter. Additional codes would be selected for the patient's other injuries, as well as any other circumstances surrounding the event, such as the location of the accident and the patient status at the time of the accident.

To look for the code for an MVA, search in the External Cause of Injuries Index, located after the ICD-10-CM Main Index. Search under the term *Accident*, and then the subterm *traffic, nontraffic, or transport,* depending on the circumstances of the accident. See figure 10.16 for the definitions related to transport accidents.

Figure 10.16. Definitions related to transport accidents

NOTE   Definitions related to transport accidents:

(a) A transport accident (V00-V99) is any accident involving a device designed primarily for, or used at the time primarily for, conveying persons or goods from one place to another.

(b) A public highway [trafficway] or street is the entire width between property lines (or other boundary lines) of land open to the public as a matter of right or custom for purposes of moving persons or property from one place to another. A roadway is that part of the public highway designed, improved and customarily used for vehicular traffic.

(c) A traffic accident is any vehicle accident occurring on the public highway [i.e. originating on, terminating on, or involving a vehicle partially on the highway]. A vehicle accident is assumed to have occurred on the public highway unless another place is specified, except i the case of accidents involving only off-road motor vehicles, which are classified as nontraffic accidents unless the contrary is stated.

(d) A nontraffic accident is any vehicle accident that occurs entirely in any place other than a public highway.

(e) A pedestrian is any person involved in an accident who was not at the time of the accident riding in or on a motor vehicle, railway train, streetcar or animal-drawn or other vehicle, or on a pedal cycle or animal. This includes, a person changing a tire, working on a parked care, or a person on foot. It also includes the user of a pedestrian conveyance such as a babystroller, ice-skates, skis, sled, roller skates, a skateboard, nonmotorized or motorized wheelchair, motorized mobility scooter, or nonmotorized scooter.

(f) A driver is an occupant of a transport vehicle who is operating or intending to operate it.

(g) A passenger is any occupant of a transport vehicle other than the driver, except a person traveling on the outside of the vehicle.

(h) A person on the outside of a vehicle is any person being transported by a vehicle but not occupying the space normally reserved for the driver or passengers, or the space intended for the transport of property. This includes a person travailing on the bodywork, bumper, fender, roof, running board or step of a vehicle, as well as, hanging on the outside of the vehicle.

(i) A pedal cycle is any land transport vehicle operated solely by nonmotorized pedals including a bicycle or tricycle.

(j) A pedal cyclist is any person riding a pedal cycle or in a sidecar or trailer attached to a pedal cycle.

(k) A motorcycle is a two-wheeled motor vehicle with one or two riding saddles and sometimes with a third wheel for the support of a sidecar. The sidecar is considered part of the motorcycle. This includes a moped, motor scooter, or motorized bicycle.

(l) A motorcycle rider is any person riding a motorcycle or in a sidecar or trailer attached to the motorcycle.

(m) A three-wheeled motor vehicle is a motorized tricycle designed primarily for on-road use. This includes a motor-driven tricycle, a motorized rickshaw, or a three-wheeled motor car.

(n) A car [automobile] is a four-wheeled motor vehicle designed primarily for carrying up to 7 persons. A trailer being towed by the car is considered par of the car. It does not include a van or minivan - see definition (o)

(o) A pick-up truck or van is a four or six-wheeled motor vehicle designed for carrying passengers as well as property or cargo weighing less than the local limit for classification as a heavy goods vehicle, and not requiring a special driver's license. this includes a minivan and a sport-utility vehicle (SUV)

(p) A heavy transport vehicle is a motor vehicle designed primarily for carrying property, meeting local criteria for classification as a heavy goods vehicle in terms of weight and requiring a special driver's license.

(q) A bus (coach) is a motor vehicle designed or adapted primarily for carrying more than 10 passengers, and requiring a special driver's license.

(r) A railway train or railway vehicle is any device, with or without freight or passenger cars couple to it, designed for traffic on a railway track. This includes subterranean (subways) or elevated trains.

(s) A streetcar, is a device designed and used primarily for transporting passengers within a municipality, running on rails, usually subject to normal traffic control signals, and operated principally on a right-of-way that forms part of the roadway. This includes a tram or trolley that runs on rails. A trailer being towed by a streetcar is considered part of the streetcar.

(t) A special vehicle mainly used on industrial premises is a motor vehicle designed primarily for use within the building and premises of industrial or commercial establishments. This includes battery-powered airport passenger vehicles or baggage/mail trucks, forklifts, coal-cars in a coal min, logging cars and trucks used in mines or quarries.

(u) A special vehicle mainly used in agriculture is a motor vehicle designed specifically for use in farming and agriculture (horticulture), to work the land, tend and harvest crops and transport materials on the farm. This includes harvesters, farm machinery and tractor and trailers.

(v) A special construction vehicle is a motor vehicle designed specifically for use on construction and demolition sites. This includes bulldozers, diggers, earth levellers, dump trucks, backhoes, front-end loaders, pavers, and mechanical shovels.

(w) A special all-terrain vehicle is a motor vehicle of special design to enable it to negotiate over rough or soft terrain, snow or sand. Examples of special design are high construction, special wheels and tires, tracks, and support on a cushion of air. This includes snow mobiles, All terrain vehicles (ATV), and dune buggies. It does not include passenger vehicle designated as Sport Utility Vehicles (SUV).

(x) A water craft is any device designed for transporting passengers or goods on water. This includes motor or sail boats, ships, and hovercraft.

(y) An aircraft is any device for transporting passengers or goods in the air. This includes hot-air balloons, gliders, helicopters and airplanes.

(z) A military vehicle is any motorized vehicle operating on a public roadway owned by the military and being operated by a member of the military.

Source: CMS 2018.

Burns

The ICD-10-CM code book differentiates between burns and corrosions. **Burn codes** are for thermal burns that come from a heat source such as fire or hot appliance. This category also includes burns from electricity or radiation, with the exception of sunburns, which are coded elsewhere in category L55, Sunburn. **Corrosion codes** are burns due to chemicals. The guidelines are the same for coding either burns or corrosions.

Burns and corrosions codes (T20 through T25) are classified by four factors:

- *Site:* This is the exact location of the burn. For multiple sites, one code should be reported for each individual burn, with the most severe sequenced before the least severe (worst comes first).

- *Depth:* Burns are classified by their depth, as first degree (erythema), second degree (blistering), or third degree (full-thickness involvement), as illustrated in figure 10.17.

Figure 10.17. Classification of burns

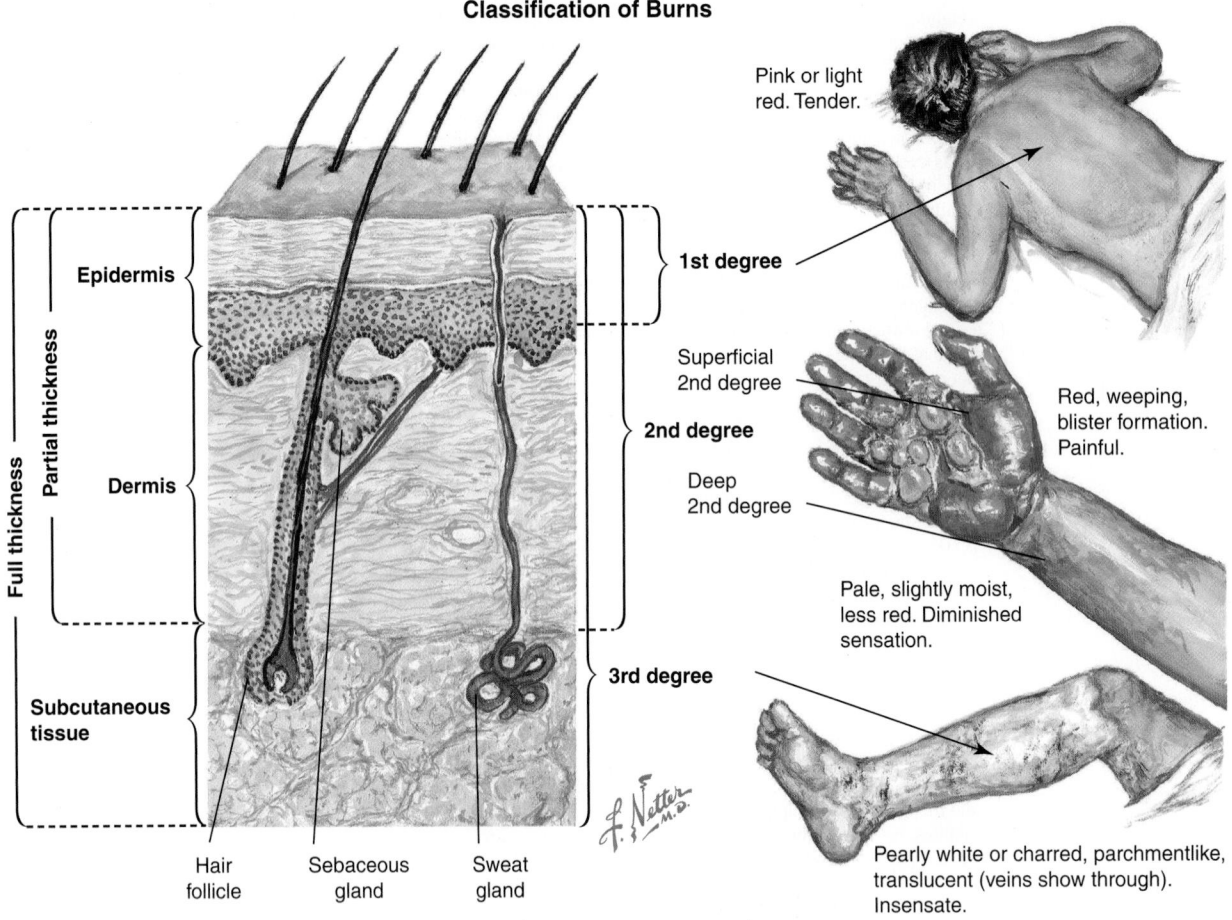

Classification of Burns

Epidermis

Partial thickness

Full thickness

Dermis

Subcutaneous tissue

Hair follicle

Sebaceous gland

Sweat gland

1st degree

2nd degree
Superficial 2nd degree
Deep 2nd degree

3rd degree

Pink or light red. Tender.

Red, weeping, blister formation. Painful.

Pale, slightly moist, less red. Diminished sensation.

Pearly white or charred, parchmentlike, translucent (veins show through). Insensate.

- *Extent:* The extent of a burn is measured by the total percentage of body surface covered by the burn. Body percentages are determined by the clinical staff treating the patient by two methods: the rule of nines and the Lund-Browder classification system, both shown in figure 10.18. The **rule of nines** divides the body's surface into percentages based on the number nine, with the groin area making up the remaining one percent of body surface. The **Lund-Browder classification** chart divides the body's surface into differing percentages, depending on the age of the patient. Because the child body is disproportionate to the adult body, the Lund-Browder classification system takes into account the varying percentage of certain body structures as the patient ages and the body becomes more proportionate to that of an adult. Although the clinical staff determines the extent of the burned area, coders must be able to identify the extent burned based on the documentation in the heath record, and assign the code(s) appropriately.

- *Agent:* The agent that caused the injury, which resulted in either a burn or a corrosion.

Because burns and corrosions are injuries, they all require a seventh-character extension to identify the encounter, and the identification of any external causes, when documented.

Coding for burns requires at least two codes—one to identify the burn, as described previously, and another to identify the extent of the body surface, from category T31

Figure 10.18. Extent of burn

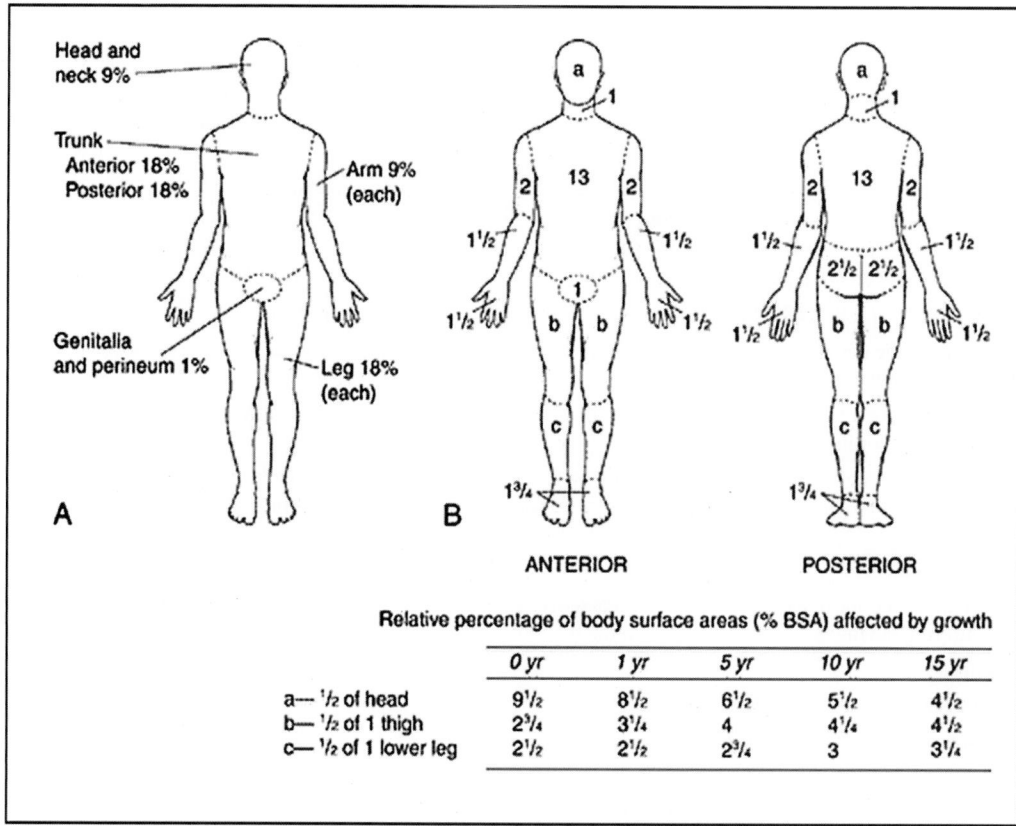

(A) Rule of "nines"
(B) Lund-Browder diagram for estimating extent of burns
Source: HHS 2013.

or T32. Codes for body surface identify the *total body surface burned* and then the *percent involved in the third-degree burn*. Read the following example and selected codes:

> *A 40-year-old patient was lighting a trash fire in his yard with lighter fluid, when the fluid splashed back onto his pants and lit his clothes on fire. He suffered second degree burns on his right and left legs (18 percent body surface), and a third-degree burn on his right foot (1 percent body surface).*

The codes selected for the injury would be the following:

- T24.291A, Burn of second degree of multiple sites of right lower limb, except ankle and foot, initial encounter
- T24.292A, Burn of second degree of multiple sites of left lower limb, except ankle and foot, initial encounter
- T25.321A, Burn of third degree of right foot, initial encounter
- T31.10, Burns involving 10-19% of body surface with 0% to 9% third degree burns

In this example, the three burn codes identify the body sites and the degree of the burns. The fourth code identified the total body surface involved (in this case 19 percent), and the amount of the burn that was third degree (in this case 1 percent). See figure 10.19 for the OGCR related to coding burns and related conditions.

Figure 10.19. OGCR I.C.19.d

---

d. Coding of Burns and Corrosions

The ICD-10-CM makes a distinction between burns and corrosions. The burn codes are for thermal burns, except sunburns, that come from a heat source, such as a fire or hot appliance. The burn codes are also for burns resulting from electricity and radiation. Corrosions are burns due to chemicals. The guidelines are the same for burns and corrosions.

Current burns (T20-T25) are classified by depth, extent and by agent (X code). Burns are classified by depth as first degree (erythema), second degree (blistering), and third degree (full-thickness involvement). Burns of the eye and internal organs (T26-T28) are classified by site, but not by degree.

1) **Sequencing of burn and related condition codes**

   Sequence first the code that reflects the highest degree of burn when more than one burn is present.

   a. When the reason for the admission or encounter is for treatment of external multiple burns, sequence first the code that reflects the burn of the highest degree.

   b. When a patient has both internal and external burns, the circumstances of admission govern the selection of the principal diagnosis or first-listed diagnosis.

   c. When a patient is admitted for burn injuries and other related conditions such as smoke inhalation and/ or respiratory failure, the circumstances of admission govern the selection of the principal or first-listed diagnosis.

2) **Burns of the same local site**

   Classify burns of the same local site (three-character category level, T20-T28) but of different degrees to the subcategory identifying the highest degree recorded in the diagnosis.

3) **Non-healing burns**

   Non-healing burns are coded as acute burns.

   Necrosis of burned skin should be coded as a non-healed burn.

4) **Infected Burn**

   For any documented infected burn site, use an additional code for the infection.

5) **Assign separate codes for each burn site**

   When coding burns, assign separate codes for each burn site. Category T30, Burn and corrosion, body region unspecified is extremely vague and should rarely be used.

6) **Burns and Corrosions Classified According to Extent of Body Surface Involved**

   Assign codes from category T31, Burns classified according to extent of body surface involved, or T32, Corrosions classified according to extent of body surface involved, when the site of the burn is not specified or when there is a need for additional data. It is advisable to use category T31 as additional coding when needed to provide data for evaluating burn mortality, such as that needed by burn units. It is also advisable to use category T31 as an additional code for reporting purposes when there is mention of a third-degree burn involving 20 percent or more of the body surface.

   Categories T31 and T32 are based on the classic "rule of nines" in estimating body surface involved: head and neck are assigned nine percent, each arm nine percent, each leg 18 percent, the anterior trunk 18 percent, posterior trunk 18 percent, and genitalia one percent. Providers may change these percentage assignments where necessary to accommodate infants and children who have proportionately larger heads than adults, and patients who have large buttocks, thighs, or abdomen that involve burns.

7) **Encounters for treatment of sequela of burns**

   Encounters for the treatment of the late effects of burns or corrosions (i.e., scars or joint contractures) should be coded with a burn or corrosion code with the 7th character "S" for sequela.

8) **Sequelae with a late effect code and current burn**

   When appropriate, both a code for a current burn or corrosion with 7th character "A" or "D" and a burn or corrosion code with 7th character "S" may be assigned on the same record (when both a current burn and sequelae of an old burn exist). Burns and corrosions do not heal at the same rate and a current healing wound may still exist with sequela of a healed burn or corrosion.

   See Section I.B.10 Sequela (Late Effects)

9) **Use of an external cause code with burns and corrosions**

   An external cause code should be used with burns and corrosions to identify the source and intent of the burn, as well as the place where it occurred.

Source: CMS 2018.

For practice assigning diagnosis codes to emergency department cases, complete the exercises in There's a Code for That 10.4.

Emergency department diagnoses

10.4

There's a Code for That

Read the following documentation and select the appropriate diagnosis code(s).

1. Patient presents to the ED with acute STEMI of the circumflex coronary artery.

   ICD-10-CM code: _____

2. Patient presents to the ED with STEMI of the left anterior descending coronary artery. Patient had a STEMI of the left main coronary artery two months ago.

   ICD-10-CM codes: _____, _____

3. Patient presents to ED in septic shock with acute kidney failure due to MRSA septicemia.

   ICD-10-CM codes: _____, _____, _____

4. 45-year-old male suffered second degree corrosive burns of both hands (including wrists) and arms in a work-related chemical spill. Total of 32 percent body surface burned. (Code for the burns only).

   ICD-10-CM codes: _____, _____, _____,
   _____

Putting It All Together: Coding for Urgent Care and ED Services

To select the correct codes for urgent care or emergency department coding it is important to carefully read the documentation, then access each code book to find the procedure or service provided, and the corresponding diagnosis or diagnoses to support the medical necessity for the service. Procedural codes for urgent care and ED services are found in the CPT code book, and diagnosis codes are found in the ICD-10-CM code book.

Determination of the correct codes relies on the answers to the following questions.

- What services were provided to the patient?
    - Was an E/M service provided?
        - For urgent care E/M encounters use the outpatient office E/M codes 99201 through 99215.
        - For emergency department E/M encounters use 99281 through 99285.
    - Were any additional procedures performed, such as labs, x-rays, or other imaging services, or any additional medical or surgical procedures?
- Are there any applicable modifiers or add-on codes?
- Is there a definitive diagnosis for the encounter? If yes, this should be the first-listed diagnosis code. If not, then use the code for the signs or symptoms.
- For injuries, include codes to identify the external causes with the appropriate seventh-character extension to identify the encounter.

Study the following vignette that demonstrates how to select the appropriate diagnosis and procedure codes. Then complete the practice exercises in There's a Code for That 10.5.

April is coding for an urgent care encounter for a 60-year-old female new patient who presented to the clinic complaining of dizziness and slight nausea. She reports that she has recently just gotten over (two days ago) a sinusitis infection and head cold, for which she was on a Z-pack. Her last dose of antibiotics was two days ago. The physician assistant performed a detailed history and examination, with moderate complexity MDM, and diagnosed the patient with vestibular labyrinthitis, bilateral. Procedures performed in the clinic include a 50 mg IM injection of Phenergan (promethazine), and 12-lead ECG to rule out cardiac arrhythmia. Labs included cardiac enzymes (CK-MB, Myoglobin, Troponin), CBC (automated, complete), and blood glucose. CBC revealed slightly lowered WBC and RBC counts. Physician prescribed oral antihistamines and instructed patient to return as necessary if symptoms don't subside in one week.

First, April asks herself: What did the healthcare provider do? The physician assistant performed an E/M encounter for a new patient in the urgent care setting, which she will code using the appropriate E/M encounter code from 99201 to 99205 with a modifier -25, to indicate that the E/M service was a significant, separately identifiable service from the procedures performed. The provider also administered a Phenergan injection, so she will need to code for the therapeutic injection as well as the substance, using a HCPCS code. Additional procedures included an ECG, a cardiac enzyme panel, a CBC, and a glucose test. Coding for the cardiac enzymes test requires that she select one code for each of the blood components that was tested for (to find these she goes to the Pathology and Laboratory, Chemistry entry in the Index and searches for each individual component). She selects the following codes:

Phenergan injection ⎰
⎱

Cardiac enzymes ⎰
⎱

- **99203-25, *Level 3 office visit, new patient***
- **96372, *Therapeutic, prophylactic, or diagnostic injection (specify substance or drug); submuscular or intramuscular***
- **J2550, *Injection, promethazine HCL, up to 50 mg***
- **93000, *Electrocardiogram, routine ECG with at least 12 leads; with interpretation and report***
- **82550, *Creatine kinase (CK), (CPK); total***
- **82553, *Creatine kinase (CK), (CPK); MB fraction only***
- **83874, *Myoglobin***
- **84484, *Troponin, quantitative***
- **85027, *Blood count; complete (CBC), automated (Hgb, Hct, RBC, WBC and platelet count)***
- **82947, *Glucose; quantitative, blood (except reagent strip)***

Now that she has the procedure codes, April asks herself: Why did the physician assistant do it? In this case, the patient was diagnosed with vestibular labyrinthitis, which was the definitive diagnosis, so it includes the additional symptoms of dizziness and nausea. April searches under the term Labyrinthitis *in the Main Index of the ICD-10-CM code book, and references subcategory H83.0- for the code, and she chooses the following:*

- *H83.03, Labyrinthitis, bilateral*

She then rechecks the documentation to make sure she has coded everything for the encounter, and reports the chosen codes on the claim for the service.

Coding for urgent care and emergency department services

Read the following documentation and select the appropriate CPT, HCPCS, and ICD-10-CM code(s).

1. Patient presents to the ED with right lower quadrant pain. Abdominopelvic CT (computed tomography) performed without contrast revealed acute unperforated appendicitis. After IV antibiotics administered in the ED, symptoms, WBC, and fever resolved satisfactorily and patient was discharged home, with a delayed (interval) appendectomy scheduled in 6 weeks. Comprehensive history and examination, with high complexity MDM in the ED setting. (Hint: do not code for the IV antibiotics or WBC).

   CPT codes: _____, _____,

   ICD-10-CM code: _____

2. 15-year-old male established patient presented to the urgent care clinic in the evening hours with moderate persistent asthma with acute exacerbation. Pulse oximetry revealed oxygen level of 89 percent, pressurized nebulizer treatment provided in the office. Provider performed an expanded problem-focused examination with moderate complexity MDM. Flu shot (IIV3) 0.5mL also administered in the office intramuscularly without counseling.

   CPT codes: _____ - _____, _____,

   _____, _____, _____,

   _____, _____

   ICD-10-CM code: _____

3. Patient received in the ED after MVA with traumatic pneumothorax. She was driving her pick-up truck when she began hydroplaning on a wet patch of road, hit a median, and flipped over, pinning her between her seat and the steering wheel. Tube thoracostomy performed in the ED and patient was transferred to the hospital for continued observation and treatment.

   CPT codes: _____

   ICD-10-CM code (code for the injury and the MVA only):
   _____, _____

End of Chapter Content

Instructions: Indicate whether the following statements are true or false (T or F). For false statements, rewrite the statement on the line below to make the statement true.

1. In an emergent situation, a patient is suffering from a life- or limb-threatening injury.

   _____

   _____

(Continued on next page)

(Continued)

2. The place of service code is optional for medical claims.

_____

_____

3. Box 24.C of the CMS-1500 claim form is used to identify the place of service for the claim.

_____

_____

4. Outpatient office E/M codes are used to report encounters in the urgent care setting

_____

_____

5. A complete x-ray has at least the minimum number of views described in the CPT code for the complete service.

_____

_____

6. The professional component of an ECG consists of the healthcare provider reading and interpreting the test results.

_____

_____

7. Semi-permanent casts are often performed in the urgent care setting as a treatment for fractures until the patient can be seen by an orthopedist for definitive treatment.

_____

_____

8. There are three categories of complexity for would repair codes.

_____

_____

9. Coding for wound repair requires adding up the same lengths of the same sites and the same complexity.

_____

_____

10. An ED encounter is coded with inpatient observation codes from the E/M chapter.

_____

_____

Instructions: Choose the best answer.

1. In which of the following situations would a patient present to an urgent care clinic?

   a. After a severe car accident, having suffered traumatic, life-threatening injury

   b. When he has a high fever and his regular doctor is not available

   c. After falling from a tree and suffering a compound (open) fracture

   d. When he needs a routine physical examination

2. Which place of service code should be used for ED coding?

   a. 20

   b. 21

   c. 22

   d. 23

3. Which of the following is true regarding coding for urgent care and ED services?

   a. Only a small selection of CPT codes is used

   b. Many CPT codes are used, but not many ICD-10-CM codes

   c. It requires a good working knowledge of all sections of the CPT and ICD-10-CM code books

   d. E/M codes are the same for both settings

4. Which of the following type of procedures are used to determine the patient diagnosis for infectious diseases?

   a. X-rays and imaging services

   b. E/M encounters

   c. Surgical procedures

   d. Laboratory tests

5. Which of the following is a simple test that can diagnose a cardiac arrhythmia?

   a. Pulse oximetry

   b. Nebulizer treatment

   c. Electrocardiogram

   d. Incision and drainage

6. Which of the following describes an orthosis?

   a. An external device designed to immobilize a body part

   b. An internal device used to assist in surgical procedures

   c. A procedure to open airways allowing the patient to breathe more easily

   d. An injection of a therapeutic substance

7. Wound repairs are coded in which of the following?

   a. in

   b. cm

   c. mg

   d. mL

8. The time reported for moderate (conscious) sedation is for which component of the procedure?

   a. Preservice work

   b. Intraservice work

   c. Postservice work

   d. The entire procedure from start to finish

9. Which of the following is a procedure used to open the airways using instrumentation inserted into the mouth?

   a. Tracheostomy

   b. Tracheotomy

   c. Needle thoracotomy

   d. Endotracheal intubation

10. Codes for penetrating wound exploration include which of the following?

    a. Exploration and extension of the wound

    b. Major repair to blood vessels

    c. Repair of internal organs

    d. Extensive scar revision

11. When sequencing codes for injuries, which code should go first?

    a. The code for the least severe injury

    b. Sequencing does not matter

    c. The code for the most severe injury

    d. The codes should be sent on separate claims

12. Which of the following could cause systemic inflammatory response syndrome (SIRS)?

    a. An underlying infection
    b. A traumatic injury
    c. A routine physical examination
    d. Septicemia

Instructions: Answer the following question with the appropriate code(s) and modifier(s).

13. A 35-year-old male patient presents to the ED with anterior dislocation of left shoulder. He was wrestling (horseplay) while at work at a heavy truck body shop and his arm was twisted out of its socket by his opponent. He appears in good spirits but is in pain, and would like to undergo moderate sedation for the reduction procedure. Risks and benefits of the procedure explained. Moderate sedation was achieved using Ketamine, and the dislocation reduction took approximately 30 minutes due to difficulty in determining if the joint was back in place. E/M encounter involved comprehensive history and examination with high complexity MDM performed. (Tip: moderate sedation does not count as an anesthesia service.)

    CPT codes: _____ - ____, _____,

    _____, _____

    ICD-10-CM code: _____, _____

References

Ahmadinejad, M., S. Karamouzian, and M. Lashkarizadeh. 2011. Use of Glasgow Coma Scale as an Indicator for Early Tracheostomy in Patients with Severe Head Injury. *Tannafos* 10(1): 26–30. https://www.ncbi.nlm.nih.gov/pmc/articles/PMC4153128/.

American Medical Association. 2017 (January). *Current Procedural Terminology (CPT)*. Chicago: AMA.

Blausen.com staff. 2013. "Lumbar Puncture." Digital Image. Wikimedia Commons. Accessed December, 2017. https://en.wikipedia.org/wiki/Lumbar_puncture#/media/File:Blausen_0617_LumbarPuncture.png.

Centers for Medicare and Medicaid Services. 2018. ICD-10-CM Official Guidelines for Coding and Reporting FY 2018. https://www.cms.gov/Medicare/Coding/ICD10/Downloads/2018-ICD-10-CM-Coding-Guidelines.pdf.

Centers for Medicare and Medicaid Services. 2017. Details for title: CMS 1500. https://www.cms.gov/Medicare/CMS-Forms/CMS-Forms/CMS-Forms-Items/CMS1188854.html.

Hackethal, V. 2017 (August 16). Skip Pulse Oximetry in Bronchiolitis, Experts Say. https://www.medscape.com/viewarticle/884396.

US Department of Health and Human Services. 2013. "Lund-Browder chart." Radiation Emergency Medical Management. Digital Image. Accessed December, 2017. https://www.remm.nlm.gov/burns.htm.

US National Library of Medicine Medline Plus. 2017. Chest Tube Insertion. https://medlineplus.gov/ency/article/002947.htm.

Resources

Agency for Healthcare Research and Quality. 2014 (June). Healthcare Cost and Utilization Project Statistical Brief #174. https://www.hcup-us.ahrq.gov/reports/statbriefs/sb174-Emergency-Department-Visits-Overview.pdf.

American College of Emergency Physicians. 2016. ED Facility Level Coding Guidelines. https://www.acep.org/content.aspx?id=30428.

Journal of Urgent Care Medicine. 2008 (July). National Urgent Care Chart Survey. http://jucm.com/pdf/JUCM_Urgent_Care_Chart_Research.pdf.

University of Texas Health Science Center at Houston School of Public Health. 2011 (July). Top Twenty Primary Discharge Diagnoses in the Emergency Room in Harris County, Texas in 2009: Breakdown by Age and Payer Source. https://sph.uth.edu/content/uploads/2011/12/Top-2009-ER-diagnoses-by-age-and-payer-source.pdf.

Surgical Services

Learning Objectives

- Understand the basics of billing and coding for surgical services performed in the inpatient hospital, outpatient hospital, and ambulatory surgical center (ASC) settings.
- Examine the basics of coding for surgical procedures from the CPT Surgery section.

- Examine procedural codes, diagnosis codes, and guidelines for surgical services performed in the inpatient hospital, outpatient hospital, and ASC settings.
- Determine and apply ICD-10-CM, CPT, and HCPCS codes to surgical services.

Key Terms

Ablation
Admitting provider
Allograft
Ambulatory surgical center (ASC)
Appendectomy
Appendicitis
Autograft
Block
Cadaver donor
Cholangiography
Cholangitis
Cholecystectomy
Cholecystitis
Choledocholithiasis
Cholelithiasis
Code edit
Comorbid condition
Complication of care
Debridement
Destruction
Diagnostic procedure
Diaphragm

Endoscopy
Excised diameter
Excision
Global period
Global surgical package
Homograft
Incidental appendectomy
Incision
Introduction
Laparoscopy
Living donor
Manipulation
Margin
Mediastinum
Mohs micrographic surgery
National Correct Coding Initiative
 (NCCI)
Never events
Non-pressure ulcer
Outpatient
Outpatient hospital
Paring

Performing provider
Peritonitis
Postoperative diagnosis
Preoperative diagnosis
Pressure ulcer
Removal
Repair
Resection
Rhinoplasty
Robot-assisted surgery
Separate procedure
Shaving
Skin lesion
Skin ulcer
Stage
Surgical procedure
Therapeutic procedure
Transplantation
Unbundling
Xenograft

The complexities of coding in the surgical setting are fundamental to and challenging for novice coders. A surgical procedure is any single, separate, systematic process upon or within the body that can be complete in itself; is normally performed by a physician, dentist, or other licensed practitioner; can be performed either with or without instruments; and is performed to restore disunited or deficient parts, remove diseased or injured tissues, extract foreign matter, assist in obstetrical delivery, or aid in diagnosis. Surgical procedures require a skilled practitioner to use manual and instrumental techniques to treat, investigate, or diagnose a patient's healthcare condition. Surgical procedures may also be performed to improve bodily function, change appearance, and repair body structures and organs.

Surgeries are, by definition, invasive procedures that usually involve breaking the skin in order to perform the procedure. (Medical procedures, on the other hand, are less invasive, and rarely break the skin, if only minimally). They range from highly invasive and risky, such as transplant surgeries and internal organ repairs, to minimally or practically noninvasive like wart cryosurgery. Thus, the settings in which surgeries are performed depend greatly on the *type* of surgery performed. This chapter discusses various types of surgeries and the different settings in which they are performed (inpatient hospital, outpatient hospital, and ambulatory surgical centers). It does not discuss minimally invasive surgeries that are often performed in the outpatient office setting, such as those performed in primary care (discussed in chapter 8). This chapter also discusses the different surgical specialists who provide these services and the basics of coding for surgeries, including changes in the place of service and procedural and diagnostic coding for surgeries.

Surgical Billing and Coding Basics

Coding for surgical services requires a solid understanding of human anatomy and physiology, including medical terminology, the way surgical procedures are performed, and the terminology used to describe them. There are numerous settings in which surgeries are performed, determined by the complexity and riskiness of the procedure; also there are specific procedures approved for certain settings. This chapter also addresses surgical coding and billing in general, as well as the different types of surgical specialists.

Surgical Settings

Given the various types of surgical procedures and the resources required to perform them, only certain surgical procedures may be performed in particular healthcare settings. Depending on the resources required and risks involved in performing the procedures, some minimally invasive surgeries, such as a biopsy, may be performed in the outpatient office setting. However, the majority of surgical procedures are performed in an inpatient hospital, outpatient hospital, or ambulatory surgical center.

Inpatient Hospital

Inpatients are patients that have been formally admitted to a hospital. Inpatient hospital surgeries typically involve a patient that has been admitted to a specific floor or unit, where they reside before or after the surgery. For example, a patient may be admitted to an inpatient facility for a surgery that involves admission to a room in the hospital where a preoperative evaluation and pre-procedural treatments are performed, after which the surgery is performed in the surgical suite or operating room. The patient then stays in the hospital until he or she has recovered from the surgery enough to be discharged either to the patient's home or to another facility (such as a rehabilitation hospital). This process is usually at least overnight but can also be a longer period of time, lasting weeks or more. It depends on the type of surgery performed, severity of the patient's condition, and any other comorbidities or complications that may develop (discussed later in this chapter).

When a surgery is performed in an inpatient facility, like an inpatient hospital, the doctor that performs the surgery reports the CPT code as well as any other procedural codes, such as E/M services; and the hospital facility reports the service the provider performed using ICD-10-PCS codes, which are inpatient procedural codes. This allows the healthcare provider to bill for the services that he or she performed, such as a surgery or anesthesia service, and also allows the hospital to identify the service performed to justify the cost of the hospital resources for the patient while the services were being provided. Both the surgeon and the facility report ICD-10-CM (diagnosis) codes to identify the medical necessity for the service. This chapter only discusses the ICD-10-CM and CPT codes that are involved in performing surgical procedures, as would be billed by the performing surgeon. The inpatient facility (hospital) would report the ICD-10-CM and ICD-10-PCS codes involved in the procedure. Inpatient facility coding (using ICD-10-PCS codes) is discussed in chapter 20 (Inpatient Hospital Services) (see figure 11.1). Note, however, that the codes used to report procedures (either CPT/HCPCS or ICD-10-PCS) will depend on each individual facility. For example, some hospital outpatient facilities may report ICD-10-PCS codes, while others will report only CPT and HCPCS for procedures.

Figure 11.1. Facility inpatient versus professional outpatient coding

Codes Used to Identify	Inpatient Facility Services	Outpatient Professional Services
Diagnosis	ICD-10 **CM**	ICD-10 **CM**
Procedure	ICD-10 **PCS**	CPT
Supplies and Services	Hospital Service Codes	HCPCS
	↑	↑
	Reported by the hospital	Reported by the surgeon

When coding for services performed in the inpatient setting, like surgeries, it is easy to get confused between inpatient and outpatient coding. Inpatient facilities provide the room, board, equipment, and other supplies and services so the healthcare provider can perform the procedure, so the facilities bill for these items. They are like a medical hotel. The healthcare provider who performed the service bills only for the service that he or she performed, such as a surgery or anesthesia service. Therefore, the codes reported by the healthcare provider who performed the service are CPT codes that identify the specific procedures performed.

Inpatient hospital services reported by the physician (including observation stays and discharges) are billed with a special set of evaluation and management (E/M) codes, 99221 to 99239 (refer to chapters 7 and 8 for a discussion of E/M codes). These codes are used for a patient who has been formally admitted to a hospital as an inpatient, and a healthcare provider performs an E/M encounter with this patient. This healthcare provider does not have to be the admitting provider (the provider who admitted the patient to the hospital) nor the **performing** (or rendering) **provider** (the provider performing the surgery or other service), it can be any provider who performs an E/M encounter.

When billing for services provided in the inpatient hospital setting, it is necessary to use the place of service (POS) code 21, Inpatient Hospital, on the CMS-1500 form in box 24.B to identify that the procedure was performed in "a facility, other than psychiatric, which primarily provides diagnostic, therapeutic (both surgical and nonsurgical), and rehabilitation services by, or under, the supervision of physicians to patients admitted for a variety of medical conditions" (AMA 2017) (see figure 11.2).

Figure 11.2. CMS-1500 box 24.B: Place of service code 21-Inpatient Hospital

Source: CMS 2017a.

Outpatient Hospital

An **outpatient hospital** is a part of the hospital facility designed to treat patients who do not need to be admitted as an inpatient or a bed for overnight care. It may be an actual part of the hospital or a separate building that provides outpatient services to patients such as diagnostic tests, screenings, and minor surgical procedures. An **outpatient** is a patient who has not been admitted as an inpatient, but is still receiving services from the hospital facility. A patient who is staying in the main building of the hospital might be an outpatient because the physicians do not expect the patient to stay overnight or for an extended period of time, and thus he or she has not been formally admitted as an inpatient of the facility.

Because the patient has not been admitted and is considered outpatient, the E/M cods used to bill for these services are the same as those used for outpatient office encounters: 99201 to 99215 (first discussed in chapter 7). The place of service code indicates that the outpatient service was performed in the outpatient hospital setting, rather than the outpatient office setting (POS 11). Outpatient hospital codes are reported with POS code 22, On Campus-Outpatient Hospital. This POS location code is for "a portion of a hospital's main campus which provides diagnostic, therapeutic (both surgical and nonsurgical), and rehabilitation services to sick or injured persons who do not require hospitalization or institutionalization" (AMA 2017). See figure 11.3.

Figure 11.3. CMS-1500 box 24.B: Place of service code 22-On Campus Outpatient Hospital

Source: 2017a.

Ambulatory Surgical Center (ASC)

An **ambulatory surgical center (ASC)** is an outpatient healthcare facility not affiliated with a hospital that specializes in diagnostic, preventive, and surgical procedures. As a well-equipped healthcare facility that can offer surgical interventions, ASCs perform surgical procedures outside of the hospital setting (either inpatient or outpatient). Often ASCs are owned by a group of physicians and some specialize in the type of services that are performed. For example, a group of ophthalmologists (eye surgeons) may open an ASC together in which they can perform surgical procedures on their own patients.

ASCs can thus provide the surgical services that a hospital can provide, but at a much lower cost to patients. This lower cost is because an ASC does not have to maintain the same overhead (in terms of staff and facility resources) that a large inpatient facility does. Furthermore, because an ASC can operate as an outpatient hospital, it may not have to charge the additional inpatient facility fees (ICD-10-PCS and hospital service codes, addressed in chapter 20) that an inpatient hospital charges. However, not *all* surgical procedures can be performed in the ASC setting, as only approved procedures may be safely performed at an ASC. Approved procedures are determined by the third-party payer according to the patient's insurance policy. ASCs do not have all the life-saving equipment and staff on hand (like a hospital) to handle large-scale operations that involve several medical and surgical specialists. Furthermore, because they are outpatient facilities, the procedures performed at the ASC must not require an overnight stay.

As an outpatient facility, the outpatient office E/M codes are used for evaluation and management encounters in the ASC setting: 99201 to 99215. The place of service code indicates that the procedure took place in an ASC, rather than the outpatient office setting (POS 11); ASC codes are reported with POS 24, Ambulatory Surgical Center. This POS location code is for "a free-standing facility, other than a physician's office, where surgical and diagnostic services are provided on an ambulatory basis" (AMA 2017). See figure 11.4.

Figure 11.4. CMS-1500 box 24.B: Place of service code 23-Ambulatory Surgical Center

Source: CMS 2017a.

Approved Procedures by Site

Surgeries differ significantly depending on how invasive they are, how medically risky they are, how long they take, and what resources (staff, equipment) are required to perform the surgery. Therefore, certain healthcare settings are restricted to a set of approved procedures. Typically, these restrictions are set by third-party payers, who may or may not approve certain procedures at specific types of facilities depending on the facility's available resources. Other restrictions may be in place because of a lack of resources, such as the absence of an intensive care unit or the lack of available clinical staff (for example, a cardiothoracic surgeon in the area). Generally, inpatient hospitals are not restricted to a certain set of approved procedures because these facilities are equipped to perform more complex, resource-intensive surgeries (such as high-risk and trauma surgeries). That being said, if a hospital does not have the required resources in order to perform a complex or high-risk procedure (such as a heart transplant on a pediatric patient), then the patient will likely be transferred to a hospital with the necessary resources.

Outpatient hospitals and ASCs may perform minor surgeries like biopsies, endoscopies, injections, cataract surgeries, arthrocentesis, hernia repair, tonsillectomies and adenoidectomies, arthroscopies, carpal tunnel and trigger release, and bunionectomies, as well as laparoscopic surgical procedures.

Services that may be provided by ASCs and outpatient clinics are also limited by payer regulations. For example, Medicare will not pay for just any service that is performed at an ASC; it must be included on the list of approved services in the ASC setting. These procedures have been determined by Medicare to not pose a significant safety risk, and they are not expected to result in an overnight stay following the procedure. For example, surgical procedures performed at an ASC must meet the following criteria to be covered by Medicare:

- It must not pose a significant safety risk to the patient
- It cannot require an overnight stay or monitoring past midnight
- It cannot be reported using an unlisted services code (CMS 2016)

These criteria differ annually and from payer to payer, depending on the circumstances. It is always a good idea to verify if any planned service would be covered in the ASC setting with the patient's individual insurance policy.

ASC coding is also much more complicated than simply complying with a list of approved procedures. It requires an understanding of facility and professional fee coding, sometimes referred to as "pro-fee" coding, as ASCs typically perform both. The way an ASC bills for services depends on the way the ASC is set up. Some use the CMS-1500 form for outpatient billing and report CPT and HCPCS codes for services performed; others use the UB-04 form for inpatient billing (discussed in chapter 20, Inpatient Hospital Services) and report ICD-10-PCS codes to identify the services performed. For the purposes of this chapter, it is assumed that the ASC reports ICD-10-CM, CPT, and HCPCS codes and bills services on the CMS-1500 claim form. ASCs also have a specific set of CPT modifiers to be used exclusively for the ASC setting. These modifiers are discussed later in this chapter.

Surgical Packages and Billing for Services

Imagine leaving a grocery store with a bag of groceries, inside of which is everything needed to make a specific recipe. At home, you use all of the ingredients together to make that one dish. Coding for surgeries is similar to cooking a specific recipe. Instead of coding for each item—such as a preoperative evaluation and preparation, then an incision, then a surgical procedure, then the skin repair, followed by the postoperative evaluation, and a two-week follow-up examination and the removal of stitches or staples—the coder only reports *one* code that identifies all of these components.

The global surgical package is a set of services included within a single code that identifies the surgery performed, other services integral to the procedure, and a specific amount of time after the surgery. This amount of time included in the surgical package is referred to as the global period, and is defined by each individual insurance carrier. For example, Insurance A may have a 14-day global period for a specific procedure, while Insurance B has a 20-day global period for a specific procedure. It is important to verify the specific length of the global period with the insurance payer for each procedure performed on the patient. There are three types of global surgical packages that fit the Medicare definitions of each type of global period, depending on the type of surgical procedure performed.

- *Simple procedures, zero global period.* These are simple procedures, like an endoscopy, without any preoperative or postoperative procedures; the global period is only the day of the procedure.

- *Minor surgical procedures, 10-day global period.* For minor surgeries, such as wound repairs, the global period starts on the day of the procedure. This global period includes 11 total days (the day of the procedure and the additional 10-day global period).

- *Major surgical procedures, 90-day global period.* This type of surgery includes one day of preoperative care, so the global period starts the day before the surgery, unless the decision to perform the surgery was made on the day of the surgery. This global period includes 92 total days (the day before the procedure, the day of the procedure, and then the additional 90-day global period). An example of a major surgical procedure would be the insertion of a pacemaker or major organ transplant.

As a coder, it is important to understand surgical packages and what is included within the package because it will impact the modifiers and any additional services reported for the surgery. An evaluation and management encounter that results in the decision for surgery should be reported with modifier -57 to identify it as a separate encounter that excludes it from the surgical package, so it is reimbursed separately.

Each surgical package includes a bundle of procedures, which are all identified by one code:

- Pre-treatment (either the day before a major procedure or the day of a minor procedure)

- Preoperative care

- Surgical services including local infiltration or topical anesthesia, the surgery itself, immediate postoperative care, dictation of operative notes, and meetings or discussions with the patient or family and other physicians

- Evaluation of the patient in the recovery or post-anesthesia care unit (PACU)

- Writing orders for the patient

- Some surgeries also include conscious sedation within the global package

- Postoperative follow-up care (for up to 10 or 90 days, depending on the procedure)

- All services in the postoperative period, other than a return to the operating room (see figure 11.5) (CMS 2017b)

Figure 11.5. Surgical package

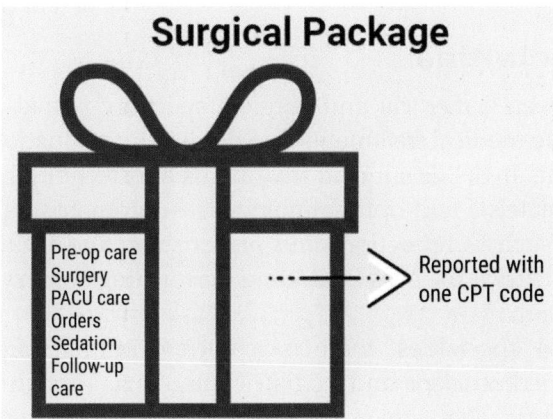

If the patient returns for an encounter for something *unrelated* to the surgery, then it may be billed separately, using the appropriate modifier.

It is possible to separate the surgical package and bill for only portions of the service using the appropriate modifier. Breaking up a surgical package is called **unbundling**, the practice of using multiple codes to bill for the individual steps in a single procedure rather than using a single code that includes all the steps of the comprehensive procedure. Unbundling may be considered unnecessary or improper coding, and codes that have been unbundled from a surgical package may be denied by the third-party payer. However, in some instances it may be necessary to report individual codes to identify procedures that are distinct from the primary surgical procedure. These individual services are referred to as separate procedures (refer to chapter 5), and are identified in the CPT code descriptions with the statement "separate procedure" in parentheses. As discussed in chapter 5, a **separate procedure** is one that is commonly part of another, more complex procedure, but which may be performed independently or be otherwise unrelated to the procedure. For example, code 44850, Suture of mesentery (separate procedure).

According to CPT guidelines, codes that are identified as separate procedures may be reported with a primary service when the separate procedure reports a service unrelated to or independent of the other procedure(s) performed. The separate procedure code should be appended with modifier -59 to indicate that it was a distinct procedural service from the other procedure(s) performed. Separate procedure codes should be reported with a modifier -59 when they are performed at a different operative session, during a different procedure or surgery, in a different anatomical site or organ system; or with a separate incision, excision, lesion, or injury (AMA 2017).

When reporting multiple surgeries or procedures performed on the same date, it may be necessary to check for code edits with the insurance payer. A **code edit** is an accuracy checkpoint in the claims-processing software that ensures all codes are valid and may be reported in conjunction with each other, and if any modifiers are necessary. An example of an accuracy edit may be to check that a female procedure (like a hysterectomy) was performed only on a female patient.

CMS has instituted a national code editing system called **National Correct Coding Initiative (NCCI)** edits. NCCI was developed to promote national correct coding methodologies and to control improper coding leading to inappropriate payment in Part B Medicare claims. CMS developed its coding policies based on coding conventions defined in the CPT code book, national and local policies and edits, coding guidelines developed by national societies, analysis of standard medical and surgical practices, and a review of current coding practices (AHIMA 2017). NCCI edits are an important part of coding for surgical procedures because they identify when certain procedures may be reported together, when they may not be reported together, and when a modifier is required.

Surgical Specialties

The difference between a medical and surgical specialty is that a medical specialty performs noninvasive medical treatments and diagnostic evaluations, whereas a surgical specialty performs invasive surgical treatments and techniques. This is the difference between optometrists and ophthalmologists—optometrists perform procedures related to eyesight, such as refractions and prescription and fitting of contact lenses; and ophthalmologists treat the eyes (including performing surgery), such as the repair of a retinal detachment.

For most medical specialties, there is a corresponding surgical specialty. For example, there are pediatricians and pediatric surgeons. There are cardiologists and cardiothoracic surgeons. There are orthopedists and orthopedic surgeons. While both providers focus on the same medical specialty, surgeons receive additional training in surgical techniques and treatments. This chapter discusses surgical procedures, many of which are performed by surgical specialists; services such as those performed by a urologist or a gastroenterologist are discussed throughout this text.

The surgeries discussed within this chapter include those performed by colorectal, general, oral/maxillofacial, plastic and reconstructive, thoracic, vascular, bariatric, pediatric, burn/trauma and wound care, transplant, and foot and ankle surgeons. Orthopedic, neurological and spine, obstetrics and gynecology (OB/GYN) and cardiovascular surgeries are discussed individually in later chapters.

Coding correctly for surgical procedures requires a thorough understanding of the Surgery section of the CPT code book, how the Surgery subsections are organized, and how to select and interpret CPT coding guidelines for surgical services.

Understanding Coding for Surgical Services

Understanding how to code for surgical procedures requires an in-depth understanding of the Surgery section of the CPT code book and its subsections, as well as the ability to interpret and apply CPT guidelines and rules. It also requires an understanding of the different types of surgical procedures.

Exploring the Surgery Subsections

There are 15 subsections within the Surgery section of the CPT code book, each one organized around a certain organ system or body area; they are listed as follows.

- Integumentary
- Musculoskeletal
- Respiratory
- Cardiovascular
- Hemic and Lymphatic
- Mediastinum and Diaphragm
- Digestive
- Urinary
- Male Genital
- Female Genital
- Maternity Care and Delivery
- Endocrine System
- Nervous System
- Eye and Ocular Adnexa
- Auditory System

Each one of these subsections, organized by organ system/body area, contains a number of surgical procedures that are applicable to that specific body system. For example, the Integumentary subsection includes surgical procedures on the skin and accessory structures, such as excision of malignant lesions, skin grafting, burn debridement, and mastectomy procedures.

Each subsection is further subdivided into subheadings that combine surgeries performed on a specific body area or surgeries of the same type. Each subheading contains smaller groups of surgical procedures, called categories. For example, in figure 11.6 the Section name is *Surgery*, the subsection is the *Cardiovascular System*, the first subheading is *Heart and Pericardium*, and the first category is *Pericardium*.

Figure 11.6. Divisions of Cardiovascular subsection

Surgery

Cardiovascular System* (33010–37799)..**201**

The following is a listing of heading and subheadings that pair within the Cardiovascular System section of the CPT codebook. The subheadings or subsections denoted with asterisks (*) below have special instructions unique to that section. Where these are indicated, special "notes" or guidelines will be presented preceding those procedural terminology listings, referring to that subsection specifically.

Heart and Pericardium (33010–33999)..**201**
    Pericardium (33010–33050) 201
    Cardiac Tumor (33120–33130) 201
    Transmyocardial Revascularization (33140–33141)..201
    Pacemaker or Implantable Defibrillator* (33202–33273)..201

Source: AMA 2018, 197.

Subsections of the Surgery section are all divided based on the specific types of procedures performed on each respective body area or organ system. For example, the Cardiovascular subsection is divided first by organ system (Heart and Pericardium, Arteries and Veins), and then by procedure type, specific organ, or condition (Pericardium, Cardiac Tumor, Transmyocardial Revascularization). The Musculoskeletal subsection, on the other hand, contains subheadings for organs (Hand and Fingers, Pelvis and Hip Joint), and subheadings by type of procedure (Application of Casts and Strapping, Endoscopy/Arthroscopy).

Understanding the way that these subsections are organized is integral to coding for surgical procedures. For example, if a coder was looking up a procedure that was performed to treat a cardiac tumor, then he or she could refer to the table of contents at the beginning of the Cardiovascular subsection, find the subheading for Heart and Pericardium, and then the category of codes for Cardiac Tumor (33120 to 33130) (see figure 11.6). Then the coder would refer to that code range to find the code.

Take the time to review the table of contents for each Surgery subsection within the CPT code book, as this will help with understanding the different types of procedures performed in these sections and how they are coded.

Key to Success

Do not overlook the organization of surgical subsections! It is easy to get lost in the CPT code book, especially if you are unfamiliar with the procedure you are looking up. When you are stuck, go back to the beginning of the subsection and look at the table of contents. Make a note of how the subsection is arranged, and find the section for the procedure you are searching for. Does this section of codes match the procedure code that you thought was right in the first place? If so, you are probably in the right place. If not, where did you go wrong?

For practice exploring the surgical subsections of the CPT manual, complete the exercises in There's a Code for That 11.1.

Exploring the surgery subsections

Using the table of contents at the beginning of each subsection in the Surgery section, identify the code range for the following services (the first one has been done for you).

Example: Incision procedures on the pharynx, adenoids, and tonsils (digestive subsection).

CPT code range: *42700–42725*

1. Injection, drainage, or aspiration procedures on the skull, meninges, and brain (nervous system subsection).

CPT code range: _____

2. Arthrodesis procedures on the humerus (upper arm and elbow) (musculoskeletal subsection).

CPT code range: _____

3. Incision procedure on the tunica vaginalis (male genital subsection).

CPT code range: _____

4. Repair procedures on the urethra (urinary subsection).

CPT code range: _____

5. Endoscopy of the cervix uteri (female genital subsection).

CPT code range: _____

Surgical Coding Guidelines

At the beginning of the surgery section in the CPT code book and within each of the Surgery subsections are important guidelines that give instructions on how to use the codes in each of those sections. The guidelines at the beginning of the Surgery section apply to all the codes in that section (10021 through 69990). Additional guidelines are found within each subsection.

Guidelines at the beginning of the Surgery section include the CPT Description of Surgical Package, Follow-Up Care for Diagnostic Procedures, Follow-Up Care for Therapeutic Surgical Procedures, Supplied Materials, Reporting More Than One Procedure/Service, Separate Procedures, Unlisted Services or Procedures, Special Reports, Imaging Guidance, and Surgical Destruction. Coders should refer to these guidelines for definitions and instructions on assigning CPT codes in the Surgery section.

When guidelines are present in the Tabular List of codes (within a subsection), it is important to read through them before assigning a code, as these guidelines discuss when a specific code should be reported versus a different one, as well as is and when specific modifiers should be used. Guidelines also offer descriptions of services and definitions of terms used within the code descriptions. See figure 11.7 for an example of guidelines found in the Surgery section.

Any notes under a subheading (the heading in red in figure 11.7) pertain to all the codes within that subheading. All the notes under a category heading (the heading in blue in figure 11.7), pertain to all the codes within that category only. Any notes under individual codes or sets of codes (standalone and indented codes) pertain to the codes *above* the notes. For example, if an arthrotomy of the temporomandibular joint was done on both sides (bilaterally), then the coder would need to report modifier -50 to identify it as a bilateral service.

Figure 11.7. Guidelines within the Surgery subsection

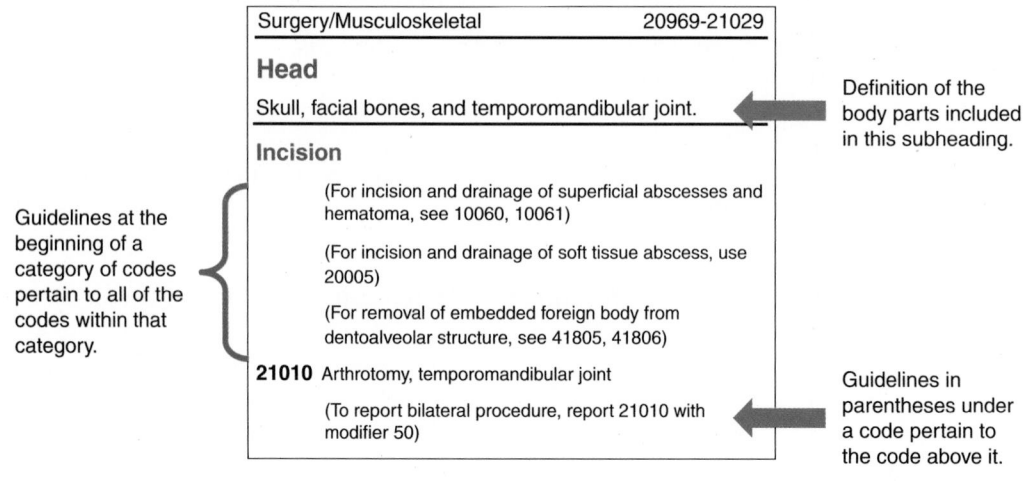

Source: AMA 2018.

Key to Success

It is easy to overlook the parenthetical notes in the Tabular List of the Surgery section, but it is extremely important to read them and follow their instructions. If you have difficulty remembering that the notes are there, it might be a good idea to place a star, underline, or highlight important notes, so you do not forget them.

Types of Surgical Procedures

Categories of codes in the Surgery subsections are groups of procedures that are similar in nature. They are all procedures that use the same instrumentation, surgical technique, or treat a specific condition. Some of these categories are used across all of the subsections of surgical codes. For example, the category Excision is found in all the subsections. The Excision category groups together all of the surgical procedures that are performed to excise a specific organ, body part, or foreign body.

The following procedures include the common surgical categories found in the CPT Surgery section. Note that this is not an all-inclusive list. Additional categories of codes are found in each subsection that are specific to that subsection and may not be found anywhere else in the CPT code book. For example, the Incision and Drainage category is listed in the Integumentary subsection, but not in the Cardiovascular subsection.

- *Incision.* An **incision** is a cut made on a body part or organ. Codes found within an incision category include incision and drainage (I&D) codes and surgical incision codes for exploration, removal of foreign bodies, biopsies, or other surgical service. For example, code 39000, Mediastinotomy with exploration, drainage, removal of foreign body, or biopsy; cervical approach is an incision code. Note that sometimes an entire category is reserved for Incision and Drainage codes, and I&D codes are excluded from the Incision category.

- *Excision.* An **excision** is the surgical removal of an organ, body tissue, lesion, or other body part or foreign object. Note that any excision code is an *open* removal, using a scalpel. For example, an open biopsy of an intranasal lesion includes cutting into the nose to excise the tissue sample (see code 30100, Biopsy, intranasal). On occasion, the term **resection** is used to identify the excision of tissue. In CPT coding, *resection* is the removal of all or part of an organ or body tissue. For example, a resection of the small intestine would be an excision of a portion of tissue from the small intestine (see code 44202, Laparoscopy, surgical; enterectomy, resection of small intestine, single resection and anastomosis).

- *Introduction.* An **introduction** is the insertion of a device, object, or substance into a body part or organ. Introduction codes may sometimes be classified as Injections, in which a therapeutic or diagnostic substance is injected into the patient. An example of an introduction code is 58300, Insertion of intrauterine device (IUD).

- *Removal.* A **removal** is taking out a device, object, or substance from a body part or area. Because removal procedures are sometimes related or performed in conjunction to introduction procedures, some removal codes are included in the same category of codes for Introduction procedures. For example, 58301, Removal of intrauterine device (IUD).

- *Repair.* A **repair** is a procedure performed to return an organ or body part to its original function, or to improve functioning or improve a cosmetic outcome. For example, a rhinoplasty is performed to repair the shape and/or function of the nose, and it may also be done for cosmetic purposes. See code 30400, Rhinoplasty, primary; lateral and alar cartilages and/or elevation of nasal tip.

- *Destruction.* A **destruction**, or **ablation**, is a procedure that destroys tissue. It may be done in several different ways including laser surgery, electrosurgery, cryosurgery, chemosurgery, surgical curettement, radiocautery, radiofrequency ablation, or tissue volume reduction. Note that an ablation differs from an excision, as no tissue remains after a destruction procedure because the tissue is destroyed during the procedure. An excision, however, preserves the tissue but removes it from the body (in this way, many biopsies are excision procedures because the tissue is not destroyed). An example of a destruction procedure is 54050, Destruction of lesion(s), penis (e.g., condyloma, papilloma, molluscum contagiosum, herpetic vesicle), simple; chemical (this is a destruction of penile tissue using chemical destruction).

- *Other Procedures.* The Other Procedures category of codes often lists a specific type of repair or a range of different types of procedures that do not belong in any other category. For example, nasal packing codes are in the Other Procedures category of codes in the Nose subheading of the Respiratory System subsection (see codes 30901 to 30999).

- *Endoscopy.* An **endoscopy** is a procedure performed with the aid of an endoscope. This device has a small camera attached to the end of a long, thin, lighted tube, which is inserted through a natural opening or stoma. The healthcare provider can maneuver the endoscope through a body passage, such as the gastrointestinal tract, to see inside the organ for diagnostic or therapeutic services. The endoscopy is named after the body passageway that is viewed during the procedure. For example, a bronchoscopy is an endoscopic examination of the bronchus, and a cystoscopy is an endoscopic examination of the urinary bladder. Figure 11.8 displays a healthcare provider using a bronchoscope to perform an endoscopic examination of the bronchus and lungs, which would be coded with 31622, Bronchoscopy, rigid or flexible, including fluoroscopic guidance, when performed; diagnostic, with cell washing, when performed (separate procedure).

Figure 11.8. Bronchoscopy

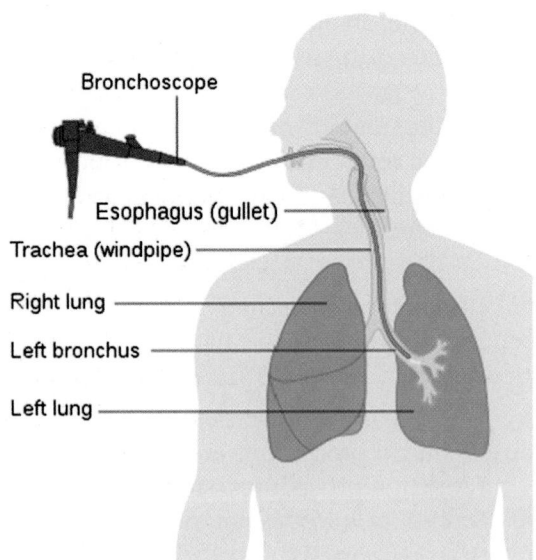

Source: Cancer Research UK, 2014.

Endoscopes are highly specialized instruments and may be used in numerous procedures, such as biopsies and removal of foreign bodies. When coding for endoscopies, it is important to keep in mind that there are three components to endoscopy coding—approach, extent, and surgical versus diagnostic services.

- *Approach*. When coding for an endoscopy, it is necessary to select the code for the correct approach to the procedure. Coders should ask themselves: Where was the endoscope inserted? Note that not all endoscopy codes differ by approach, so this may not always impact code selection.
- *Extent*. The code used to identify the endoscopy differs based on how far the endoscope was inserted in the patient. For example, an endoscopy inserted through the mouth, through the pharynx and larynx, and then stopped at the trachea would be considered a tracheoscopy. If it was inserted all the way into the bronchus, then it would be considered a bronchoscopy. Coders should ask themselves: How far did the endoscopy go? Code to the furthest extent of the endoscopy.
- *Surgical versus diagnostic services*. Endoscopic procedures can be either diagnostic or surgical. A *diagnostic* endoscopy is one that is performed to determine a diagnosis. A *surgical* procedure is one that is performed to treat a diagnosis. Some endoscopy codes are purely diagnostic, whereas others describe an endoscopic procedure in which a surgical treatment was performed, like the removal of a foreign body, biopsy, or placement of a stent. When an endoscopy is done to determine a diagnosis and a surgical procedure is performed during the same endoscopy, then the coder should only report the surgical endoscopy. (More on the difference between diagnostic and surgical, or therapeutic, procedures is discussed in the next section of this chapter). If a surgical endoscopy is performed, code only for the surgical procedure and not the diagnostic endoscopy as well, as the surgery code includes the diagnostic service. When multiple surgical procedures are performed during the same endoscopy, append modifier -51, Multiple procedures, to the codes for the additional procedures performed. Note that modifier -51 is not approved for use by the outpatient hospital

(the facility), but may be reported on the physician's claim for the service. (See figure 11.9 for illustrations of surgical endoscopic procedures.)

Figure 11.9. Surgical endoscopic procedures

Band ligation of esophageal varices

Endoscopic removal of gastric polyp

Snare with fulgurating current

Laser treatment for bleeding ulcer

Snare capture of foreign object

Exposure to laser beam

Sphincterotomy for release of stone in ampulla of Vater

Fulguration

K. Carter

A variety of surgical procedures can be performed endoscopically. If a surgical procedure is performed during the endoscopy, report the code for the surgical procedure, not the diagnostic procedure. Use one code for each surgical procedure performed, with additional codes appended with modifier -51.

- *Laparoscopy.* A **laparoscopy** is similar in nature to an endoscopy, as it uses a lighted scope that is inserted into the body through several small incisions to perform a diagnostic or therapeutic procedure. In this procedure, a fiber-optic laparoscope is inserted through the skin of the abdominal wall, after which air is injected into the abdominal cavity so the surgeon can see and access the internal organs (see figure 11.10). Although they have the same suffix (*-oscopy*), do not confuse a laparoscopic procedure with an endoscopic procedure, as they are two different types of services. Laparoscopic procedures are less invasive than and provide alternatives to open surgeries. So when coding for any type of surgery pay close attention to whether it was performed openly or laparoscopically. Open procedures are found in the Excision category of codes, while laparoscopic procedures are found in the Laparoscopy category of codes. For example, see 51990, Laparoscopy, surgical; urethral suspension for stress incontinence.

A technologically advanced and increasingly utilized type of laparoscopic procedure is **robotic-assisted surgery**, performed with the aid of a robot with miniature instruments controlled by the surgeon (see figure 11.11). Robotic surgeries allow a maximum range of motion and precision and help in reducing surgeon

Figure 11.10. Laparoscopy

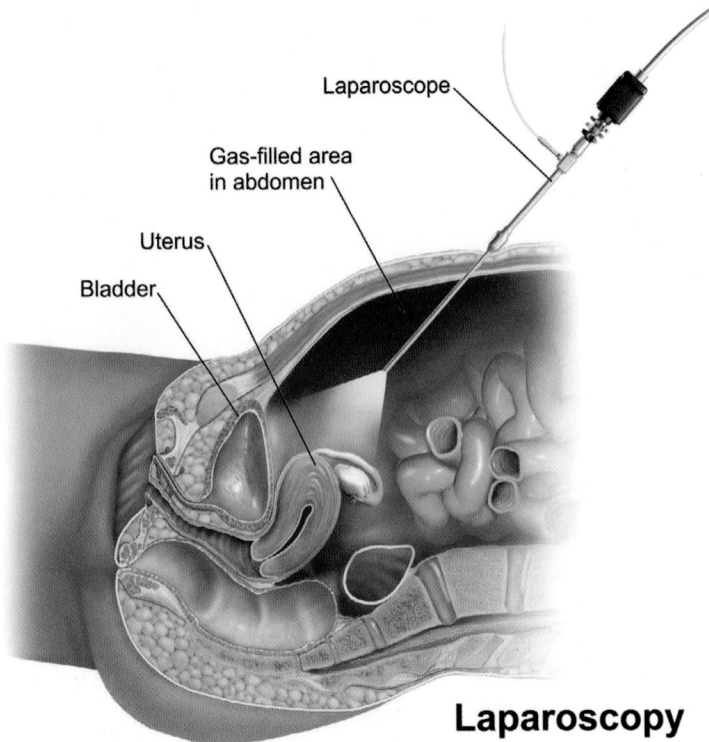

A laparoscopic examination of the peritoneum.
Source: Blausen.com staff, 2014.

Figure 11.11. Robotic-assisted surgery

Source: mathisworks/iStockphoto.com.

fatigue. When coding for a procedure that was performed via robotic-assisted surgery, such as a robotic-assisted laparoscopic hysterectomy, the coder should select the code for the laparoscopic version of the procedure, and append modifier -22, Increased procedural services (more on this modifier in the next section of this chapter). An additional HCPCS code may also be used to identify the service performed with the help of a robotic surgical system: S2900, Surgical techniques requiring use of robotic surgical system. This code should be reported in addition to the code for the primary procedure. However, note that this code is not considered payable by Medicare, and it is unlikely to be reimbursed by a third-party payer. Thus, it is likely to be reported to justify any additional charges (as identified by modifier -22) for the procedure.

Key to Success

Laparoscopic procedures are minimally invasive. They are performed using several small incisions into the body cavity, through which instruments are inserted to perform the surgical procedure (a closed procedure). Any procedure performed laparoscopically ending with the suffix -scopy (or -scopic) are located under the Laparoscopy category in the CPT code book, within each subheading. Open procedures that involve a direct incision into the body cavity through which the surgeon performs the procedure using his or her hands, scalpels, and other tools (an open procedure) are located in the Incision, Excision, Removal, or Repair categories (among others). Keep this important distinction in mind when coding for surgical services. Any procedural description ending in -scopy should be coded as a laparoscopic procedure, *not* an open procedure (see figure 11.12 for more surgical terminology). Note that this does not pertain to endoscopic procedures, which also end with the suffix -oscopy.

- *Transplantation.* A transplantation procedure removes a damaged, diseased, or otherwise nonfunctioning organ from the body and replaces it with a donated organ in its place. Often the new organ is from a donor (either a live or cadaver donor), and sometimes the original organ is left in place. Only a handful of organs in the human body may be transplanted, so the Transplantation category is not found in each of the Surgery subsections. For example, liver transplantations are found in codes 47133 to 47147.

Figure 11.12. Surgical terminology

Surgical Terminology

Surgical Suffix	Meaning	Example
• -otomy	• incision	• laparotomy (incision into abdominal cavity)
• -ectomy	• excision	• nephrectomy (excision of the kidney)
• -plasty	• repair	• rhinoplasty (surgical repair of the nose)
• -pexy	• fixation	• orchiopexy (surgical fixation of the testes)
• -scopy	• performed with endoscope	• bronchoscopy (endoscopic exam of bronchus)
• -ostomy	• creation of surgical opening	• colostomy (opening from colon to external body)
• -graphy	• process of recording	• cholangiography (x-ray recording of bile ducts)

- *Manipulation*. **Manipulation** is manually moving one body part into its original location or into another location. For example, an orthopedist may manually move a fractured radius back into its original location before placing a cast on the outside of the arm to immobilize the extremity. The majority of all manipulation codes are located in the Musculoskeletal System subsection, but a few other manipulation categories are found elsewhere in the Surgery section. See code 27275, Manipulation, hip joint, requiring general anesthesia, as an example of a manipulation code.

Key to Success

There are a number of additional categories of codes found in the Surgery subsections, so as you learn more about surgical coding and become more familiar with surgeries and the CPT codes they represent, you will notice more categories of procedures. When you encounter a category of codes for a procedure for which you are unfamiliar, search for any guidelines that may describe the procedure and utilize a medical dictionary and other reference items to obtain more information about the procedures in that category. This text introduces the beginning coder to some of these procedures, but as medicine and surgical techniques evolve, these categories are sure to change. Being flexible and knowing how to access and use your resources is a helpful way to stay ahead of these changes.

The next section of this chapter discusses the actual CPT codes for surgical services, as well as related diagnosis codes for many different surgical specialties.

Procedural and Diagnostic Coding for Surgical Services

Coding for surgeries requires an understanding of the difference between diagnostic and therapeutic procedures and preoperative and postoperative diagnoses, as well as the ability to correctly report any complication or comorbidities. It further requires the ability to interpret precise procedural descriptions and report them accurately, with the appropriate modifier (if necessary) and a diagnosis code or codes that fully support the medical necessity for the service.

Therapeutic versus Diagnostic Procedures

Procedures can be either therapeutic or diagnostic. A **diagnostic procedure** is one that is performed to determine a diagnosis. For example, a diagnostic bronchoscopy is performed to determine if there is a medical condition within the bronchus or lungs. A **therapeutic procedure** is one that is performed to treat a diagnosis. For example, if a bronchoscopy was performed to remove a foreign body, then this is a therapeutic procedure because it treated the medical condition (removal of the foreign body). Surgical procedures may be either diagnostic or therapeutic.

In some cases, a diagnostic procedure is transformed into a therapeutic procedure. For example, if a diagnostic bronchoscopy was performed due to hemoptysis (coughing up blood) to determine the cause of the condition, and then it was found that a foreign body was present in the bronchus and removed, then the definitive procedure was therapeutic (the removal of the foreign body to treat the diagnosis).

It is important to understand the difference between diagnostic and therapeutic procedures, as some surgical code descriptions include these terms. Although the difference between diagnostic and therapeutic procedures is present throughout the CPT code book, the difference between these two types of procedures is especially important when coding for endoscopies. Endoscopy codes are divided based on if the procedure was diagnostic or therapeutic. For example, 31231, Nasal endoscopy, *diagnostic, unilateral or bilateral (separate procedure)* versus 31237, Nasal endoscopy, *surgical; with biopsy, polypectomy or debridement (separate procedure).*

Pay attention to this type of difference between CPT code descriptions in the surgery section. Any procedure that is performed to determine a diagnosis is a diagnostic procedure; any procedure performed to treat a known diagnosis is a surgical procedure. If the diagnosis is determined during the diagnostic procedure and it is then transformed into a therapeutic procedure, select the code for the therapeutic (or surgical) service.

Preoperative and Postoperative Diagnoses

When a diagnostic procedure is performed and converted into a therapeutic procedure, it is likely done because a medical condition was encountered during the diagnostic procedure and treated at that time. In this case, the preoperative diagnosis was either for a medical screening, or sign or symptom, and the postoperative diagnosis was a definitive diagnosis—the condition that required treatment. Therefore, there are two diagnoses—the preoperative and postoperative diagnoses.

A preoperative diagnosis is the diagnosis given to the patient at the beginning of a procedure. For example, if a patient is coughing up blood and requires a bronchoscopy, then the preoperative diagnosis is hemoptysis. The postoperative diagnosis is the definitive medical condition of the patient either diagnosed or treated during the procedure. For example, if the bronchoscopy discovers a foreign body in the bronchus that was the cause of the hemoptysis, then the postoperative diagnosis is foreign body in the bronchial tube, rather than hemoptysis.

Sometimes the preoperative and postoperative diagnoses are the same, and other times they are different. When these two diagnoses differ, the postoperative diagnosis is the one that should be reported on the claim as the medical necessity for the service. According to the guidelines for outpatient surgical coding, the postoperative diagnosis is the most definitive, which is why it should be reported, rather than the preoperative diagnosis (see figure 11.13).

Using the given example, the preoperative diagnosis for the patient coughing up blood would be R04.2, Hemoptysis, and the postoperative diagnosis would be T17.508A, Unspecified foreign body in bronchus causing other injury, initial encounter. The diagnosis code reported for the procedure would be the latter code, as illustrated in figure 11.14.

In this example, the hemoptysis code would not be reported because it is a symptom of the definitive diagnosis (the foreign body). However, if there were additional,

Figure 11.13. OGCR IV.N

> **N. Ambulatory Surgery**
>
> For ambulatory surgery, code the diagnosis for which the surgery was performed. If the postoperative diagnosis is known to be different from the preoperative diagnosis at the time the diagnosis is confirmed, select the postoperative diagnosis for coding, since it is the most definitive.

Source: CMS 2018.

Figure 11.14. Preoperative versus postoperative diagnosis

> PREOPERATIVE DIAGNOSIS: Hemoptysis
> POSTOPERATIVE DIAGNOSIS: FB in bronchus
> ICD-10-CM Code: T17.508A, Unspecified foreign body in bronchus causing other injury, initial encounter

unrelated signs, symptoms, or comorbid conditions or complications, then those should be reported in addition to the primary diagnosis.

Complications and Comorbidities

As previously mentioned in this chapter, the surgical process from admission to discharge can sometimes be brief and last less than 24 hours, or long and lasting days, weeks, or more. This all depends on the patient's comorbid conditions and any complications of care.

A **comorbid condition** is a chronic or long-term condition that presents along with another chronic or long-term condition; for example, diabetes mellitus and epilepsy. Comorbidities can make recovery from a surgery more difficult or lengthy. When a patient presents with multiple comorbid conditions, each condition should be represented with an individual ICD-10-CM code, with the diagnosis code for the condition that required treatment sequenced first.

An additional consideration for diagnosis coding in the surgical setting is complications of care. A **complication of care** is a condition that occurs as a result of the medical care or surgery. For example, an organ transplant may result in the body rejecting the transplanted organ. This would be a complication of the transplant. To report a condition as a complication of care, the documentation must clearly identify the cause and effect relationship between the surgery (or medical treatment provided) and the resulting complication. If there are any questions about the relationship, the coder should ask the healthcare provider for clarification (see figure 11.15).

Figure 11.15. OGCR I.B.16

---

16. **Documentation of Complications of Care**
   Code assignment is based on the provider's documentation of the relationship between the condition and the care or procedure, unless otherwise instructed by the classification. The guideline extends to any complications of care, regardless of the chapter the code is located in. It is important to note that not all conditions that occur during or following medical care or surgery are classified as complications. There must be a cause-and-effect relationship between the care provided and the condition, and an indication in the documentation that it is a complication. Query the provider for clarification, if the complication is not clearly documented.

Source: CMS 2018.

Codes for complications of care are found in each respective body system chapter in the ICD-10-CM code book, and are often listed as either intraoperative (during the procedure) or postprocedural (after the procedure) complications. For example, code E89.0, Postprocedural hypothyroidism, is listed in chapter 4: Endocrine, Nutritional and Metabolic Diseases, and is the result of a medical procedure.

Coding for complications of care are listed in various areas of the ICD-10-CM code book, and identify complications that may result from surgical procedures throughout the body. When searching for a complication of care, search for the term *Complication* in the ICD-10-CM Index, and then refer to either the specific body system, type of procedure, or resulting medical condition. There are many pages of subterms and cross-references under the term *Complication*, so it is important to pay attention to the main entries and follow all subterms and cross-references carefully.

Key to Success

When searching through long lists of main terms, subterms, and cross-references in the ICD-10-CM Main Index, pay attention to the lines on the far side of each column. These help to orient coders to the main terms and indented terms.

For example, prosthetic left knee joint instability in a patient who underwent a knee transplant two years ago may be coded as a complication of the previous knee joint prosthesis. In this case, the coder would look up *Complication* in the Index, then refer to the subterm *joint prosthesis*, then *mechanical,* and then the specific type of mechanical problem—in this case *instability,* which refers the coder to the code T84.02-. Once the code is identified, it needs to be verified in the Tabular List, and all necessary characters added to make a valid code. In this case, code options identify the laterality and specific joint. The correct code for this example would be T84.023A, Instability of internal left knee prosthesis, initial encounter. Figure 11.16 lists the additional OGCR related to complications of care.

Figure 11.16. OGCR I.C.19.g

---

g. Complications of care

1) General guidelines for complications of care

(a) Documentation of complications of care

See Section I.B.16. for information on documentation of complications of care.

2) Pain due to medical devices

Pain associated with devices, implants or grafts left in a surgical site (for example painful hip prosthesis) is assigned to the appropriate code(s) found in Chapter 19, Injury, poisoning, and certain other consequences of external causes. Specific codes for pain due to medical devices are found in the T code section of the ICD-10-CM. Use additional code(s) from category G89 to identify acute or chronic pain due to presence of the device, implant or graft (G89.18 or G89.28).

3) Transplant complications

(a) Transplant complications other than kidney

Codes under category T86, Complications of transplanted organs and tissues, are for use for both complications and rejection of transplanted organs. A transplant complication code is only assigned if the complication affects the function of the transplanted organ. Two codes are required to fully describe a transplant complication: the appropriate code from category T86 and a secondary code that identifies the complication.

Pre-existing conditions or conditions that develop after the transplant are not coded as complications unless they affect the function of the transplanted organs.

See I.C.21. for transplant organ removal status.

See I.C.2. for malignant neoplasm associated with transplanted organ.

(b) Kidney transplant complications

Patients who have undergone kidney transplant may still have some form of chronic kidney disease (CKD) because the kidney transplant may not fully restore kidney function. Code T86.1- should be assigned for documented complications of a kidney transplant, such as transplant failure or rejection or other transplant complication. Code T86.1- should not be assigned for post kidney transplant patients who have chronic kidney (CKD) unless a transplant complication such as transplant failure or rejection is documented. If the documentation is unclear as to whether the patient has a complication of the transplant, query the provider.

Conditions that affect the function of the transplanted kidney, other than CKD, should be assigned a code from subcategory T86.1, Complications of transplanted organ, Kidney, and a secondary code that identifies the complication.

For patients with CKD following a kidney transplant, but who do not have a complication such as failure or rejection, *see section I.C.14. Chronic kidney disease and kidney transplant status.*

4) Complication codes that include the external cause

As with certain other T codes, some of the complications of care codes have the external cause included in the code. The code includes the nature of the complication as well as the type of procedure that caused the complication. No external cause code indicating the type of procedure is necessary for these codes.

5) Complications of care codes within the body system chapters

Intraoperative and postprocedural complication codes are found within the body system chapters with codes specific to the organs and structures of that body system. These codes should be sequenced first, followed by a code(s) for the specific complication, if applicable.

Surgery Modifiers

There are numerous CPT modifiers that are applicable for surgical services, an additional set of modifiers that are designed specifically for ASC and outpatient hospital use, and others that are used to report never events. For this reason, knowing the modifiers applicable to surgical services is especially important for accurately reporting surgical procedures and optimizing payment for them.

CPT Modifiers

CPT modifiers that are applicable to surgical services are the following:

- *Modifier -22, Increased procedural services.* This modifier should be used when the work required to perform a service was above and beyond that which is typically required. The documentation for the service must clearly identify why the service was considered increased, by describing the additional time, intensity, technical difficulty, severity of the patient's condition, or physical or mental effort involved in the procedure.

- *Modifier -47, Anesthesia by surgeon.* This modifier should be appended to the code for the medical procedure, to indicate that the anesthesia was administered directly by the surgeon who performed the procedure.

- *Modifier -50, Bilateral procedure.* This modifier should be appended to the code for a primary procedure when that procedure was performed bilaterally (on both sides), and the CPT code description is for a unilateral procedure. If the code for the primary procedure was for a unilateral service, and that procedure was performed bilaterally, then modifier -50 should be appended to the procedure code to identify it as bilateral. For example, code 69210, Removal impacted cerumen requiring instrumentation, unilateral is a unilateral code. If this procedure was performed on both ears (bilaterally), then it would be reported as follows: 69210-50. If, on the other hand, the CPT code descriptor notes that it is either unilateral or bilateral, and the procedure was performed bilaterally, then modifier -50 would not need to be appended to the code for the service.

- *Modifier -51, Multiple procedures.* This modifier is used when a provider performs multiple procedures of the same type. For example, if a podiatry surgeon performs a partial ostectomy on two metatarsal heads, then he would report code 28288, Ostectomy, partial, exostectomy or condylectomy, metatarsal head, each metatarsal head twice, with the second code appended with modifier -51, as follows: 28288, and 28288-51. This modifier indicates to the payer that the procedure was performed multiple times. Insurance will usually pay 100 percent for the primary procedure, and then reduce the amount of payment for the second or subsequent procedures, paying at a downward scale of 75 percent, 50 percent, and 25 percent. The exact amount of reimbursement depends on the agreement with the insurance payer. Note that this modifier should not be used with add-on codes, E/M codes, physical medicine or rehabilitation, or provision of supplies such as vaccines. As discussed previously, note that modifier -51 is not approved for use by the outpatient hospital facility. It may only be reported by an independent provider billing for services performed.

- *Modifier -52, Reduced services.* This modifier should be used to identify that a procedure was partially reduced or eliminated at the discretion of the healthcare provider. For example, if a code description is for a bilateral service, but only the unilateral service was performed.

- *Modifier -53, Discontinued procedure.* This modifier should be used to identify that a procedure was discontinued due to extenuating circumstances that threaten the well-being of the patient. For example, if a patient undergoing a procedure becomes hypotensive or experiences respiratory distress, and the procedure is discontinued. The normal procedure code would be reported with modifier -53.

Modifiers -52 and -53 are very similar, but are used in two very different situations, so be careful! Modifier -52 is used when the procedure is not completed to the full extent of the code description, based on the provider's judgment. Modifier -53 is used when the procedure is discontinued due to the patient's health or other extenuating circumstance that threatens the well-being of the patient.

MOD

- *Modifier -54, Surgical care only.* This modifier should be used when the provider performs only the *surgical* portion of a service. It is used to break up the surgical package so that the provider is only paid for the portion of the procedure performed; in this case the surgery itself, about 70 percent of the charge (depending on the insurance). For example, a general surgeon working in an emergency department may perform only the surgical portion of an appendectomy, which involves only the incision and removal of the appendix in the operating room.
- *Modifier -55, Postoperative management only.* This modifier should be used when the provider performs only the *postoperative* portion of the service. Like modifier -54, it is used to break up the surgical package so that the provider is only paid for the portion of the procedure that was performed; in this case the postoperative management of the patient, about 20 percent of the charge (depending on the insurance). For example, if a physician in an emergency department had to complete the postoperative followup of an appendectomy patient because the general surgeon was unable to, then the appendectomy procedure would be reported with a modifier -55 (the surgeon would report his or her portion of the procedure with the same appendectomy code appended with modifier -54).
- *Modifier -56, Preoperative management only.* This modifier should be used when the provider performs only the *preoperative* portion of the service. Like modifiers -54 and -55, it is used to break up the surgical package so that the provider is only paid for the portion of the procedure that was performed; in this case the preoperative management of the patient, about 10 percent of the charge (depending on the insurance). For example, if one provider completed the preoperative evaluation and preoperative preparation of a surgical appendectomy patient, but was called out to perform a different procedure and a different provider performed both the surgical and postoperative portions of the service, then he or she would report the appendectomy procedure appended with modifier -56. (See figure 11.17 for an example of how these modifiers may impact payment).
- *Modifier -62, Two surgeons.* This modifier should be used when a procedure is performed by two surgeons. In this case, each surgeon would report the procedure, both appended with modifier -62, and each would only get paid for half of the service performed.
- *Modifier -63, Procedure performed on infants less than 4 kg.* This modifier should be appended to any service performed on a neonate or infant who weighs less than 4 kg. It is used to identify the increased complexity and work required for patients of this size. Note that it may only be reported with codes within the range

Figure 11.17. Example of modifiers -54, -55, and -56 impacting payment

20005 through 69990, and cannot be used on E/M, anesthesia, radiology, pathology and laboratory, or medicine services.

- *Modifier -66, Surgical team.* This modifier should be used when a team of surgeons perform a highly complex medical procedure. These surgeries require the concomitant services of several providers, often of different medical specialties, with the addition of other highly trained personnel or complex equipment. Each participating healthcare provider should report the code for the procedure appended with modifier -66. In terms of payment, each provider receives payment for the service according to a predetermined agreement made between the surgeons and the insurance company.

- *Modifier -76, Repeat procedure or service by same physician or other qualified health care professional.* This modifier should be used when a procedure or service is repeated by the same healthcare provider after the original procedure or service. For example, if an endoscopy is performed twice in one day by the same healthcare provider. Both procedures would be reported by the same physician, with the second procedure appended with the modifier. Note that is should not be used with E/M services.

- *Modifier -77, Repeat procedure by another physician or other qualified health care professional.* This modifier should be used when a procedure or service is repeated in the same day, but performed by a different healthcare provider. For example, if an endoscopy was performed in the morning by one provider, and then the same procedure is performed by a different provider later in the day; this subsequent procedure would be reported with the modifier -77.

- *Modifier -78, Unplanned return to the operating/procedure room by the same physician or other qualified health care professional following initial procedure for a related procedure during the postoperative period.* This modifier should be used when a procedure is performed in an operating room or surgical suite, and is an unplanned procedure following the initial procedure, related to the original procedure. It is used when a patient experiences a complication after the primary procedure and must return to the operating room or surgical suite for an additional procedure. The subsequent procedure should be appended with modifier -78.

- *Modifier -79, Unrelated procedure or service by the same physician or other qualified health care professional during the postoperative period.* This modifier is used to indicate that the procedure performed is unrelated to the primary surgical procedure. It is used while the patient is within the global package timeframe for the primary procedure, and allows reimbursement for the unrelated procedure. If this modifier is not used for the unrelated procedure, then it will be considered part of the surgical package for the primary procedure and will not be paid separately.

- *Modifier -80, Assistant surgeon.* This modifier is used to indicate that the procedure is performed by an assistant surgeon. This occurs when one surgeon assists another surgeon in the performance of a procedure, and the assisting surgeon is present for most of the procedure. The primary operating surgeon would report the procedure without a modifier, and the assistant surgeon would report the procedure with modifier -88 to indicate that he or she was the assistant surgeon for the procedure.

- *Modifier -AS, Physician assistant, nurse practitioner, or clinical nurse specialist services for assistant at surgery.* This modifier is essentially the same as modifier -80, except that it is used when the assistant surgeon is a mid-level provider such as a physician assistant (PA), clinical nurse specialist (CNS), or nurse practitioner (NP). Note that this is a HCPCS modifier, and it is not listed in the CPT code book. Instead it is found in the modifiers listing in the HCPCS code book.

- *Modifier -81, Minimum assistant surgeon.* This modifier is similar to modifier -80, but is used when the assistant surgeon is only present for a relatively short period of time and provides only minimal assistance to the primary surgeon. The primary surgeon would report the service without a modifier, and the minimum assistant surgeon would report the service with modifier -81.

- *Modifier -82, Assistant surgeon (when qualified resident surgeon not available).* This modifier is used in teaching hospitals and should be used when a qualified resident surgeon is not available to assist at surgery, and minimal assistance at surgery is required. The assistant surgeon would report the procedure code with modifier -82.

Note that there are four codes that identify when a surgeon assisted at surgery: 80, 81, 82, and AS. These modifiers are used by the surgeon who performed the assistance and are paid at a reduced amount. For example, appending modifier -82 to a service reported to Medicare might mean that the payment is only 16 percent of the full-service amount. Modifier -62, Two surgeons, and modifier -66, Surgical team, also identify circumstances where more than one surgeon performs a procedure, but here they are working together rather than assisting one primary surgeon. In these cases, payment for the services performed is usually predetermined between the surgeons and insurance providers prior to the surgery.

MOD

These modifiers should be used for medical procedures used in the inpatient hospital setting. Procedures performed in the outpatient hospital or ASC setting have a different set of applicable modifiers.

ASC or Hospital Outpatient Modifiers

There are several modifiers that are used specifically for services performed in the ASC or outpatient hospital settings. Although some of them are similar to those used for inpatient services, there are a handful of completely separate modifiers that are used specifically for services in these settings. The list of ASC modifiers is located in Appendix A of the CPT code book.

Note that not all ASC modifiers are listed here, only those that are significantly different than those described in the previous section (CPT modifiers).

- *Modifier -27, Multiple outpatient hospital E/M encounters on the same date.* This modifier should be used when the patient receives multiple E/M encounters on the same date of service, performed in different outpatient hospital settings. The E/M services may be performed by either the same or two different healthcare providers, but the E/M encounters both must be performed at different outpatient settings. For example, if a patient had an E/M encounter and then endoscopy performed in an ASC for trouble swallowing in the morning, and then had to go to the emergency department later in the day where another E/M procedure was performed, then the E/M encounter would be appended with modifier -27.

- *Modifier -73, Discontinued out-patient hospital/ambulatory surgical center (ASC) procedure prior to the administration of anesthesia.* This modifier should be used to identify that a procedure was discontinued due to extenuating circumstances that threaten the well-being of the patient, and that the procedure was discontinued *prior* to the administration of anesthesia. This includes local, regional block, or general anesthesia.

- *Modifier -74, Discontinued out-patient hospital/ambulatory surgical center (ASC) procedure after administration of anesthesia.* This modifier is very similar to modifier -73, except that it is used to identify that a procedure was discontinued due to extenuating circumstances *after* administration of the anesthesia (local, regional block, or general), or after the procedure was started (incision was made, intubation started, scope inserted).

> Note that modifiers -73 and -74 are both very similar to modifier -53, Discontinued procedure, which is used for physician billing. The difference (besides that fact that these modifiers may only be used in the outpatient hospital or ASC setting), is that they describe *when* the procedure was discontinued—either before or after the administration of anesthesia or the beginning of the procedure.

MOD

The existence of these ASC and outpatient hospital modifiers is one of the reasons why ASC coding and billing is so different from other traditional coding and billing. Coding for ASC and outpatient hospital services requires more insight into the special nature of the outpatient/inpatient relationship, and specific knowledge on how each individual facility charges for services. For example, some ASCs may be classified as outpatient facilities, in which case they would report outpatient codes only. On the other hand, some ASCs may be affiliated with an inpatient hospital, in which case they may be required to report inpatient codes (such as ICD-10-PCS) as well as outpatient (CPT) codes. This all depends on each individual ASC and the way in which the facility is organized.

Never Events

In rare instances a mistake is made in treatment that is erroneously performed by the healthcare provider. These are called never events, a term coined in 2001 by Ken Kizer of the National Quality Forum (NCF) to identify serious errors in medical treatment that should never happen (AHRQ 2017). Never events are classified as the following: surgery performed on the wrong body part, surgery performed on the wrong patient, and wrong surgery performed on the patient. These are rare events that are not considered payable by the insurance company. Because the healthcare provider made the error in treatment, he or she is expected to write off the cost of that treatment. It may not be charged to either the patient or the patient's third-party payer. To report a never event, the procedure code should be appended with the appropriate HCPCS modifier:

- PA, Surgical or other invasive procedure on wrong body part
- PB, Surgical or other invasive procedure on wrong patient
- PC, Wrong surgery or other invasive procedure on patient

Never events may happen in either the inpatient or the outpatient setting, and no matter the setting they are not reimbursable services. This includes services performed by other providers during the same visit that are related to the never event. However, after the patient has been discharged, any medically necessary services are covered by the patient's third-party payer, regardless of whether or not they are related to the never event.

Complete the following There's a Code for That 11.2 to test your knowledge of surgical modifiers.

Surgical modifiers

11.2

There's a Code for That

Read the description of the surgical procedure and assign the appropriate modifier for the case (code only for the modifier, not the procedure performed).

1. Patient was sedated and prepped and colonoscope was inserted for screening examination. 10 minutes into the procedure, the patient began experiencing respiratory distress. Procedure was discontinued, and the colonoscope was removed. Patient was awoken and placed under observation.

   Modifier: _____

2. Surgeon destroyed three malignant lesions using cryosurgery: one on the left arm, one on right leg, and one on right foot.

   Modifier: _____

3. Dr. A performed an exploratory laparotomy on the patient, but was unable to perform the postoperative care and follow-up services, as he was called out to an emergency. Dr. B was called in to perform the postoperative care. Which modifier should be appended to Dr. B's service?

   Modifier: _____

4. In the ASC setting, a surgical procedure was discontinued due to extenuating medical circumstances after patient anesthesia was administered.

   Modifier: _____

5. Surgical procedure was begun but was quickly discontinued when it was discovered that the procedure was performed on the wrong patient.

   Modifier: _____

6. Complex surgical procedure performed by team of surgeons consisting of an oral maxillofacial surgeon, a plastic reconstructive surgeon and neurosurgeon.

   Modifier: _____

Coding for Surgical Services

The surgeries discussed in this section include those performed by general, transplant, plastic and reconstructive, and burn and trauma surgeon, and include skin, general, and transplant surgeries. Additional surgical procedures are discussed throughout the rest of this text within their respective specialties such as orthopedic, female genital, neurological and spine, and such.

These surgeries may be performed in several different settings—from inpatient hospital to outpatient hospital, as well as ambulatory surgical center. Some procedures (such as excision or destruction of lesions) may also be performed in the outpatient office setting. The setting in which the procedure is performed depends on the complexity of the surgery, whether the patient needs general anesthesia, and the resources needed for the surgery. In some cases, a group of surgical specialists may decide to open their own ASC to have a place to perform their own surgeries. Again, this depends on the highly variable nature of what services and resources are needed and available, as well as the interests of the healthcare providers.

It is important to understand that the specific type of surgery that a doctor performs depends on his or her interest, expertise, and regional resources. For example, a general surgeon may decide to focus on abdominal procedures, like appendectomies or herniorrhaphy (repair of hernia), or neck procedures like thyroidectomies. Because of these differences, a coder should be flexible and knowledgeable about the codes that must be reported to correctly identify all of the services performed by the healthcare provider.

Skin Surgeries

Dermatological specialists deal with the integumentary system, which includes the skin, nails, hair, and breasts. Surgical dermatological procedures involve surgical interventions in the integumentary system, the most common of which is the excision or destruction of benign, pre-malignant, or malignant lesions.

Plastic and reconstructive surgeons may also perform the same procedures as dermatologists, such as excisions, skin flaps, and scar revisions. Wound and burn or trauma surgeons may also treat complex wounds, such as burns. All of these specialists focus on the surgical treatment of conditions of the skin and integumentary system.

The following sections identify specific integumentary system surgical procedures, including excision and destruction of lesions, plastic and reconstructive surgeries, and burn and wound treatments.

Excision and Destruction of Lesions

A **skin lesion** is any abnormality of the skin. This is a wide definition and includes freckles and moles, precancerous and malignant areas, skin tags, and scrapes or cuts. Lesions may be removed or destroyed for various reasons, which include improving cosmetic appearance, improving function of an area, or removing irritation or pain. In certain circumstances, lesions suspected to be cancerous or precancerous, and lesions that have already been determined to be cancerous are removed from the skin.

The kind of removal or treatment of the lesion depends on the type of lesion that the patient has, and the procedure codes vary accordingly. These CPT procedure codes include the following.

- Paring or Cutting (11055 to 11057) codes are for the paring or cutting of a benign hyperkeratotic lesion, such as a corn or callus. Code selection is based on the number of lesions treated. **Paring** is the process of cutting or trimming away the outer edges of a skin growth to make it smaller, remove pressure points, or remove it completely. It is often an outpatient procedure performed in the office setting. Because corns often occur on the feet, this is a common procedure for specialists in podiatry.

- Removal of Skin Tags (11200 and 11201) codes are for the physical removal of skin tags, by scissors or any other sharp method. Removal includes ligature strangulation, electrosurgical destruction, chemical destruction, or combination of methods. In this case, removal is different than previously described in this chapter—for example, , the removal category typically includes procedures that involve taking out a device, object, or substance from a body part or area. In this case, the removal of skin tags is the excision (surgical removal) of the skin tag.

- Shaving of Epidermal or Dermal Lesions (11300 to 11313) codes report the removal via shaving of benign lesions of the skin. Shaving is the act of sharp removal by transverse incision or horizontal slicing. Shaving may require local anesthesia or cauterization, but it does not require suture closure. Codes for shaving of lesions vary based on the site of the lesion and the size of the excised lesion.

- Excision-Benign Lesions (11400 to 11471) codes identify the excision of lesions that have been determined to be benign in nature. Excision is the full-thickness removal (through the dermis) of the lesion, and includes a margin of skin that is excised around the lesion in addition to the lesion itself. Excision codes include a simple, nonlayered closure of the skin (when required). Any repair over and above simple repair should be reported with the appropriate intermediate (12031 to 12057) or complex (13100 to 13153) repair codes. Reconstructive closure of the wound should be coded with the appropriate skin replacement surgery (15002 to 15261, 15570 and 15571) codes. If adjacent tissue transfer (14000 to 14302) is used to repair the defect, then the excision of the benign lesion is not coded separately, code only for the adjacent tissue transfer. Codes for excision of benign lesions rely on the site and type of the lesion as well as the excised diameter of the lesion. The excised diameter is the size of the lesion in addition to the margins around the lesion that were removed. Unlike shaving of epidermal or dermal lesion codes, excision of benign lesion codes includes a margin of excised skin. This margin is the area around a lesion that is excised in addition to the lesion. For example, if a surgeon removes a 0.5 cm lesion with 0.2 cm margins on each side, then the total excised diameter is 0.9 cm (0.5 cm lesion + 0.2 cm margin on right + 0.2 margin on left = 0.9 cm total excised diameter). See figure 11.18.

- Excision-Malignant Lesions (11600 to 11646) codes identify the excision of lesions that have been determined to be malignant. These excision codes identify the full-thickness excision of lesions and include local anesthesia. Simple repair (single-layer) is included but intermediate, complex, reconstructive, or adjacent tissue transfer is not included within the code description. Intermediate (12031 to 12057), complex (13100 to 13153), and reconstructive skin procedures (15002 to 15261, 15570 to 15770) should be reported in addition to the lesion excision codes, whereas adjacent tissue transfer codes include the lesion excision and the two should not be coded separately (code only for the adjacent tissue transfer). Code selection relies on the site of the excision and the excised diameter, which includes the size of the lesion and the excised skin margins.

- Destruction, Benign or Premalignant Lesions (17000 to 17250) codes are for the ablation of benign, or premalignant skin lesions by any method.

Figure 11.18. Measuring lesion removal

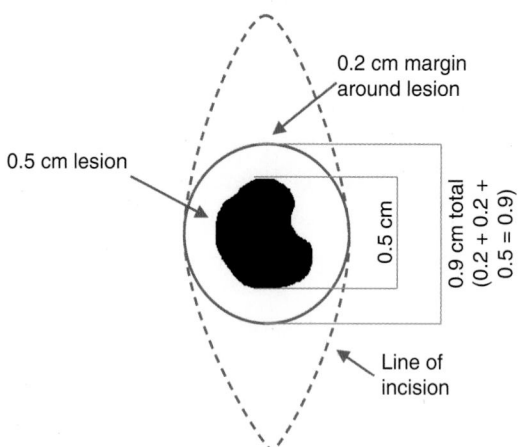

Source: Adapted from AMA 2018.

These codes include local anesthesia (when performed), but do not usually require sutures closure. Ablation is the destruction of tissue using any of the following methods: electrosurgery, cryosurgery, laser treatment, and chemical treatment. Note that the difference between excision and destruction codes is that excision removes intact tissue, while ablation destroys tissue and nothing is removed. Codes for destruction of benign or premalignant lesions depend on the type of lesion (premalignant, cutaneous vascular proliferative, benign other than skin tags, granulation tissue), as well as either the size or the number of lesions removed.

- Destruction, Malignant Lesions, Any Method (17260 to 17286) codes are for the destruction (ablation) of lesions which have been determined to be malignant. These codes rely on the site of the lesion and the lesion diameter. Note that destruction of lesion codes identify the size of the lesion, not the excised diameter; this is because no skin is excised. The code reported should identify only the size of the lesion destroyed.

- Mohs Micrographic Surgery (17311 to 17315) codes identify the removal of lesions using the Mohs micrographic technique. **Mohs micrographic surgery** is used for the removal of complex and ill-defined skin malignancies, and includes the examination of all the excised margins. In this way, the surgeon acts as both surgeon and pathologist. If a surgeon performs the excision and a pathologist performs the histologic examination, then Mohs codes should not be used. Rather, use individual codes for the excision and for the pathologic examination. It requires two parts—excision of the lesion and pathological examination. In this process, the surgeon removes one layer of the lesion and breaks it into pieces that are frozen and embedded into **blocks** (the frozen specimens being examined by the surgeon). Each block is examined for evidence of malignancy. Additional layers of skin are removed and studied in this way until no further evidence of the malignancy remains (see figure 11.19). Each layer excised is referred to as a **stage**. For example, if the surgeon removed one layer, then this is the first stage; the next layer would be the second stage, and so on. Figure 11.19 shows four stages of removal.

Figure 11.19. Mohs micrographic surgery

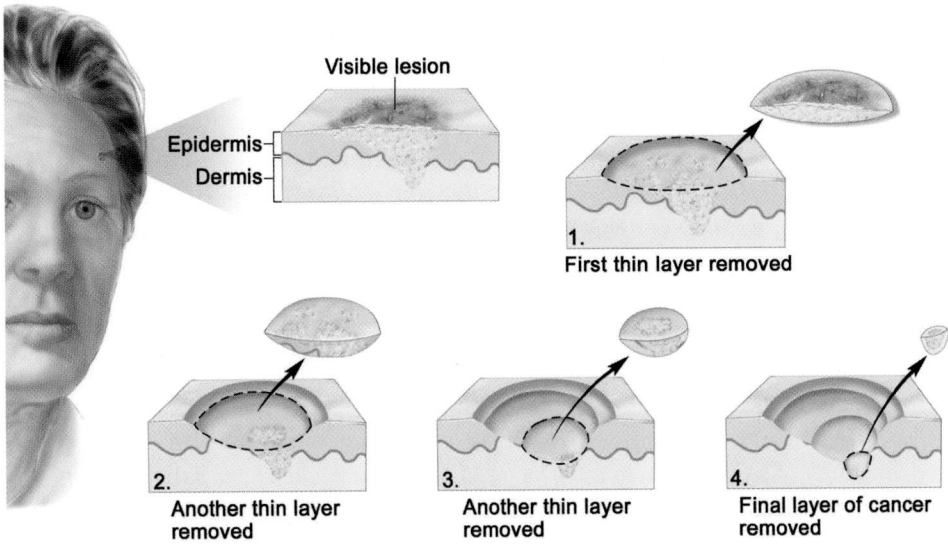

Mohs Surgery

Source: © 2009 Terese Winslow, U.S. Govt has certain rights.

Codes for Mohs surgery do not include repair and therefore if a repair is done, then the appropriate repair, flap, or skin graft code should be used. Coding for Mohs micrographic surgery is detailed. First of all, there are two primary codes based on the site of the lesion excision (17311, Mohs micrographic technique, including removal of all gross tumor, surgical excision of tissue specimens, mapping color coding or specimens, microscopic examination of specimens by the surgeon, and histopathologic preparation including routine stains(s) (e.g., hematoxylin and eosin, toluidine blue), *head, neck, hands, feet, genitalia, or any location with surgery directly involving muscle, cartilage, bone, tendon, major nerves, or vessels*; first stage, up to 5 tissue blocks, and 17313, Mohs micrographic technique, including removal of all gross tumor, surgical excision of tissue specimens, mapping color coding or specimens, microscopic examination of specimens by the surgeon, and histopathologic preparation including routine stains(s) (e.g., hematoxylin and eosin, toluidine blue), *of the trunk, arms or legs*; first stage, up to 5 tissue blocks), for the first stage of the procedure. If a surgeon performing Mohs removes one layer and divides that layer into five blocks for examination, then the code would be either 17311 or 17313 depending on the site of the lesion. If the surgeon removes more than one layer (each additional stage after the first stage) and divides that second (or third, or fourth, or fifth) layer into blocks for examination, then each additional *stage* (with up to five blocks per stage) is coded using the add-on codes 17312, Mohs micrographic technique, including removal of all gross tumor, surgical excision of tissue specimens, mapping color coding or specimens, microscopic examination of specimens by the surgeon, and histopathologic preparation including routine stains(s) (e.g., hematoxylin and eosin, toluidine blue), head, neck, hands, feet, genitalia, or any location with surgery directly involving muscle, cartilage, bone, tendon, major nerves, or vessels; *each additional stage after the first stage, up to 5 tissue blocks* or 17314, Mohs micrographic technique, including removal of all gross tumor, surgical excision of tissue specimens, mapping color coding or specimens, microscopic examination of specimens by the surgeon, and histopathologic preparation including routine stains(s) (e.g., hematoxylin and eosin, toluidine blue), of the trunk, arms or legs; *each additional stage after the first stage, up to 5 tissue blocks.* Note that 17312 should only be used with 17311, and 17314 should only be used with 17313. If any stage (layer) is divided into more than five blocks, then the add-on code 17315, Mohs micrographic technique, including removal of all gross tumor, surgical excision of tissue specimens, mapping color coding or specimens, microscopic examination of specimens by the surgeon, and histopathologic preparation including routine stains(s) (e.g., hematoxylin and eosin, toluidine blue), *each additional block after the first 5 tissue blocks, any stage* should be used, to identify each additional block after the first five blocks.

If more than one lesion is excised using the Mohs technique, then they should be coded separately, using modifier -59 to identify that the procedures are distinct from each other. Read the following example to see how these codes are reported:

Surgeon excised a lesion from the forehead of a 35-year-old female patient. The first layer is excised and divided into seven blocks. Surgeon determined that there are positive margins for malignancy on four of the blocks, and thus removed a second layer, which was divided into five blocks. After pathological examination, the surgeon determined that none of the blocks were positive for further malignancies.

In this example, there are two stages of excision. In the first stage, the layer was divided into seven blocks. This results in the selection of code 17311 for the first stage, up to five blocks, and then 17315 X 2 for the additional blocks from stage one. The last code needed is 17312, to identify the second stage of excision, up to five blocks. Since there were only four blocks examined in stage two, and there were no other stages of the procedure, then these three codes are all needed to code this scenario completely:

- o 17311, Mohs micrographic technique…head, neck, hands, feet, genitalia, or any location with surgery directly involving muscle, cartilage, bone, tendon, major nerves, or vessels; first stage, up to 5 tissue blocks
- o 17312, Mohs micrographic technique…head, neck, hands, feet, genitalia, or any location with surgery directly involving muscle, cartilage, bone, tendon, major nerves, or vessels; each additional stage after the first stage, up to 5 tissue blocks
- o 17315 X 2, Mohs micrographic technique…each additional block after the first 5 tissue blocks, any stage

Key to Success

Look carefully at the codes for Mohs surgery. Codes 17311 and 17312 identify the *stages* of the procedure (either the first stage or each additional stage). Code 17315, however, identifies each additional *block* examined during the procedure. This is an excellent example of why it is so important to read code descriptions carefully. When you come across small differences like these, it is easy to overlook them—especially when trying to complete a timed certification exam. Make sure to place a star, arrow, or highlight these small differences to make them stand out when it really matters!

When multiple lesion excision or destructions are performed during the same operative session, list each lesion excision or destruction code separately with modifier -51 to indicate they were multiple procedures all performed in the same surgical session. If multiple lesions of the same anatomical site were destroyed at the same operative session, then report the appropriate CPT code for the size and site of the destruction or excision, each listed individually to identify that they were separate procedures from each other, and append the additional excisions or destructions with modifier -59 to identify them as distinct from each other.

The codes discussed are for the excision or destruction of lesions on the skin, *not* the deeper structures underlying the skin. Excision or destruction of deeper tissues are coded in their respective subsections (musculoskeletal, male genital, and such).

Diagnostic Coding for Skin Lesions

The two main types of skin lesions are benign and malignant. Benign skin lesions are non-cancerous and generally slow-growing, although they can be painful, cause irritation, and may be an indicator of a precancerous condition. Malignant skin lesions are considered cancerous, can invade other cells within the body, and may be dangerous and sometimes fatal. In some instances, lesions may be pre-malignant or suspicious in nature if a healthcare expert suspects that the lesion is depicting behavior indicating it will become malignant.

When coding for skin lesion diagnoses, coders should rely on the provider's documentation of the type of lesion. Lesions can range from freckles and moles to cancerous growths, corns and calluses, and congenital anomalies of the skin (see figure 11.20).

Figure 11.20. Neoplasms of skin

Malignant melanoma of the skin
Source: National Cancer Institute 1985b.

Kaposi's Sarcoma
Source: National Cancer Institute 1985a.

Basal cell carcinoma
Source: Nelson 2012a.

Squamous cell carcinoma
Source: Nelson 2012b.

Coders should reference the type of lesion in the Main Index of the ICD-10-CM code book, and then follow all subterms and cross-references until the correct code is found. For example, if the provider documented the skin condition as a melanocytic nevus on the right breast, then the coder should look up the term *nevus* in the Index, then refer to the subterm *skin* (because the nevus is located on the skin), then find the subterm for the location of the nevus, in this case *breast*, leading the coder to D22.5, Melanocytic nevi of trunk.

When the lesion is any type of cancer or malignancy, refer to the histologic type of the condition in the Index. If the histologic type is not known, or if the condition is not listed in the Index, then refer to the Table of Neoplasms. For example, if the provider documents that the patient has a basal cell carcinoma of the skin of the breast, then the coder should reference the term *carcinoma* in the Index, then search for the subterm *basal cell*. In this case, there are no subterms that identify a basal cell carcinoma of the skin of the breast, so it is necessary to refer to the cross-reference *see also* Neoplasm, skin, malignant. In the Table of Neoplasms, the coder should search for the heading for *breast*, then the site of the lesion, *skin of the breast*, and then find the additional subterm for *basal cell carcinoma*. This leads the coder to C44.511, Basal cell carcinoma of skin of breast. (For a reminder on how to use the Table of Neoplasms, refer to chapter 4, Learning the ICD-10-CM Code Book).

Key to Success

Remember that the diagnosis code identifies the medical necessity for the procedure performed. This is important in the excision of benign lesions, as the removal of such may be considered cosmetic and not medically necessary. If the excision of a benign lesion—such as a mole—is purely cosmetic, insurance may not pay for the procedure and financial responsibility falls solely on the patient. However, if an unsightly mole is also causing pain or irritation, it may be enough to make a removal of the mole medically necessary. If so, a code is needed for the benign lesion and the other symptoms experienced by the patient to fully identify the medical necessity for the service performed.

For practice assigning procedure and diagnosis codes for skin lesions, complete the exercises in There's a Code for That 11.3.

11.3

There's a Code for That

Diagnostic and procedural coding for skin lesions

Read the description of the procedure and assign the appropriate ICD-10-CM and/or CPT codes.

1. 2 cm squamous cell carcinoma was excised from the right side of the nose of a 50-year-old male patient. Excised diameter was 2.5 cm.

   CPT code: _____

   ICD-10-CM code: _____

2. Removal of seven skin tags from the right axillary region of a 35-year-old female.

   CPT code: _____

   ICD-10-CM code: _____

3. Destruction of five flat warts via cryosurgery on the right foot.

   CPT code: _____

   ICD-10-CM code: _____

4. Dermatologist destroyed the following malignant melanomas from the skin of a 67-year-old male patient using chemosurgery: 0.5 cm and 1.4 cm lesions on the right arm; 0.8 cm lesion on the left forearm; and 2.2 cm lesion on the right scapular region.

   CPT code(s): _____, _____, _____,

   _____

   ICD-10-CM code: _____, _____

5. Mohs micrographic surgery performed on patient with basal cell carcinoma of the forehead. Surgeon removed the first stage and divided the specimen into four blocks of tissue. Upon pathological examination, it is evident that the margins are clear of any further malignant cells.

   CPT code: _____

   ICD-10-CM code: _____

Plastic and Reconstructive Surgeries

Plastic and reconstructive surgeons specialize in surgical procedures that aim to enhance and reshape the body to improve appearance, and treat structures of the body to repair disabilities in function due to congenital defects, developmental abnormalities, trauma, infection, tumors, or disease. Although some plastic and reconstructive surgeons may specialize in elective procedures, others perform a vast array of medically necessary surgeries that help the body to return to normal function and appearance. However, because sometimes the line between cosmetic and medically necessary is difficult to discern, some procedures may be covered for some patients for certain diagnoses, whereas others are not. Ultimately, when selecting codes for plastic and reconstructive surgeries, pay close attention to diagnosis codes to ensure that they fully support the procedure code selected.

Plastic and reconstructive surgeries on the breast include Mastectomy Procedures (19300 to 19307) and Repair and/or Reconstruction (19316 to 19396) of the breast. When coding mastectomies, coders should identify the reason for the mastectomy, the extent of the mastectomy (partial/lumpectomy, with lymphadenectomy, radical, modified radical), and any additional procedures performed. Note that all mastectomy codes are unilateral codes. If the procedure is performed bilaterally, append modifier -50 to the code. Breast repair and reconstruction codes identify several different procedures that are performed to repair and/or reconstruct the breast(s), either due to a congenital defect, traumatic injury, or previous mastectomy.

The majority of mastectomy procedures are due to breast cancer. Breast cancer diagnosis codes are detailed and identify the gender of the patient (male or female), laterality of the condition (right or left), and exact location of the malignancy (where in the breast does the condition occur). They are located in category C50, Malignant neoplasm of breast. If there are multiple neoplasms in different sites, use one code per neoplasm. Remember, as discussed in chapter 4, a neoplasm is an abnormal growth of tissue and can be fast-growing and invasive like malignant cancer, or a benign mass or tumor. Note that codes in category C50 do not include malignancies on the skin of the breast. Category C50, Malignant neoplasms of breast, includes codes for the deeper structures of the breast, rather than of the skin of the breast. This is an important distinction, as neoplasms of the skin are reported with different codes. In addition to the breast cancer code, report a supplementary code to identify the patient's estrogen receptor status, if known (Z17.0, Estrogen receptor positive status [ER+], or Z17.1, Estrogen receptor negative status [ER-]). If the patient has already undergone a mastectomy procedure, which removes the breast tissue, then the appropriate code from category Z90.1-, Acquired absence of breast and nipple, should be reported. For example, a patient that is status post right mastectomy would be coded with Z90.11, Acquired absence of right breast and nipple.

Key to Success

The difference between the skin of the breast and the deeper structures of the breast is an important distinction when coding, as it will change the subsection or chapter of code used to report the condition or the procedure. If the malignancy is on the *skin* of a structure or body part, this is different than it being *in* the body part. For example, the excision of a skin lesion on the leg is different than the excision of a lesion within the deep tissues of the leg.

Rhinoplasties are also commonly performed by plastic and reconstructive surgeons. A **rhinoplasty** is the surgical repair or revision of the nose, either for cosmetic or functional and medical purposes. Codes for rhinoplasties are located in the Respiratory system subsection under the Repair category (30400 to 30630). Note that these procedures do involve the deeper structures of the nose, and not just the skin on the outside of the nose.

Skin flap, graft, and tissue transfer procedures may be performed by dermatologists, wound specialists, or plastic and reconstructive surgeons. These procedures place a portion of skin or synthetic skin substitute over a damaged or diseased area of skin for repair. Skin replacement procedures include the surgical preparation of the graft site, which may include cleaning, debridement, extension of the wound surface, or removal of nonviable tissue. After the site is prepared, a skin graft is placed on the area for repair and anchored into place. Skin grafts and replacements may be temporary or permanent depending on the type of graft or wound and the patient's individual healing process.

Depending on the circumstance, there are different graft substances that may be used to complete the procedure. An **autograft** is a skin graft from a different site from the patient's own body. An **allograft** is a skin graft from tissue from a donor. A **xenograft** is a skin graft made from a different species (commonly pig skin). A **homograft** is a skin graft taken from a donor of the same species. Autografts and allografts are both homografts, except that an autograft is from the patient and an allograft is from a donor of the same species. Because allografts and xenografts are made from tissues that are recognized as foreign by the patient's body, they will eventually be rejected. Therefore, these two types of skin grafts are temporary and must eventually be replaced with an autograft.

Coding for skin flaps and tissue transfers is complex and requires an understanding of the type of flap, graft, or tissue transfer; site of the procedure; size of the graft or skin replacement; and any additional procedures performed. They include the following:

- Adjacent Tissue Transfer or Rearrangement (14000 to 14350). Tissue transfers or rearrangements are not technically skin grafts, although they do use a portion

Figure 11.21. Skin flap designs

Advancement flap	Rotation flap	Transposition flap
Source: Taylornate 2011a.	Source: Taylornate 2011b.	Source: Taylornate 2011c.

of the patient's own skin to cover a defect area. These procedures involve rearranging an area of tissue to cover an area that needs to be covered. This is done by incising the tissue in a specific pattern, and stretching it over the defect. The size of the skin transfer or rearrangement is based on the size of the primary defect (for example, a 1.5 cm wound), plus the size of the secondary defect (a 3 cm advancement flap created), which are added to calculate the total skin defect size (1.5 cm primary defect + 3 cm secondary defect = 4.5 cm total defect size). Codes for adjacent tissue transfers *include* the excision of a defect or lesion, and the excision of a benign (11400 to 11446) or malignant (11600 to 11646) lesion should not be coded separately. Coding for these procedures relies on the site and size (measured in square centimeters) of the tissue transfer or rearrangement (see figure 11.21).

- Skin Replacement Surgery (15002 to 15278). Skin replacement surgeries include free grafts of skin and skin substitutes, used to cover a defect in the skin. A free graft is one that has been completely removed from the surrounding tissue and does not remain connected to any type of blood supply, but is completely excised from the donor site and placed on the site of the graft. Before a skin graft can be placed on a site, the site must be prepared to receive the graft. This surgical preparation of the area includes excision of an open wound, burn eschar, scar, or incisional release of scar contracture. In some cases, after the site is prepared, it may be closed using adjacent tissue transfer (described previously) or complex repair codes. Surgical preparation codes (15002 to 15005) are not to be used for debridement of tissue, wound management, or for the removal of nonviable tissue in a chronic wound (such as venous or diabetic wounds). Codes for autografts, tissue cultured autografts, and skin substitute grafts (15040 to 15278) identify the application of skin grafts. Code selection requires the identification of the type of graft used, such a split-thickness, dermal autograft, or full-thickness, as well as the site and size of the graft. A split-thickness graft is one in which the epidermis and only part of the dermis is used for the graft. A dermal autograft is a skin graft from a donor. A full-thickness skin graft is one in which the epidermis and the entire thickness of the dermis is included in the graft. Pay close attention to the add-on codes in this selection of codes. These codes may be added to the code for the primary procedure and should total the full size of the graft that was performed. Multiple add-on codes may be necessary. For example, if a patient received a 200 sq cm tissue cultured skin autograft of the trunk, the codes would be as follows:

- 15150, Tissue cultured skin autograft, trunk, arms, legs; *first 25 sq cm or less*
- 15151, Tissue cultured skin autograft, trunk, arms, legs; *additional 1 sq cm to 75 sq cm*
- 15152, Tissue cultured skin autograft, trunk, arms, legs; *each additional 100 sq cm, or each additional 1% of body area of infants and children, or part thereof*

Code 15150 accounts for the first 25 sq cm; 15151 accounts for the next 75 sq cm, which together with the previous code equals 100 sq cm. The last code, 15152, accounts for the remaining 100 sq cm. So, the correct reporting of a 200 sq cm tissue cultured skin autograft would be 15150, 15151, and 15152 (25 cm + 75 cm + 100 cm = 200 cm).

- Flaps (Skin and/or Deep Tissues) (15570 to 15738). Skin and deep tissue flaps identify planned, staged procedures that may be completed over a period of time. This is because either the procedure is delayed, or the tissue is formed into a tube and kept connected to a blood supply and slowly walked to the recipient site. This allows the skin graft to stay viable as it is slowly maneuvered into place over a period of time. Codes for skin and deep tissue grafts are identified based on the service performed—either the formation of the graft (direct or tubed pedicle), delay or sectioning of the flap, or transfer of the flap. When assigning these codes, pay attention to the type of tissue used in the procedure and the site of the graft. Codes identify the recipient site, not the donor site.

- Other Flaps and Grafts (15740 to 15777). These codes identify a range of other skin flaps and grafts that do not fit into any other category, such as 15758, Free fascial flap with microvascular anastomosis, which is a free graft (not attached to a blood supply) of fascia connected at the graft site with microvascular anastomosis. Code selection requires identification of the type of graft as well as any additional services performed.

Burn Surgeries and Wound Treatments

Wounds may be complex, non-healing, chronic, and necrotizing; and wound treatment surgeries and procedures are closely monitored, staged services that may require various elements before the wound is ultimately healed. Procedures to treat burns, open wounds, and chronic wounds may include repair or grafting, as discussed previously, or other special procedures like debridement, burn and pressure ulcer treatment, and wound care management services.

- Debridement (11042 to 11047) is the removal of dead, diseased, infected, or otherwise nonviable tissue from a wound to improve the healing ability of the area. After debridement of a wound, only healthy tissue is left remaining, and bandaged or treated to promote healing. Codes for debridement rely not only on the size of the wound, but on the depth of the debridement. When coding for a debridement, select the code for the deepest level of tissue removed during the debridement session such as skin, subcutaneous tissue muscle fascia, muscle, or bone. Note that some of the debridement codes report a specific site or type of skin condition, while others do not. Debridement of nails are coded with (11720 and 11721), depending on the number of nails debrided. Note that these debridement codes are not to be used for the debridement of burn wounds.

- Active Wound Care Management (97597 to 97610) codes report debridement of dermal or epidermal tissue only, as well as wound care procedures including negative pressure wound therapy services. These codes are not to be used with debridement codes from the Integumentary subsection (11042 to 11047) nor are they to be used to report the debridement of burn wounds.

- Burns, Local Treatment (16000 to 16036) codes refer to the treatment of the burned surface only, and include the application of materials such as dressings to the wound. These codes do not, however, include any other necessary related medical services such as E/M encounters or skin grafting/replacement (both are reported separately). Code selection requires the identification of the percentage of body surface involved in the burn and the depth of the burn. The CPT code book relies on the Lund-Browder Classification for burn percentages, as discussed in chapter 10 (Urgent Care and Emergency Department Services). Burn debridement codes are classified as first-degree, second-degree (partial thickness), or as an escharotomy (to treat full-thickness, third-degree burns).

- Pressure Ulcers (Decubitus Ulcers) (15920 to 15999). These codes identify the treatment of pressure, or decubitus, ulcers. Code selection relies on the site of the ulcer and additional removal such as an ostectomy (removal of bone) and type of closure (when identified). Note that these codes are only to be used with pressure ulcers and not with wounds identified as non-pressure or venous ulcers. Treatment of non-pressure ulcers, such as venous ulcers, is coded with the appropriate debridement, skin closure, or skin flap code, as applicable.

Diagnostic Coding for Burns and Skin Ulcers

Diagnostic codes for repairs of the skin should detail the area and extent of the wound, burn, or ulcer. Diagnostic coding for burns is discussed in chapter 10 (Urgent Care and Emergency Department Services). Remember, burn codes identify the *site* of the burn, the *extent* of the burn, the *depth* of the burn, and the *agent* that caused the burn.

A skin ulcer is an open wound on the skin that may be caused by infection, pressure, or venous problems. When coding for ulcers of the skin, coders must be able to identify that the ulcer is indeed on the skin, and not in any underlying structures or organs. For example, a stomach ulcer or corneal ulcer are both located within those organs. There are two main types of skin ulcers—pressure and non-pressure. A pressure ulcer, also known as a bedsore or decubitus ulcer, is an ulcer that has occurred on the skin because of prolonged pressure on the skin. They most commonly develop on areas with an underlying bone such as heels, ankles, hips, and tailbone (see figure 11.22.) A non-pressure ulcer is an ulcer on the skin caused by anything other than pressure, such as one caused by atherosclerosis of the extremities (and loss of blood circulation), chronic venous hypertension, diabetes mellitus, postthrombotic syndrome, postphlebitic syndrome, or varicose veins. They are often chronic problems that are difficult to heal.

Diagnostic coding for skin ulcers requires the healthcare provider to identify the ulcer as either pressure or non-pressure. Codes further mandate the identification of the site of the ulcer such as heel, ankle, or thigh, as well as the laterality of the condition. Pressure ulcers are located in category L89, Pressure ulcer. For pressure ulcers, the severity of the ulcer should be identified as stage one through four, as follows:

1. Stage 1: skin changes limited to persistent focal edema
2. Stage 2: with abrasion, blister, partial thickness skin loss involving epidermis and/or dermis
3. Stage 3: full-thickness skin loss involving damage or necrosis of subcutaneous tissue
4. Stage 4: with necrosis of soft tissues through to underlying muscle, tendon, or bone (AHIMA 2016)

Figure 11.22. Pressure ulcer sites

First Image: Common sites of pressure ulcers, which occur on areas with underlying bone.
Second image: Inflammation around the sacrum. Third image: A sacral pressure ulcer.
Source: ©2017. Used with permission of Elsevier. All rights reserved.

In some cases an ulcer cannot be staged, such as when it is covered with a skin graft or covered with eschar tissue. In this case, the coder should report the *unstageable* option. Any associated gangrene should also be identified using code I96, Gangrene, not elsewhere classified. The gangrene code should be sequenced before the code for the pressure ulcer.

Non-pressure ulcers are located in category L97, Non-pressure chronic ulcer of lower limb, not elsewhere classified, and L98.4, Non-pressure chronic ulcer of skin, not elsewhere classified. Coding for non-pressure ulcers is similar to coding for pressure ulcers. Codes identify the severity of the ulcer in terms of depth and whether the condition presents with or without necrosis:

1. Limited to breakdown of skin
2. With fat layer exposed
3. With necrosis of muscle
4. With necrosis of bone
5. Unspecified severity
6. Muscle involvement without evidence of necrosis
7. Bone involvement without evidence of necrosis
8. Other specified severity
9. Unspecified severity

The underlying cause of the ulcer should also be documented with causal language. For example, "non-pressure ulcer of the right heel *due to* atherosclerosis of the lower extremities." This clearly shows that the ulcer is a result of the atherosclerosis. In this case, two codes should be selected: one for the underlying cause (atherosclerosis of the extremities), and one for the non-pressure ulcer (category L97 code).

Note that skin ulcer codes are all HCC codes, and so the documentation of these conditions should be as specific as possible, as should code selection. See figure 11.23 for the OGCR related to coding pressure ulcers.

Figure 11.23. OGCR I.C.12

---

12. Chapter 12: Diseases of the Skin and Subcutaneous Tissue (L00-L99)

a. Pressure ulcer stage codes

1) Pressure ulcer stages

Codes from category L89, Pressure ulcer, are combination codes that identify the site of the pressure ulcer as well as the stage of the ulcer.

The ICD-10-CM classifies pressure ulcer stages based on severity, which is designated by stages 1-4, unspecified stage and unstageable.

Assign as many codes from category L89 as needed to identify all the pressure ulcers the patient has, if applicable.

2) Unstageable pressure ulcers

Assignment of the code for unstageable pressure ulcer (L89.--0) should be based on the clinical documentation. These codes are used for pressure ulcers whose stage cannot be clinically determined (e.g., the ulcer is covered by eschar or has been treated with a skin or muscle graft) and pressure ulcers that are documented as deep tissue injury but not documented as due to trauma. This code should not be confused with the codes for unspecified stage (L89.--9). When there is no documentation regarding the stage of the pressure ulcer, assign the appropriate code for unspecified stage (L89.--9).

3) Documented pressure ulcer stage

Assignment of the pressure ulcer stage code should be guided by clinical documentation of the stage or documentation of the terms found in the Alphabetic Index. For clinical terms describing the stage that are not found in the Alphabetic Index, and there is no documentation of the stage, the provider should be queried.

4) Patients admitted with pressure ulcers documented as healed

No code is assigned if the documentation states that the pressure ulcer is completely healed.

5) Patients admitted with pressure ulcers documented as healing

Pressure ulcers described as healing should be assigned the appropriate pressure ulcer stage code based on the documentation in the medical record. If the documentation does not provide information about the stage of the healing pressure ulcer, assign the appropriate code for unspecified stage.

If the documentation is unclear as to whether the patient has a current (new) pressure ulcer or if the patient is being treated for a healing pressure ulcer, query the provider.

For ulcers that were present on admission but healed at the time of discharge, assign the code for the site and stage of the pressure ulcer at the time of admission.

6) Patient admitted with pressure ulcer evolving into another stage during the admission

If a patient is admitted **to an inpatient hospital** with a pressure ulcer at one stage and it progresses to a higher stage, two separate codes should be assigned: one code for the site and stage of the ulcer on admission and a second code for the same ulcer site and the highest stage reported during the stay.

b. Non-Pressure Chronic Ulcers

1) Patients admitted with non-pressure ulcers documented as healed

No code is assigned if the documentation states that the non-pressure ulcer is completely healed.

2) Patients admitted with non-pressure ulcers documented as healing

Non-pressure ulcers described as healing should be assigned the appropriate non-pressure ulcer code based on the documentation in the medical record. If the documentation does not provide information about the severity of the healing non-pressure ulcer, assign the appropriate code unspecified severity.

If the documentation is unclear as to whether the patient has a current (new) non-pressure ulcer or if the patient is being treated for a healing non-pressure ulcer, query the provider.

For ulcers that were present on admission but healed at the time of discharge, assign the code for the site and severity of the non-pressure ulcer at the time of admission.

3) Patient admitted with non-pressure ulcer that progresses to another severity level during the admission

If a patient is admitted to an inpatient hospital with a non-pressure ulcer at one severity level and it progresses to a higher severity level, two separate codes should be assigned; one code for the site and severity level of the ulcer on admission and a second code for the same ulcer site and the highest severity level reported during the stay.

Source: CMS 2018.

For practice assigning diagnosis and procedure codes for skin flaps and wound treatments, complete the exercises in There's a Code for That 11.4.

Diagnostic and procedural coding for skin flaps and wound treatments

Read the description of the procedure and assign the appropriate ICD-10-CM and/or CPT codes.

1. Excision of 2.5 cm benign nevus on the anterior abdomen of a 54-year-old male patient. Wound site covered with 5.0 cm advancement flap.

   CPT code: _____

   ICD-10-CM code: _____

2. Debridement of second degree burn on left lower leg (8 percent of body surface).

   CPT code: _____

   ICD-10-CM code: _____

3. Excision of stage 4 sacral pressure ulcer with involvement of bone. Partial ostectomy performed and excision site was covered with skin flap closure.

   CPT code: _____

   ICD-10-CM code: _____

General Surgery

General surgery is a surgical specialty that focuses on surgical procedures all over the human body, with an emphasis on the abdominal area, including procedures on the esophagus, stomach, small and large intestines, liver, pancreas, and the gallbladder and bile ducts. General surgeons may also perform surgeries on the thyroid gland, peripheral vascular conditions, hernias, soft tissue and traumatic injuries, and conditions affecting the skin and breast. The exact procedures that a general surgeon performs depend on his or her level of expertise, interest, and regional resources. For example, a general surgeon working in the same vicinity as a surgical endocrinologist is less likely to perform a thyroidectomy than a general surgeon working in a region in which there are no other surgical specialists more qualified to perform the procedure.

Coding for general surgery requires an overall knowledge of surgical procedures and how to report them with CPT codes. Furthermore, depending on the specialized training or interests of the general surgeon, he or she might specialize in certain types of procedures. Typically general surgeons focus on surgeries of the abdomen (including appendectomy), cholecystectomy, herniorrhaphy, and other procedures performed on the mediastinum and diaphragm and the abdomen, peritoneum, and omentum.

Mediastinum and Diaphragm

The mediastinum is the area in the thorax in-between the lungs. It is the compartment that contains the heart and great vessels, esophagus, trachea, phrenic and cardiac

Figure 11.24. Mediastinum and diaphragm

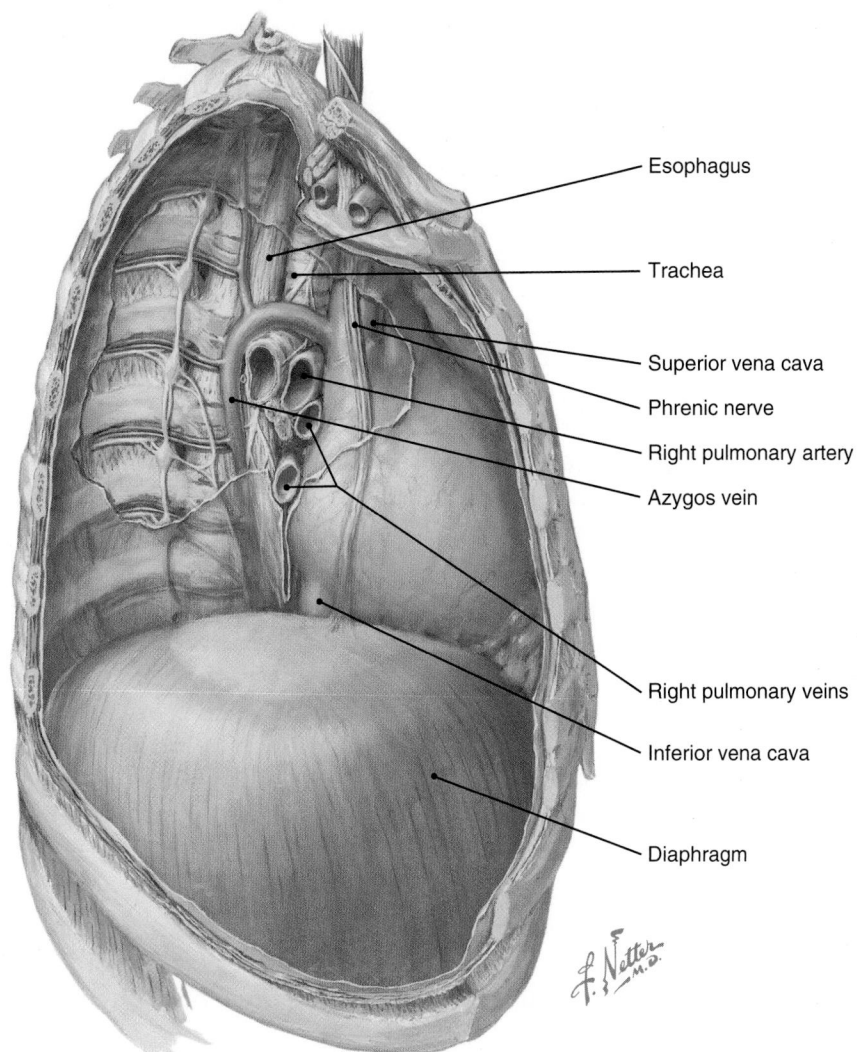

- Esophagus
- Trachea
- Superior vena cava
- Phrenic nerve
- Right pulmonary artery
- Azygos vein
- Right pulmonary veins
- Inferior vena cava
- Diaphragm

nerves, thoracic duct, thymus, and chest lymph nodes (see figure 11.24). Procedures on the mediastinum are limited, as this structure is a compartment for other organs in the chest. They are located in the Mediastinum and Diaphragm subsection (39000 to 39499) and include mediastinotomy (an incision into the mediastinum for exploration or drainage), resection (excision) of a mediastinal cyst or tumor, and mediastinoscopy with biopsy (when performed). Note that because the mediastinum is located within the thoracic cavity, in close vicinity to the heart and lungs, procedures on this area are more likely to be performed by a thoracic surgeon.

The **diaphragm** is a muscle that lies underneath the thoracic cavity, separating the heart and lungs from the abdominal contents. This muscle also performs an important function in breathing as it contracts and expands, allowing the lungs to drawn in and expel air. Procedures performed on the diaphragm are limited as well. They are located in the Mediastinum and Diaphragm subsection (39000 to 39599). They include repair of lacerations or diaphragmatic hernias, imbrication for eventration (a procedure to reshape an abnormally elevated diaphragm), and resection of diaphragmatic tumors.

Appendectomy and Appendicitis

Appendicitis is a problem that is commonly treated surgically by removing the appendix, a procedure often performed by general surgeons in the inpatient hospital setting. Appendectomy (removal of the appendix) codes are straightforward:

- 44950, Appendectomy. This procedure is performed on a patient with appendicitis, an inflammation of the appendix. If left untreated, an inflamed appendix may rupture, causing a dangerous infection of the peritoneal cavity. This code may also be used to report an incidental appendectomy, which is performed in addition to a primary procedure within the abdomen. For example, a surgeon performing a cholecystectomy (removal of the gallbladder) may choose to also perform an incidental appendectomy at the time of the primary procedure (the cholecystectomy) as a preventive procedure to prevent future appendicitis and the need for another surgery. Incidental appendectomies are usually not coded, as they are minor procedures. However, if it is necessary to report an incidental appendectomy that was performed along with a primary procedure, append modifier -52, Reduced services, to the code for the appendectomy and the code for the primary procedure.

- 44955, Appendectomy; *when done for indicated purpose at time of other procedure (not as separate procedure).* In some instances, when a surgeon is performing an abdominal procedure, he or she may notice that the appendix is inflamed or calcified, and perform an appendectomy at the time of the primary procedure. In this case, the appendix is not removed as an incidental procedure but rather due to an *"indicated purpose"* at the time of the primary procedure. Note that this is an add-on code that should be used in addition to the code for the primary procedure. When reporting this procedure code, the diagnosis code for the "indicated purpose" is needed to identify that the appendectomy was medically necessary.

- 44960, Appendectomy; *for ruptured appendix with abscess or generalized peritonitis.* This appendectomy code is to report the removal of an appendix that has already ruptured or resulted in generalized peritonitis (infection within the peritoneal cavity).

- 44970, Laparoscopy, surgical, appendectomy. This code should be used for an appendectomy that was performed laparoscopically and may be performed in the hospital outpatient setting.

Diagnosis codes for conditions of the appendix are located in categories K35 to K38, Diseases of the Appendix. Codes should identify the condition as Acute appendicitis (K35), Other appendicitis (K36), or Unspecified appendicitis (K37). Codes for acute appendicitis further identify if the appendix has ruptured and resulted in peritonitis. If peritonitis is present, coders should identify the peritonitis as either generalized or localized peritonitis. The code for unspecified appendicitis (K37) should only be used when the documentation does not identify the appendicitis as either acute (K35) or chronic/recurrent (K36). Additional codes for diseases of the appendix (category K38) identify conditions of the appendix, which may or may not require removal of the appendix, such as hyperplasia, diverticulum, and fistula of the appendix.

Cholecystectomy, Cholelithiasis, and Cholecystitis

Cholecystitis is the inflammation of the gallbladder and is usually related to a complication of stones in the gallbladder—a condition called cholelithiasis. A cholecystectomy is a procedure performed to remove the gallbladder, commonly done in the

Figure 11.25. Cholelithiasis and choledocholithiasis

Gallstone blocking
common bile duct

Gallbladder

Gallstones

Source: BruceBlaus 2015.

inpatient setting. Codes for cholecystectomies identify the type of removal (laparoscopic or open/excisional) and any additional procedures performed along with the removal of the gallbladder.

- Laparoscopic procedures (47562 to 47579) are less invasive procedures that involve the use of thin instruments inserted through small incisions, aided by the use of a video camera, and may be performed in the outpatient hospital setting.

- Open/Excisional procedures (47600 to 47715) are more invasive and are likely to be performed in the inpatient hospital setting.

Note that many of these code descriptions include cholangiography, which is an examination of the bile ducts used to identify an obstruction. A cholangiography may be performed in addition to a cholecystectomy to detect any further obstructions that may require an additional procedure.

Obstructions within the gallbladder and bile ducts are commonly caused by cholelithiasis, the presence of gallstones. Choledocholithiasis is the presence of one of more gallstones within the common bile duct. If the bile duct is obstructed by the gallstones, it may result in cholecystitis—an inflammation of the gallbladder. This is a painful condition that may require surgical removal of the gallbladder (cholecystectomy), as described previously. See figure 11.25 for an illustration of both conditions.

Diagnosis codes for gallstone and biliary tract conditions (K80, K81, K82, K83) identify the condition as either the presence of calculi (lithiases), including the location of the calculus (the gallbladder or the bile ducts), or that the gallstones have resulted in an inflammation of the gallbladder (cholecystitis). Cholecystitis may also present without the presence of gallstones.

Cholelithiasis (K80) codes require careful reading of the components included in the codes (see figure 11.26). Reporting the correct code relies on identification of the following:

- *The location of the stone*, either the gallbladder, bile ducts, or both the gallbladder and bile ducts.

Figure 11.26. Cholelithiasis code components

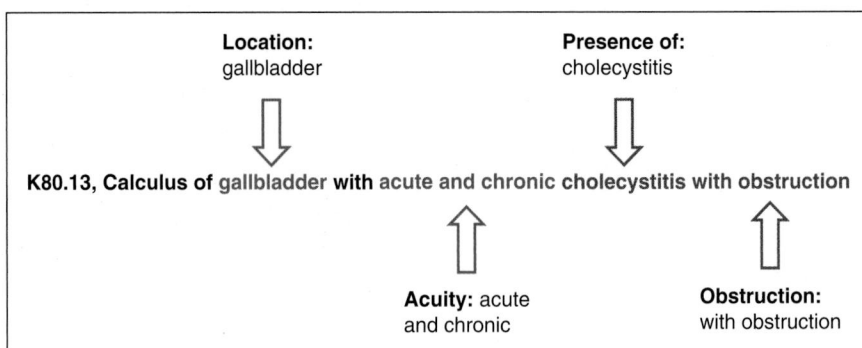

- *The presence or absence of cholecystitis or cholangitis* (inflammation of the bile ducts). Identify whether the condition presents with cholecystitis, without cholecystitis, with cholangitis, without cholangitis, or without cholangitis and cholecystitis. Note that if the patient has cholecystitis due to cholelithiasis, documentation should specify that the patient has both conditions. If the patient has acute cholecystitis without cholelithiasis, report code K81.0.
- *The acuity of the condition.* If cholecystitis or cholangitis is present, it should be identified as acute, chronic, or acute and chronic.
- *The presence or absence of obstruction* (with or without obstruction).

Abdomen, Peritoneum, and Omentum, and Herniorrhaphy

The last heading in the Gastrointestinal subsection in the CPT code book includes codes for procedures performed on the Abdomen, Peritoneum, and Omentum (49000 to 49999). Unlike the rest of the procedures in the gastrointestinal subsection, these codes identify procedures that are performed on the structures within the abdomen or on the abdomen itself. They include exploratory, drainage, and lavage of the peritoneal cavity; biopsy; excision and destruction of tumors within the peritoneal cavity; removal of peritoneal foreign bodies and insertion and removal of devices or obstructive material; and herniorrhaphies (repair of hernias).

There are four components to repair of hernia codes (hernioplasty, herniorrhaphy, herniotomy 49491 to 49659). Note that not all of these components are present in every hernia code.

- *Type.* The type of hernia identifies the area or structures involved in the herniation. They include inguinal, lumbar, femoral, incisional/ventral, epigastric, umbilical, and spigelian.
- *Recurrence.* Hernias may be identified as either initial (the first instance of the hernia) or recurrent (the hernia has recurred more than once in the same location).
- *Clinical presentation.* The clinical presentation of the hernia identifies it as either reducible (meaning that the structure can be easily moved back into its original location), or incarcerated/strangulated (meaning that the structure cannot be moved back into its original location). Incarcerated or strangulated hernias may be dangerous, leading to restriction of blood flow, death of the structure, or gangrene.
- *Age of the patient.* Some hernia codes differ based on the age of the patient. If the code description does not describe the patient's age, then this component will not change the code selection.

Note that codes for the repair of diaphragmatic hernias are located in the diaphragm subsection of the CPT code book, codes 39503 to 39541.

Diagnosis codes for hernias are in categories K40 to K46 and contain many of the same components of hernia procedure codes.

- *Type of hernia.* These include inguinal (K40), femoral (K41), umbilical (K42), ventral (K43), diaphragmatic (K44), other (K45), and unspecified abdominal hernia (K46).

- *Laterality.* Inguinal and femoral hernias should be identified as either unilateral (one sided) or bilateral (both sides). Note that codes for unilateral hernias do not specify the side of the hernia, just that it presents unilaterally.

- *Recurrence.* Hernias should be specified as either recurrent or not. If the documentation does not specify that the hernia is recurrent, then select the code for the "not specified as recurrent" option.

- *Presence of obstruction.* Codes identify whether the hernia is obstructed or not, as with or without obstruction. Note that in procedural coding for hernia repairs the clinical terminology is incarcerated or strangulated, whereas in diagnostic coding the terminology is obstructed. They should be used for the same condition.

- *Presence of gangrene.* The presence of gangrene should also be identified. Note that gangrene may present with or without obstruction.

When coding for hernias and hernia repairs, it is important to make sure that the hernia diagnosis code matches the procedure, so that it fully supports the medical necessity for the service. For example, if the coder selected diagnosis code K40.21, Bilateral inguinal hernia, without obstruction or gangrene, recurrent, with procedure code 49555, Repair recurrent femoral hernia; reducible, the service would be considered not medically necessary and would not be paid. This is because the types of hernia do not match; the diagnosis code identifies the condition as an inguinal hernia, while the procedure code identifies the hernia as a femoral hernia.

For practice identifying the procedure and diagnosis codes for general surgery procedures, complete the exercises in There's a Code for That 11.5.

Coding for general surgery

11.5

There's a Code for That

Read the description of the procedure and assign the appropriate ICD-10-CM and/or CPT codes.

1. Herniorrhaphy with hydrocelectomy performed on 4-year-old male patient with initial, reducible inguinal hernia.

   CPT code: _____

   ICD-10-CM code: _____

2. Cholecystectomy without cholangiography performed laparoscopically on 30-year-old female patient with cholelithiasis and acute cholecystitis without obstruction.

   CPT code: _____

   ICD-10-CM code: _____

(Continued on next page)

11.5

Continued

3. Laparoscopic appendectomy completed on a 60-year-old male patient with ruptured appendix with localized peritonitis.

CPT code: _____

ICD-10-CM code: _____

Transplant Surgery

Transplant surgeries may be performed by a healthcare specialist trained in a specific field of medicine (such as a cardiovascular surgeon), or one who specializes in transplants specifically (a cardiac transplant specialist). Any type of transplant is a complex, major procedure, and as such is performed in the inpatient hospital setting. Organs and tissues that can be transplanted include the heart, lungs, intestines, islet cells (from the pancreas), kidneys, liver, pancreas, corneas, thymus, stomach, testis, bone, skin, stem cells, and hands. However, some of these procedures are rare (such as hand transplants) and performed only in specialized settings with trained surgeons and clinical technicians. In these infrequent cases, it may be necessary to use the unlisted services code to report the procedure performed, or a combination of codes to report each service performed.

Transplants that have a specific set of transplant codes in the CPT code book include the heart (33930 to 33945), intestines (included in the range 44100 to 44160), liver (47133 to 47147), lung (32850 to 32856), pancreas (48550 to 48556), and kidney (50300 to 50380). When coding for transplant procedures, there are three components of the procedure that should be clearly identified and reported for the service performed.

- *Removal of the donated organ.* This includes the harvesting of the organ from the donor. In some cases, the donor of the organ is a **cadaver donor** (brain dead patient from whom organs are being harvested), or the donor may be a **living donor** (when the organ being donated is one that can be harvested from a living patient).

- *Backbench work to prepare the organ.* Backbench work involves the preparation of the organ for transplantation, including dissection of the organ from soft tissues and preparation of the valves and vessels for transplantation.

- *Transplantation of the organ.* Transplantation of the donated organ may include the removal of the recipient's organ(s) prior to the transplantation, or not. Once the recipient area is prepared for the organ transplantation, then the transplantation code identifies the placement of the organ in the patient, with or without the removal of the recipient's organ.

The coder should report only the service that was performed by his or her provider. For example, if the provider performed a cadaver donor pneumonectomy (removal of the lungs), and then the lungs were transported to another facility for the transplant, performed by a different surgeon, then the coder would only report the code for the removal of the donated organ, 32850, Donor pneumonectomy(s) (including cold preservation), from cadaver donor.

Putting It All Together: Coding for Surgical Services

When coding for surgical services, keep in mind that multiple procedure codes may be necessary to report the service fully. Do not code for services that are included in the surgical package or the code description for the primary procedure. See figure 11.27 for steps to coding for surgical services.

Figure 11.27. Steps to coding for surgical services

Procedure Code(s)

1. Carefully read the documentation of the surgical procedure.
2. Locate the procedural terms (verbs) that describe the procedure performed, as well as any specifics that might indicate the need for a modifier.
3. Locate the codes for the procedures by looking them up in the CPT Index and referencing the Tabular List.
4. Check that the specifics of the code selected match the procedure that was performed. Is it the right site? Is it the right type of procedure (for example, open versus laparoscopic)? Does the code description include everything that was performed during the procedure?
5. Check CPT guidelines and parenthetical notes for additional information and make sure the code is reported correctly .
6. Check for any applicable modifiers or additional CPT codes.

Diagnosis Code(s)

7. Determine the postoperative diagnosis and any comorbid conditions or complications.
8. Locate all necessary diagnosis codes in the ICD -10-CM Index.
9. Verify each ICD -10-CM code in the Tabular List and check for any applicable guidelines or additional required codes.
10. Return to the documentation of the procedure to verify that the codes selected are correct and that all services and diagnoses were reported.

End of Chapter Content

Instructions: Indicate whether the following statements are true or false (T or F). For false statements, rewrite the statement on the line below to make the statement true.

1. An invasive procedure rarely involves breaking the skin in order to perform the procedure.

_____

_____

2. An inpatient is one that has been formally admitted to a hospital.

_____

_____

3. POS code 21 would be used to report services performed in the inpatient hospital setting.

_____

_____

(Continued on next page)

(Continued)

4. Outpatients in a hospital must be confined to the outpatient unit and may never stay in the main building of the hospital.

_____

_____

5. E/M codes 99201 to 99215 should be used for encounters in the ASC setting.

_____

_____

6. A minor surgical procedure typically includes a 90-day global period.

_____

_____

7. Surgical procedures are found in the Medicine section of the CPT code book.

_____

_____

8. An excision is an open procedure.

_____

_____

9. A therapeutic procedure is one that is performed to treat a diagnosis.

_____

_____

10. Modifier -47 should be appended to the code for an anesthesia procedure that was performed by an anesthesiologist.

_____

_____

Instructions: Match the terms with the appropriate descriptions.

1. _____ Incision

2. _____ Excision

3. _____ Introduction

4. _____ Removal

5. _____ Repair

6. _____ Destruction

A. The insertion of a device, object, or substance into a body part or organ

B. Procedure to destroy tissue, also known as ablation

C. Taking out a device, object, or substance from a body part or area

D. Manually moving a body part into its original location or into another location

E. A cut made on a body part or organ

F. Procedure performed to return an organ or body part to its original function, to improve function, or to improve cosmetic appearance

7. _____ Endoscopy   G. Procedure that uses a lighted scope, inserted through incisions into the body to perform a diagnostic or therapeutic procedure

8. _____ Laparoscopy   H. The surgical removal of an organ, body tissue, lesion, or other body part or foreign object

9. _____ Transplantation   I. Removal of a damaged, diseased, or nonfunctioning organ and replacing it with a donated organ

10. _____ Manipulation   J. Procedure performed with the aid of an endoscope inserted through a natural opening or stoma

Instructions: Choose the best answer.

1. Which of the following is a noninvasive, non-surgical procedure?
   a. Cryosurgery
   b. Organ transplant
   c. Nebulizer treatment
   d. Internal organ repair

2. In which setting would a major or risky surgery be performed?
   a. Inpatient hospital
   b. Outpatient hospital
   c. Ambulatory surgical center
   d. Outpatient office

3. Which set of E/M codes are used for hospital inpatient E/M encounters?
   a. 99201 to 99215
   b. 99217 to 99226
   c. 99221 to 99239
   d. E/M services are not billed for inpatients

4. What does ASC stand for?
   a. Acute setting for care
   b. Ambulatory surgical care
   c. Ambulatory surgical center
   d. Acute surgery center

5. Which of the following is a facility in which the patient would remain overnight?
   a. Urgent care clinic
   b. Ambulatory surgical center
   c. Inpatient hospital
   d. Office

6. Which of the following rules apply to procedures performed at an ASC?
   a. The procedure cannot pose a significant safety risk to the patient
   b. The procedure may be emergent or life threatening in nature
   c. The procedure must involve an overnight stay for the patient
   d. The procedure may be performed in anywhere, including in the physician's office

7. How many days are included in the global period for a major surgical procedure?
   a. 10 days
   b. 90 days
   c. 30 days
   d. 45 days

8. Where can the guidelines for CPT surgical codes be found?
   a. At the beginning of the Surgery section
   b. Within each subsection of medicine codes
   c. Before specific codes located in parentheses
   d. After the diagnosis description

9. A robot-assisted surgery is which type of procedure?
   a. Laparoscopy
   b. Endoscopy
   c. Excision
   d. Introduction

10. If the pre- and postoperative diagnoses differ, which diagnosis should be reported to identify the medical necessity for the procedure?

    a. The preoperative diagnosis

    b. Both preoperative and postoperative diagnoses

    c. The postoperative diagnosis

    d. Neither—send in a special report to explain the lack of ICD-10-CM code

11. A surgical procedure was performed by a team of two surgeons. Each of the surgeons had an equal share of responsibility in the procedure. Which modifier should be appended to the procedure?

    a. -62

    b. -82

    c. -66

    d. -AS

12. Each layer of skin excised in Mohs surgery is referred to as a what?

    a. Block

    b. Specimen

    c. Stage

    d. Lesion

13. Which of the following grafts would come from a donor of a different species?

    a. Autograft

    b. Allograft

    c. Xenograft

    d. Homograft

Instructions: Answer the following questions with the appropriate code(s) and modifier(s).

1. Healthy liver was harvested from a 32-year-old female patient declared brain dead.

    CPT code: _____

2. Transplantation of kidney, without recipient nephrectomy.

    CPT code: _____

3. Cholangiography reveals choledocholithiasis with acute cholecystitis, with obstruction. Emergent cholecystectomy performed at the same session.

    CPT code: _____

    ICD-10-CM code: _____

4. Debridement of all five toenails on the left foot and three toenails on the right foot due to onychomycosis.

    CPT code: _____

    ICD-10-CM code: _____

5. 42-year-old female with malignant neoplasm of the right upper outer breast underwent lumpectomy procedure of the right breast with axillary lymphadenectomy.

    CPT code: _____

    ICD-10-CM code: _____

References

Agency for Healthcare Research and Quality. 2017 (June). Never Events. https://psnet.ahrq.gov/primers/primer/3/never-events.

American Health Information Management Association. 2017. *Pocket Glossary of Health Information Management and Technology*, 5th ed. Chicago: AHIMA.

American Health Information Management Association. 2016. *ICD-10-CM Code Book: 2017*. Chicago: AHIMA.

American Medical Association. 2018. *CPT© 2018 Professional Edition*. Chicago: AMA.

Blausen.com staff. 2014. "Laproscopy." Digital Image. Wikimedia Commons. Accessed December, 2017. https://commons.wikimedia.org/wiki/File:Blausen_0602_Laparoscopy_02.png.

BruceBlaus. 2015. "Gallstones.png." Digital Image. Wikimedia Commons. Accessed December, 2017. https://commons.wikimedia.org/wiki/File:Gallstones.png.

Centers for Medicare and Medicaid Services. 2018. ICD-10-CM Official Guidelines for Coding and Reporting FY 2018. https://www.cms.gov/Medicare/Coding/ICD10/Downloads/2018-ICD-10-CM-Coding-Guidelines.pdf.

Centers for Medicare and Medicaid Services. 2017a. Details for title: CMS 1500. https://www.cms.gov/Medicare/CMS-Forms/CMS-Forms/CMS-Forms-Items/CMS1188854.html.

Centers for Medicare and Medicaid Services. 2017b (April 14). Medicare Claims Processing Manual Chapter 12 - Physicians/Nonphysician Practitioners. https://www .cms.gov/Regulations-and-Guidance/Guidance /Manuals/downloads/clm104c12.pdf.

Centers for Medicare and Medicaid Services. 2016 (November 10). Medicare Claims Processing Manual, Chapter 14-Ambulatory Surgical Centers. https://www .cms.gov/Regulations-and-Guidance/Guidance /Manuals/downloads/clm104c14.pdf.

National Cancer Institute. 1985a. "Kaposi's Sarcoma." Digital image. National Cancer Institute. Accessed December, 2017. https://visualsonline.cancer.gov /details.cfm?imageid=2168.

National Cancer Institute. 1985b. "Melanoma.jpg." Digital image. Wikimedia Commons. Accessed December, 2017. https://commons.wikimedia.org/wiki/File:Melanoma.jpg.

Nelson, Kelly. 2012a. "Skin Cancer, Basal Cell Carcinoma, Superficial." Digital image. National Cancer Institute. Accessed December, 2017. https://visualsonline.cancer .gov/details.cfm?imageid=9236.

Nelson, Kelly. 2012b. "Skin Cancer, Squamous Cell Carcinoma, Leg." Digital image. National Cancer Institute. Accessed December, 2017. https:// visualsonline.cancer.gov/details.cfm?imageid=9249.

Taylornate. 2011a. "Advancement flap.svg." Digital image. Wikimedia Commons. Accessed December, 2017. https://commons.wikimedia.org/wiki/File: Advancement_flap.svg.

Taylornate. 2011b. "Rotation flap.svg." Digital image. Wikimedia Commons. Accessed December, 2017. https:// commons.wikimedia.org/wiki/File:Rotation_flap.svg.

Taylornate. 2011c. "Transposition flap.svg." Digital image. Wikimedia Commons. Accessed December, 2017. https://commons.wikimedia.org/wiki/File: Transposition_flap.svg.

Resources

American Academy of Professional Coders. 2014 (October 15). Coding Robot-assisted Surgery. https://www.aapc.com/blog/28266-coding-robot -assisted-surgery/.

American Association of Oral and Maxillofacial Surgeons. 2013. Ambulatory Surgical Center Coding and Billing. http://www.aaoms.org/images/uploads/pdfs/asc _coding_and_billing.pdf.

American Medical Association. 2018. CPT© 2018 Professional Edition. Chicago: American Medical Association.

Cancer Research UK. 2014. "Diagram showing a bronchoscopy." Digial Image. Wikimedia Commons. Accessed December, 2017. https://commons.wikimedia .org/wiki/File:Diagram_showing_a_bronchoscopy _CRUK_053.svg.

Centers for Medicare and Medicaid Services. 2015 (March). Global Surgery Fact Sheet. https://www.cms.gov /Outreach-and-Education/Medicare-Learning-Network -MLN/MLNProducts/downloads/GloballSurgery -ICN907166.pdf.

Centers for Medicare and Medicaid Services. 2005 (January 14). Pub. 100–04 Medicare Claims Processing. https://www.cms.gov/Regulations-and-Guidance /Guidance/Transmittals/downloads/R434CP.pdf.

Chrysopoulo, M.T. 2017 (August 7). Tissue Flap Classification. https://emedicine.medscape.com /article/1284474-overview#a1.

Smith, G. 2017. *Basic Current Procedural Terminology and HCPCS Coding, 2018*. Chicago: AHIMA.

CHAPTER

Anesthesia and Pain Management Services

Learning Objectives

- Understand the basics of billing and coding within the specialty of anesthesia and pain management services.
- Examine procedural codes and guidelines for anesthesia and pain management services.

- Examine diagnosis coding and medical necessity for anesthesia and pain management services.
- Determine and apply ICD-10-CM, CPT, and HCPCS codes to anesthesia and pain management services.

Key Terms

Acupuncture
Analgesia
Anesthesia services
Anesthesiology
ASA crosswalk
Base units
Cervicalgia
Chronic pain
Conversion factor (CF)
Electrodiagnostic studies
Electromyography (EMG)
Enthesopathy
Epidural steroid injection

Facet joint injection
Fibromyalgia
General anesthesia
Integrative medicine
Interventional pain procedures
Kyphoplasty
Local anesthesia
Lumbago
Moderate (conscious) sedation
Modifying factors
Monitored anesthesia care (MAC)
Myalgia
Myositis

Nerve condition study (NCS)
Occipital nerve block
Osteoarthritis
Pain management services
Peripheral nerve stimulation
Physical status modifier
Qualifying circumstance CPT codes
Radiculopathy
Radiofrequency nerve ablation
Regional anesthesia
Sciatica
Spinal cord stimulation (SCS)
Time units

Anesthesia and pain management specialties both aim to reduce sensation (typically the sensation of pain); however, **anesthesia services** are procedures that create analgesia—the absence of pain—and are provided for a brief amount of time in order to facilitate a medical procedure, such as a surgery. Unlike anesthesia procedures, which are performed as part of a medical or surgical procedure to anesthetize the patient, **pain management services** are given as a treatment for chronic pain in patients who are not undergoing any type of surgical procedure. Pain management services are often aimed at reducing discomfort for patients suffering from chronic pain. **Chronic pain** is the constant or long-term sensation of pain that may be due to postoperative complications, past injuries, or nerve conditions. Pain management procedures are designed to improve quality of life for patients by alleviating chronic pain. The goal of pain management is not to cure the pain or underlying cause of the pain, but to treat or reduce the pain to a level considered manageable by the patient.

This chapter discusses both anesthesia and pain management coding—first examining the intricacies of anesthesia billing and its impact on the codes reported for anesthesia services, followed by a discussion of pain management basics, and then applying procedural and diagnostic coding for both specialties.

Anesthesia Billing and Coding Basics

Anesthesiology is the healthcare specialty of relieving patient pain before, during, and after surgery. The aim of anesthesia services is to provide **analgesia**, or the inability to feel pain. Anesthesiologists perform the majority of their services in the inpatient hospital, outpatient hospital, or ASC settings, in which patients are undergoing invasive, painful surgeries.

Anesthesia coding is quite different from medical evaluation and management or surgical procedure coding. Instead of coding for the procedure performed by the doctor, anesthesia codes identify the anesthesia service provided while the doctor was performing the procedure. Anesthesia codes do not specify the exact substance administered to induce anesthesia or the specifics of the anesthesia service itself. Rather, anesthesia codes identify the surgical procedure that the patient was undergoing, which necessitated the anesthesia in the first place. Anesthesia codes are located in a special (Anesthesia) section of codes in the CPT code book. Furthermore, billing for anesthesia services requires a special calculation to determine how much to charge for the service performed, depending on the circumstances surrounding each particular service. Pain management, on the other hand, is more similar to surgical and medical coding, as it uses codes from the Surgery section of the CPT code book. Pain management procedures are more like surgical interventions that treat either the cause of the pain (such as removing a herniated disc) or the symptom of pain (such as an injection of anesthetic into a joint or nerve).

Beginning coders must understand the basics of anesthesia services, including how services were billed, how the services are coded, and the difference between anesthesia and pain management procedures. Anesthesia and pain management specialists perform services to reduce sensation, either during a medical procedure or as a treatment for chronic pain.

There are three main types of providers that may provide anesthesia services—anesthesiologists, anesthesiology assistants (AAs), and certified registered nurse anesthetists (CRNAs). Anesthesiologists are medical doctors who specialize in anesthesiology. AAs are similar to physician assistants (PAs), in that they have completed a graduate program in medical training, with an emphasis in anesthesia. CRNAs, on the other hand, are registered nurses (RNs) who have completed a graduate program with an emphasis in anesthesia. AAs and CRNAs are both mid-level providers who are able to perform anesthesiology procedures only under the supervision of an anesthesiologist. It is important to understand the differences between anesthesiology providers, as the codes billed may differ depending on which provider performed the service (discussed later in this chapter).

Billing for anesthesia services is further complicated by the varying nature of anesthesia procedures. Anesthesia services are performed in order to create analgesia, the absence of the sensation of pain, in a number of different ways such as by the intravenous or inhaled administration of drugs or other substances to induce unconsciousness and analgesia. The anesthesiologist is the practitioner who determines which type of anesthesia is best according to the patient's specific needs and what is needed for the surgical or medical procedure. The anesthesiologist administers the anesthesia and monitors the patient during the surgical procedure to ensure that the anesthesia is working and the patient's vital signs are stable.

Therefore the actual anesthesia service, including the time spent on the service, varies greatly depending on the patient, the medical procedure, and any complications that may occur during the surgery. For example, an anesthesiologist administering anesthesia to a patient for a routine appendectomy may spend less overall time monitoring the patient during the anesthesia procedure than if the surgeon was performing a complicated appendectomy that took an inordinate amount of time, or if it was a very young or very old patient. The next sections discuss the unique nature of billing and coding for anesthesia services, which combine many of these elements including the basic service, the time it took to perform the service, and any modifying factors involved in the service. It also discusses the detailed documentation required for anesthesia services.

Billing and Coding for Anesthesia Services

Billing for anesthesia services is not as simple as reporting a specific CPT code and linking to an ICD-10-CM code to identify the medical necessity for the service. These two items are still required, but additional information is needed to be able to bill for anesthesia services appropriately.

Correct billing of anesthesia services is based on three things: base units, time, and modifying factors. Base units are numerical values given to each anesthesia service, time units identify the amount of time spent on the anesthesia service, and modifying factors identify any additional complications or extra work needed to perform the procedure (discussed fully later in this section). These three components are combined according to each anesthesia service and multiplied by a conversion factor, which is a dollar amount, to calculate the amount of payment for the anesthesia service. Although CMS annually publishes a conversion factor for anesthesia services, keep in mind that this conversion factor may vary across insurance policies and often changes each year. The conversion factor determines the dollar amount billed per service, and is discussed in further detail later in this section.

This is vastly different from typical billing for medical or surgical services. For example, a primary care physician bills for a preventive medical examination by submitting the CPT code along with the ICD-10-CM code. An anesthesiologist, on the other hand, bills for a service by reporting the CPT code for the service that was performed (which carries the base units for the procedure), then adds the amount of time involved in the procedure (time units), as well as any modifying factors that identify additional work or complexity that the procedure involved (modifying units). Each of

Figure 12.1. Anesthesia billing formula

these components are combined and then multiplied by a conversion factor that ultimately determines the amount of payment for the service rendered. In this manner, if a service was less complicated or took less time, then the reimbursement amount for the service would be smaller than if the procedure took more time or was more complicated or risky to perform.

In a simplified format, the formula for anesthesia billing is as follows:

$$(B + T + M) \times CF = \text{Amount billed}$$

In this formula, B is base units, T is time, M is modifying factors, and CF is conversion factor (see figure 12.1).

Base Units

Base units, a set of numerical values created and maintained by the American Society of Anesthesiologists (ASA), give each anesthesiology service a numerical relative value in relation to how complicated or risky a procedure is, and are used to set the relative cost of each procedures. The higher base values of an anesthesia procedure, the higher the charge for the procedure; the lower the base units, the lower the charge for the procedure. Base unit values assigned by CMS range from 0 to 2 (unlisted procedures and add-on codes) to 30 (00796, Anesthesia for all intraperitoneal procedures in upper abdomen including laparoscopy; liver transplant (recipient)) (CMS 2014).

A simple procedure may be assigned 1 base unit, a moderate procedure may be assigned 3 base units, and a complicated procedure may be assigned 5 base units. So a more complicated or risky procedure holds more value (in terms of billing) than a simpler procedure, and anesthesiologists may be reimbursed more for complex procedures and less for simpler procedures. For example, CPT code 00524, Anesthesia for closed chest procedures; pneumocentesis, is assigned 4 base units. Code 00528, Anesthesia for closed chest procedures; mediastinoscopy and diagnostic thoracoscopy not utilizing 1 lung ventilation, is assigned 8 units, as this is a more complex closed chest procedure than the pneumocentesis. Code 00529, Anesthesia for closed chest procedures; mediastinoscopy and diagnostic thoracoscopy utilizing 1 lung ventilation, is assigned 11 base units, as this procedure is more complex than the mediastinoscopy without lung ventilation.

Base unit values are published on the CMS website each year for reference (see figure 12.2); note that these base unit values have not been updated since 2014. Base unit values are also published in the ASA Relative Value Guide (ASA RVG), which contains more than 300 CPT codes, all of which have a relative value assigned. When billing for services covered by Medicare, coders should refer to the base units published

Figure 12.2. CMS anesthesia base units

Code	2014 Base Unit
00100	5
00102	6
00103	5
00104	4
00120	5
00124	4
00126	4
00140	5
00142	4
00144	6
00145	6
00147	4
00148	4
00160	5
00162	7
00164	4
00170	5

Source: Adapted from CMS 2014.

by CMS. However, some commercial payers use the base unit values published by the ASA. So coders should use the ASA RVG when coding for commercial payers (unless otherwise stated by the contract with the payer) to determine the base unit values for procedures performed, and use the Medicare base unit values when coding claims for Medicare patients.

Though base unit values are reviewed and updated by either CMS or the ASA on an annual basis, this sometimes results in little to no changes in these values. For example, figure 12.2 shows the 2014 base unit values published by Medicare. Note that these values have not been changed since they were published in 2014. The services included within the base unit include

- All usual anesthesia services, such as the determination of the anesthesia dose and substance, preparation of the patient and administration of the anesthesia, and monitoring during the procedure (except the time involved in the procedure and any modifying factors)
- Usual pre- and postoperative visits
- Administration of fluids or blood products
- Interpretation and monitoring of noninvasive monitoring procedures, such as ECG, temperature, blood pressure, oximetry, capnography, and mass spectrometry (AMA 2018)

Base unit values do not include the placement of arterial, central venous, or pulmonary arterial catheters or the use of transesophageal echocardiography (TEE) (among other procedures, as discussed in the following Procedural Coding section). Any additional procedures (other than those identified previously) are included in the base units for the anesthesia service reported and may not be reported separately.

When coding for anesthesia services, knowing the base unit value of each procedure is important because when an anesthesiologist is providing anesthesia to a patient who is undergoing more than one procedure, then only the anesthesia procedure with the *highest* base units should be billed. For example, if the surgeon is performing a liver transplant and an appendectomy, then only the anesthesia for the liver transplant should be reported, because it has the higher number of base units. According to CMS, the base unit values for an appendectomy (code 00790, Anesthesia for intraperitoneal procedures in upper abdomen including laparoscopy; not otherwise specified) are 7, whereas the base unit values for a patient receiving anesthesia for a liver transplant (code 00796, Anesthesia for intraperitoneal procedures in upper abdomen including laparoscopy; liver transplant (recipient)) are 30. In this case, the base unit values for the liver transplant procedure outweigh those for the appendectomy procedure, so only the liver transplant anesthesia code should be reported. The anesthesia service for the appendectomy would be included in the base units for the more complex procedure (liver transplant). Any additional procedures that the provider performed above and beyond either anesthesia service may be reported separately. Anesthesia coders must therefore know and understand the relative values of each of the services performed by the provider for whom they bill to correctly report the service(s) provided.

To test your understanding of base unit values, complete the exercises in There's a Code for That 12.1.

12.1

There's a Code for That

Base unit values

Using the following table, identify either the number of base unit values for the given anesthesia code, or determine which anesthesia code should be reported.

Code	Units	Code	Units	Code	Units	Code	Units
00100	5	00164	4	00222	6	00470	6
00102	6	00170	5	00300	5	00472	10
00103	5	00172	6	00320	6	00474	13
00104	4	00174	6	00322	3	00500	15
00120	5	00176	7	00326	7	00520	6
00124	4	00190	5	00350	10	00522	4
00126	4	00192	7	00352	5	00524	4
00140	5	00210	11	00400	3	00528	8
00142	4	00211	10	00402	5	00529	11
00144	6	00212	5	00404	5	00530	4
00145	6	00214	9	00406	13	00532	4
00147	4	00215	9	00410	4	00534	7
00148	4	00216	15	00450	5	00537	7
00160	5	00218	13	00452	6	00539	18
00162	7	00220	10	00454	3	00540	12

Source: Adapted from CMS 2014.

1. Which anesthesia service holds the highest number of base units: 00454 or 00402? _____

2. The surgeon performed a radical mastectomy of the bilateral female breasts, with internal mammary node dissection. Which anesthesia code would be reported for the service: 00404 or 00406? _____

3. The surgeon performed multiple intracranial procedures while the patient was under anesthesia, including a craniotomy for evacuation of hematoma (00211) and a cranioplasty of depressed skull fracture (00215). Which anesthesia service should be reported?

   CPT code: _____

4. The surgeon performed a bronchoscopy (00520) as well as a biopsy of the soft tissue of the accessory sinuses (00164). Which anesthesia code should be reported?

   CPT code: _____

Time

The **time units** for anesthesia services take into account the duration of the procedure, from the beginning of the anesthesia service until the patient is released to a postoperative or post-anesthesia care unit. Time units are based on the standard time measurements in guidelines determined by either the ASA or per the patient's third-party payer. The anesthesia time starts when the anesthesiologist (or AA or CRNA) begins to prepare the patient for the anesthesia service. This can take place in the operating room or other designated area. The time calculated does not include a preoperative evaluation performed by the anesthesiologist, which may be completed before the patient is even in the operating suite, but varies depending on when the service is begun by the provider performing the medical procedure; for example, the moment when the provider starts an intravenous line, begins to place monitors on the patient, administers sedation, or begins to physically prepare the patient for the anesthesia service in any other manner and remains in constant attendance.

Anesthesia time ends when the anesthesiology provider has transferred care of the patient to a postoperative area or in a post-anesthesia care unit (PACU). The end time never occurs in the operating room. The time reported is continuous, encompassing the entire time of the service from start to finish.

Time is reported in 15-minute increments, so a service that lasted 60 minutes would total 4 time units (60 minutes divided by 15 minute increments = 4 units). Any additional time less than 7.5 minutes should be rounded down and not counted in the total time reported, and any additional time over 7.5 minutes should be rounded up to the next unit. For example, if the provider spent 67 minutes on the service (60 minutes = 4 time units, plus 7 extra minutes), the total time units reported would be 4. On the other hand, if the provider spent 68 minutes on the service (60 minutes = 4 time units, plus 8 extra minutes = 1 time unit), the total time units reported would be 5.

These are the standard time ASA and AMA reporting guidelines. However, keep in mind that Medicare has different time reporting rules, as other insurance carriers might. For example, Medicare requires that the total time spent on a procedure be divided by 15, and then the units reported in increments of one decimal point. For example, 5 minutes total would be 0.3 units (5 minutes / 15 = 0.3 units), 6 minutes would be 0.4 units (6 minutes / 15 = 0.4 units), and so on. For the purposes of this text, time reported should be in full integers, rounding down anything under 7.5 minutes and rounding up anything over 7.5 minutes.

Time units are entered in box 24.G on the CMS-1500 claim form (see figure 12.3).

Time units are yet another example of how the intricacies of billing affect the coding of claims, and how understanding the differences between payer guidelines and requirements is an integral part of correctly reporting codes and additional information entered on claims.

Figure 12.3. Time units in box 24.G

4 units = 60 minutes total anesthesia time

Source: CMS 2017a.

Modifying Factors

Modifying factors are similar to CPT modifiers, in that they provide additional information in the anesthesia procedure description, and describe an anesthesia procedure that was more complex than it would have been if it had been performed on a normal, healthy patient, or one that required additional skill to complete. Modifying factors come in two forms: CPT modifiers, called physical status modifiers, added to the CPT code for the anesthesia service; and qualifying circumstances codes, which are supplementary CPT codes that may be reported in addition to the anesthesia service codes to identify further complexity involved in the anesthesia procedure. Modifying factors are published as part of the CPT code set and may be updated annually. They assign additional units to the base and time units for the procedure, according to a preset amount per modifying factor. Note that the exact number of additional units or values assigned to the modifying factor depend on the values assigned by the patient's insurance payer. For example, some insurance plans may assign additional units to qualifying circumstances codes, while others bundle these codes into the primary service and do not provide any additional payment. There are two types of modifying factors—physical status modifiers and qualifying circumstances add-on codes.

Physical Status Modifiers

Physical status modifiers are modifiers that should be appended to the end of the anesthesia procedure code for a given service to identify the physical status of the patient and capture any additional complexity that may be present due to the patient's physical condition. They begin with the letter P and end with a number (1 through 6), and identify the physical status of the patient, as follows:

- P1: A normal, healthy patient. For example, a healthy non-smoking patient with minimal or no alcohol use.
- P2: A patient with mild systemic disease. A patient with a mild systemic disease, without any functional limitations, such as a current smoker (without problems); social drinker; pregnant without complications; mild obesity (BMI between 30 and 40); or controlled diabetes or hypertension.

- P3: A patient with severe systemic disease. A patient that has one or more moderate or severe diseases with functional limitations, such as uncontrolled or poorly controlled diabetes or hypertension; morbid obesity (BMI over 40); hepatitis; alcohol abuse or dependence; an end-stage renal disease (ESRD) patient undergoing dialysis; an implanted pacemaker; a premature infant; a myocardial infarction (MI) more than three months ago; or history of cerebrovascular accident (CVA/stroke) or transient ischemic attack (TIA).

- P4: A patient with severe systemic disease that is a constant threat to life. A patient who has a moderate or severe condition with functional limitations (as described previously), which presents a constant threat to life, such as recent MI (less than three months ago); CVA/stroke; TIA; coronary atherosclerosis; sepsis; or ESRD not undergoing regularly scheduled dialysis.

- P5: A moribund patient who is not expected to survive without the operation. A patient whose medical condition presents an immediate threat to life, and as such must undergo immediate operation. For example, ruptured aneurysm, massive traumatic injury, or intracranial bleeding.

- P6: A declared brain-dead patient whose organs are being removed for donor purposes. This patient has been declared brain dead and is receiving anesthesia during the procedures to harvest internal organs for donation. (ASA 2014)

Physical status modifiers usually hold a unit value that should be added to the total units for the anesthesia service. However, this depends on the patient's insurance payer. For example, some insurance policies assign additional time units for physical status modifiers, rather than additional base units. This is yet one more reason why coders must be vigilant about the patient's insurance payer when entering codes for claims. For example, the anesthesia service for a patient with controlled diabetes would be appended with modifier -P2. Alternatively, the anesthesia procedure code for a patient with uncontrolled diabetes, stage 5 chronic kidney disease, and hypertension would be appended with -P3. See figure 12.4 for an example of unit values for physical status modifiers.

Figure 12.4. Physical status modifier unit values

Physical Status Modifier	Unit Value
P1	0
P2	0
P3	1
P4	2
P5	3
P6	0

Qualifying Circumstances

Qualifying circumstances CPT codes are add-on codes that should be used in addition to the code for the anesthesia service (as well as any applicable physical status modifier). They describe a particularly difficult service due to the extraordinary condition of the patient, notable operative conditions, or unusual risk factors. They are all designated add-on codes that must be reported with the primary code for the anesthesia service, and may never be reported alone. Qualifying circumstance codes are listed in the CPT code book at the beginning of the Anesthesia section in the guidelines, and also in the Medicine section. They are as follows:

- 99100, Anesthesia for patient of extreme age, younger than 1 year and older than 70. This code identifies patients that are either very young or very old, and should be used in addition to the code for the anesthesia service. However, pay attention to the code description for anesthesia services, as some describe a procedure on a pediatric patient. If this is the case, then the add-on code to identify the patient as of extreme young age is not necessary. For example, code 00326, Anesthesia for all procedures on the larynx and *trachea in children younger than 1 year of age* already identifies the patient as under the age of 1 year, so the qualifying circumstance code 99100 is not necessary.

- 99116, Anesthesia complicated by utilization of total body hypothermia. Hypothermia may be induced for some anesthesia procedures because of its ability to protect the heart and brain during certain procedures. When hypothermia is induced during the procedure, this qualifying circumstance code should be used, except if the code for the anesthesia procedure includes hypothermia in the code description (such as 00563, Anesthesia for procedures on heart pericardial sac, and great vessels of chest; with pump oxygenator *with hypothermic circulatory arrest*).

- 99135, Anesthesia complicated by utilization of controlled hypotension. Hypotension (low blood pressure) is used during surgical procedures to reduce the need for blood transfusions and to help with patient outcomes by reducing bleeding as well as helping to maintain a bloodless surgical field.

- 99140, Anesthesia complicated by emergency conditions (specify). A procedure is considered an emergency when a delay in treatment would lead to an increase in the threat to the patient's life or limb. The specific emergency conditions must be clearly identified in the documentation for the procedure.

More than one qualifying circumstance code may be used, if necessary, to fully describe the circumstances of the anesthesia service. For example, anesthesia for a pneumocentesis on a 9-month-old patient complicated by emergency conditions would be coded as follows: 00524, Anesthesia for closed chest procedures; pneumocentesis, plus 99100, Anesthesia for patient of extreme age, younger than 1 year and older than 70, and 99140, Anesthesia complicated by emergency conditions.

Each qualifying circumstance code holds a unit value that should be added to the rest of the units for the procedure. For example, the 9-month-old undergoing a pneumocentesis procedure would have an additional 1 unit value added for the qualifying circumstance code 99100, and an additional 2 unit values for the qualifying circumstances code 99140. Note again that the exact amount of values added by each qualifying circumstance code depends on the insurance payer. Some third-party payers bundle qualifying circumstance codes into the payment for the anesthesia procedure, while others may add only one extra value point per qualifying circumstance code. Yet others use a scale in which each qualifying circumstance code holds a unique value. See figure 12.5 for an example of the unit values of qualifying circumstance codes.

Medicare does not take into account modifying factors, and it does not pay for any additional work (as identified by modifying factor units) for anesthesia procedures. Medicare only accounts for the base and time units for each procedure.

Figure 12.5. Qualifying circumstance unit values

Qualifying Circumstance Code	Unit Value
99100	1
99116	5
99135	5
99140	2

Figure 12.6. Selected CMS conversion factors for anesthesia services, 2017

Locality	Locality Name	National Anes CF of 22.0454
00	ALABAMA	21.06
01	ALASKA	30.69
00	ARIZONA	21.80
13	ARKANSAS	21.00
54	BAKERSFIELD, CA	22.19

Source: Adapted from CMS 2017b.

Conversion Factor

Once the units for the procedure have been totaled, this number must be multiplied by the **conversion factor (CF)** rate, which is the dollar amount per unit for the reimbursement of anesthesia services. The conversion factor depends on the insurance payer being billed, so it is important to understand which payer is being billed for the service when calculating the amount of payment expected from the insurance. The dollar amount is negotiated in a private contract between the anesthesia office and the insurance payer. For example, the conversion factor between an anesthesia provider and a third-party payer may be negotiated to a dollar amount of $25.00 per unit value.

Medicare, on the other hand, has an annually published conversion factor used to calculate anesthesia payment amounts for each service. Medicare CFs change according to the region in which the anesthesia service was billed, which creates a discrepancy in payments depending on where the anesthesia procedure was performed. See figure 12.6 for an excerpt of the 2017 CMS conversion factors for anesthesia services. Note that the CF for services provided in Alabama is 21.06, whereas the CF for services performed in Alaska is 30.69. An anesthesia provider in Alaska would be paid almost $9.00 more per unit than an anesthesia provider in Alabama (CMS 2017b).

Documentation of Anesthesia Services

Documentation for anesthesia services should include the details of the pre-anesthesia evaluation, the record of the intraoperative or procedural anesthesia (in a time-based record of events), and a record of the post-anesthesia transfer of care and end time of the procedure. Anesthesia health records are complicated forms that include numerous details. Figure 12.7 is an example of a paper anesthesia record.

Pain management is a healthcare specialty similar to anesthesia, as they both perform procedures to reduce or eliminate sensation; but pain management is less complicated in terms of reimbursement and more complicated in terms of CPT coding.

Figure 12.7. Paper anesthesia record

DA FORM 7389, FEB 1998   COPY 1 - PATIENT'S MEDICAL RECORD   APD LC v1.00

Source: APD 2017.

Pain Management Billing and Coding Basics

Pain management is a specialty in which healthcare providers employ various procedures to improve the quality of life and ease the suffering of patients with chronic pain.

It is a unique specialty, because it is a treatment-based—not cure-based—medical specialty. In other words, pain management treats the symptom of pain and not the underlying cause of the pain. However, some pain management procedures may be focused on eliminating the causes of pain, such as performing a spinal surgery to decompress a pinched nerve or herniated disc. In many instances, there is no possible cure for the chronic pain and so pain management is the only option patients have to live a normally functioning life.

Because pain management is a long-term process, billing for pain management may be complicated by payer requirements and approvals for procedures, which may be done only once per specified timeframe. For example, radiofrequency ablation, a procedure performed to treat chronic pain, may only be allowed once a year by the patient's insurance company. However, it may be necessary to perform the procedure more often than every 12 months. If this is the case, then the provider's office may request a prior authorization for the procedure from the patient's insurance. If the insurance does not authorize the procedure, then the patient either must pay for the service out of his or her pocket or go without the service until the 12 months has passed. At the very least this means that billers and coders in pain management need to be careful about what procedure is being performed, whether or not it is a payable procedure, and if it needs a prior authorization from the patient's insurance.

Unlike anesthesia procedures, pain management services are reported with procedure codes from the Surgery section of the CPT code book. Anesthesia procedure codes identify the procedure that was performed on the patient that necessitated the anesthesia. Pain management procedures are performed by the healthcare provider and codes reflect the actual procedure performed. Sometimes the patient may require anesthesia during the surgical procedure, in which case the pain management provider would report the codes for the pain management procedure, while the anesthesiologist reports the CPT code for the anesthesia service provided to the patient during the pain management procedure. Because pain management codes are surgical CPT codes, they may be reported like any other surgical or medical service. They do not require the identification of base units, time units, or modifying factors, and do not rely on anesthesia conversion factors. Rather, they are paid on the medical fee schedule typical for all other healthcare specialties (coding for other healthcare specialties is discussed throughout the rest of this text).

Procedural Coding for Anesthesia and Pain Management Services

Anesthesia and pain management procedure codes are located in two distinct locations within the CPT code book: the Anesthesia section and the Surgery section. The Anesthesia section of the CPT code book is devoted only to codes that represent anesthesia services, and pain management codes are found in various subsections throughout the Surgery section according to the type of procedure performed.

Coding for anesthesia or pain management procedures depends on the method of analgesia used and how it was administered. Some codes are dependent on the patient's condition, and code selection differs depending on the reason why the patient was treated.

Types of Anesthesia

There are four main types of anesthesia, the usage of which depends on the type of surgery performed on the patient, the expected duration of the surgery, the health of the patient, and the preferences of the patient and the anesthesiology provider. The four types of anesthesia are local, regional, general, and moderate sedation.

Moderate (Conscious) Sedation

Moderate (conscious) sedation is a type of anesthesia given either orally or via an injection. This method allows the patient to be sedated but awake so he or she can respond to commands if necessary. Moderate sedation is discussed in further detail in chapter 10 (Urgent Care and Emergency Department Services). Moderate (conscious) sedation is coded with CPT codes 99151 to 99157.

Local Anesthesia

Local anesthesia blocks a small amount of nerves using an injection or a topical cream or spray that numbs a specific amount of the body. It is usually initiated by the healthcare provider performing the procedure, rather than an anesthesiologist. For example, an anesthetic cream can be injected into a patient's skin by the provider to excise a lesion of the chest without the patient experiencing any pain. Local anesthesia is often used for minor surgeries or to perform small wound repairs. Patients receiving local anesthesia may also receive moderate sedation at varying levels to help them relax and induce drowsiness, and to make the injection of the local anesthetic and ensuing procedure more tolerable. Once the procedure is complete, local anesthesia is allowed to gradually wear off naturally until the patient receives full sensation. This process may take a few hours or up to a day, depending on the type of anesthesia administered and procedure performed.

There is no CPT code for the administration of local anesthesia, as this service is bundled into the payment for the surgical procedure. However, if the patient did receive moderate sedation in addition to the local anesthesia, then the moderate sedation may be coded. See figure 12.8.

Figure 12.8. Types of anesthesia

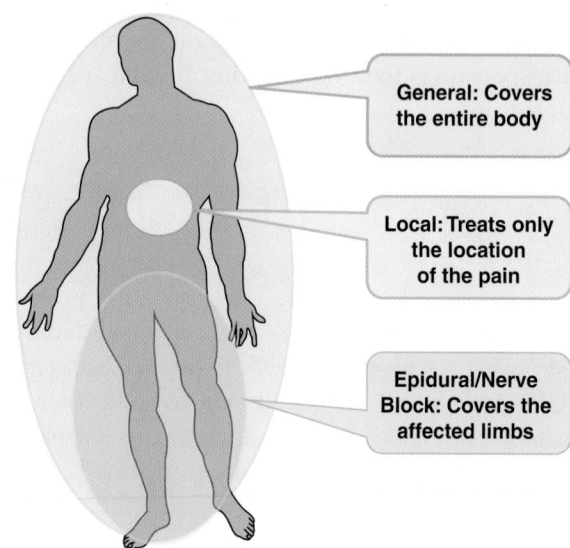

Regional Anesthesia

Regional anesthesia employs an injection to block a large amount of nerves, numb a more extensive body area, and prepare the patient for an extensive surgery or procedure. Regional anesthesia is commonly used for procedures involving the lower part of the body—on the legs, during vaginal delivery and cesarean sections, or during urogenital surgery. Regional anesthesia may entail one single injection of anesthetic, or may be a continuous administration of an anesthetic through a catheter or tube that is left in place throughout a surgical procedure or hospital stay. Codes for regional anesthesia are located in the Surgery section of codes within the CPT manual.

Common regional anesthesia procedures are spinal and epidural injections. A sedative may also be used with regional anesthesia to help the patient relax and better endure the injection of the regional anesthetics. Once the procedure is complete, the regional anesthesia is stopped (as in the case of an epidural), and allowed to gradually wear off until the patient has regained full sensation and function of the body area that was anesthetized.

Note that in both local and regional anesthesia, the patient is awake and aware of the procedures. This is unless moderate sedation is used to help the patient relax and undergo the procedure. Local and regional anesthesia procedure codes may be found within the Surgery section of the CPT code book, as they are considered surgical procedures in which the anesthesiologist must actually perform the injection of the anesthetic substance into the patient. However, if the regional anesthesia service was performed in order to anesthetize the patient to facilitate a *different* healthcare procedure, then the appropriate code from the Anesthesia section of the CPT code book is assigned. To find anesthetic injections, search for the term *Injection*, and then *Anesthetic Agent*, and find the subterm for the area being anesthetized. For nerve injections, search for the term *Injection*, and then *Nerve,* and find the subterm for *Anesthetic.*

General Anesthesia Care

General anesthesia is the administration of a substance that results in a complete loss of consciousness in order to produce analgesia to facilitate a surgical or other healthcare procedure (Palmetto 2013). It may be given intravenously, inhaled through a mask, or both intravenously and inhaled. It results in the patient being completely unconscious, with no memory of the surgical procedure when they wake up. General anesthesia is the riskiest form of anesthesia because the patient is rendered completely unconscious, requiring close monitoring of breathing and heart rate, and as such it is only used for procedures that cannot be performed with either local or regional anesthetic or moderate sedation. Patients may also be sedated before the general anesthesia is administered.

Monitored anesthesia care (MAC) is a similar procedure that produces analgesia in a patient and may be performed along with or in lieu of general anesthesia. MAC is an anesthesia service that is consists of a conscious sedation, control of patient anxiety, and pain control. MAC services result in a more rapid post-anesthesia recovery, which make MAC services suitable for outpatient procedures (Das and Gosh 2015). MAC services are similar to moderate sedation (refer to chapter 10), however, a MAC provider must be a qualified anesthesiologist because he or she must be ready to convert to a full general anesthesia service in the case of an adverse event. In moderate sedation, the healthcare provider performing the anesthesia service is the provider performing the procedure, and not a certified anesthesiologist provider. Both general anesthesia and MAC services are reported with codes from the Anesthesia section of the CPT code book.

General anesthesia results in the need to assist the patient's respiration to ensure adequate ventilation, which is done via an oral airway (a small plastic tube that keeps the airway open by keeping the tongue in place so that it does not cover the epiglottis), or a mask that fits over the nose and mouth. Due to its reliability in ensuring adequate breathing, endotracheal intubation is commonly used to assist the patient's breathing during the surgical procedure and is often used in procedures that are lengthy or if the patient is receiving large amounts of anesthesia.

Throughout the general anesthesia procedure, the patient's vital signs are closely monitored by the anesthesiologist. This includes the patient's heart rate, blood pressure, and blood oxygen levels, which are recorded continuously in the provider's documentation of the entire procedure. Once the procedure is complete, the anesthesiologist will reverse the anesthesia using a medicinal agent, which stops the effects of the anesthesia, allowing the patient to wake up and regain sensation; the patient is taken to the post-anesthesia care unit. General anesthesia services are reported with CPT codes 00100 through 01999. They can be found by searching under the term *Anesthesia* in the CPT Index.

Understanding the different types of anesthesia services is integral to coding for them appropriately, as the different types of anesthesia services are located in different sections of the CPT code book.

Procedural Coding for Anesthesia Services

Anesthesia services are reported with codes 00100 to 01999. Note that not all anesthesia procedures are included within this code range, as some local and regional injections are located in the Surgery section codes.

As with the other five CPT sections, the Anesthesia section begins with a selection of guidelines applicable to anesthesia codes. These guidelines provide important information on anesthesia services and what is included within the code descriptions, as well as guidelines for time reporting, supplied materials, separate or multiple procedures, and special reports (special reports are discussed in detail in chapter 5). This section also includes the anesthesia physical status modifiers and qualifying circumstances add-on codes for reference. For example, coders with questions on how time is reported for anesthesia codes may refer to the guidelines at the beginning of the Anesthesia section to read the CPT guidelines related to time reporting: "Time for anesthesia procedures may be reported as customary in the local area. Anesthesia time begins when the anesthesiologist begins to prepare the patient for the induction of anesthesia in the operating room (or in an equivalent area) and ends when the anesthesiologist is no longer in personal attendance, that is, when the patient may be safely placed under postoperative supervision" (AMA 2018).

Key to Success

The beginning of each section in the CPT code book begins with a selection of important guidelines applicable to all of the codes within that section. This is a good place to write notes, reminders, and other codes or modifiers that are important for this section of codes. This is especially a beneficial strategy to help you succeed in taking certification exams. Most exams will allow you to write notes and highlight important items in the code books, as long as you do not tape anything to the pages or write down sample test questions. Ask your instructor or check the website for the certification exam for which you are preparing to see what you are allowed to write in your books.

Coding for anesthesia services can be a bit confusing because the codes are different than surgical, medical, or evaluation and management codes. However, it is easier to find the correct CPT codes for anesthesia codes once you know how they work.

The anesthesia section of the CPT code book is divided by body area or condition. For example, the first subheading is Head, then Neck, then Thorax (Chest Wall and Shoulder Girdle). Under these headings is a list of the anesthesia services for patients undergoing a procedure on those specific areas. For example, under the subheading Head, the first code, 00100, Anesthesia for procedures on salivary glands, including biopsy, covers any anesthesia service performed on a patient undergoing any kind of procedure on his or her salivary glands (including a biopsy).

In this way, anesthesia codes are not too much more complicated than surgical or medical CPT codes, they just require a change of thinking. When coding for anesthesia services, coders must identify the main procedure that the healthcare provider performed in order to correctly select the code for the anesthesia service. The anesthesia provider is not performing the surgery on the salivary glands, just anesthetizing the patient for the procedure, and the anesthesia code is what is reported by the anesthesiologist. The provider reports the code for the procedure performed using a CPT code from elsewhere in the CPT manual and bills it separately.

Note that there are four subsections at the end of the Anesthesia section that describe anesthesia procedures performed for specific conditions or specific types of procedures. Rather than a specific body system, these three sections describe anesthesia procedures for specific types of procedures that may occur throughout the body: Radiological Procedures (01916 to 01936), Burn Excisions or Debridement (01951 to 01953), Obstetric (01958 to 01969), and Other Procedures (01990 to 01999).

When a patient is anesthetized and the healthcare provider performs more than one procedure, the anesthesiologist should report only the anesthesia code representing the most complex procedure, represented by the highest number of base units (as discussed previously). For example, if the patient received a liver transplant and an appendectomy in the same operative session, then the anesthesiologist would only report one anesthesia code—in this case code 00796, Anesthesia for intraperitoneal procedures in upper abdomen including laparoscopy; liver transplant, and *not* report code 00840, Anesthesia for intraperitoneal procedures on lower abdomen including laparoscopy; not otherwise specified (for the appendectomy). When determining which code to report (the most complex procedure), report the code with the highest base units, as determined by ASA RVG or CMS RVG.

The American Society of Anesthesiologists also publishes a valuable tool in anesthesia coding, the ASA Crosswalk—a book that bridges all applicable CPT surgical and therapeutic procedure codes to the appropriate anesthesia codes. The crosswalk lists the CPT surgical or therapeutic code, and then crosswalks, or maps, the surgical code to the appropriate anesthesia code to report the procedure. This is helpful for anesthesia coders, as they can look up the surgical CPT code for the procedure performed by the surgeon, and the book refers the them to the anesthesia code that should be reported for the accompanying anesthesia service. For example, code 44970, Laparoscopy, surgical, appendectomy, would crosswalk to anesthesia code 00840, Anesthesia for intraperitoneal procedures on lower abdomen including laparoscopy; not otherwise specified. The crosswalk is a valuable resource for anesthesia coders to ensure that the anesthesia code selected is appropriate for the surgical procedure performed.

Key to Success

Anesthesia coding requires additional resources other than the ICD-10-CM, CPT, and HCPCS manuals. These are the relative value guides (both ASA and CMS versions, for Medicare patients) and the anesthesia crosswalk. These resources help coders correctly determine the base units per procedure and identify the correct anesthesia code for the medical procedure performed.

When coding for anesthesia services, there are a number of HCPCS modifiers that may be appended depending on the provider of the anesthesia service. It may also be necessary to report additional procedures that were performed with the anesthesia service.

Anesthesia Providers and Modifiers

There are three providers that are qualified to perform an anesthesia service: anesthesiologists, anesthesiology assistants (AA), and certified registered nurse anesthetists (CRNA). Anesthesiologists are medical doctors who may perform services at their own discretion, whereas AAs and CRNAs are mid-level providers who must work under the supervision of an anesthesiologist. It is necessary to identify the provider of anesthesia service using the appropriate HCPCS modifier:

- AA, Anesthesiology services performed personally by anesthesiologist
- AD, Medical supervision by a physician; more than four concurrent anesthesia procedures
- QK, Medical direction of two, three, or four concurrent anesthesia procedures involving qualified professionals
- QY, Medical direction of one certified registered nurse anesthetist (CRNA) by an anesthesiologist
- QX, CRNA service: with medical direction by a physician
- QZ, CRNA service: without medical direction by a physician

Modifier -AA should be used to identify that the service was provided directly by the anesthesiologist. Modifiers -AD, -QK, and -QY should be used by an anesthesiologist to report that he or she supervised the anesthesiology procedure performed by an AA or CRNA. The mid-level provider bills for his or her service using the same anesthesia code, but appended with -QX to indicate that the anesthesiologist supervised the procedure. When this happens, both the supervising anesthesiologist and the CRNA performing the procedure receive a percentage of the anesthesia reimbursement. Modifier -QZ is used when the CRNA performs the anesthesia service without the supervision of an anesthesiologist (see figure 12.9).

Figure 12.9. Anesthesia provider modifiers

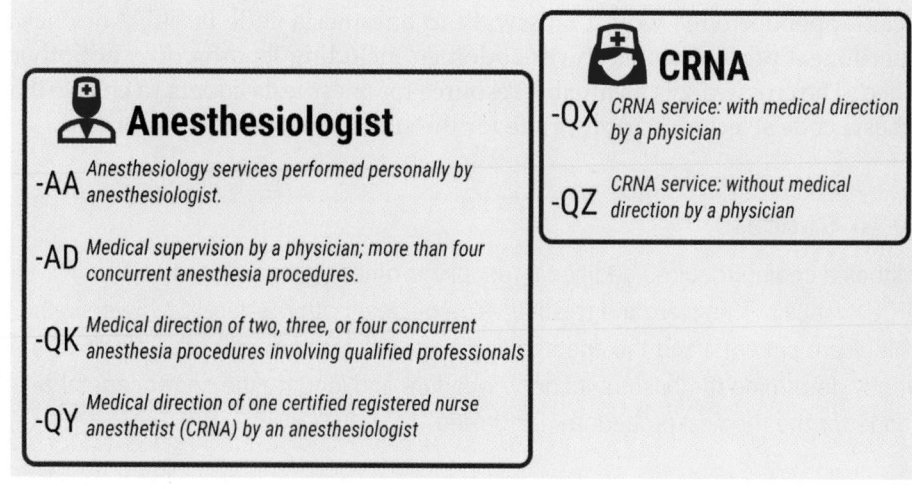

Additional modifiers used for anesthesia services include:

- G8, Monitored anesthesia care (MAC) for deep complex, complicated, or markedly invasive surgical procedure
- G9, Monitored anesthesia care for patient who has history of severe cardiopulmonary condition
- QS, Monitored anesthesia care service

These modifiers all report specific circumstances in which monitored anesthesia care is administered by an anesthesiologist, in some cases to help justify why the sedation was performed by an anesthesiologist, rather than the physician.

Multiple modifiers might be necessary in order to correctly report anesthesia services. For example, a modifier to identify the provider of service as the anesthesiologist, -AA; another modifier to identify the service as monitored anesthesia care, -QS; and yet another modifier to identify the patient's status as having a severe systemic disease, -P3. Coding correctly for anesthesia services requires identification of all the factors involved in reporting these services correctly: identification of the procedure code, identification of the provider of service, identification of the patient's physical status, the amount of time involved in the procedure, and whether any qualifying circumstances were involved. Remember that sometimes multiple qualifying circumstance codes may be necessary too!

Additional Procedures and Bundled Services

There are many procedures bundled into the anesthesia service that may not be coded elsewhere. These include

- the administration of fluids and/or blood
- usual monitoring services (patient vitals, temperature, blood pressure, ECG/EKG [93000 to 93010], oxygen level, capnography, and mass spectrometry)

When these procedures are performed with the anesthesia service they are considered part of the service and cannot be reported elsewhere. The anesthesiologist may perform additional procedures throughout the service, such as cardiopulmonary resuscitation, interpretation of lab tests, blood transfusions, bronchoscopy, or laryngoscopy. Several additional procedures may be considered bundled into the primary code for the anesthesia service and not separately payable. Therefore it is a good practice to always check insurance policy regarding which services may or may not be reported separately for payment. However, the following additional procedures are commonly paid separately and may be necessary to report in certain circumstances.

- Insertion of central venous catheter (36555 to 36558, 36568 and 36569)
- Insertion of intra-arterial catheter (36620 to 36625)
- Insertion of Swan-Ganz catheter (93503)

When any of these services are performed in addition to the anesthesia service, they may be reported by appending them with modifier -59, Distinct procedural service, along with the code for the anesthesia procedure. Catheters are commonly inserted to allow for the infusion of substances or products, and may be inserted by the anesthesia provider before or during the anesthesia procedure. In order for the anesthesia provider to be able to code for the catheter (or line) placement, it must have been performed by the anesthesia provider (and not the healthcare provider) and the procedure must be fully documented with a diagnosis to identify the medical necessity for the service.

In addition to the list given, any procedures that are performed to control postoperative pain may also be coded in addition to the code for the primary anesthesia service. Note that these procedures are performed only when the original procedure is complete and the patient has fully recovered from the anesthesia and operation, but still requires anesthesia services for pain management. These include

- Epidural spinal injections (62320 to 62323 for single injections, 62324 to 62327 for continuous infusion or intermittent bolus). For subsequent daily hospital management of postoperative pain, report code 01996, Daily hospital management of epidural or subarachnoid continuous drug administration. Do not calculate time units for code 01996; instead report one unit per day.
- Nerve blocks. Codes for nerve blocks are based on the nerve being blocked, and identify either a single injection or continuous infusion by catheter. The nerve being blocked must be identified in the documentation (brachial plexus, sciatic nerve, femoral nerve, lumbar plexus).

Do not include the time for performing the given procedure within the total anesthesia time. These codes are reported in addition to the anesthesia service, appended with modifier -59. Note that these procedures are separately reportable for *postoperative pain management only*. Postoperative pain management is anesthesia provided to the patient after the surgery or procedure is performed and the patient has been transferred to the postoperative unit, but still requires some sort of anesthesia service to control pain in the postoperative period. This means that the procedure has been completed, including the original anesthesia service, but the patient is still in pain and needs additional pain management procedures in order to manage his or her comfort level.

For practice assigning procedure codes to anesthesia services, complete the exercise in There's a Code for That 12.2.

12.2 Procedural coding for anesthesia services

There's a Code for That

Read the following documentation and select the appropriate CPT code for the anesthesia service. Remember to include the appropriate modifier(s) for physical status and anesthesia provider, as well as any qualifying circumstances code(s).

1. Anesthesiologist provided anesthesia for diagnostic arthroscopy on right knee joint of a normal, healthy patient.

   CPT code: _____ - _____ , -_____

2. CRNA (under direct supervision by anesthesiologist) provided anesthesia for open osteotomy of humerus on a patient with uncomplicated pregnancy.

   CPT code: _____ - _____ , -_____

3. Without supervision by anesthesiologist, CRNA provided physiological support for the harvesting of a declared brain-dead patient.

   CPT code: _____ - _____ , -_____

4. Anesthesiologist provided anesthesia for a 76-year-old male patient receiving a coronary artery bypass graft with pump oxygenator. Patient has poorly controlled diabetes and has a history of MI approximately one year ago.

   CPT codes: _____ - _____ , -_____ , _____

Procedural Coding for Pain Management Services

Pain management procedure codes are located within the Surgery section of the CPT code book, mostly in the Nervous System subsection. There are many different pain management methods, which depend on the type of practitioner, and his or her specialty and level of interest. Methods include electrodiagnostic studies to help find the cause of the pain, integrative medicine like acupuncture and yoga, interventional pain procedures, muscle and joint injections, peripheral nerve stimulation, and spinal cord stimulation.

Electrodiagnostic Studies

Electrodiagnostic studies are a way of measuring the electrical activity in muscles and nerves, and can help diagnose the cause or specific area from which pain is originating. There are two types of electrodiagnostic studies—electromyography and nerve conduction study.

Electromyography (EMG) evaluates the condition of muscle and nerves to determine the cause of pain, such as a pinched nerve or a diseased muscle. Electromyography codes may be found in the range 95860 to 95887, and in other locations in the CPT manual. To find the code for the EMG service performed, access the CPT Index and search for the term *Electromyography*, then refer to the type of EMG (fine wire, needle, surface), and the subterm for the area being evaluated (cranial nerve supplied muscle, extremities, face and neck muscles) (Mount Sinai Hospital 2017a).

A **nerve conduction study (NCS)** is a test that activates nerves and gauges their responses as a way of determining if there is a problem with the functioning of the nerve. Nerve conduction tests are often performed alongside EMG evaluations to provide a complete picture of the patient's nerves and to determine the cause of the patient's pain. Codes for NCS (95905 to 95913) identify the number of studies performed. For example, code 95907, Nerve conduction studies; 1-2 studies, or 95912, Nerve conduction studies, 11-12 studies (Mount Sinai Hospital 2017a).

Key to Success

Remember that Appendix J, Electrodiagnostic Medicine Listing of Sensory, Motor, and Mixed Nerves, includes a summary of sensory, motor, and mixed nerves with the appropriate nerve conduction study (NCS) code. Write a reminder next to codes 95905 to 95913 in the CPT Tabular List to refer to Appendix J if you need help assigning codes to specific nerves.

Integrative Medicine

Integrative medicine consists of complementary and alternative therapies that may be used to treat chronic pain. Integrative medicine combines traditional medical treatments with alternative therapies such as acupuncture, yoga, cupping, and nutritional integration. **Acupuncture** is an ancient method of treating a variety of medical ailments like headaches, low back pain, anxiety, inflammation, constipation, insomnia, joint pain, nerve pain, stress, and tinnitus. The practice of acupuncture consists of inserting thin, flexible needles into specific areas of the body to restore the body's balance and relieve discomfort. Medical acupuncture codes (97810 to 97814) are based on time spent with the patient performing the procedure, and whether or not the procedure was performed with electrical stimulation.

Interventional Pain Procedures

Interventional pain procedures are a range of different procedures that utilize invasive interventions to treat the patient's pain. They include epidural injections, medial branch blocks and facet joint injections, radiofrequency nerve ablations, joint injections, occipital nerve blocks, and kyphoplasty.

Epidural Steroid Injections

An **epidural steroid injection** is a minimally invasive procedure that can treat pain in the neck, shoulders, arms, back, buttocks, and legs, resulting from irritation of spinal nerves due to conditions such as herniated discs, degenerative disc disease, and arthritis (Mount Sinai Hospital 2017b). Note that an epidural steroid injection is an injection of long-lasting corticosteroid, which is an anti-inflammatory agent and *not* an anesthetic substance. An anesthetic substance can be injected through an epidural site, but this is usually done as part of an anesthesia procedure, or to alleviate postoperative pain (see figure 12.10).

Figure 12.10. Epidural injection

Source: Blausen.com staff 2013a.

When coding for epidural injections, know the substance involved, the site of the epidural injection (cervical, thoracic, lumbar, or sacral), and whether or not imaging guidance was used. Imaging guidance is the use of imaging, such as x-ray, CT scan, ultrasound, or fluoroscopy, during the procedure to help guide the surgeon during the surgery. For example, code 62320, Injection(s), of diagnostic or therapeutic substance(s) (e.g., anesthetic, antispasmodic, opioid, steroid, other solution), not including neurolytic substances, including needle or catheter placement, interlaminar epidural or subarachnoid, cervical or thoracic; without imaging guidance, identifies the substance involved, *diagnostic or therapeutic substance not including neurolytic substance*; the site of the injection, *cervical or thoracic*; and if imaging guidance was used, *without imaging guidance*. In this case, the procedure is performed without imaging guidance, so the healthcare provider injected the area without the use of any imaging services to help see the exact injection site.

To find the code for an epidural injection, search for the term *Epidural* in the CPT Index, then reference the type of epidural procedure. For epidural anesthesia procedures, reference the main term *Epidural Anesthesia* in the CPT Index.

Medial Branch Nerve Blocks and Facet Joint Injections

Facet joint injections are injections made into the facet joint of the vertebra (see figure 12.11) that are used to treat pain coming from the small joints of the spine. Injections made into this area deliver low doses of long-lasting corticosteroids or local anesthetics directly to the source of the pain (the joint) to alleviate discomfort. Medial nerves connect to the facet joints and are injected concurrently with the facet joint injection (Mount Sinai Hospital 2017b).

Figure 12.11. Facet joints of the vertebra

Source: ©AHIMA

Codes for facet joint injections, 64490 to 64495, are based on the area of the injection—either cervical or thoracic, or lumbar or sacral. Add-on codes identify additional levels of the vertebra that were injected (see figure 12.12). A level is each individual vertebral level injected. For example, the injections at the first level might be L2 to L3, a second level L3 to L4, and a third level L4 to L5. Code 64493, Injection(s), diagnostic or therapeutic agent, paravertebral facet (zygapophyseal) joint (or nerves innervating that joint) with image guidance (fluoroscopy or CT), lumbar or sacral; *single level*, for the first level injected (L2 to L3), and then the add-on codes for the second level and then the other add-on code for the third (or any other additional) level: 64494, Injection(s), diagnostic or therapeutic agent, paravertebral facet (zygapophyseal) joint (or nerves innervating that joint) with image guidance (fluoroscopy or CT), lumbar or sacral; *second level*, and 64495, Injection(s), diagnostic or therapeutic agent, paravertebral facet (zygapophyseal) joint (or nerves innervating that joint) with image guidance (fluoroscopy or CT), lumbar or sacral; *third and any additional level(s)* (see figure 12.13). Note that the add-on code 64495 may only be reported once per day, even if the provider performed more than three facet joint injections.

Figure 12.12. Levels of the spine

Source: ©AHIMA

Figure 12.13. Facet joint injection coding

CPT Code	Facet Joint Injected
64493	L2 to L3
64494	L3 to L4
64495	L4 to L5

If the facet joint injection was performed bilaterally, append modifier -50, Bilateral procedure to each injection that was performed bilaterally.

Radiofrequency Nerve Ablations

Radiofrequency nerve ablation is a procedure used to treat back and neck pain by using a controlled heat source to disable nerves responsible for causing pain. The procedure is performed using a small needle with a heated tip placed near the nerve causing the pain, to disrupt the nerve's ability to send a pain signal (Mount Sinai Hospital 2017b).

Codes for radio frequency nerve ablation are found under the Destruction by Neurolytic Agent (e.g, Chemical, Thermal, Electrical, or Radiofrequency), Chemodenervation section of codes, 64600 through 64681. To find the correct code, it is necessary to identify the area or nerve destroyed by the procedure. Be careful to read parenthetical notes and guidelines in this section of codes to ensure correct code selection. For example, code 64616, Chemodenervation of muscle(s); neck muscle(s), excluding muscles of the larynx, unilateral (e.g., for cervical dystonia, spasmodic torticollis) is followed by important guidelines located in parentheses after the code: *For bilateral procedure, report 64616 with modifier 50*; and *for chemodenervation guided by needle electromyography or muscle electrical stimulation, see 95873, 95874. Do not report more than one guidance code for ay unit of 64616.*

Joint Injections

A joint injection is an injection of a therapeutic substance, such as corticosteroid, local anesthetics, or hyaluronan, into a joint to relieve pain caused by painful joint conditions such as osteoarthritis, synovitis, or inflammatory arthritis.

Coding for joint injections requires the identification of the joint, the substance injected, and whether or not the procedure was performed with ultrasound or imaging guidance. Note that joint injection codes are included in the Musculoskeletal System subsection of the CPT code book, not the Nervous System subsection. This is because the injections are given directly into the patient's affected joint. To search for the code, refer to the main term *Injection* in the CPT Index, then find the subterm for either the area of the injection, such as *Joint, Nerve,* or *Trigger Point* (a small, tight area of muscle tissue), or the type of substance injected, such as *Anesthetic Agent,* as applicable.

Occipital Nerve Blocks

An occipital nerve block is an injection directly into the greater and lesser occipital nerves, used to treat headaches and migraines (Mount Sinai Hospital 2017b). There is one code for occipital nerve block, 64405, Injection, anesthetic agent; greater occipital nerve.

Key to Success

Turn to code 64405, Injection, anesthetic agent; greater occipital nerve, in your CPT code book. Note that this code is located with the subheading for Extracranial Nerves, Peripheral Nerves, and Autonomic Nervous System, and within the category of codes that identify procedures on the facial, vagus, and phrenic nerves (among others). These are all *peripheral* nerves located within the cranium. They are not part of the *central* nervous system. Keep this in mind when coding for services performed on nerves in the cranial and cervical area. Even though they are close to the central nervous system in distance, they are still part of the peripheral nervous system.

Kyphoplasty

A **kyphoplasty** is a treatment for vertebral compression fractures and the pain they cause. In this procedure, a balloon is threaded through an incision in the back, to the site of the compression fracture, where it is slowly inflated to push the compressed bone back into place. Once in place, cement is injected into the area to hold the bone in the proper position. This is a more invasive procedure than most injections for pain management, and is usually done in an operating room under general anesthesia (Mount Sinai Hospital 2017b).

Kyphoplasty codes, 22513 to 22515, identify the site of the procedure—either lumbar or thoracic. The add-on code 22515 should be used for each additional thoracic or lumbar vertebral body involved in the procedure. For example, if the provider performed a kyphoplasty on two lumbar vertebrae, then the codes selected would be 22514, Percutaneous vertebral augmentation, including cavity creation (fracture reduction and bone biopsy included wen performed), using mechanical device (e.g., kyphoplasty), 1 vertebral body, unilateral or bilateral cannulation, inclusive of all imaging guidance; *lumbar*, and 22515, Percutaneous vertebral augmentation, including cavity creation (fracture reduction and bone biopsy included when performed), using mechanical device (e.g., kyphoplasty), 1 vertebral body, unilateral or bilateral cannulation, inclusive of all imaging guidance; *each additional thoracic or lumbar vertebral body*.

Peripheral Nerve Stimulation

Peripheral nerve stimulation is a way to help treat pain that results from traumatic injury or dysfunction of the peripheral nerves. The procedure is performed by placing small electrodes next to peripheral nerves to ensure that the correct nerves have been identified for the procedure. Once the nerves causing the pain are found, the trial leads are removed and a neurostimulator is placed, with permanent leads and a small battery pack, to continuously stimulate the nerves and relieve pain (Mount Sinai Hospital 2017c).

Codes for peripheral nerve stimulation procedures are in the range for Neurostimulators (Peripheral Nerve), 64550 to 64595. Code selection relies on the procedure performed (such as percutaneous implantation through a small incision in the skin, an open incision for implantation, revision or replacement of the device, or complete removal of the device) and the nerve involved in the procedure (cranial, peripheral, or such).

Once the device is in place, it may be necessary to analyze the functioning of the neurostimulators and program the stimulator for optimal function. These services are reported with codes from the Medicine section, Neurostimulators, Analysis-Programming (95970 to 95982). These codes identify the nerves treated by the neurostimulators and various services related to the analysis and programming of the neurostimulator. Pay close attention to these codes, as some of them identify the time spent on the analysis and programming service (95974, 95978), while others do not. Furthermore, a handful of add-on codes (95975, 95979) exist to identify additional time (in increments of 30 minutes) spent on the procedure.

Spinal Cord Stimulation

Spinal cord stimulation (SCS) is similar to peripheral nerve stimulation, except this procedure is performed on the spinal nerves. Once the exact spinal nerves causing the pain are identified, a permanent battery and lead wires are placed to alleviate pain. Spinal cord stimulation can also be programmed with a remote control to work at certain times, such as when the patient is walking, and then turn the leads off before lying down for bed (Mount Sinai Hospital 2017c).

Codes for spinal cord stimulation are also similar to those for peripheral nerve stimulation. Located in the range for Neurostimulators (Spinal), 63650 to 63688, codes identify the procedure performed (percutaneous implantation, laminectomy for implantation, removal, or revision), as well as any imaging guidance (fluoroscopy).

The decision to treat chronic pain using any one of these surgically invasive procedures is based on a number of factors, and must be medically necessary. Diagnostic coding for anesthesia services requires the indication for the operation and indications of medical necessity for any additional procedures that were performed during the anesthesia session. Pain management, on the other hand, relies on more specific diagnoses that must be placed in a specific order to identify the reason why the patient was being seen for pain management, and to justify the pain management procedure with an indication of medical necessity for the service.

For practice reporting procedure codes for pain management services, complete the exercises in the There's a Code for That 12.3.

Procedural coding for pain management services

12.3

There's a Code for That

Read the following documentation and select the appropriate CPT code for the pain management service.

1. Needle EMG of the thoracic paraspinal muscles.

   CPT code: _____

2. Thoracic epidural anesthesia injection with fluoroscopic guidance.

   CPT code: _____

3. Radiofrequency ablation of bilateral cervical spinal and accessory nerves with electrical stimulation for guidance on a patient with chronic migraine.

   CPT codes: _____, _____

4. Laminectomy performed to gain open access to the spinal column, and electrode plate with simple receiver is placed in the epidural space for spinal neurostimulation.

   CPT code: _____

Diagnosis Coding for Anesthesia and Pain Management Services

Diagnostic coding for anesthesia procedures must identify the medical necessity for the procedure performed, for which the patient was placed under anesthesia. Pain management diagnosis coding is a bit more complicated, as it requires an indication for medical necessity for the pain management procedure (that is, the diagnosis of pain), as well as the underlying diagnosis that is causing the pain, if known. There are also a number of guidelines that identify the correct reporting of pain diagnoses.

Diagnostic Coding for Anesthesia Services

Diagnostic coding for anesthesia procedures requires the identification of the indication for the procedure(s) performed. In other words, anesthesiologists do not diagnose patients; they rely on the documentation of the diagnosis from the healthcare provider performing the procedure. In this case, diagnostic coding for anesthesia services is relatively straightforward. Remember, if the preoperative and postoperative diagnoses for a patient differ from each other, select the postoperative diagnosis as the diagnosis code for the service.

The only exception to this is if the patient experiences some kind of medical condition or reaction to the anesthesia, for which the anesthesiologist has to perform additional procedures, such as inserting an arterial catheter or transesophageal echocardiography.

If the patient has a reaction to the anesthesia procedure, the appropriate complication of anesthesia code should be reported. These include

- T88.2, Shock due to anesthesia
- T88.3, Malignant hyperthermia due to anesthesia
- T88.4, Failed or difficult intubation
- T88.5, Other complications of anesthesia:
  - T88.51, Hypothermia following anesthesia
  - T88.52, Failed moderate sedation during procedure
  - T88.53, Unintended awareness under general anesthesia during procedure
  - T88.59, Other complications of anesthesia

For any of the codes categories T88.2, T88.3, or T88.5, use an additional code for adverse effect to identify the drug administered. For example, if a patient was administered ketamine, a drug used in moderate sedation, and the drug wore off and the patient regained full consciousness during the procedure, code T88.52, Failed moderate sedation during procedure, should be reported, as well as code T41.295A, Adverse effect of other general anesthetics, initial encounter.

Do not confuse complications of anesthesia codes with *history* of complications to anesthesia codes. A history code identifies a condition that the patient reports having experienced in the past, but which he or she is not currently experiencing. For example, if the patient had been anesthetized in the past (either moderate sedation or general anesthesia), and the anesthesia did not work as intended, then one of the following codes would be reported: Z92.83, Personal history of failed moderate sedation, or Z92.84, Personal history of unintended awareness under general anesthesia. These codes should be used if the patient has a personal history of these reactions, but is not currently experiencing said reaction.

Diagnostic Coding for Pain Management Procedures

As previously mentioned, coding for pain management is slightly more complicated than coding for anesthesia services, due to the numerous guidelines (discussed as follows) that govern code selection and sequencing for pain management procedures. This sequencing of codes for anesthesia and pain management conditions is important. Remember to check for notes in the ICD-10-CM Tabular List to *use additional code, code first,* and *code also.* When you see *use additional code,* report the additional code *after* the code you are referencing. When you see *code first,* report the additional code *before* the code you are referencing. When you see *code also,* you can place the additional code either before or after the code you are referencing, depending on the circumstances of the encounter.

Additional diagnoses that may require pain management procedures are also listed as follows. These include acute and chronic pain, post-thoracotomy and postprocedural pain, neoplasm related pain, and additional relevant diagnoses.

Acute and Chronic Pain

Chronic pain is the constant or long-term sensation of pain and, among other causes, may be a result of postoperative complications, past injuries, or nerve conditions. Acute pain is the short-term sensation of pain, which may last from just moments to a matter of months and is typically due to an injury, soft tissue damage, or acute condition. Correctly coding for acute and chronic pain relies on close reading of the guidelines pertaining to these conditions, as well as the reason for the patient's healthcare encounter (whether it is to treat the underlying cause of the pain or to treat the pain itself). When a patient presents with the symptom of pain, such as right knee pain, and there is no definitive diagnosis, the coder should report the unspecified code for the pain—code M25.561, Pain in right knee. (Find the code for knee pain, reference the term *pain* in the ICD-10-CM Index, and then the site of the pain.)

However, if the knee pain is identified as acute, chronic, post-thoracotomy/postprocedural, or neoplasm-related, an additional code from category G89, Pain, not elsewhere classified, should be reported in addition to the knee pain code. So if the condition was chronic right knee pain due to a traumatic injury, then two codes would be needed to identify the condition: M25.561, Pain in right knee, and G89.21, Chronic pain due to trauma. Note that sequencing of these two codes will depend on the circumstances of the encounter. If the patient's pain is a symptom of an underlying condition, such as osteoarthritis, and the patient is being seen for a treatment of the underlying condition, then it is not necessary to use a code from category G89 to identify the pain and the underlying condition.

However, if the patient has an underlying condition that is causing the pain (like osteoarthritis), and the patient is being seen for treatment of the pain (rather than the underlying condition), then a code from category G89 should be reported, and sequenced before the code for the underlying condition. For example, if the patient is being seen for a pain management procedure (an injection of the knee joint) due to chronic pain in the knee from osteoarthritis, then the codes selected should be as follows:

1. G89.29, Other chronic pain

2. M25.561, Pain in right knee

3. M17.11, Unilateral primary osteoarthritis, right knee

Note that the code identifying the specific site of the pain is also included to fully identify the condition (see figure 12.14).

Figure 12.14. Sequence of diagnosis codes for pain management

21. DIAGNOSIS OR NATURE OF ILLNESS OR INJURY Relate A-L to service line below (24E)			ICD Ind.	
A. ⌐ G89.29	B. ⌐ M25.561	C. ⌐ M17.11	D. ⌐	
E. ⌐	F. ⌐	G. ⌐	H. ⌐	
I. ⌐	J. ⌐	K. ⌐	L. ⌐	

24. A. DATE(S) OF SERVICE		B. PLACE OF SERVICE	C. EMG	D. PROCEDURES, SERVICES, OR SUPPLIES (Explain Unusual Circumstances) CPT/HCPCS MODIFIER	E. DIAGNOSIS POINTER
From MM DD YY	To MM DD YY				

Source: CMS 2017a.

According to OGCR, the only time a code from category G89 should be sequenced first is if the patient is being seen for a pain management procedure, intended to treat the patient's pain. If the treatment is aimed at the underlying condition, then the code for the underlying condition should be coded first (see figure 12.15). For example, if the

Figure 12.15. OGCR I.C.6.b through I.C.6.b.ii

---

b. Pain-Category G89

1) General coding information

Codes in category G89, Pain, not elsewhere classified, may be used in conjunction with codes from other categories and chapters to provide more detail about acute or chronic pain and neoplasm-related pain, unless otherwise indicated below.

If the pain is not specified as acute or chronic, post- thoracotomy, post procedural, or neoplasm-related, do not assign codes from category G89.

A code from category G89 should not be assigned if the underlying (definitive) diagnosis is known, unless the reason for the encounter is pain control/management and not management of the underlying condition.

When an admission or encounter is for a procedure aimed at treating the underlying condition (e.g., spinal fusion, kyphoplasty), a code for the underlying condition (e.g., vertebral fracture, spinal stenosis) should be assigned as the principal diagnosis. No code from category G89 should be assigned.

(a) Category G89 Codes as Principal or First-Listed Diagnosis

Category G89 codes are acceptable as principal diagnosis or the first-listed code:

- When pain control or pain management is the reason for the admission/encounter (e.g., a patient with displaced intervertebral disc, nerve impingement and severe back pain presents for injection of steroid into the spinal canal). The underlying cause of the pain should be reported as an additional diagnosis, if known.

- When a patient is admitted for the insertion of a neurostimulator for pain control, assign the appropriate pain code as the principal or first-listed diagnosis. When an admission or encounter is for a procedure aimed at treating the underlying condition and a neurostimulator is inserted for pain control during the same admission/encounter, a code for the underlying condition should be assigned as the principal diagnosis and the appropriate pain code should be assigned as a secondary diagnosis.

(b) Use of Category G89 Codes in Conjunction with Site Specific Pain Codes

(i) Assigning Category G89 and Site-Specific Pain Codes

Codes from category G89 may be used in conjunction with codes that identify the site of pain (including codes from chapter 18) if the category G89 code provides additional information. For example, if the code describes the site of the pain, but does not fully describe whether the pain is acute or chronic, then both codes should be assigned.

(ii) Sequencing of Category G89 Codes with Site- Specific Pain Codes

The sequencing of category G89 codes with site-specific pain codes (including chapter 18 codes), is dependent on the circumstances of the encounter/admission as follows:

- If the encounter is for pain control or pain management, assign the code from category G89 followed by the code identifying the specific site of pain (e.g., encounter for pain management for acute neck pain from trauma is assigned code G89.11, Acute pain due to trauma, followed by code M54.2, Cervicalgia, to identify the site of pain).

- If the encounter is for any other reason except pain control or pain management, and a related definitive diagnosis has not been established (confirmed) by the provider, assign the code for the specific site of pain first, followed by the appropriate code from category G89.

Source: CMS 2018.

patient is being seen for medication management of osteoarthritis, then the primary code for the encounter would be M17.11, Unilateral primary osteoarthritis, right knee. The codes for chronic pain and knee pain would not be assigned, as these are included within the primary diagnosis of osteoarthritis of the knee.

Post-thoracotomy and Postprocedural Pain

Post-thoracotomy and postprocedural pain is not reported if the pain is experienced immediately after surgery because of the procedure. However, if the pain remains and requires treatment, then codes from category G89 may be reported to identify the condition (see figure 12.16).

Figure 12.16. OGCR I.C.6.3

---

3) Postoperative Pain

The provider's documentation should be used to guide the coding of postoperative pain, as well *as Section III. Reporting Additional Diagnoses and Section IV. Diagnostic Coding* and *Reporting in the Outpatient Setting.*

The default for post-thoracotomy and other postoperative pain not specified as acute or chronic is the code for the acute form.

Routine or expected postoperative pain immediately after surgery should not be coded.

(a) Postoperative pain not associated with specific postoperative complication

Postoperative pain not associated with a specific postoperative complication is assigned to the appropriate postoperative pain code in category G89.

(b) Postoperative pain associated with specific postoperative complication

Postoperative pain associated with a specific postoperative complication (such as painful wire sutures) is assigned to the appropriate code(s) found in Chapter 19, Injury, poisoning, and certain other consequences of external causes. If appropriate, use additional code(s) from category G89 to identify acute or chronic pain (G89.18 or G89.28).

Source: CMS 2018.

There are two scenarios for which there are guidelines for reporting post-thoracotomy or postprocedural pain:

- If the pain is not related to any specific postoperative complication, then use the appropriate pain code from category G89. For example, pain in the knee three months after a knee joint prosthesis insertion, would not be reported as postprocedural pain, as the pain is experienced after the healing phase of the prosthesis insertion surgery is complete.

- If the postoperative pain is associated with any specific complication, such as painful wire sutures, then report the code for the complication. Coders may also report a code from category G89, if it is necessary to identify the pain as acute or chronic.

Neoplasm-Related Pain

Code G89.3, Neoplasm-related pain (acute) (chronic), should be reported when any pain is documented because of a cancer, primary or secondary malignancy, or tumor. For example, pain due to an osteosarcoma (cancer of the bone) of the lower leg would be reported with the appropriate ICD-10-CM pain code (site specific), as well as the G89 code for the neoplasm-related pain. When a patient presents for a pain management encounter for the treatment of the pain, sequence the neoplasm-related pain code first, with an additional code to identify the malignancy.

When the patient presents for treatment of the malignancy, then the code for the malignancy should be sequenced first, with an additional code to identify the neoplasm-related pain, if necessary. In this case, it is not necessary to include an additional code to identify the specific site of the pain (see figure 12.17).

Additional Diagnoses for Pain Management

There are numerous underlying causes of pain, ranging from psychological factors to underlying diseases such as osteoarthritis, to traumatic injuries. Many of the pain management procedures discussed are used to treat musculoskeletal conditions, such as osteoarthritis, muscle pain and inflammation, back pain and sciatica, and spinal and intervertebral disc disorders.

Figure 12.17. OGCR I.C.6.5

---

5) Neoplasm Related Pain

Code G89.3 is assigned to pain documented as being related, associated or due to cancer, primary or secondary malignancy, or tumor. This code is assigned regardless of whether the pain is acute or chronic.

This code may be assigned as the principal or first- listed code when the stated reason for the admission/encounter is documented as pain control/pain management. The underlying neoplasm should be reported as an additional diagnosis.

When the reason for the admission/encounter is management of the neoplasm and the pain associated with the neoplasm is also documented, code G89.3 may be assigned as an additional diagnosis. It is not necessary to assign an additional code for the site of the pain.

See Section I.C.2 for instructions on the sequencing of neoplasms for all other stated reasons for the admission/ encounter (except for pain control/pain management).

Source: CMS 2018.

Osteoarthritis

Osteoarthritis is a degenerative condition of the joints that results from wear and tear of the cartilage between joints; and causes pain, swelling, and problems with range of motion of the joint. Diagnosis codes for osteoarthritis are found in categories M15 to M19, Osteoarthritis, and depend on the identification of the type and site of the condition, including laterality. For example, M19.171, Post-traumatic osteoarthritis, right ankle and foot, identifies the type of osteoarthritis, *post-traumatic*; the site, *ankle and foot*; and the laterality, *right*.

Muscle Pain and Inflammation

Muscle pain and inflammation can take many forms, such as enthesopathies, myositis, and myalgias.

An enthesopathy is an inflammation of the tendon or ligament at the site of attachment to the bone that causes pain, tenderness, stiffness, and swelling. Enthesopathies include ankylosing spondylitis (inflammation of the joints of the spine), plantar fasciitis (which results in pain in the heel and bottom of the foot), and Achilles tendinitis.

Myositis is an inflammation of the muscle that can be caused by an infection, injury, medicine, or a chronic disease, and causes muscle weakness and pain, along with other symptoms.

Myalgia is muscle pain, which may be a symptom of many medical conditions including overuse of the muscle, overstretching, infection, or disease process. Fibromyalgia (M79.7) is a myalgia that is characterized by chronic, full-body pain, with a sensitivity to pressure. Fibromyalgia also causes fatigue, problems sleeping, memory problems, restless leg syndrome, numbness or tingling, and other psychological factors such as depression and anxiety.

When coding for muscle pain and inflammation, identify the specific type of condition (tendinitis, spondylosis, fasciitis, fibromyalgia), and then the specific site, if necessary. For paired organs, report the code for the correct laterality of the condition. For spinal conditions, it is necessary to identify the specific site of the condition according to spinal region, as follows: occipito-atlanto-axial, cervical, cervicothoracic, thoracic, thoracolumbar, lumbar, lumbosacral, sacral and sacrococcygeal, or multiple sites in the spine.

Back Pain and Sciatica

Back pain is typically experienced at a specific area along the spine, such as cervicalgia (neck pain), M54.2, or lumbago (low back pain), M54.5.

Sciatica (M54.3-) is a combination of pain, numbness, and weakness along the sciatic nerve from the lower back area, radiating to the buttocks and the leg. It is usually caused by a lower back problem putting pressure on the sciatic nerve.

Figure 12.18. Clinical manifestations of lumbar disc herniation

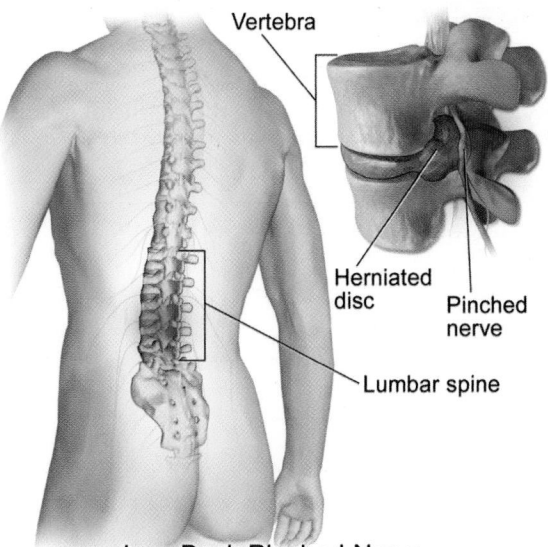

Source: Blausen.com staff 2013b.

Diagnosis codes for back pain identify the specific region of the pain. Codes for sciatica identify the laterality of the condition. Note that there is an additional subcategory of codes for lumbago with sciatica (M54.4-), which should be used when a patient experiences both conditions concurrently. Also note that if any of these conditions are due to an intervertebral disc disorder, then the coder should report the code for the disc disorder that includes the symptoms of pain or sciatica.

Intervertebral Disc Disorders

Intervertebral disc disorders are common causes of pain due to spinal issues. They include intervertebral disc deterioration, herniation, and prolapse of an intervertebral disc. These problems can cause chronic or radiating pain, numbness, tingling, and loss of strength and range of motion of movement; and can also result in **radiculopathy**, a nerve-related pain (see figure 12.18 for an illustration of a herniated disc causing a pinched nerve).

Codes for intervertebral disc disorders (M50 and M51) identify the region (and in some cases the exact vertebra) involved in the pain, as well as any additional conditions that may present with the disc disorder like sciatica pain, radiculopathy, or myelopathy.

For practice identifying diagnosis codes for anesthesia and pain management services, complete the exercises in There's a Code for That 12.4.

Diagnostic coding for anesthesia and pain management services

12.4

There's a Code for That

Read the following documentation and select the appropriate ICD-10-CM diagnosis code(s) for the anesthesia or pain management service.

1. Patient undergoing open herniorrhaphy manifested malignant hyperthermia due to inhalation anesthesia.

ICD-10-CM codes: _____ , _____

(Continued on next page)

12.4

Continued

2. Patient undergoing inhaled anesthesia for open repair of open traumatic femur shaft fracture of the right leg.

   ICD-10-CM code: _____

3. Patient with ankylosing spondylitis of the thoracolumbar spine presents for management of his chronic pain.

   ICD-10-CM code: _____, _____

4. 45-year-old male presents with lumbago and sciatica due to thoracic disc prolapse.

   ICD-10-CM code: _____

5. Interstitial myositis of the left shoulder.

   ICD-10-CM code: _____

Putting It All Together: Coding for Anesthesia and Pain Management Services

In order to select the correct codes for an anesthesia or pain management service, it is important to carefully read the documentation then access each code book to find the procedure or service provided and the corresponding diagnosis or diagnoses to support the medical necessity for the service. Procedural codes for anesthesia services are found in the Anesthesia section of the CPT code book, and diagnosis codes are found in the ICD-10-CM code book. Some anesthesia services may also be found in the Surgery section of the CPT code book, such as postoperative epidurals or pain management procedures. Pain management procedures are found in the Surgery section of the CPT code book.

Determining the correct codes relies on the answers to the following questions.

- What service was provided to the patient—was it an anesthesia service or pain management service?
  - For anesthesia services, you need the following information:
    - The base unit values for the anesthesia service
    - The time spent on the anesthesia service
    - Any applicable modifying factors:
      - Physical status of the patient
      - Qualifying circumstances surrounding the service
    - Were any additional services performed that are not included in the anesthesia service, such as TEE or PICC line insertion? (If so, code for the additional service with modifier -59.)
    - Add any applicable HCPCS modifiers to identify the provider of the anesthesia service or any specific circumstances surrounding the service.
  - For pain management procedures, check coding guidelines for any applicable add-on codes or modifiers for additional or bilateral procedures.

- What is the primary condition being treated?
  - In anesthesia coding, this is the reason why the patient is having the procedure.
  - For pain management encounters, pay close attention to the sequencing of the diagnosis codes (remember to check the coding guidelines in the ICD-10-CM code book).
- Are there any additional diagnoses that need to be included to justify the medical necessity of the services?

Study the following vignette that demonstrates how to select the appropriate diagnosis and procedure codes. Then complete the practice exercises in There's a Code for That 12.5.

Carson is completing the coding for an anesthesia case for a patient that received anesthesia services related to the delivery of her child. The normal, healthy patient, at 39 weeks gestation, was brought into the delivery room and labor was induced at 0850 hours. The patient's labor progressed until the anesthesiologist was called into perform an epidural for management of the patient's pain at 1500 hours. After the administration of the epidural, the patient's labor progressed less rapidly, and eventually the patient was taken for cesarean section due to prolonged second stage of labor. The patient's epidural was transferred to epidural anesthesia for cesarean section, after which a single live born child was delivered without further incident. After the procedure was complete, epidural was removed and care of the patient was transferred to the delivery nurse. Total time for the epidural for labor was 3.5 hours (210 minutes), and the total time for the cesarean anesthesia was 30 minutes.

First, Carson asks himself: What did the anesthesiologist do? The anesthesiologist performed an neuraxial labor anesthesia (epidural) procedure for a planned vaginal delivery, which was converted to a cesarean delivery. He looks up the procedures in the CPT Index under the main term Anesthesia, *then references the subterm* Neuraxial, *and then* Cesarean Delivery, *and finds two codes: 01968 and 01969. Code 01968 is for anesthesia for cesarean delivery, and code 01969 is for cesarean hysterectomy, so in this case the correct code is 01968 as no hysterectomy was performed. Carson notes that 01968 is an add-on code, and according to the parenthetical note in the CPT code book should be used in conjunction with 01967, to identify the anesthesia for the planned vaginal delivery.*

- *01967, Neuraxial labor analgesia/anesthesia for planned vaginal delivery.*
- *01968, Anesthesia for cesarean delivery following neuraxial labor analgesia/ anesthesia*

Now, Carson needs to identify the base units for the anesthesia service. He refers to the CMS RVGs for anesthesia services and determines that the base units for 01967 are 5 and the base units for 01968 are 2 (see figure 12.19).

Figure 12.19. Base unit values for CPT range 01967 through 01991

CPT code	Base Unit Value
01967	5
01968	2
01969	5
01990	7
01991	3

Now he needs to determine the time units that he will report for the service. Time units for the patient's insurance company are reported in 15-minute increments, and the total time spent on the epidural service was 210 minutes, so he reports 14 units (210 minutes divided by 15-minute increments = 14 units), which is reported for CPT code 01967. The total time spent for the cesarean anesthesia was 30 minutes, which would be reported with 2 units on procedure code 01968.

Finally, Carson needs to identify any modifying factors for the anesthesia service. In this case, the patient was a normal, healthy patient, so he can append physical status modifier -P1. No qualifying circumstances are relevant and need to be reported on the claim. He will also add modifier -AA to indicate that the procedure was performed personally by the anesthesiologist.

Carson also needs to calculate the amount of money to charge for the service, and to do this he must add all of the units for the service and multiply them by the conversion factor for the area in which the procedure was performed. The anesthesia was performed in Arizona, so he refers to the CMS locality-adjusted conversion factor tables (accessed via the CMS website), the conversion factor is 21.80 (see figure 12.20), and he enters this amount in the charges for the claim.

Figure 12.20. Calculating anesthesia charges

CPT code	Base Units	Time Units	Modifying Factors	Conversion Factor	Total Charge Amount
01967	5	14	0	$21.80	$1,456.00
01968	2	2	0	$21.80	$ 87.20

His calculations are as follows: (B + T + M) × CF = Total charge amount

Now that Carson has the procedure codes, modifiers, and the charge amount, he needs to identify the ICD-10-CM code(s) for the diagnosis. He asks himself: Why did the doctor do it? In this case, the patient was anesthetized for a cesarean section, which was necessary due to prolonged second stage of labor. Carson finds this by searching under the term Delivery *in the ICD-10-CM Index, and then references the subterm* complicated by, *and then* prolonged labor, *and finds the code for* second stage, O63.1. *When a delivery occurs, an additional code should also be reported to identify the outcome of the delivery, in this case a single live born infant, Z37.0, as well as the weeks of gestation, Z3A.39.*

- *O63.1, Prolonged second stage (of labor)*
- *Z37.0, Single live birth*
- *Z3A.39, 39 weeks gestation of pregnancy*

Carson enters the codes and charges on the claim and looks at the claim to ensure everything was entered correctly (see figure 12.21).

Figure 12.21. Reporting anesthesia services

Source: CMS 2017a.

Key to Success

Coding for anesthesia services may or may not require performing the calculations to add the base units, time units, modifying factors, and then multiplying the sum by the conversion factor. Many anesthesia electronic health record systems have these functions built in, so that the calculations are performed automatically. However, is it still important to understand these calculations, as not all anesthesia providers have the same software, and you may find yourself in the rare situation in which these calculations must be done by hand.

Coding for anesthesia and pain management services

12.5

There's a Code for That

Read the following documentation and select the appropriate CPT and ICD-10-CM code(s) for the anesthesia or pain management service.

1. 78-year-old female experiencing chronic pain underwent balloon kyphoplasty to repair vertebral compression fractures at the T5 and T6 levels.

   CPT codes: _____, _____

   ICD-10-CM code: _____

2. Anesthesia administered by CRNA without anesthesiologist supervision for patient undergoing kyphoplasty of the T5 and T6 vertebrae for compression fractures at those levels in a 78-year-old female with mild hypertension.

   CPT codes: _____ - _____ - _____, _____

   ICD-10-CM code: _____

3. Anesthesia provided for 4-year-old female with receiving heart/lung transplant for myxoma of the heart, CHF, and cardiomyopathy, which are a constant threat to her life.

   CPT codes: _____ - _____

   ICD-10-CM code: _____

4. Bilateral facet joint injections with fluoroscopic guidance of the C6, C7, and C8 vertebrae performed on 48-year-old male with chronic pain in the neck, bilateral shoulders, and bilateral arms.

   CPT codes: _____ - _____, _____ - _____,

   _____ - _____

   ICD-10-CM codes: _____, _____, _____,

   _____, _____, _____

End of Chapter Content

Instructions: Indicate whether the following statements are true or false (T or F). For false statements, rewrite the statement on the line below to make the statement true.

1. Analgesia is the inability to feel pain.

_____

_____

2. The modifier used for services provided by anesthesiology assistants is -AA.

_____

_____

3. Coders may use the CMS or ASA RVG to find the base units for anesthesia services.

_____

_____

4. When an anesthesiologist provides an anesthesia service for more than one procedure at the same operative session only one anesthesia code is billed: the one with the highest base units.

_____

_____

5. Physical status modifiers describe a particularly difficult anesthesia service due to the condition of the patient, notable operative conditions, or unusual risk factors.

_____

_____

6. Pain management specialists employ various procedures to improve the quality of life for patients suffering from chronic pain.

_____

_____

7. Anesthesia services are located within the Surgery section of the CPT code book.

_____

_____

8. Anesthesia codes identify the general procedure performed by the surgeon for which the patient was anesthetized.

_____

_____

9. Medical acupuncture may be performed for pain management purposes but these services may not be coded on the health record.

_____

_____

10. A peripheral nerve stimulation device is implanted directly in the spinal column for pain management.

_____

_____

Instructions: Choose the best answer.

1. Which of the following components takes into account how long an anesthesia procedure took to complete, from start to finish?
   a. Base units
   b. Time units
   c. Physical status
   d. CPT code

2. Which of the following is the correct formula for calculating the amount billed for anesthesia services?
   a. $B + T + CF = M$
   b. $(B + T + M) = CF$
   c. $CF \times (B + T + M)$
   d. $B + T + M + CF$

3. Which of the following units takes into consideration the relative value for each anesthesia service?
   a. Base
   b. Time
   c. Physical status modifiers
   d. Conversion factor

4. Time units for most commercial payers are reported in increments of how many minutes?
   a. 1 minute
   b. 7.5 minutes
   c. 30 minutes
   d. 15 minutes

5. Which physical status modifiers would be used for a patient with a severe systemic disease that is a constant threat to life?
   a. P6
   b. P5
   c. P4
   d. P3

6. Which qualifying circumstance code should be reported for a patient who received anesthesia under controlled hypothermia?
   a. 99100
   b. 99116
   c. 99135
   d. 99140

7. How many unit values are assigned for qualifying circumstance code 99140?
   a. 1
   b. 2
   c. 5
   d. 4

8. Which type of anesthesia blocks a small amount of nerves using an injection, topical cream, or spray?
   a. Local
   b. Regional
   c. General
   d. Moderate (conscious) sedation

9. In which of the following types of anesthesia is the patient completely unconscious?

a. Local

b. Regional

c. General

d. Moderate (conscious) sedation

10. Which of the following anesthesia codes should be appended to a service performed by a CRNA with anesthesiologist supervision?

a. -AA

b. -QY

c. -QZ

d. -QX

11. Which of the following pain management procedures utilizes invasive interventions to treat the patient's pain?

a. Integrative medicine

b. Electrodiagnostic studies

c. Medical management

d. Interventional pain procedures

12. Which type of pain management procedure injects a steroid or anesthetic directly into the patient's spinal joints?

a. Epidural steroid injections

b. Facet joint injections

c. Trigger point injections

d. Occipital nerve blocks

13. A patient with a history of failed anesthesia underwent a surgical procedure under general anesthesia. Which of the following ICD-10-CM diagnosis codes should be assigned?

a. Z92.83

b. T88.53

c. T88.4

d. Z92.84

14. A patient with neoplasm-related pain presented for a pain management procedure. Which code should be sequenced as the first-listed diagnosis?

a. The code for the neoplasm

b. The code for acute pain

c. The code for the pain management procedure

d. The code for chronic pain

Instructions: Answer the following questions with the appropriate code(s) and modifier(s).

1. An anesthesiologist performed anesthesia for a patient with ESRD on a regular dialysis schedule, receiving a kidney transplant. The patient was transferred to the PACU and care transferred to PACU nurse. Two hours later, anesthesiologist was called back in to perform a single injection epidural without imaging guidance in the thoracic area, to manage the patient's postprocedural pain.

CPT codes: _____ - ___, - ___,

_____ - ___

ICD-10-CM codes: _____, _____

2. 65-year-old female with idiopathic peripheral neuropathy presented for monthly acupuncture treatment. 30 minutes of medical acupuncture with 20 needles provided without electrical stimulation.

CPT codes: _____ , _____

ICD-10-CM code: _____

References

American Medical Association. 2018. *CPT 2018 Professional Edition*. Chicago: AMA.

American Society of Anesthesiologists. 2014 (October 15). ASA Physical Status Classification System. https://www.asahq.org/search?q=physical%20status%20classification%20system#q=physical%20status%20classification%20system&sort=relevancy.

Army Publishing Directorate. 2017. DA Forms: Medical Record Anesthesia. http://www.apd.army.mil/ProductMaps/PubForm/DAForms_Details.aspx?ID=0902c85180011267&PUBNO=DA+FORM+7389.

Blausen.com staff. 2013a. "Blausen 0354 EpiduralSteroidInjection.png." Digital image. Wikimedia Commons. Accessed December, 2017. https://commons.wikimedia.org/wiki/File:Blausen_0354_EpiduralSteroidInjection.png.

Blausen.com staff. 2013b. "Blausen 0484 HerniatedLumbarDisc.png." Digital image. Wikimedia Commons. Accessed December, 2017. https://commons.wikimedia.org/wiki/File:Blausen_0484_HerniatedLumbarDisc.png.

Centers for Medicare and Medicaid Services. 2018. ICD-10-CM Official Guidelines for Coding and Reporting FY 2018. https://www.cms.gov/Medicare/Coding/ICD10/Downloads/2018-ICD-10-CM-Coding-Guidelines.pdf.

Centers for Medicare and Medicaid Services. 2017a. Details for title: CMS 1500. https://www.cms.gov/Medicare/CMS-Forms/CMS-Forms/CMS-Forms-Items/CMS1188854.html.

Centers for Medicare and Medicaid Services. 2017b (July 6). Locality-Adjusted Anesthesia Conversion Factors as a result of the CY 2017 Final Rule. https://www.cms.gov/Center/Provider-Type/Anesthesiologists-Center.html.

Centers for Medicare and Medicaid Services. 2014. 2014 Anesthesia Base Units by CPT Code. https://www.cms.gov/Medicare/Medicare-Fee-for-Service-Payment/PhysicianFeeSched/Downloads/2014-Anesthesia-BaseUnits-CPT.zip.

Das, S. and S. Ghosh. 2015 (January-March). Monitored anesthesia care: An overview. J Anaesthesiol Clin Pharmacol 31(1): 27–29. https://www.ncbi.nlm.nih.gov/pmc/articles/PMC4353148/.

Mount Sinai Hospital. 2017a. Electromyography. http://www.mountsinai.org/patient-care/service-areas/pain-management/pain-management-services/electrodiagnostic-studies.

Mount Sinai Hospital. 2017b. Interventional Pain Procedures Under X-Ray Guidance. http://www.mountsinai.org/patient-care/service-areas/pain-management/pain-management-services/interventional-spinal-procedures-under-x-ray-guidance.

Mount Sinai Hospital. 2017c. Peripheral Nerve Stimulation. http://www.mountsinai.org/patient-care/service-areas/pain-management/pain-management-services/peripheral-nerve-stimulation.

Palmetto GBA. 2013 (July). Anesthesia Billing Guide. https://engage.ahima.org/HigherLogic/System/DownloadDocumentFile.ashx?DocumentFileKey=9af2a07d-26e1-4694-b1de-a4c59d0dbc30.

Resources

abeo. 2016 (February 15). Specialty Tip #15 Anesthesiology. http://abeo.com/wp-content/uploads/2016/02/15-ICD10_SpecialtyTips_Anesthesiology.pdf.

Centers for Medicare and Medicaid Services. 2016 (August). Medicare Claims Processing Manual Chapter 12 - Physicians/Nonphysician Practitioners. https://www.cms.gov/Regulations-and-Guidance/Guidance/Manuals/Downloads/clm104c12.pdf.

Mount Sinai Hospital. 2017. Pain Management Services and Treatments. http://www.mountsinai.org/patient-care/service-areas/pain-management/pain-management-services.

CHAPTER 13

Radiology and Imaging Services

Learning Objectives

- Understand the basics of billing and coding for independent radiology and imaging centers.
- Examine procedural codes and guidelines for independent radiology and imaging services.
- Examine diagnosis coding and medical necessity for independent radiology and imaging services.
- Determine and apply ICD-10-CM, CPT, and HCPCS codes to independent radiology and imaging services.

Key Terms

Anterior
Antero-posterior
Axial plane
Computed tomography (CT)
Contralateral
Contrast material
Coronal plane
Distal
Doppler ultrasound
Global radiology service
Imaging services
Independent radiology and
   imaging center
Inferior

Ipsilateral
Lateral
Lateral (view)
Magnetic resonance imaging (MRI)
Mammography
Medial
Nuclear medicine
Oblique
Pleural effusion
Posterior
Postero-anterior
Professional component (PC)
Projection
Proximal

Pulmonary edema
Radiologic guidance
Radiological supervision and
   interpretation (S&I)
Radiologist
Radiology services
Sagittal plane
Superior
Technical component (TC)
Transverse plane
Ultrasound
X-ray

Radiology and imaging services are medical procedures that use a variation of techniques to view the inner structures of the body for diagnostic or therapeutic purposes. **Radiology services**, x-rays and CT scans (discussed in this chapter), use radiation to produce images of the inside of the body, such as bones and organs. **Imaging services** is a more inclusive term used for the wide array of types of techniques used to produce images of the inside of the body, including radiology services, ultrasounds, fluoroscopy, and nuclear imaging.

This chapter discusses radiology and imaging techniques including basics of radiology and imaging services, billing for radiology and imaging procedures, and substantiating radiology and imaging services with the appropriate diagnosis codes.

Radiology and Imaging Basics

When coding for radiology services, knowledge of the different settings and providers, components of the services, and the medical terminology is important, including the terms used for body plans, body positions, movement, and projections of radiology services. Coders must also remember the importance of the professional and technical components of radiology procedures, and that they must bill only for the portion of the service performed by each medical provider.

Radiology and Imaging Settings and Providers

Radiology and imaging services are performed in various medical settings—independent facilities that focus on only imaging procedures, inpatient and outpatient hospitals, or individual clinics that use certain imaging services relevant to their specialty services.

An **independent radiology and imaging center** is an office that specializes in only radiology and imaging techniques. These offices receive requests from physicians to perform a specific imaging service or services on a patient, and then send the result of the imaging study to the requesting provider. For example, if a patient went to her primary care physician (PCP) and complained of pelvic pain, the PCP might choose to have an ultrasound of the patient's abdomen performed to rule out ovarian cysts. In some cases, depending on the type of provider and resources, an in-house ultrasound machine to perform the imaging may be available. If not, then the provider would likely send the patient to an imaging center that would perform the imaging service. The imaging center would receive the request from the patient's PCP, perform the ultrasound, and then send a written report of the findings to the PCP. This report may be provided through an electronic health record (EHR) system, emailed, or faxed. Often, depending on the type of imaging service performed, the actual images from the service are also sent with the report of the findings via the EHR system, emailed, or saved to a data storage device for transport to the requesting provider.

Radiology services may also be performed in the facility setting (inpatient or outpatient hospital). In these settings, the imaging or radiology service is often performed for an acute problem or as part of a surgical procedure. For example, a patient complaining of severe abdominal pain that presents to the emergency department may have an ultrasound of the abdomen done to rule out appendicitis. In the outpatient setting, imaging guidance may be used to help lead an outpatient surgical procedure; for example, fluoroscopic guidance used during a facet joint injection for the administration of a corticosteroid for pain management.

Some medical specialist offices may invest in their own imaging equipment so that certain radiology or imaging studies may be performed directly in the office. For example, a maternal-fetal medicine specialist may invest in a number of ultrasound machines, so that patients can receive ultrasounds in the office and the results are read immediately. Orthopedists also often have x-ray equipment so they can diagnose patient conditions and the healing status of fractures.

When a medical office has its own imaging equipment, the images produced are typically read by the ordering physician. For example, the maternal-fetal medicine specialist orders an ultrasound for a high-risk patient and then reads the ultrasound results, or the orthopedist reads the x-rays and determines if a fracture is present or not. However, when the ordering provider is not present, the image is usually read by a radiologist.

A radiologist is a medical doctor who specializes in the diagnosis and treatment of medical conditions using radiology and imaging techniques. These include x-rays, ultrasounds, computed tomography (CT), magnetic resonance imaging (MRI), nuclear medicine, and positron emission tomography (PET) scans. Radiologists are further trained in radiation safety, protection, and the effects of radiation on the human body, as well as imaging techniques and interpretation of imaging studies.

A radiology technician is the staff member trained to perform the imaging procedure. This person has received specialized training in how to operate the imaging machine, such as x-ray or ultrasound machine, and knows how to position the patient at the optimum angle for the image so the radiologist can get a clear view of the body area, organ, or other internal component involved in the imaging service. Radiology technicians are usually certified in their field of expertise, and have completed formal schooling such as diagnostic medical sonography or radiology technician program.

These differences become significant when coding for radiology services, as there are two components to imaging procedures—the technical component and the professional component.

Components of Radiology Services

In any typical imaging service—such as an ultrasound, x-ray, or MRI scan—a technician uses the appropriate machine to take images of the patient, according to the directions of the ordering provider. Once these images are captured, the radiologist or ordering provider reads the images to determine the patient's diagnosis. This doctor then provides a written report of the findings of the imaging service (for instance, a fracture, gallstones, or tumor).

This example illustrates the two components of an imaging service, each capturing a portion of the service provided. The technical component (TC) of a service includes the equipment, supplies, clinical personnel, and any other costs needed to perform the imaging procedure. For example, the technical component of an x-ray would include the x-ray machine, any supplies used to take the x-ray, and the salary for the x-ray technician who captured the image.

The professional component (PC) of a service includes the professional supervision, interpretation, and written report of the findings from the imaging service. For example, the professional component of an x-ray would be the radiologist reading the x-ray and determining that a fracture is present (interpreting the results), and then submitting a written report of his or her findings to the ordering provider.

Billing for imaging services depends on the portion of the service that was provided by the office. For example, if an ultrasound was performed at an imaging center and the images were sent directly to the ordering doctor without interpretation, then the imaging center would bill only for the *technical* component of the service—because only the technical component was provided (machine and any supplies used, and the clinical staff required to operate the machine and perform the ultrasound). The doctor receiving the images, however, would bill only for the *professional* component of the service (interpretation of the images and a written report of the findings). In this way, imaging centers, radiologists, and any other provider who performs and reads imaging services can divide the components of an imaging service, and bill only for the portion of the service they performed.

Billing for either of these portions is done by adding the appropriate modifier to the CPT code for the radiology procedure. Modifier -26, Professional component, is used to indicate that only the professional component of the procedure was performed. So, using the previous example, an ultrasound was performed and sent to the provider's office, who then read, interpreted, and delivered a written report of the findings. The CPT code reported by the provider's office would be appended with modifier -26 to indicate that only the professional component of the service was performed.

Billing for the technical component of the procedure is done by appending modifier -TC, Technical component, to the code. Again using the previous example, the imaging center performing the ultrasound would report the CPT code for the ultrasound procedure, and append it with modifier -TC to indicate that only the technical part of the procedure was performed. Modifier -TC should only be used when the reporting facility owns the equipment and pays for the performance of the imaging service, as well as the salary for the clinical staff needed to perform the service. However, there may be a caveat to the reporting of modifier -TC and imaging services for some types of medical settings. For example, in the inpatient hospital setting, if the inpatient hospital facility performed the radiology procedure, then this would not be reported with a CPT code (rather, it would be reported with an ICD-10-PCS code to identify the procedure performed, as discussed in chapter 20). In the outpatient hospital setting (submitting professional fee codes), the third-party payer may assume that the hospital owns the radiology equipment, and so the use of modifier -TC is not necessary (Verhovshek 2015). As with other areas of medical coding, it is necessary to check with payer policy to ensure that the patient's insurance accepts modifier -TC and verify the rate at which they pay for the service.

Using either of these modifiers divides the CPT code into two parts—one technical and one professional—so the provider who performed the service can bill for that portion of the service. Appending either of these modifiers means that the reimbursement for the procedure is broken into two parts. The exact amount depends on the insurance but, typically, performing the technical component of the procedure pays more than performing the professional component of the procedure. For example, the technical component of the procedure might pay 60 percent of the allowable amount of payment for the code, whereas the professional component might pay 40 percent of the allowable amount of payment for the code. Note, however, that these payment percentages depend on the third-party payer for the service.

When a provider performs both the technical and professional components of a code, it is not necessary to append any modifier to the code. For example, if the ultrasound is performed in the office of an obstetrician where the practice owns the ultrasound machine, pays the clinical staff to perform the procedure, and also pays the doctor to read the ultrasound and interpret the results, then the practice would bill for *each* component of the imaging service (both professional and technical). In this case, the same CPT code would be reported, once per date of service, *without any modifiers*. This is called billing for the **global radiology service**. A global radiology service is the performance of both components of the procedure—professional and technical—by the same facility. Billing for the global service requires simply the reporting of the CPT code for the

Figure 13.1. Components of radiology services

Technical Component
equipment, supplies, clinical personnel
▶ **-TC**

Professional Component
supervision, interpretation, and report
▶ **-26**

Global Service
both technical and professional components
▶ **None**

service, appended without either the -26 or -TC modifier (see figure 13.1 for an illustration of the components of a radiology service).

Key to Success

Think about surgery billing and global surgery packages discussed in chapter 11. A global surgical package includes all of the little procedures needed to perform the surgery. Billing for the global radiology service is very similar. When neither the -26 nor the -TC modifiers are used, it indicates that the provider performed the global radiology procedure, which included both the professional and technical components of the service.

Services that include both the professional and technical components are found in sections other than the Radiology section of the CPT code book. Some codes in the Medicine section as well as the Pathology and Laboratory sections also identify either component of the code. For example, code 93005, Electrocardiogram, routine ECG with at least 12 leads; tracing only, without interpretation and report, is a Medicine section code that identifies only the technical components of the procedure (tracing only without interpretation and report). On the other hand, code 93010, Electrocardiogram, routine ECG with at least 12 leads; interpretation and report only, identifies only the professional component of the service (interpretation and report only). Neither of these codes requires either modifier -26 or -TC because the component is identified in the code description. It is important to pay close attention to code descriptions, as some identify either portion of the service performed with different codes, rather than needing to use modifier -TC or -26. The wording to look out for here is **radiological supervision and interpretation (S&I)**, which is the professional component of the study, and includes the supervision of the radiology service as well as interpretation of the results. For example, code 74445, Corpora cavernosography, *radiological supervision and interpretation*, already describes the procedure as the professional component. It is not necessary to include modifier -26 with this code, as this code *only* applies for the professional component.

For practice identifying the components of a radiology service, complete the exercises in There's a Code for That 13.1.

13.1

There's a Code for That

Radiology components

Read the following documentation of the radiology service and determine if it should be reported as the technical service only (-TC), professional service only (-26), or global service (no modifier).

1. A chest x-ray is performed at a freestanding radiology center. The films are sent to the office of a physician who is employed at a private practice for interpretation and report. Which component of the radiology service should the radiology center bill for?
   a. Technical
   b. Professional
   c. Global

2. A chest x-ray is performed at a freestanding radiology center. The films are sent to the office of a physician who is employed at a private practice for interpretation and report. Which component of the radiology service should the physician that reads the report bill for?
   a. Technical
   b. Professional
   c. Global

3. A spinal x-ray is performed at an orthopedic clinic that employs the physician who reads and interprets the x-ray films. Which component will the orthopedic clinic bill for?
   a. Technical
   b. Professional
   c. Global

4. A hospital performs an abdominal imaging service for a patient with severe abdominal pain. A physician who is not employed by the hospital reads the images and determines that the patient has a ruptured appendix. Which component would the physician bill for?
   a. Technical
   b. Professional
   c. Global

5. An imaging center performs a series of scans on a patient with suspected cancer. The in-house radiologist reads the scans and determines that there are a number of metastases present throughout the body. Which component would the imaging center bill for?
   a. Technical
   b. Professional
   c. Global

Medical Terminology for Radiology and Imaging Procedures

Reporting the correct radiology code requires a solid knowledge of the basic directional terms, planes of the body, and projection terminology. These terms help coders to understand the documentation of the radiology or imaging service, so that the correct CPT code may be reported for the service.

Basic Directional Terms

Basic directional terms are often used to describe the general direction of a body part or area. Although these terms are useful in coding across all medical specialties, they are especially important when coding for radiological procedures. For example, diagnosis coding relies frequently on identification of the exact location of the condition, such as of the proximal arm versus the distal arm. Radiology and imaging service coders must be able to decipher the provider's documentation, which may include these terms, to determine which code should be reported for the service. They include:

- Anterior: situated toward the front of the body (such as the face or the breasts)
- Posterior: situated toward the back of the body (such as the buttocks or heels)
- Superior: toward the top of the body (the head)
- Inferior: toward the bottom of the body (the feet)
- Medial: toward the midline of the body (the belly button)
- Lateral: away from the midline of the body (the sides)
- Proximal: toward the center of the body (the upper arm)
- Distal: away from the body (the fingertips)
- Ipsilateral: the same side of the body (the right upper and lower extremities)
- Contralateral: the opposite side of the body (the right arm and the left arm)

Planes of the Body

The planes of the body are imaginary lines that dissect the body into sections. Just as with directional terms, the planes of the body are often used in health record documentation to identify the general area of a medical condition or procedure and include the following (see figure 13.2).

- The axial plane is a horizontal line perpendicular to the long axis of the body that divides the body into superior and inferior portions (top and bottom halves). The axial plane is also known as the transverse or transaxial plane.
- The sagittal plane is a vertical line that divides the body into right and left halves.
- The coronal plane is also a vertical line, but divides the body into anterior and posterior halves (front and back).

Projection

The projection of an imaging service is the direction in which the imaging rays pass through the body. For example, an x-ray machine is positioned at the front of the bod, and the ray passes in through the anterior (the front of the body) and out through the posterior (the back of the body). The projection of an imaging service is also known

Figure 13.2. Planes of the body and basic directional terms

as the view, so if there are two projections during an imaging service, this means the service consisted of two views and include:

- Antero-posterior, which passes through the front to the back of the body
- Postero-anterior, which passes through the back to the front of the body
- Lateral, which passes from one side of the body to the other (for example, from the right to the left)
- Oblique, which passes through the body at a diagonal angle

Key to Success

Knowing basic directional terms, planes of the body, and terms for projections is an important part of being able to decipher a health record and determine the correct procedure or diagnosis code. As you read through procedural notes or descriptions of surgical or radiology procedures, it helps to picture the procedure in your mind as the steps of the procedure are being described in the documentation. Knowing the planes of the body, directional terms, and projections, is a good place to start.

Procedural Coding for Radiology and Imaging Services

Procedural coding for radiology and imaging services requires an understanding of how the Radiology section of the CPT code book is organized, the different types of imaging services included in the Radiology section, guidelines for coding radiology services (including how to code for contrast material), and modifiers used in radiology coding.

All radiology and imaging services are located in the Radiology section of the CPT code book, which is organized first by the type of radiology service provided and then subcategorized by the area that was included in the study, or the specific type of study or service provided. These services include diagnostic radiology services, diagnostic ultrasound, radiologic guidance, mammography, bone and joint studies, radiation oncology, and nuclear medicine. It is also important to understand the modifiers other than -26 and -TC that are used in radiology coding.

Diagnostic Radiology Services

The first and largest subsection of the Radiology section of the CPT code book is Diagnostic Radiology (Diagnostic Imaging) (70010 to 76499). This section includes codes for a number of different radiology and imaging services, arranged by general body area. Codes for several different imaging studies may be listed within each body area, such as radiologic examinations, special imaging studies, magnetic resonance imaging, and computed tomography scans. Diagnostic radiology services also include the administration of contrast materials.

Radiologic Examination (X-ray)

An **x-ray** examination is a form of imaging that produces a beam of x-rays, a form of electromagnetic radiation, that pass through the body. As the rays pass through the body, denser objects, like bones, absorb less of the radiation than less dense objects like internal organs or blood vessels. The rays that are not absorbed are captured behind the image, creating a negative image of the dense structures within the body (see figure 13.3). The human body is made up of many structures of varying densities, which makes x-ray imaging a painless and noninvasive method for diagnosing a range of medical conditions such as fractures, pneumonia, and cysts or tumors (NIBIB 2017). Code descriptions in the CPT code book refer to x-rays as radiologic examinations.

Figure 13.3. Posteroanterior chest x-ray

Source: ©2017. Used with permission of Elsevier. All rights reserved.

Key to Success

Code descriptions in the CPT code book refer to x-rays as radiologic examinations. So do not be surprised when you do not see any CPT codes for "x-rays." For example, code 72100, Radiologic examination, spine, lumbosacral; 2 or 3 views, is for an x-ray of the lumbosacral spine. On the other hand, health record documentation may read that the patient received an x-ray or radiographic examination of the spine. In this case, the coder must realize that an x-ray or radiographic examination in the health record is the same procedure described in the CPT code description as a radiologic examination.

Codes for x-rays often describe the number of views included in the procedure. A view is the angle at which the x-ray was taken. Multiple x-ray angles help to diagnose a medical condition with certainty. So if a patient with a possible wrist fracture received an anteroposterior x-ray, a lateral x-ray, and an oblique x-ray of the wrist, then the x-ray of the wrist entailed three views (anteroposterior, lateral, and oblique).

When searching for the code for an x-ray in the CPT code book, reference either the term *X-ray* or *Radiology* in the Index, and then locate the subterm for the type of procedure and the area that was viewed in the procedure. In this case, if the patient had an x-ray of the wrist, the coder should reference the subterm *Wrist,* which leads to code range 73100 to 73110. Code options include 73100, Radiologic examination, wrist; *2 views,* or 73110, Radiologic examination, wrist; *complete, minimum of 3 views.* In this example, the x-ray consisted of three views, so the correct code would be 73110. If the x-ray had only consisted of one or two views, then the correct code would be 73100. Note that code 73110 describes a complete x-ray of the wrist, with a minimum of three views. This means that if more than three views were taken, such as five or six views, the correct code would still be 73110, as it describes a *minimum* of three views.

Key to Success

Notice that when you are searching for an x-ray in the Index, you can look up the term "x-ray," but when you verify the code(s) in the Tabular List, they are all listed as "Radiologic examinations." Don't let this confuse you! X-rays and radiologic examinations are the same procedure.

Special Radiological Studies

There are a number of special radiological studies listed in the Diagnostic Radiology subsection of the CPT code book. These are a special set of x-rays used to diagnose specific medical conditions. They are found throughout the Diagnostic Radiology section, and instead of describing an x-ray of a specific body area or organ, they are listed by the name of the study itself. For example, a dacryocystography is a radiologic examination of the lacrimal sacs and associated structures within the orbital area of the eyes. It is performed by injecting a contrast material (discussed later in this section) into the nasolacrimal ducts and then a series of x-rays are taken. To look up a special radiological study, search for the term directly in the CPT Index (in this case the coder should look up *Dacryocystography*).

Key to Success

If you are coding for a special radiological study and you are having problems locating the code, use a medical dictionary and your knowledge of anatomy and physiology to determine the body area or organ system involved in the study. Then use this information to search for the radiologic examination of that particular body part, or scan through the table of contents for the Diagnostic Radiology subsection of codes.

Note that in this example, and for many special radiological studies, the code describes the *radiological supervision and interpretation* of the study: 70170, Dacryocystography, nasolacrimal duct, *radiological supervision and interpretation.* In this case, the imaging study is performed by injecting a contrast material into the patient's nasolacrimal ducts, and then taking the x-ray images. The entire procedure would be reported with two codes—one for the injection and one for the x-ray supervision and interpretation. The injection is coded within the appropriate surgery section of the CPT code book (in this case 68850, Injection of contrast medium for dacryocystography).

The coder should report *only* the portion of the service that was performed by their medical provider. For example, if both the injection and the imaging study were performed by the same physician, then both codes should be reported. If the two components were performed by different providers, then each provider should code only for the service that he or she performed. Note that because the x-ray code in this example identifies the radiological supervision and interpretation of the study, modifier -26 should not be appended to the code to identify the professional component.

Computed Tomography (CT)

A computed tomography (CT), also known as computed axial tomography (CAT) scan is an imaging study that combines x-ray images from different angles to produce a virtual cross-section of the area being studied. CT scans are noninvasive and painless procedures, which may be used to diagnose patients suffering from acute traumatic events or patients with acute symptoms such as chest or abdominal pain, or difficulty breathing. It is also often used to create images of the chest, head, abdomen, and pelvis, because it can provide a cross-sectional view of all types of body tissues (see figure 13.4).

Figure 13.4. Axial CT scan of the head

Source: ©2010. Used with permission of Elsevier. All rights reserved.

Codes for CT scans are located in the Diagnostic Radiology subsection of codes, and are usually listed after radiologic examination codes within each respective body area. Code selection depends on the site of the CT scan and whether or not any contrast material was used. For example, code 72192, Computed tomography, pelvis; without contrast material, identifies the area of the study (pelvis), as well as whether or not contrast material was used (without contrast material).

Magnetic Resonance Imaging (MRI)

Magnetic resonance imaging (MRI) is a form of imaging that uses strong magnetic fields and radio waves to produce detailed images of the anatomy and physiology of the internal structures of a patient's body, and can be used to diagnose a range of medical conditions. MRI images include more detail of vascular structures and soft tissues than those produced by x-ray imaging. MRI studies are noninvasive and painless, and may be used to diagnose neurologic conditions like dementia and cerebrovascular diseases, cardiovascular conditions, cancer staging, and assessment of joint diseases, and countless other conditions (see figure 13.5).

Figure 13.5. MRI of a lumbosacral herniated disc

Codes for MRI studies are located in the Diagnostic Radiology subsection, usually listed after radiologic examination and computed tomography scan codes. Code selection depends on the site of the MRI, and whether or not any contrast material was used. For example, code 72198, Magnetic resonance imaging, pelvis, with or without contrast material(s), identifies the site of the study (pelvis) and whether contrast material was used (with or without contrast).

Contrast Materials

Contrast material, or contrast medium, is a substance that is injected into the patient to enhance the contrast of certain structures in the body while performing x-rays and imaging procedures. Contrast material may be given to the patient orally, rectally, or via injection, depending on the imaging procedure and intent of the study. For example, some imaging studies of the gastrointestinal tract may require a swallowed contrast material, and an x-ray of the lung may require an inhaled contrast material. However, note that according to CPT guidelines, only contrast that is given intravascularly (into a blood vessel), intra-articularly (into a joint), or intrathecally (into the spinal canal) counts as "with contrast" for CPT code selection. In other words, if the contrast material is not given via an injection it does not count as contrast. This is due to the fact that the administration of the contrast material (as built into the code description) is only reported when it requires the physician's skill to do so.

The use of contrast material produces images that may be more or less detailed in certain areas and, as a result, it is common that diagnostic radiology studies may be performed with contrast, without contrast, or with and without contrast, depending on the needs of the study. When coding for contrast, there are three code options:

- without contrast
- with contrast
- without contrast material(s) followed by contrast material(s) and further sequences

This last option identifies procedures that are performed with and without contrast. The imaging study is done without contrast material first, then contrast material is

Figure 13.6. Contrast in abdominal imaging

CTs Demonstrating Time Sequence from Organs Without Contrast to Clearance of Contrast By Kidneys

A. Noncontrast CT study. Note the subtle differences between the shades of grey in the solid viscera. Blood vessels in the liver are not well seen.

B. Arterial phase image. After 30 seconds of the injection, the contrast is predominantly in the arteries, which are seen as white rounded and linear structures.

C. Portal-venous phase image. The liver is better visualized, and both the portal veins and the hepatic veins are opacified *(white)*. Contrast has also reached both the renal cortex and the medulla.

D. Contrast clearance by the kidneys and ureters at approximately 120 seconds. Contrast in the organs is "washing out" and is excreted by the kidneys. The renal calices, renal pelvis, and ureters become white with the concentrated contrast.

administered, and then the imaging study is performed again. Figure 13.6 shows an abdominal imaging CT with varying stages of contrast material. The top left image shows the abdominal CT without contrast and the other three images show varying stages of the contrast material working its way through the organs and abdominal structures.

When a contrast agent is used, it is also necessary to report the contrast material used with the appropriate supply code (HCPCS code). These HCPCS codes identify the specific contrast material used. Codes for contrast materials can be found in the Supplies for Radiology Procedures (Radiopharmaceuticals) (A9500 to A9700) and in Contrast (Q9951 to Q9983) in the HCPCS code book. For example, if an MRI of the brain was performed with and without contrast (contrast material used was Gadolinium), the codes reported would be 70553, Magnetic resonance (e.g., proton) imaging, brain (including brain stem); without contrast material followed by contrast material(s) and further sequences, and A9579, Injection, gadolinium-based magnetic resonance contrast agent, not otherwise specified (NOA), per ml.

Review figure 13.7 to see the multiple components of coding for diagnostic radiology services and then complete There's a Code for That 13.2 for practice assigning codes for diagnostic radiology procedures.

Figure 13.7. Diagnostic radiology components

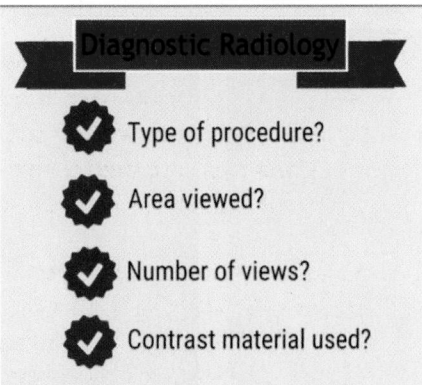

13.2

There's a Code for That

Diagnostic radiology procedures

Read the following documentation of the Diagnostic Radiology service and identify the correct Radiology procedure code(s).

1. CT of the abdomen with oral contrast.

   CPT code: _____

2. CT of the abdomen and pelvic without contrast.

   CPT code: _____

3. Antero-posterior and lateral radiographs of the chest taken on a patient with atypical chest pain.

   CPT code: _____

4. X-ray of the cervical spine, antero-posterior, lateral, and both oblique views were obtained.

   CPT code: _____

5. MRI of the right shoulder with 100 ml low osmolar contrast.

   CPT code: _____

   HCPCS code: _____ x _____

6. Physician was called into ED to read x-ray films of patient involved in MVA. Films included complete x-ray of left ankle and complete x-ray examination of left foot.

   CPT codes: _____ - _____, _____ - _____

Diagnostic Ultrasound

The next subsection of codes in the Radiology section of the CPT code book is Diagnostic Ultrasound (76506 to 76776), which includes codes for ultrasound evaluations. The format of this subsection is similar to the Diagnostic Radiology subsection, as codes are listed according to body area. An **ultrasound**, also known as a sonogram, uses high-frequency sound waves through the use of a transducer applied to a specific area of the body. The sound waves bounce off internal structures within the body, creating an image on a computer screen. Ultrasounds are noninvasive, painless, and do not require the patient to undergo any type of radiation; and are commonly used to view the real-time structure and movement of the internal organs of the body, as well as blood vessels and blood flow. Ultrasounds can be specialized using 3D technology, which transforms the sounds waves into a 3D image projected to the computer screen. A **Doppler ultrasound** is a special technique that uses color-coded mapping during the ultrasound procedure that allows the viewer to see oxygenated and de-oxygenated blood flow through body organs in real time (see figure 13.8) (NIBIB 2016).

Figure 13.8. Ultrasound imaging

Gallbladder

Gallstone

Acoustic shadow under the stone

A. Ultrasound image of a gallstone. Note the bright echogenicity of the stone and the lack of echoes beneath the stone. The gallbladder is otherwise anechoic because it is filled with fluid.

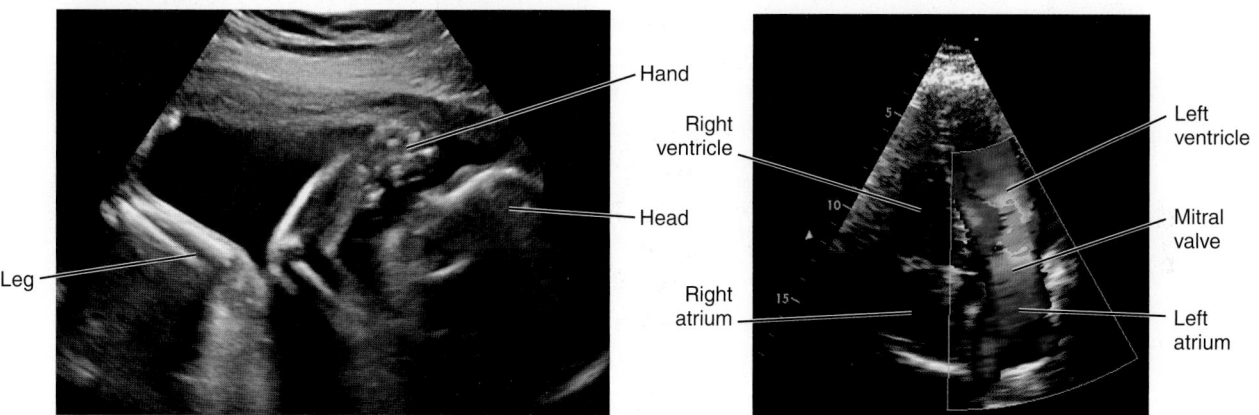

Hand

Right ventricle

Head

Leg

Right atrium

Left ventricle

Mitral valve

Left atrium

B. Ultrasound image of a second-trimester fetus. Ultrasound is used to monitor prenatal development, detect congenital defects, and determine sex.

C. Color Doppler ultrasound image of blood flowing from left atrium into the left ventricle. By convention, red color is blood flowing toward the transducer on the skin; blue is flow away from the transducer.

Codes for ultrasound studies identify the type of ultrasound technique used, the area viewed in the study, and whether the study was limited or complete. There are a number of different ultrasound techniques. Note that in some cases the ultrasound technique impacts code selection. For example, code 76511, Ophthalmic ultrasound, diagnostic; quantitative A-scan only, identifies an A-scan of the eyes, whereas code 76512, Ophthalmic ultrasound, diagnostic; B-scan (with or without superimposed non-quantitative A-scan) identifies a B-scan, that may or may not be performed with an A-scan. On the other hand, code 76800, Ultrasound, spinal canal and contents, does not identify the type of scan that was used to perform the imaging procedure. Ultimately, if the type of scan is not listed in the code description (as in the spinal canal ultrasound), then it does not impact code selection. The types of scans are as follows:

- A-mode scan produces a one-dimensional ultrasonic measurement.
- M-mode scan produces a one-dimensional ultrasonic measurement with tracing of the amplitude and velocity of echo-producing structures.
- B-scan ultrasounds include a two-dimensional ultrasound scan, which produces a two-dimensional display.
- Real-time scan produces a two-dimensional display along with movement in real-time.
- Doppler ultrasound evaluates the integrity of vascular structures and blood flow. Note that the Doppler imaging that is included in ultrasound codes is for anatomic structure identification in conjunction with the ultrasound. For Doppler studies that evaluate the vascular structures using both color and spectral, Doppler is separately reportable using Noninvasive Vascular Diagnostic Studies codes (93880 to 93990).

When coding for pelvic ultrasounds, note the difference between codes for Obstetrical pelvic ultrasounds (76801 to 76828), versus those for Non-obstetrical ultrasound (76830 to 76857). Obstetrical ultrasounds are performed on the fetus in a pregnant female patient, and codes depend on the type of ultrasounds and any additional procedures performed. Non-obstetrical ultrasounds are performed on the pelvic of non-pregnant females and males. Note also that there are a number of add-on codes through this section, to identify each additional gestation for patients with a multiple pregnancy. If the ultrasound was performed with 3D imaging, report the service with either 76376, 3D rendering with interpretation and reporting of computed tomography, magnetic resonance imaging, ultrasound, or other tomographic modality with image postprocessing under concurrent supervision; not requiring postprocessing on an independent workstation, or 76377, 3D rendering with interpretation and reporting of computed tomography, magnetic resonance imaging, ultrasound, of other tomographic modality with image postprocessing under concurrent supervision; requiring image postprocessing on an independent workstation, in addition to the obstetric ultrasound code.

Radiologic Guidance

The next subsection in the Radiology section of the CPT code book is Radiologic Guidance (77001 to 77022). **Radiologic guidance** procedures are performed together with an invasive or minimally invasive procedure to help guide the provider performing the procedure to the correct anatomical location. There are three types of radiologic guidance: fluoroscopic, computed tomography (CT), and magnetic resonance (MR) guidance. Code selection depends on the type of guidance performed and the primary surgical procedure. Fluoroscopic guidance codes are all add-on codes that should be used in conjunction with the code for the primary surgical procedure. For example, code 77003, Fluoroscopic guidance and localization of needle or catheter tip for spine or paraspinous diagnostic or therapeutic injection procedures (epidural or subarachnoid) is an add-on code for fluoroscopic guidance.

Because guidance procedures are performed in conjunction with another procedure, there are many parenthetical notes (discussed first in chapter 5) within this section of codes that identify when each code may or may not be used in conjunction with the code for the surgical procedure. For example, in parentheses under code 77003 is a list of the surgical codes that it may be reported with: (*Use 77003 in conjunction with 61050,*

61055, 62267, 62270, 62272, 62273, 62280, 62281, 62282, 62284, 64510, 64517, 64520, 64610). It also identifies specific codes with which 77003 may not be reported: (*Do not report 77003 in conjunction with 62320, 62321, 62322, 62323, 62324, 62325, 62326, 62327*).

Mammography

The next subsection contains codes for Breast, Mammography studies (77053 to 77067). Mammography, or a mammogram, is an x-ray image of the breast used to diagnose breast conditions such as tumors or fibrocystic diseases (see figure 13.9). Note that even though a mammography is a diagnostic x-ray procedure, it is located in its own special subsection of codes.

Figure 13.9. Mammographic imaging

Mammogram

Source: Blausen.com staff 2014.

Code selection depends on the specific type of procedure and if the mammography was bilateral or unilateral. It is important to note the difference between a diagnostic mammography (77065 and 77066) and a screening mammography. A diagnostic mammography is performed when a patient has some sort of clinical sign or symptom, such as a lump in the breast or nipple discharge. A screening mammography (77067) is performed on a regular basis when no symptoms are present to detect early changes in the breast, which may indicate breast cancer. This is a preventive examination and is typically covered by most insurance companies, as long as it is performed according to schedule. Note that mammograms for Medicare patients should be reported with the appropriate HCPCS code (G0202 to G0206).

A number of mammography codes include the use of computer-aided detection (CAD), a recognition software used to decrease the rates of false-negatives in mammography studies, and this increases the detection of breast cancer via mammography. Codes for both diagnostic and screening mammographies include CAD when performed; for example, 77065, Diagnostic mammography, including computer-aided detection (CAD) when performed; unilateral (Castellino 2005).

Bone and Joint Studies

The next subsection of the Radiology section of the CPT code book is for Bone/Joint Studies (77071 to 77086). These are special studies on the bones and joints designed to help diagnose conditions of the bones, such as osteoporosis, as well as specialized studies for bone age, bone growth, and bone tumors. For example, code 77072, Bone age studies, and 77073, Bone length studies (orthoentgenogram, scanogram), both identify different types of bone studies.

Radiation Oncology

The next subsection of the Radiology section of the CPT code book is unique from the others in this section. Whereas the majority of Radiology codes are used to diagnose medical conditions, Radiation Oncology codes (77261 to 77799) are used to treat oncological conditions. These codes identify services to manage, plan, and deliver radiation treatments to patients with cancer.

Because radiation oncology is performed on patients with cancer and metastatic diseases, it is better discussed within the specialty context of Hematology and Oncology (see chapter 18, under the Hematology and Oncology section). This section of codes is mentioned only in passing in this chapter.

Nuclear Medicine

Nuclear medicine is the practice of using small radioactive elements that are introduced into the patient through an intravenous injection. These elements are designed to travel to a specific organ or type of tissue. Then their radioactive emissions are captured with a nuclear medicine scan, such as a positron emission tomography (PET) or single-photon emission computerized tomography (SPECT) scan, to produce a detailed image of the patient's internal structures and organs. These images can help locate

Figure 13.10. Nuclear medicine imaging

Source: Rauscher et al. 2016.

and diagnose the metabolic rates of cancerous tumors and the functioning of internal organs or body tissues (see figure 13.10).

Codes for nuclear medicine studies depend on the body area or organ involved in the study, the extent of the study (limited area, multiple areas, whole body), and special nature of the test, such as with or without vascular flow, or with or without intrinsic factor. When coding for nuclear medicine procedures, pay close attention to the code descriptions, as multiple codes that differ from each other only slightly may exist within the same body area. For example, code 78700, Kidney imaging morphology, has five different variations of the same procedure indented beneath it, including *with vascular flow* (78701), *with vascular flow and function, single study without pharmacological intervention* (78707), *with vascular flow and function, single study, with pharmacological intervention (e.g., angiotensin converting enzyme inhibitor and/or diuretic)* (78708), *with vascular flow and function, multiple studies, with and without pharmacological intervention (e.g., angiotensin converting enzyme inhibitor and/or diuretic)* (78709), and *tomographic* (78710).

Modifiers in Radiology Coding

There are a handful of modifiers used in radiology coding that identify special aspects of the procedure and that may have a significant impact on reimbursement.

- *Modifiers -26, Professional component* and *-TC, Technical component*, identify the professional and technical components of a radiological service, as previously discussed in this chapter.
- *Modifier -LT, Left side*, and *Modifier -RT, Right side*, identify the laterality of the radiology procedure, and are used for imaging procedures that may be done on either side of the body, such as x-ray of the elbow (right or left).
- *Modifier -59, Distinct procedural service*, may also be necessary when additional imaging services are performed on different sites.
- *Modifier -76, Repeat procedure or service by same physician or other health care professional*, and *Modifier -77, Repeat procedure or service by another physician or health care professional*, may be necessary to append to services that were repeated. For example, an x-ray was taken to diagnose a dislocated shoulder that the surgeon then reduced back into the joint, and an additional x-ray was taken to ensure that the shoulder joint was properly back in place. Modifiers -76 and -77 are discussed in more detail in chapter 11 (Surgical Services).

For practice assigning codes for radiology procedures, complete the exercises in There's a Code for That 13.3.

Radiology procedures 〔13.3〕

There's a Code for That

Read the following documentation of the Radiology service and identify the correct Radiology procedure code(s).

1. Complete renal ultrasound, suspect kidney stones.
   CPT code: _____

2. Nuclear medicine parathyroid scan with SPECT.
   CPT code: _____

(Continued on next page)

13.3

Continued

3. Follow-up pelvic ultrasound on patient with PCOS.

CPT code: _____

4. Complete osseous survey of the axial and appendicular skeleton.

CPT code: _____

5. Bilateral MRI of breasts.

CPT code: _____

6. SPECT scan of liver with measurement of vascular flow.

CPT code: _____

Diagnosis Coding for Radiology and Imaging Services

Diagnosis coding for radiology services depends on whether it is a diagnostic imaging service performed to determine a diagnosis, or if the patient already has a diagnosis and the image is used to determine healing status, tumor progression or remission, or fetal growth, for example. Signs and symptoms are commonly coded, especially when an imaging procedure is performed and a definitive diagnosis cannot be determined. When diagnoses are definitively determined, they may include a variety of lung conditions, breast conditions, uterine fibroids or cysts, gallstones, and kidney stones. Fracture coding is also important in reporting radiology procedures correctly.

Diagnostic Imaging Services

Diagnostic imaging services are performed to determine a diagnosis. In many cases, a patient has suffered an injury or illness or is experiencing symptoms that may indicate an internal medical condition, such as a fracture or pneumonia. Diagnostic imaging services are requested by an ordering physician who has determined that an imaging study is necessary in order to definitively determine the patient's diagnosis. The radiologist receives the orders, performs the imaging procedure, and reads the images and determines the diagnosis, if possible. In some cases, it is not possible to determine a diagnosis, while a definitive diagnosis is easily known in other cases.

Images with No Definitive Diagnosis

Just as in coding for physical examinations and office visits in which no definitive diagnosis is determined, the coder should only report the signs or symptoms that prompted the imaging service. For example, if a patient with a severe productive cough receives a chest x-ray to rule out pneumonia, and the x-ray results do not clearly show that a pneumonia is present, then the coder must only report the sign or symptom that prompted the x-ray procedure (the cough).

In many cases, the radiologist may write that a specific condition is "suspected," "possible," "questionable," or that it needs to be "ruled-out." If any of these questionable terms are present, then the questionable diagnosis must not be coded. Again, only the signs or symptoms that prompted the imaging service in the first place can be coded. For instance, if the patient received a chest x-ray for shortness of breath and the radiologist's impression of the x-ray was "suspected pleural effusion," then the code that should be reported for the case would be shortness of breath. The pleural effusion was only suspected and was not determined as the diagnosis, therefore it cannot be coded. If necessary, query the healthcare provider regarding the patient's diagnosis (as mentioned in chapters 4 and 5) before reporting the diagnosis code.

Common signs and symptoms that require imaging services are chest pain, limb pain, abdominal pain, joint pain, and cough. Remember, when coding for pain it is necessary to search for the term *pain* in the ICD-10-CM Index and then the specific site of the pain.

Images with a Definitive Diagnosis

When an imaging service is ordered and a definitive diagnosis is determined, then the coder should report the definitive diagnosis and not the signs or symptoms of the disease. Common diagnoses that may be seen on x-rays include conditions of the lungs, breast conditions, and the presence of stones in the urinary tract (including the kidneys) and gallbladder and bile ducts.

Conditions of the Lungs

Imaging services such as x-rays and CTs are commonly used to diagnose a number of different conditions affecting the lungs and pleura. These include:

- Pneumonia (J12 to J18). Most pneumonia codes identify the infectious organism or specific type of pneumonia. If this information is known, then code to the highest level of specificity for the code. If no other information is known other than the fact that pneumonia is present, use the unspecified version of the code: J18.9, Pneumonia, unspecified organism.
- Pleural effusion (J90 to J92). **Pleural effusion** is a collection of fluid in the pleural space between the pleural sac, which lines the lung, and the lung itself. This fluid places pressure on the lung and does not allow it to expand completely, causing shortness of breath or chest pain. Pleural effusion is found in a range of conditions—cardiovascular and pulmonary conditions, inflammatory diseases, and malignancies (see figure 13.11). When coding for pleural effusions, if the cause of the condition is known, use category J91, Pleural effusion in conditions

Figure 13.11. Pleural effusion on x-ray and CT

Source: Konijn et al. 2008.

classified elsewhere, and further specify if the effusion is due to a malignancy or other condition classified elsewhere. An additional code should be used to identify the underlying condition (either the malignancy or the underlying condition coded elsewhere). If the underlying cause of the effusion is not known, use the unspecified code J90, Pleural effusion, not elsewhere classified.

- Pulmonary edema (J81). **Pulmonary edema** is a fluid collection in the lungs themselves caused by heart failure, myocardial infarction, cardiac ischemia, and other heart problems, as well as sepsis and severe anemia. Symptoms of pulmonary edema include respiratory fatigue, chest pain, and cough. Codes for pulmonary edema identify the condition as either acute (J81.0, Acute pulmonary edema), or chronic (J18.1, Chronic pulmonary edema). According to the Tabular note at the beginning of chapter 10: Diseases of the Respiratory System, if the patient has any known history or current use of tobacco or tobacco products, an additional code should be selected to identify the tobacco use or history, as necessary. These include Z77.22, Contact with and (suspected) exposure to environmental tobacco smoke (acute) (chronic), P96.81, Exposure to (parental) (environmental) tobacco smoke in the perinatal period, Z87.891, Personal history of nicotine dependence, Z57.31, Occupational exposure to environmental tobacco smoke, F17.-, Tobacco dependednce, or Z72.0,Tobacco use. If the pulmonary edema is due to chemical exposure, radiation, drowning, high altitude, or other external agent, do not use the code from category J81. Search for the term *Edema* in the ICD-10-CM Index, then refer to the subterm *lung*, and then the appropriate type of pulmonary edema. Be sure to verify the code in the Tabular.

- Abnormal findings that are not otherwise classified can be reported with codes from category R91, Abnormal findings on diagnostic imaging of lung. These include the presence of a solitary pulmonary nodule, or other nonspecific finding of lung field.

Additional lung conditions such as pulmonary nodules, embolisms, and cysts or tumors may also be found using imaging techniques. These codes can be found by referencing the Main Index of the ICD-10-CM code book and following the main terms, subterms, and cross references, then verifying the code in the Tabular List.

Conditions of the Breasts

Breast imaging studies may be useful in finding a number of different breast conditions. These include cysts, malignancies, fibrocystic changes, hematomas, lipomas, and mastitis (see figure 13.12). Many breast disorders are coded within categories N60 to N65, Disorders of breast, including mammary dysplasia (cysts and fibrocystic changes), inflammatory disorders of the breast (mastitis and abscess), hypertrophy, lump in breast, and other disorders (signs and symptoms of the breast).

When an imaging study of the breast is done due to a lump in the breast and a tumor is found, it is not possible to determine whether or not the lump is malignant from the imaging study alone. A biopsy of the lump must be performed in order to identify if the lump is benign or malignant. Remember, if a diagnostic imaging study cannot determine the definitive diagnosis, then code only for the sign or symptom. If the patient already has a diagnosis of either a benign or malignant neoplasm of the breast and the imaging study is done to determine the location or growth or decline of the tumor, then report the code for the diagnosis that has already been determined.

There are two codes to report that a patient presented for a breast imaging study to screen for breast malignancies. Z12.31, Encounter or screening mammogram for

Figure 13.12. Findings on mammography

Source: National Cancer Institute 1991.

malignant neoplasm of breast should be used when a patient presents for a screening mammogram. Screening mammograms are a common breast imaging procedure and are performed as a preventative service when the patient has no symptoms, such as a breast lump. If a patient presents for a screening mammogram and no abnormalities are present, report code Z12.31. If an abnormality is present, then report the code for the screening mammogram first, followed by the code for the abnormality, such as a mass or lump. Code Z12.39, Encounter for other screening for malignant neoplasm of breast, should be used when an imaging service other than a mammogram is used to perform the breast screening. Note that these two screening codes should only be used when the patient presents for a routine screening.

If a breast abnormality is found on a diagnostic imaging of the breast, the finding should be reported with a code from category R92, Abnormal and inconclusive findings of diagnostic imaging of breast. These include mammographic microcalcification, mammographic calcification, and inconclusive mammogram (dense breasts), or other abnormal or inconclusive finding.

Cholelithiasis and Nephrolithiasis

Imaging services are commonly used to find stones in the gallbladder and bile ducts as well as in the kidneys. Coding for cholelithiasis, or gallstones, requires detailed reading of the code descriptions to ensure that the code selected correctly reports the documented condition. For example, K80.60, Calculus of gallbladder and bile duct with cholecystitis, unspecified, without obstruction. For a refresher on coding for cholelithiasis, refer to chapter 10 (Urgent Care and Emergency Department Services).

A nephrolithiasis, otherwise known as kidney stone, is also diagnosed with the use of imaging, such as x-ray or CT scan. Coding for nephrolithiasis is decidedly simpler than coding for cholelithiasis, as codes rely on the site of the stone. For example, code

N20.1, Calculus of ureter. Category N20, Calculus of kidney and ureter, includes codes for calculus of the kidney, calculus of the ureter, calculus of both kidney and ureter, and unspecified urinary calculus.

Fracture Coding

When a patient presents to a healthcare provider with a possible fracture, an x-ray is usually ordered to confirm if indeed a fracture is present, determine exactly which bone or bones are fractured, and identify the clinical aspects of that fracture. Coding for fractures is complicated and reporting the correct code depends on a number of factors.

Orthopedic specialists (bone doctors, also called orthopods) are trained to diagnose, treat, and manage the healing of fractures. As such, orthopods are more likely to perform diagnostic imaging for fractures, read the images, and specify the patient's exact type of fracture. Orthopedic services are discussed in chapter 15 (Orthopedic Services), with a more thorough discussion of fracture diagnosis coding. At the very least, diagnosis codes for fractures identify the site of the fracture (the specific bone that is fractured), the laterality, whether the fracture is open (pierces the skin) or closed (does not pierce the skin), and the encounter (initial, subsequent, or sequela). For example, S42.001A, Fracture of unspecified part of right clavicle, initial encounter for closed fracture.

To search for a fracture in the Index, look up the term *Fracture*, and then refer to the section for either pathological or traumatic fractures. Pathological fractures are caused by a disease process, such as osteoporosis. Traumatic fractures are caused by a traumatic injury, such as a fall. Then find the subterm for the site of the fracture. Follow all additional subterms and cross-references, and verify the code in the Tabular List. All fracture codes are seven-character codes, which means that a seventh character should be assigned to identify the encounter for the fracture. For a refresher of seventh-character extensions, refer to chapter 4. For practice assigning diagnostic codes for radiology procedures, complete the exercises in There's a Code for That 13.4.

13.4

There's a Code for That

Diagnostic coding for radiology procedures

Read the following documentation of the radiology service and identify the correct diagnosis code(s).

1. Complete renal ultrasound, suspect kidney stones in patient with flank pain.

   ICD-10-CM code: _____

2. Patient with hypercalcemia received parathyroid SPECT scan. Impression: probable parathyroid adenoma of the upper pole of the left thyroid bed.

   ICD-10-CM code: _____

3. Encounter for bilateral screening mammogram revealed lump in left breast. Patient has a significant family history of breast cancer.

   ICD-10-CM codes: _____, _____, _____

4. Impression from renal ultrasound: calculus of kidney and ureter.

   ICD-10-CM code: _____

5. 56-year-old patient with congestive heart failure presents for x-ray of the chest. Patient is experiencing shortness of breath, chest pain, and a feeling of fullness in the chest. X-ray positive for acute pulmonary edema.

   ICD-10-CM code: _____, _____

Putting It All Together: Coding for Radiology and Imaging Services

Coding correctly for radiology and imaging services requires an understanding of the different types of studies, coding components for each type of code, and an understanding of the professional and technical components of each service, and also how to differentiate between a service that has a definitive diagnosis and one that does not.

Determination of the correct codes relies on the answers to the following questions.

- What type of imaging procedure was performed (x-ray, MRI, CT, ultrasound)?
- What body area, organ, or organ system was visualized by the imaging procedure?
    - How many views were included in the procedure?
    - Was contrast material used?
    - Was the procedure limited or complete?
    - Was the procedure bilateral or unilateral? If unilateral, which side was imaged?
- Which component should you code for?
    - Code for the global fee (no modifiers) if the office owns the imaging equipment, and the provider also works for the same clinic.
    - Code for the technical component (modifier -TC) if the clinic or facility owns the equipment but does not employ the medical provider that read the films.
    - Code for the professional component (modifier -26) if the provider interpreted and provided a report for images that were produced by an independent facility.
- Were there any additional procedures or imaging services that should be coded as well?
    - If so, check for the need for modifiers.
- Is there a definitive diagnosis for the imaging service?
    - If yes, then code the definitive diagnosis.
    - If no, then code for the signs, symptoms, or abnormal finding code.
    - If the image is for a screening service, report the screening diagnosis code.

Study the following vignette that demonstrates how to select the appropriate diagnosis and procedure codes. Then complete the practice exercises in There's a Code for That 13.5.

Bethany is a recent graduate from a medical billing and coding program and she just landed a job in a local independent radiology and imaging center. Now that Bethany is ready to begin coding in her position at the imaging center, she remembers that she needs to ask herself two questions: What did the doctor do? and Why did the doctor do it? She is coding the following imaging report.

Study Name: Mammography
Description: Diagnostic mammography of the right female breast with computer-aided detection (CAD)
Clinical indication: Lump in right breast
Image Report: 1.5 cm mass on right breast seen in the right upper outer quadrant, consistent with ductal carcinoma in situ. Recommend ultrasound-guided biopsy of lump to confirm diagnosis.
Impression: 1.5 cm mass in right breast

First, Bethany asks herself: What did the doctor do? In this case, the procedure was a diagnostic mammography of the right female breast with computer-aided detection. There were no additional procedures performed. Also, there is no mention of whether only the professional component or the technical components were performed, so she will code for the global service, without modifiers. She refers to the CPT Index and finds the term Mammography, *and then with* Computer-Aided Detection (CAD), *which leads her to the code range 77065 to 77067. She turns to this section in the Tabular List of codes and determines that her correct imaging code is:*

77065-RT, Diagnostic mammography, including computer-aided detection (CAD), when performed; unilateral

Note that Bethany appended modifier -RT to the code to indicate the laterality of the procedure.

Now that she has her procedure code, she asks herself: Why did the doctor do it? In this case, the clinical indication, which is the reason why the imaging study was performed, was due to a lump in the breast. This is different than the imaging report that indicates the findings are consistent with ductal carcinoma in situ. However, the impression at the end of the report, which is the final impression that the radiologist got from the study, was a 1.5 cm mass in the right breast. Bethany remembers that she can only code for a definitive diagnosis, so she cannot code for the ductal carcinoma in situ. The provider wrote that the findings were "consistent with" ductal carcinoma in situ, not that the patient has ductal carcinoma in situ. In this case, she must code for the signs or symptoms, which is the lump/mass in the right breast. She looks up the term lump *in the ICD-10 Index, and the cross-reference is to see Mass. She then refers to the term* Mass *in the Index, and then* Breast, *which refers her to code N63. She verifies the code in the Tabular and determines that it is correct:*

N63, Unspecified lump in breast

She then rechecks the documentation to make sure she has coded everything for the encounter, and reports the chosen codes on the claim for the service.

Diagnostic and procedural coding for radiology and imaging services

13.5

There's a Code for That

Read the following documentation and assign the appropriate CPT, HCPCS, and ICD-10-CM code(s) for the encounter.

1. Study: X-ray of left foot

   Indication: Pain

   Technique: Three views

   Findings: Bones of the foot are intact, no stress fractures noted. Mild swelling is noted along the dorsal aspect of the foot.

   Impression: No acute fracture or injury noted.

   CPT code: _____ - _____

   ICD-10-CM codes: _____

2. MRI of the internal auditory canals with and without contrast material. Contrast administered was 50 mL of Gadavist (gadobutrol). Patient has right-sided hearing loss and a clinical history of acoustic neuroma. Impression from today's study: Slight increase in right cerebellopontine angle mass compatible with vestibular schwannoma.

   CPT code: _____, _____ x _____

   ICD-10-CM codes: _____, _____

3. CT of the abdomen without contrast and CT of the pelvis with contrast on patient with abdominal pain. Patient's clinical history is significant for post-cholecystectomy 8 months ago. Impression: CT of the abdomen and pelvis is without findings to explain the patient's symptoms. Post-cholecystectomy.

   CPT code: _____

   ICD-10-CM codes: _____, _____

End of Chapter Content

Instructions: Indicate whether the following statements are true or false (T or F). For false statements, rewrite the statement on the line below to make the statement true.

1. Radiology services may be performed in the inpatient or outpatient settings.

   _____

   _____

2. Radiological supervision and interpretation is the professional component of a procedure.

   _____

   _____

(Continued on next page)

(Continued)

3. Modifier -26 is used to identify the global radiology service.

   _____

   _____

4. When a provider performs both the technical and professional components of a service, do not append a modifier.

   _____

   _____

5. The plane of an imaging service is the direction in which the imaging rays pass through the body.

   _____

   _____

6. MRI uses strong ultrasonic waves to produce detailed images of the internal structures of the patient.

   _____

   _____

7. Contrast material may be injected intravenously, intrathecally, or intra-articularly.

   _____

   _____

8. There is no difference between obstetric and non-obstetric pelvic ultrasound codes.

   _____

   _____

9. When a definitive diagnosis is not determined by the imaging procedure, it is ok to report the probable diagnosis.

   _____

   _____

10. Pleural effusion is fluid buildup within the lungs themselves.

    _____

    _____

Instructions: Match the terms with the appropriate descriptions.

1. _____ Anterior		A. Away from the body
2. _____ Posterior		B. The same side of the body
3. _____ Superior		C. Toward the mid-line of the body
4. _____ Inferior		D. Toward the top of the body
5. _____ Medial		E. Toward the back of the body
6. _____ Lateral		F. The opposite side of the body
7. _____ Proximal		G. Toward the center of the body
8. _____ Distal		H. Away from the midline of the body
9. _____ Ipsilateral		I. Toward the front of the body
10. _____ Contralateral		J. Toward the bottom of the body

Instructions: Choose the best answer.

1. Which type of medical doctor specializes in the diagnosis and treatment of medical conditions using radiology and imaging techniques?
   a. Imaging technician
   b. Radiologist
   c. Inpatient hospitalist
   d. Certified radiological supervisor

2. A physician on-call read an x-ray report for a study that was performed at the hospital. Which component of the radiology service was performed?
   a. Professional
   b. Technical
   c. Global
   d. None, this would not be billable

3. Which component of a radiology service represents the equipment, supplies, and clinical staff that took the image?
   a. Professional
   b. Technical
   c. Global
   d. Both professional and technical components

4. Which modifier is used to identify the global radiology service?
   a. -26
   b. -TC
   c. -GB
   d. No modifier

5. Which plane of the body is a vertical line that divides the body into anterior and posterior halves?
   a. Axial
   b. Transverse
   c. Sagittal
   d. Coronal

6. Which subsection of the Radiology section contains codes for PET and SPECT scans?
   a. Diagnostic Radiology
   b. Radiologic Guidance
   c. Ultrasound
   d. Nuclear Medicine

7. Which imaging type combines a number of x-ray images to produce a virtual cross-section of the area being studied?
   a. X-ray
   b. CT
   c. MRI
   d. PET

8. When coding for a radiology service that was performed with and without contrast, how is the service reported?
   a. Use the code for with contrast
   b. Use the code for without contrast
   c. Use the code for without contrast followed by with contrast
   d. Use one code for with contrast, and another code for without contrast

9. Which imaging technique allows the viewer to see blood flow through body organs in real time?

    a. Doppler ultrasound
    b. Nuclear imaging
    c. Radiologic guidance
    d. MRI

10. What type of imaging service is performed on a scheduled basis as a preventative measure to rule out breast cancer?

    a. Diagnostic mammogram
    b. MRI of the breast
    c. Screening mammogram
    d. Screening ultrasound of the breast

11. Which modifier should be used when multiple x-rays were performed by the same doctor on the same site on the same day?

    a. -59
    b. -77
    c. -76
    d. No modifier would be necessary

Instructions: Answer the following questions with the appropriate code(s) and modifier(s).

1. Diagnostic mammogram on a female patient with a lump in her right breast confirmed the presence of fibroadenosis of the right breast.

    CPT code: _____

    ICD-10-CM code: _____

2. Diagnostic x-ray examination of the right clavicle confirms displaced fracture (closed fracture, initial encounter).

    CPT code: _____

    ICD-10-CM code: _____

3. Clinical indication: Left neck and shoulder pain × 2 months

    Contrast material: None

    Technique: MRI of the cervical spine

    Findings: Moderate narrowing of disc space from C4 – 5 with spondylosis.

    Impression: Spondylosis of the cervical spine with radiculopathy

    CPT code: _____

    ICD-10-CM code: _____

4. Nuclear medicine PET scan, whole body, on patient with known lung cancer. Findings from the study include a lesion in the left upper lobe of the lung, representing the patient's known lung carcinoma. No evidence of any metastases. Findings also significant for diverticulosis.

    CPT code: _____

    ICD-10-CM code: _____

References

Blausen.com staff. 2014. "Blausen 0628 Mammogram. png." Digital image. Wikimedia Commons. Accessed December, 2017. https://commons.wikimedia.org/wiki/File:Blausen_0628_Mammogram.png.

Castellino, R. 2005 (August 23). Computer Aided Detection (CAD): An Overview. https://www.ncbi.nlm.nih.gov/pmc/articles/PMC1665219/.

Konijn, A. J. M., P. H. M. Egbers, and M. A. Kuiper. 2008. "Pneumothorax hemothorax pneumomediastinum contusion.JPG." Digital image. Journal of Medical Case Reports. Accessed December, 2017. https://jmedicalcasereports.biomedcentral.com/articles/10.1186/1752-1947-2-100.

National Cancer Institute. 1991. "Mammogram Showing Small Lesion." Digital image. National Cancer Institute. Accessed December, 2017. https://visualsonline.cancer.gov/details.cfm?imageid=2553.

National Institute of Biomedical Imaging and Bioengineering. 2017. Ultrasounds. https://www.nibib.nih.gov/science-education/science-topics/ultrasound.

National Institute of Biomedical Imaging and Bioengineering. 2016. X-rays. https://www.nibib.nih.gov/science-education/science-topics/x-rays.

Rauscher, I., T. Maurer, W. P. Fendler, W. H. Sommer, M. Schwaiger, and M. Eiber. 2016. "Gallium PSMA PET scan. png ." Digital image. Accessed December, 2017. https://www.ncbi.nlm.nih.gov/pmc/articles/PMC4898465/.

Verhovshek, G.J. 2015 (November). Radiology Billing and Coding: Professional and Technical Components. http://www.radiologytoday.net/archive/rt1115p7.shtml.

Resources

American College of Radiology. 2017. What is a Radiologist? https://www.acr.org/Quality-Safety/Radiology-Safety/Patient-Resources/About-Radiology.

NYU Langone Health. 2017. Nuclear Medicine. https://med.nyu.edu/radiology/about-nyulmc-radiology/subspecialty-sections/nuclear-section.

CHAPTER

Laboratory and Pathology Services

Learning Objectives

- Understand the basics of billing and coding for independent laboratory and pathology services.
- Examine procedural codes and guidelines for independent laboratory and pathology services.

- Examine diagnosis coding and medical necessity for independent laboratory and pathology services.
- Determine and apply ICD-10-CM, CPT, and HCPCS codes to independent laboratory and pathology services.

Key Terms

Bacteriology
Cytopathology
Frozen block
Frozen section
Gross examination
Independent laboratory
Laboratory and pathology services
Methicillin-resistant *Staphylococcus aureus* (MRSA)

Methicillin-susceptible *Staphylococcus aureus* (MSSA)
Microscopic examination
Mycology
Nonspecific test
Panel
Parasitology
Pass-through billing
Permanent block

Permanent section
Qualitative examination
Quantitative examination
Smear
Specific test
Specimen
Virology

Coding for laboratory and pathology services is a bit different than any other type of coding in the CPT code book. First, instead of performing procedures on the patient, **laboratory and pathology services** are diagnostic analyses of bodily tissue samples, such as urine, blood, or tissue. Often abbreviated as lab and path, laboratory and pathology services are designed to examine these specimens to determine a diagnosis, evaluate the quality of a specimen, or to assist in a surgical process. A **specimen** is a bodily tissue sample from the patient. Specimens come from all parts of the body—from blood, urine, and saliva to muscle tissues, stool, and even breath.

Coding for laboratory and pathology services requires an in-depth knowledge of the types of tests performed, the ways in which they are performed, and their many differences. It also requires a basic knowledge of the various practices that perform laboratory and pathology services, how these services are performed and billed, and the diagnosis codes that support the medical necessity for these services. This chapter discusses the basics of coding for laboratory and pathology services and covers the procedural and diagnostic guidelines for laboratory and pathology procedures.

Laboratory and Pathology Basics

Laboratory and pathology tests are a special type of service. While a handful of them may be performed in the healthcare office, such as Clinical Laboratory Improvement Amendments of 1988 (CLIA)-waived tests, many are performed in independent laboratories without the patient present. Billing and coding laboratory and pathology services require an understanding of the types of laboratory providers and how they bill and code for their services.

Key to Success

Rather than performing actual procedures on patients, laboratory and pathology services are only performing tests on specimens acquired from the patient. So these codes are unique when compared to other CPT codes that identify procedures performed on patients. Indeed, the code structure and uses of the codes are the same, but the descriptions differ and identify only the test that was performed, not how it was obtained. It helps to keep this in mind when learning laboratory and pathology coding, as this can be confusing. Instead of performing surgical or medical procedures, evaluations, or managing patient conditions, laboratory and pathology services are only handling patient specimens—to perform a specific test on those specimens according to a doctor's request.

Laboratory and Pathology Settings and Billing for Services

In the United States, many healthcare offices have in-house CLIA-waived labs (discussed in chapter 8), which allow the clinical staff in the office to perform certain, low-complexity, low-risk laboratory tests and procedures. These include strep swabs, bacterial cultures, rapid influenza tests, mono spot cultures (for mononucleosis), blood counts, and simple urinalysis examinations. Additional CLIA-waived tests are **panels**, a group of specific tests (from the chemistry section) that are commonly performed together, such as a lipid or comprehensive metabolic panel. When a healthcare office provides the lab test themselves, the code(s) for the lab(s) are billed along with the procedure codes for all other services provided at the encounter, such as E/M encounter and any other procedures.

When a more complex laboratory procedure is necessary, the patient (or a patient's sample specimen) is sent to an independent laboratory for analysis. An **independent laboratory** is a facility that is recognized and accredited to test and evaluate patient specimens as an independent entity free from a hospital or private practice. Accreditation of an independent laboratory is achieved by meeting a certain set of standards set by an accrediting body, such as Centers for Medicare and Medicaid Services (CMS) or other accrediting organization. An independent laboratory processes patient specimens according to orders given from healthcare providers, which identify the specimen to be examined and the purpose of the examination. When an independent laboratory provides the procedure, it can either bill for the lab directly, or send the ordering provider a bill for the services and the ordering provider bills the patient's insurance on the lab's behalf. This is a process called pass-through billing, discussed in more depth in the following section.

In the hospital setting, the hospital usually has an in-house lab that can process more complex laboratory and pathology procedures. When specimen testing is needed for a patient, the hospital staff or healthcare provider takes the patient sample and sends it directly to the in-house lab for processing and examination. If a diagnosis is determined, the lab sends the results to the ordering provider, who reads the results of the test and manages the patient accordingly. For example, a sample of wound exudate from a patient with a wound infection being treated in the hospital can be evaluated in the hospital's in-house laboratory to determine the infectious organism. Once the infectious organism is identified, then the treating provider can manage the patient's condition appropriately. Depending on the hospital, lab, and available equipment, some tests (such as a complex genetic sequencing test) may have to be sent to an outside independent lab that has more specialized equipment to process the patient specimen for the exact test ordered. A common theme in healthcare, this all depends on the resources, availability, and need for the laboratory and pathology procedures. When a hospital performs the laboratory procedure in-house, the services performed are billed directly, together with other resources used during the patient's stay in the facility.

Laboratories are found in several healthcare settings, such as healthcare provider offices (which may only bill for CLIA-waived labs), inpatient and outpatient hospitals (including ASCs), and in the independent laboratory setting. The setting in which the laboratory service was provided depends on the needs of the patients and the resources available to the healthcare practice or facility. While this chapter focuses on coding for lab and path services in an independent lab, as a coder you will likely report lab or path services across a number of different settings.

Any type of laboratory or pathology procedure must be performed according to the orders of a healthcare provider. This provider has already examined or evaluated the patient and determined the need for the lab test. For example, a maternal fetal medicine specialist has performed an ultrasound on a patient and determined that there is a possibility that a chromosomal abnormality may be present. This doctor can do one of two things: either take a blood sample from the patient and send it to an independent lab, or send the patient to an independent lab to have them draw the blood sample. Either way, once the lab receives the blood sample with the orders to test the blood for the specific suspected chromosomal abnormality, the sample will be tested and results will be sent to the ordering doctor.

Sometimes laboratory procedures can be especially cost-prohibitive—very expensive—and may require special authorization from the patient's insurance before they may be performed. If the test is not paid for by the patient's insurance, then the patient will be responsible for payment. As a coder, prior authorization numbers may have to be reported on the claim (as discussed in chapter 2), together with the procedure codes for the authorized test and the diagnosis code that has been pre-approved to identify the medical necessity for the specific tests. Before learning the basics for coding for laboratory and pathology services require an understanding of pass-through billing and the technical versus professional components of laboratory services.

Pass-through Billing

Pass-through billing occurs when a laboratory performs an ordered lab test and sends the ordering provider a bill for the services (instead of billing the insurance company directly), and the ordering provider bills the patient's insurance on the lab's behalf. This is typically done when the ordering provider and the independent lab have some sort of agreement in place that identifies specific lab tests and costs for each procedure.

If an office engages in pass-through billing, the healthcare provider's office must bill for the lab test ordered, with all other procedures that were performed on the patient during the encounter. But to correctly identify that the laboratory test was not performed at the healthcare provider's office, three things must be done:

- Append modifier -90, Reference (outside) laboratory, to the laboratory procedure code. This indicates that the procedure was performed by an independent laboratory and that the healthcare office is billing for the services.
- Change the place of service code for the laboratory procedure to 81, Independent laboratory, rather than 11-Office. This indicates that the laboratory procedure was performed at an outside lab, and not in the healthcare provider's office.
- Identify the charges included in the pass-through billing in box 20 of the CMS-1500 claim form. This box further identifies that the laboratory procedures performed occurred at an outside lab, and identifies the charge amount for the labs (see figure 14.1). Note that the charge amount included in this box must correspond to the actual charges billed for the lab services—the two amounts must match.

Figure 14.1. CMS-100 box 20

20. OUTSIDE LAB?	$ CHARGES
[X] YES [ ] NO	159 00

Source: CMS 2017.

Pass-through billing is not allowed by some insurance plans and it is more common to find that independent laboratories bill directly for the procedures performed. The labs are reimbursed according to a preset fee schedule that has been negotiated by the third-party payer and the lab. However, it is important to know how to code for these services when the situation arises.

Key to Success

When reporting pass-through billing for lab services, remember: append modifier -90, reference (outside) laboratory to the lab CPT code, change the place of service to 81, Independent laboratory, and add the charges in box 20 of the CMS-1500 form.

Technical versus Professional Components

Similar to radiological procedures, some laboratory and pathology procedures may be divided into technical versus professional components. The technical component of laboratory procedures consists of the testing of a sample using specialized equipment and highly trained clinical staff. The test may also require interpretation by a specially trained pathologist, who can decipher the complicated test results and provide a report of the findings—this is the professional component of the procedure.

> Just as in coding for either component of radiological procedures, modifier -TC, Technical component or -26, Professional component, should be appended for either the technical or professional components of the procedure, respectively. When both the technical and professional components of the procedure are performed, do not append any modifier for the global service.

MOD

However, not all laboratory and pathology procedures may be broken into these two components, as some codes already identify only one component of the procedure, such as 85060, Blood smear, peripheral, interpretation by physician with written report. In this case, code 85060 already identifies the professional component and as such should not be appended with modifier -26. Furthermore, some insurance payers may choose to not recognize the two separate components for laboratory and pathology procedures, and instead pay only the global fee to the provider who performed the lab test. Again, being an effective coder requires an in-depth knowledge of the connection between coding and billing for the services performed in each specialty.

Laboratory and Pathology Testing Basics

Before discussing the codes for laboratory and pathology services, it is important to review the basic terminology and processes of laboratory tests. This includes the difference between specimen collection and specimen testing; definitions of specimens, blocks, and sections; and the difference between qualitative and quantitative examinations of specimens.

Specimen Collection versus Specimen Testing

Differentiation between the *collection* of a specimen, and the *testing* of a specimen is needed, as they are two very different procedures. To test any type of patient specimen, it must first be collected from the patient (see figure 14.2). This can be as simple as having the patient submit a urine sample in a specimen cup, or as complex as performing an invasive surgery to remove a tissue sample for a biopsy.

Reporting the code for the collection of the specimen depends on the provider who took the specimen. For example, if the doctor's office took a patient blood sample via venipuncture (code 36415, Collection of venous blood by venipuncture), and then performed a complete blood count (CBC) (85027, Blood count; complete (CBC), automated (Hgb, Hct, RBC, WBC, and platelet count) in the office, then this doctor's office should bill for both the venipuncture procedure and the CBC (36416 and 85025). Note that the venipuncture may be bundled into the CBC procedure depending on the insurance, as the insurance may determine that the blood draw is an inherent component of the CBC. Sometimes the collection of the specimen is included in the E/M encounter code for the service, such as having a patient urinate in a specimen cup or taking a sample

Figure 14.2. Specimen collection versus testing

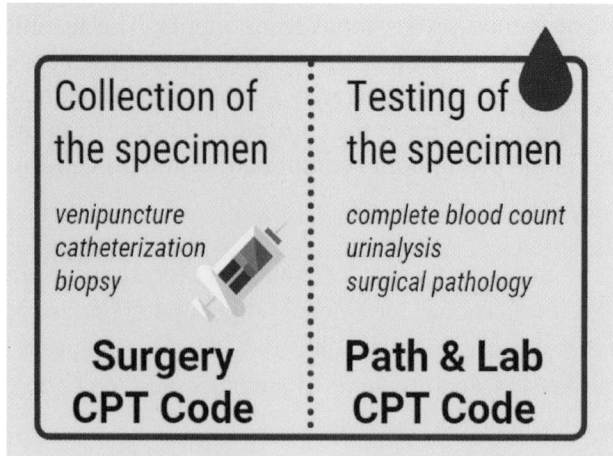

of wound exudate from an infected wound. In this case, the collection of the specimen is included in the work reported via the E/M code.

However, if the doctor's office drew the blood and then sent the sample to an independent lab, then the doctor's office would bill for the blood draw and the lab would bill for the testing of the blood. If the lab performed both the blood draw and the CBC, then it would bill for both procedures.

The collection procedure may be more invasive than a simple blood draw, as is often the case for biopsies and excision of organs or tissues examined for disease processes by a laboratory or pathologist. Remember to only report the procedure that was performed by the given office or facility. For example, if the coder is submitting codes for the independent laboratory, he or she should report only the codes that identify the services performed by the lab, and not by the doctor or surgeon who collected the specimen.

Specimens, Block, and Sections

All laboratory or pathology tests are performed on specimens, which can come from different sources. For example, a bacterial culture may be performed on a specimen obtained from wound exudate (pus from an infected wound). Or a specimen obtained from a breast lump may be examined for malignant cells (to check for breast cancer). Code selection for numerous laboratory and pathology codes depends on the type of the specimen tested in the procedure. For example, code 82565, Creatinine; blood, tests a blood sample for creatinine. Code 82570, Creatinine; other source, tests for the same substance (creatinine), but on a sample other than blood.

Once a specimen is obtained by the lab, it is prepared in several different ways, depending on the purpose of the test. Once the specimen is prepared, it is examined by the clinical laboratory and pathology staff. One type of examination is a **gross examination**—an examination of the physical characteristics of the specimen including the size, weight, consistency, and visual features such as discoloring. The laboratory technician may also place a label on the specimen to identify it, and note any additional tests that were performed on the specimen.

When a gross examination is not sufficient in determining the diagnosis, a microscopic examination is performed. A **microscopic examination** is the examination of the specimen at a minute level, which allows the pathologist to see the cells of a specimen.

These examinations are performed under a microscope on a slide that contains a small portion of the specimen, and allows the individual cells to be seen. Obtaining a clear sample for the slide is done in various ways.

- **Smear**. If the specimen is a liquid or submerged in a fluid substance, it may be smeared onto the surface of a slide and then allowed to dry. It is then secured with a fixative agent, and then stained to allow for the visualization of certain cells. The process of applying the fixative agent or otherwise preparing the specimen for examination is included in the CPT code for the lab or path test, and is not reported separately.

- **Frozen section**. For procedures that need a pathological examination quickly, the specimen may be frozen rapidly into a **frozen block** (a frozen piece of a specimen), which is cut into small slices of the tissue (a frozen section) and visualized under a microscope. This is a fast, yet impermanent method of preparing a specimen for pathological examination under a microscope. It is commonly used during surgical pathology services, in which a pathologist works together with a surgeon to evaluate tissue samples for malignancy during the surgical session.

- **Permanent section**. A permanent section procedure is similar to a frozen section, except that instead of freezing the block, it is placed in a fixative agent that immobilizes the cells so that they will not change. It is then placed in a small mold and surrounded with paraffin wax and cooled so the specimen is contained within a **permanent block**. This specimen block may be stored indefinitely for future evaluations. Once the block is formed, permanent sections may be cut from it and examined under a microscope by melting away the wax, adding water to the section, and staining it for microscopic examination.

Qualitative versus Quantitative Examinations

Laboratory and pathology procedures often differentiate between qualitative and quantitative examinations of specimens.

A **qualitative examination** is one that studies the *quality*, or characteristics and properties of a specimen. For example, is a drug or chemical present in the specimen? A qualitative examination answers the question with a yes or no. One example of qualitative examinations are Presumptive Drug Class Screenings (80305 to 80307), which only identify whether a specific drug is identified in the specimen or not. The result of a qualitative examination is either a negative or a positive result, meaning that the substance being tested is either present or absent in the specimen.

A **quantitative examination** is one that identifies the *quantity*, or amount, of a specific substance found in a specimen. A quantitative examination answers the question: How much? For example, how much of a chemical is found in the specimen? One example of quantitative examinations are Therapeutic Drug Assays (80150 to 80299), which identify the amount of the specified drug in the specimen. In this case, the result of a quantitative examination is a number or measurement. See figure 14.3 for a visual representation of the differences between qualitative and quantitative examinations.

Whether the examination is qualitative or quantitative is identified in either the guidelines before the subsection of codes or in the code description itself. For example, 84119, Porphyrins urine; qualitative, is for a qualitative examination whereas code 84120, Porphyrins, urine; quantitation and fractionation, is for a quantitative examination. If the code description does not identify the examination as either

Figure 14.3. Qualitative versus quantitative

qualitative or quantitative, refer to the guidelines at the beginning of the subsection of codes. For example, the guidelines for Therapeutic Drug Assays (80150 to 80299) read: "Therapeutic Drug Assays are performed to monitor clinical response to a known, prescribed medication. The material for examination is whole blood, serum, plasma, or cerebrospinal fluid. *Examination is quantitative.* Coding is by parent drug; measures metabolites of the drug are included in the codes, if performed" (AMA 2017). Therefore, all the procedures identified with these codes are quantitative examinations.

Some examinations can be both qualitative and quantitative, which again is described in either the code description or the guidelines before the codes in each subsection. For practice identifying qualitative versus quantitative examinations, complete the exercises in There's a Code for That 14.1.

There's a Code for That

Qualitative versus quantitative

Refer to the following codes in the CPT code book and determine if the test is qualitative or quantitative. Tip: To find this information, read the guidelines at the beginning of each subsection of codes and code descriptions carefully.

1. Code 80150, Amikacin. This test is:

  a. Qualitative

  b. Quantitative

  c. Both qualitative and quantitative

2. Code 80202, Vancomycin. This test is:

  a. Qualitative

  b. Quantitative

  c. Both qualitative and quantitative

3. Code 83045, Hemoglobin; methemoglobin, qualitative. This test is:

  a. Qualitative

  b. Quantitative

  c. Both qualitative and quantitative

4. Code 84512, Troponin, qualitative. This test is:

a. Qualitative

b. Quantitative

c. Both qualitative and quantitative

5. Code 88741, Hemoglobin (Hgb), quantitative, transcutaneous, per day; methemoglobin. This test is:

a. Qualitative

b. Quantitative

c. Both qualitative and quantitative

Procedural Coding for Laboratory and Pathology Services

CPT procedure codes for laboratory and pathology services are all located in the Pathology and Laboratory Section of the CPT code book. They describe the test performed on the patient's specimen. Sometimes code descriptions are fairly detailed and identify the type of specimen or if the test was qualitative or quantitative; and other times code descriptions can be vague. Carefully read any subsection titles, guidelines, parenthetical notes, and any additional information included in this section to ensure complete understanding of the code descriptions. The modifiers used in reporting laboratory and pathology codes are also discussed as follows.

Key to Success

Do not forget to use your resources when coding for lab and pathology services. A medical dictionary, CPT, ICD-10-CM, and HCPCS code books, as well as any other available resources can be helpful. Remember that coding for lab and pathology services is different than coding for medical procedures performed on the patient. The code descriptions only describe the type of test performed on the specimen. If you are not aware of what the test is used for and how it is performed, it may be helpful to research the procedure to ensure that you select the correct code. As you become more familiar with coding for laboratory and pathology services (or any specialty services), you will find that understanding the codes and procedures to report become easier with practice and experience.

Laboratory and Pathology Procedure Codes

The subsections of laboratory and pathology codes depend on the type of test performed on the specimen. When more than one test is performed on the same specimen, or if multiple specimens are tested, it may be necessary to code for more than one procedure. If multiple procedures are performed for the same patient on the same date of service, it is appropriate to report the services together.

The following sections discuss the different subsections of the Laboratory and Pathology section of the CPT code book.

Chemistry Tests and Organ or Disease-Oriented Panels

The Chemistry subsection of codes (82009 to 84999) is one of the largest sections of codes within the Pathology and Laboratory section. These codes describe tests for specific substances, such as potassium or lead. A specific test is one that evaluates a specimen for an identified substance. Some chemistry tests are qualitative and identify whether the specific substance is in the specimen or not, while others are quantitative and identify the exact amount of the specific substance within the specimen. For example, code 84106, Porphobilinogen, urine; *qualitative* is to determine whether porphobilinogen is present in the urine (qualitative), and code 84110, Porphobilinogen, urine; *quantitative* is to determine the amount of porphobilinogen in the urine (quantitative). If the word qualitative or quantitative is not included in the code description, then these qualities of the test do not impact code selection. If these qualities are described in the code description, then it is necessary to match the procedure performed with either the qualitative or quantitative code for the examination.

Note that the Chemistry section is organized in alphabetical order, according to the name of the chemical substance. To search for a chemistry code, look up the term *Pathology and Laboratory* in the Index of the CPT code book, and then refer to the subterm *Chemistry.* Then find the subterm for the specific substance for which the specimen is being tested.

Key to Success

The list of subterms under the Chemistry heading spans a number of pages, so it helps start at the beginning of the *Pathology and Laboratory* heading and search for the *Chemistry* subterm from there. If you do not start at the beginning, it is easy to get lost in the multiple subterms. It may also help to highlight or underline the first subterms for pathology and laboratory procedures in the Index to make them easier to find when searching through the CPT Index.

The Organ or Disease-Oriented Panels (80047 to 80081) subsection identifies groups of laboratory tests, called panels. A panel is a group of specific tests (from the chemistry section) that are commonly performed together. They are grouped together under one code description to make the reporting of the panel easier. For example, the code description for 80047 reads:

80047	Basic metabolic panel (Calcium, ionized)
	This panel must include the following:
	Calcium, ionized (82330)
	Carbon dioxide (bicarbonate) (82374)
	Chloride (82435)
	Creatinine (82565)
	Glucose (82947)
	Potassium (84132)
	Sodium (84295)
	Urea Nitrogen (BUN) (84520)

This means that the basic metabolic panel reported by code 80047 includes the following chemistry tests: Calcium ionized, Carbon dioxide (bicarbonate), Chloride, Creatinine, Glucose, Potassium, Sodium, and Urea nitrogen (BUN).

Note that the specific procedure code for each chemistry test is included after each of the components listed in the panel. For example, in the basic metabolic panel identified previously, each chemistry test included in the panel is listed in the CPT book with the appropriate CPT code for just that chemistry test, such as Chloride (82435). This code identifies the chemistry test for that specific substance, if it was performed alone. This is a helpful reference for coders, because if not all components in the panel were performed, then the coder cannot report the panel code. The coder must report each of the components individually that were tested. For example, if a provider ordered a basic metabolic panel (code 80047), but the Potassium and Sodium components of the test were not performed because they had been performed in an earlier lab test, for example, then the coder must *not* report the panel code. In this case, the coder can only report the codes for the procedures that were performed: Calcium, Carbon dioxide, Chloride, Creatinine, Glucose, and Urea nitrogen.

Key to Success

A panel code can only be reported if *all* the components within the panel were performed. If not, then report the code for each individual test separately.

For practice assigning codes for panels and chemistry tests, complete the exercises in There's a Code for That 14.2.

Panels and chemistry tests

14.2

There's a Code for That

Read the following documentation of the laboratory test and identify the correct chemistry or disease-oriented panel code(s).

1. Comprehensive metabolic panel.

   CPT code: _____

2. Hepatic function panel without bilirubin measurements.

   CPT codes: _____, _____, _____,

   _____, _____

3. Tests completed: Lipid panel, comprehensive metabolic panel, and acute hepatitis panel.

   CPT codes: _____, _____, _____

4. Qualitative ketone test.

   CPT code: _____

5. Qualitative complete (40 acids) plasma amino acid analysis on 40-year-old female with neuropsychiatric disorder.

   CPT code: _____

6. Direct measurement of HDL, VLDL, and LDL cholesterol.

   CPT codes: _____, _____, _____

Drug Assays

Drug assays, or procedures to test for drugs, are divided into three subsections: Drug Assay, Therapeutic Drug Assay, and Chemistry procedures. The selection of the code for the test depends on the purpose and desired result of the test (qualitative or quantitative).

Presumptive Drug Class Screenings and Definitive Drug Testing

The Drug Assays subsection is divided into Presumptive Drug Class Screening (to 80307) and Definitive Drug Testing (80320 to 80377) codes. Presumptive drug class screening codes are used to report screening procedures performed to qualitatively determine if a drug is present in the specimen. These codes do not identify the drug being tested nor the purpose of the test, but rather the method in which the test was performed. There are three possible codes and only one code should be reported depending on the test type, per date of service, no matter how many drug classes are being assayed in the test.

- 80305, Drug test(s), presumptive, any number of drug classes, any number of devices or procedures; capable of being read by direct optical observation only (e.g., utilizing immunoassay [e.g., dipsticks, cups, cards, cartridges]) includes sample validation when performed, per date of service, identifies a drug test capable of being read by direct optical observation, such as dipsticks, cups, cards, or cartridges.

- 80306, Drug test(s), presumptive, any number of drug classes, any number of devices or procedures; read by instrument assisted direct optical observation (e.g., utilizing immunoassay [e.g., dipsticks, cups, card, cartridges]), includes sample validation when performed, per date of service, identifies a drug test capable of being read by instrument-assisted direct optical observation. For example, if a cartridge is inserted into a device to aid in the optical reading of the test results.

- 80307, Drug test(s), presumptive, any number of drug classes, any number of devices or procedures, by instrument chemistry analyzers (e.g., utilizing immunoassay [e.g., EIA, ELISA, EMIT, FPIA, IA, KIMS, RIA]), chromatography (e.g., GC, HPLC), and mass spectrometry either with or without chromatography, (e.g., DART, DESI, GC-MS, GC-MS/MS, LC-MS, LC-MS/MS, LDTD, MALD, TOF), includes sample validation when performed, per date of service, identifies a drug test capable of being read by any type of instrument chemical analyzers, including chromatography and mass spectrometry.

The results from any of these three tests are qualitative in nature, meaning that they only give a positive result. These are nonspecific tests that only identify if a drug class is present, rather than test for the specific type of drug. A **nonspecific test** does not test for a specific chemical or substance, but rather tests for a quality, such as whether or not any type of drug from that drug class is present.

Definitive drug testing codes are used for both qualitative and quantitative analyses for drugs. These tests are specific and codes identify the exact substance that is being tested in the sample. Note that some code descriptions differ based on the number of specific substances tested. If the specific substance being tested is not listed within this code range, it is necessary to first search for the substance in the Therapeutic Drug Assays codes and Chemistry codes before assigning one of the unlisted drugs or substances codes (80375 to 80377).

Therapeutic Drug Assays

Therapeutic Drug Assays (80150 to 80299) codes are similar in nature to Drug Assay codes, except that the drugs tested in this subsection are therapeutic drugs taken upon the advice of a medical professional. These tests are run to monitor the clinical response to the prescribed drug. In this process, a patient takes a prescribed medication and the therapeutic drug assay test is performed to determine the amount of the drug in the patient's body after a specific amount of time. This is used to clinically determine the correct amount of time between doses for specific medications and to adjust dosing accordingly.

Chemistry

If the drug being tested is not listed in either the Drug Assays or Therapeutic Drug Assays sections previously noted, then it is necessary to check for a code for the test in the Chemistry section of codes (82009 to 84999) and report the test accordingly.

For practice assigning codes for drug assays, complete the exercises in There's a Code for That 14.3.

Drug assays

14.3

There's a Code for That

Read the following documentation of the laboratory test and identify the correct drug assay code(s).

1. Presumptive drug test, five drug classes, via optically-read urine dipstick.

   CPT code: _____

2. DART mass spectrometry for three drug classes with sample validation.

   CPT code: _____

3. Patient with positive drug test results is tested for four classes of amphetamines.

   CPT code: _____

4. Alcohol breath test.

   CPT code: _____

5. Therapeutic drug assay for free phenytoin.

   CPT code: _____

6. Whole blood serum gabapentin assay.

   CPT code: _____

7. Drug assay for seven benzodiazepines.

   CPT code: _____

Evocative/Suppression Testing

Evocative/Suppression Testing (80400 to 80439) codes are used to report a test in which a substance in the body is measured both before and after the administration of another substance. For example, code 80422, Glucagon tolerance panel; for insulinoma, is an evocative/suppression evaluation that tests the patient for pancreatic tumor (insulinoma). The patient is tested for the two components in the test (as listed in the full code description): Glucose (82947) and Insulin (83525). After this initial test, a substance is administered, and after a specified amount of time the same two components are tested again (glucose and insulin). Then the results for both tests are compared. The result measure may be either evocative, meaning that the level of the first substance is stimulated, or suppressed. These tests are commonly performed to diagnose endocrine disorders, such as hypothyroidism, adrenal insufficiency, and Cushing's disease.

Codes for evocative/suppression tests identify the type of test performed. Inherent in these tests is the administration of the agents administered to the patient during the test, which should be reported separately using codes from Hydration, Therapeutic, Prophylactic, Diagnostic Injections and Infusions, and Chemotherapy and Other Highly Complex Drug or Highly Complex Biologic Agent Administration (96365 to 96368, 96372, 96374 to 96376).

Consultations (Clinical Pathology)

A clinical pathology consultation should be reported when a pathologist must render a written interpretation and report of a test result that requires additional medical interpretation, as a response to a request from the ordering healthcare provider.

There are two code options in this section: a limited clinical consultation that does not require a review of the patient's healthcare history (80500), and a comprehensive clinical consultation, which requires a review of the patient's history and healthcare records (80502).

Urinalysis

Urinalysis (81000 to 81009) codes are for nonspecific tests on urine. They do not identify the quantitative evaluation of specific substances in the urine, but rather the quality of the urine itself. Code selection depends on the type of urinalysis performed and, in some cases, the purpose of the evaluation, such as 81025, Urine pregnancy test, by visual color comparison methods.

Gene Testing Procedures

There are a number of different genetic testing procedures included in the Pathology and Laboratory section of the CPT code book. These include Molecular Pathology procedures, Genomic Sequencing Procedures and Other Molecular Multianalyte Assays, and Multianalyte Assays with Algorithmic Analyses.

Molecular Pathology procedures (81105 to 81479) are highly specialized procedures performed on nucleic acid, such as DNA and RNA, to detect genetic variations and mutations. Code selection is based on the gene being analyzed.

Codes are listed in this section according to the gene name and organized in alphabetical order with their respective tiers. There are two divisions of molecular pathology codes, according to each tier: Tier 1 and Tier 2. Tier 1 tests are for a single analyte (component being tested for), and the code descriptions identify the specific analyte for which the pathology service is testing. For example, 81327, *SEPT9 (Septin9)* (e.g., colorectal cancer) methylation analysis, identifies the specific molecular pathology exam performed to test for the colorectal cancer gene. On the other hand, Tier 2 codes are less specific, as they test for less-common genetic attributes. Thus, Tier 2 code descriptions do not specify one analyte, but are more general in nature. For example, 81400, Molecular pathology procedure, Level 1 (e.g., identification of single germline variant [e.g., SNP] by techniques such as restriction enzyme digestion or melt curve analysis). Beneath this code description is a lengthy list of specific genes that may be tested with this procedure code.

To assist coders in identifying the correct code for the gene being analyzed, the professional edition of the CPT code book includes a cross-reference section at the beginning of the Pathology and Laboratory section, which lists the genes by a claim designation, abbreviated gene name, full gene, name, and commonly associated proteins and diseases, also with the appropriate molecular pathology code for each specific gene. The CPT standard edition code book does not include this cross-reference.

Genomic Sequencing Procedures and Other Molecular Multianalyte Assays (81490 to 81599) are procedures that evaluate a selection of multiple genes or genetic regions relevant to a specific medical condition. Code selection depends on the type of genetic sequence being tested or the medical condition. Some genetic sequencing codes are similar to organ or disease-related panels, because they include a number of different molecular pathology procedures (for specific genes) into one panel of tests to evaluate for a range of genetic conditions.

Multianalyte Assays with Algorithmic Analyses (81490 to 81599) are complex procedures that identify specific biomarkers, genes, and proteins. Code selection depends on the disease type, material analyzed, number of markers included in the test, methodology of the test, number of functional domains (if indicated), specimen type, algorithm result type, and report produced from the test. For example, code 81503, Oncology (ovarian), biochemical assays of five proteins (CA-125, apolipoprotein A1, beta-2 microglobulin, transferrin, and pre-albumin), utilizing serum, algorithm reports as a risk score. Appendix O of the CPT code book includes a cross-reference of the proprietary lab that performs these tests, together with their descriptions and alpha-numeric lab requisition codes.

Hematology and Coagulation

Hematology and Coagulation (85002 to 85999) codes identify tests on blood and blood products. Code selection depends on the type of test performed, or which specific component is being tested in the blood. For example, 85007, Blood count; blood smear, microscopic examination with manual differential WBC count.

Immunology

Immunology (86000 to 86849) codes identify whether a specific immunological substance is present in the body. These procedures test for the presence of antibodies to specific infectious agents. Code selection depends on the identification of the specific antigen or antibody being tested, as well as other specifics of the procedure (for example, if it was qualitative or quantitative).

Transfusion Medicine

Transfusion Medicine (86850 to 86999) codes identify procedures performed on blood and blood products that are either collected from a blood donor or tested before storage and being given to a blood recipient. Code selection depends on the specific service performed on the blood or blood product.

Microbiology

Microbiology (87003 to 87999) codes identify procedures performed to identify specific microorganisms and infectious diseases, such as streptococcus or influenza. More specifically, the tests include bacteriology, the study of bacteria; mycology, the study of fungi; parasitology, the study of parasites; and virology, the study of viruses. Microbiology tests include swabs, smears, and cultures, all of which test a patient sample for a specific microbiological agent.

The same microorganism may be tested in several different ways, and it is possible that multiple tests may be conducted on the same date of service. For example, a lab may run streptococcal, influenza, and mononucleosis tests all on the same day, to rule out those three microorganisms as the cause of the patient's symptoms.

Coders should report each test conducted on the date of service. If the same test was performed on multiple sites (for example a bacterial culture from wound exudate on the buttock as well as one on the leg), append modifier -59 to identify the procedures as distinct from each other. If the same test was run multiple times on the same date of service, append modifier -91, Repeat clinical laboratory diagnostic test.

Coding for microbiology tests relies on the identification of the specimen, the microorganism for which the study is testing, and the type of microbiology test. For example, with code 87086, Culture, bacterial; qualitative colony count, urine, the specimen is *urine*, the microorganism is *bacteria*, and the type of test is a *culture with qualitative colony count*. The microorganism in this code is only identified as bacteria, which means any type of bacteria. Some tests specify the exact bacteria for which the study is testing, but do not specify the type of specimen. For example, code 87880, Infectious agent antigen detection by immunoassay with direct optical observation; Streptococcus, group A identifies the type of test, *immunoassay with direct optical observation*, and the specific bacteria, *group A streptococcus*, but does not specify the type of specimen.

Anatomic Pathology

Anatomic Pathology (88000 to 88099) codes identify services performed by a physician on a deceased patient for pathological examinations, such as an autopsy. These codes identify the type of examination, either gross or microscopic, and the components involved in the exam. For example, 88007, Necropsy (autopsy), gross examination only; with brain and spinal cord. Remember that a gross examination includes the physical components of the specimen, such as the size, weight, and visual characteristics, and that a microscopic examination is performed with a microscope.

Cytopathology

Cytopathology (88104 to 88199) codes identify **cytopathology** studies, which examine cells from a specimen to determine a cause or nature of a disease. The most common and widely used cytopathology study is the pap smear, developed by George Nicolas Papanicolaou in 1928 (Tan 2015). A pap smear is done by taking a sample of cells from the cervix that are then examined for cancerous cell changes.

Codes in the cytopathology section identify the test technique and the source of the specimen. For example, code 88150, Cytopathology, slides, cervical or vaginal; manual screening under physician supervision, identifies the source of the specimen, *cervical or vaginal*, as well as the test technique, *slides…manual screening under physician supervision*.

Cytogenic Studies

Cytogenic Studies (88230 to 88299), also known as cytogenetic studies, are performed on chromosomes to determine abnormalities. Code selection depends on the type and purpose of the test. For example, code 88248, Chromosome analysis for breakage syndromes; baseline breakage, score 50-100 cells, count 20 cells, 2 karyotypes (e.g., for ataxia telangiectasia, Fanconi anemia, fragile X), identifies the type of test, *chromosome analysis*, and the purpose of the test, *breakage syndromes; baseline breakage, score 50-100 cells, count 20 cells, 2 karyotypes (e.g., for ataxia telangiectasia, Fanconi anemia, fragile X)*.

Complete the exercises in There's a Code for That 14.4 for practice assigning procedure codes for laboratory procedures.

Coding laboratory services

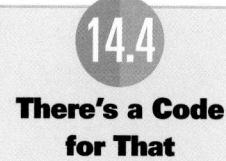

There's a Code for That

Read the following documentation of the laboratory test and identify the correct laboratory or pathology test code(s).

1. Full sequence BRCA1 with full sequence BRCA2 gene analysis for patient with family history of breast cancer.

   CPT code: _____

2. Chorionic gonadotropin stimulation panel; estradiol response.

   CPT code: _____

3. Urine pregnancy test.

   CPT code: _____

4. Bacterial urine culture with quantitative colony count.

   CPT code: _____

5. Trichomonas vaginalis detection by DNA analysis, direct probe technique.

   CPT code: _____

Surgical Pathology

Surgical Pathology (88300 to 88399) codes identify the services performed by a surgical pathologist. Surgical pathology is the study of tissues removed during surgery that are examined intraoperatively by a surgical pathologist. During the pathological examination, the surgical pathologist examines the specimen (just removed from the patient) to distinguish between malignant and non-malignant cells, detect cancerous cell changes, and identify infectious agents and pathological diseases in tissues. This process involves both gross and microscopic examination of the tissue specimen (depending on the level of surgical pathology performed).

There are six levels of surgical pathology examinations, each of which is identified with a specific CPT code.

- 88300, Level I, Surgical pathology, gross examination only. Level I examinations should be used for any specimen that is accurately diagnosed without a microscopic examination.

- 88302, Level II, Surgical pathology, gross and microscopic examination. Level II examinations require both gross and microscopic examinations of the specimen to confirm the diagnosis, or the absence of a disease.

- 88304, Level III, Surgical pathology, gross and microscopic examination.
- 88305, Level IV, Surgical pathology, gross and microscopic examination.
- 88307, Level V, Surgical pathology, gross and microscopic examination.
- 88309, Level VI, Surgical pathology, gross and microscopic examination.

Levels III through VI examinations require both gross and microscopic examinations, with the higher levels of the service representing higher levels of physician work.

Each level of surgical pathology (except for Level I) has a list of tissue specimens after the code description. When coding for surgical pathology services, a coder must identify the tissue sample that is analyzed in the service, such as carpal tunnel tissue, and then locate that specific type of tissue in the list of a specific level of surgical pathology. For example, if the tissue examined was carpal tunnel tissue, find that specific tissue type in one of the levels for the surgical pathology service. In this case, code 88304,

Level II, Surgical pathology, gross and microscopic examination would be the correct code, because *Carpal tunnel tissue* is included in the list for that level of service.

The lists of tissue types are arranged in alphabetical order, according to the type of tissue, under each code heading for Levels II through Level VI surgical pathology services. Be careful, however, as sometimes the same tissue type appears in multiple different levels. For example, breast tissue is listed under Level IV, Level V, and Level VI. This requires careful reading to ensure the selection of the correct level of surgical pathology service: Level IV is for Breast, *biopsy, not requiring microscopic evaluation of surgical margins*; Level V is for Breast, *mastectomy-partial/simple* and Breast, *excision of lesion, requiring microscopic evaluation of surgical margins*; and Level VI is for Breast, *mastectomy-with regional lymph nodes*. Selection of the correct level depends on the correct identification of the type of tissue examined.

If the same tissue sample was examined in two different areas, report the appropriate code only once. If there were two separate tissue samples from the same body area that were examined, report one code for each sample examined. For practice reporting procedure codes for surgical pathology services, complete the exercises in There's a Code for That 14.5.

14.5

There's a Code for That

Surgical pathology coding

Read the following documentation of the surgical pathology service and identify the correct surgical pathology code(s).

1. Pathological examination of two skin tags.

   CPT code: _____ × _____

2. Labial biopsy examination, surgical pathology.

   CPT code: _____

3. Surgical pathology examinations of the following tissue samples: cervical conization, endometrial biopsy, and bladder biopsy.

   CPT code: _____, _____ × _____

Other Procedures

Other procedures in the Pathology and Laboratory section include In Vivo (e.g., Transcutaneous) Laboratory Procedures (88720 to 88749), Other Procedures (89049 to 89240), and Reproductive Medicine Procedures (89250 to 89398).

In vivo procedures are tests performed on living humans, rather than on a dead or partial specimen from a patient. These procedures are performed transcutaneously, meaning that they are performed through an unbroken area of skin (such as a cardiac electrode being placed on an unbroken area of skin to read heart impulses). Code selection depends on the in vivo measurement performed. For example, code 88720, Bilirubin, total, transcutaneous, is the code reported for the in vivo examination of a patient's bilirubin level.

The Other Procedures subsection contains laboratory and pathology tests that are not classifiable into any other subsection, such as cell count of a body fluid other than blood (89050), or 89190, Nasal smear for eosinophils. Reproductive procedures are performed on both male and female reproductive products and the products of conception, such as oocytes, sperm, and embryos.

Handling of Drug Specimen

In some cases, patients may leave a specimen—such as a urine or stool sample—at their healthcare provider's office. If the needed test is not CLIA-waived, or otherwise cannot be performed at the healthcare provider's office, then the provider's office will have to send this specimen to an independent laboratory. Many independent labs collect specimens from their local area and use couriers to drive to nearby healthcare offices to pick up these samples.

Code 99000, Handling and/or conveyance of specimen for transfer from the office to a laboratory is reported when a specimen collected in the outpatient office is packed and taken to the laboratory by someone other than the patient. For example, if an outpatient office took a blood or urine sample from a patient, and this sample was picked up by a lab courier service and then delivered to an independent lab, the office would bill code 99000 to identify that the sample was taken at the office, prepared and packed by the office, and then transported to the laboratory.

If a patient dropped off the specimen directly to the lab, or of the lab drew the specimen (such as a blood draw), then code 99000 would not be reported, as the specimen was not transferred from one office to another.

Modifiers for Laboratory and Pathology Services

There are three CPT modifiers that are specifically designed for use with pathology and laboratory codes.

- Modifier -90, Reference (outside) laboratory. This modifier should be used when the healthcare office practices pass-through billing and bills for the laboratory service directly, rather than the laboratory billing for the test. This is only done when the two parties have a prior agreement to bill for services in this manner.
- Modifier -91, Repeat clinical diagnostic laboratory test. This modifier should be used when the exact same laboratory test is re-run on the same date of service for the same patient. However, it may *not* be used if the test was re-run either to confirm the previous result or if the previous test was faulty or questionable. For example:

    A patient received a CBC in the outpatient office and it was determined that the patient was fighting off a severe infection. The healthcare provider, suspecting that it was bacterial, administered an antibiotic injection in the office to immediately control the infection. The CBC was repeated after two hours to verify the effect on the patient's system.

    In this case, the test was repeated for the same patient on the same date of service, but was conducted to determine separate results. In this example, the second CBC wound be appended with modifier -91.

Note that modifier -51, Multiple procedures, may *not* be appended to laboratory and pathology procedures. This is because modifier -91, Repeat clinical diagnostic laboratory test, is more appropriate. If the same test was run multiple times, it may only be billed for in the circumstances described previously. If it was re-run because the initial test was faulty or questionable, or if the test was re-run to confirm the initial results, only one test can be reported for the date of service.

MOD

- Modifier -92, Alternative laboratory platform testing. This modifier should be appended when a laboratory test is performed using a kit or a transportable device that consists of a single-time use, disposable analytic chamber. For example, HIV tests may be performed using single, one-time use analytic chambers, so the code for the HIV test (86701, HIV-1) would be appended with modifier -92 (86701-92).

MOD

Other modifiers that may be appropriate for laboratory services include modifier -QW, CLIA-waived test, for specifically identified CLIA-waived tests, modifier -XS, Separate structure, and modifier -XU, Unusual non-overlapping service. Both -XS and -XU should be used in lieu of modifier -59, Distinct procedural service, when a laboratory test is conducted more than once and better describe the circumstances of the encounter.

Diagnostic Coding for Laboratory and Pathology Services

Diagnosis coding for pathology and laboratory services requires an in-depth knowledge of chapter 1: Certain Infectious and Parasitic Diseases in the ICD-10-CM code book. This chapter includes codes that identify certain infectious and parasitic diseases, as well as those certain infectious and parasitic diseases as the cause of conditions coded elsewhere. It contains important guidelines for coding HIV and AIDS, sepsis (discussed in chapter 10, Urgent Care and Emergency Department Services), and methicillin-resistant *Staphylococcus aureus* (MRSA).

Infectious Diseases and Infectious Diseases as the Cause of Conditions Coded Elsewhere

There are two divisions of codes in the infectious diseases chapter in the ICD-10-CM code book: codes for specific infectious diseases, including specified bacteria, viruses, fungi, and other pathogens; and codes for these infectious diseases as the cause of a condition classified elsewhere.

Codes for the infectious diseases themselves should be used when that specific infectious organism has not been confirmed as causing any specific medical condition. For example, if a lab sample runs a test on a specimen and determines that the sample is contaminated with Enterotoxigenic E. coli, then the coder should report the procedure code for the lab test along with the code for the infectious organism, in this case A04.1, Enterotoxigenic Escherichia coli infection.

However, if a healthcare office sent a urine sample to the lab to determine the infectious agent for a patient with a urinary tract infection, and it was determined that the infectious agent was E. coli, then the code selected to identify the E. coli would be B96.20, Unspecified Escherichia coli [E. coli] as the cause of diseases classified elsewhere. An additional code would also be assigned to identify the manifestation of the E. coli infection, in this case a urinary tract infection, N39.0, Urinary tract infection, site not specified. Refer to chapter 4 for a refresher of etiology and manifestation coding.

Note that in the first example, the lab is testing the specimen, identifying the infectious agent, and assigning a code to identify the organism. In the second example, the provider's office received the information from the lab and assigns a code from category B95 to B97, Bacterial and viral infectious agents (as the cause of disease classified elsewhere). The codes in these categories identify that the infectious agent has caused a specific manifestation, condition, or disease.

Because labs identify the infectious organism, when present, they are more likely to use the infectious and parasitic agent codes. On the other hand, because healthcare providers diagnose and treat known healthcare conditions, they are more likely to report codes for bacterial and viral infectious agents as the cause of a disease classified elsewhere. See figure 14.4 for the OGCR related to infectious agents as the cause of diseases classified elsewhere.

Figure 14.4. OGCR I.C.1.b

---

b. Infectious agents as the cause of diseases classified to other chapters

Certain infections are classified in chapters other than Chapter 1 and no organism is identified as part of the infection code. In these instances, it is necessary to use an additional code from Chapter 1 to identify the organism. A code from category B95, Streptococcus, Staphylococcus, and Enterococcus as the cause of diseases classified to other chapters, B96, Other bacterial agents as the cause of diseases classified to other chapters, or B97, Viral agents as the cause of diseases classified to other chapters, is to be used as an additional code to identify the organism. An instructional note will be found at the infection code advising that an additional organism code is required.

Source: CMS 2018.

Coding for HIV and AIDS

Coding for HIV and AIDS must be done with the utmost caution, as this condition is closely tracked by public health agencies, health insurance providers, and third-party payers. There are also several ICD-10-CM guidelines that specify which and how HIV codes should be used.

When a patient presents for HIV testing, report code Z11.4, Encounter for screening for human immunodeficiency virus [HIV]. If HIV counseling is performed at this visit, then report the additional code Z71.7, Human immunodeficiency virus [HIV] counseling. If the patient engages in high-risk sexual behavior, then the appropriate code from category Z72.5-, High-risk sexual behavior, should also be reported. For example, a patient with multiple heterosexual partners presents because he is worried about contracting HIV. An HIV test is performed after the provider counsels the patient on HIV risks and testing. The codes for this encounter would be as follows:

* Z11.4, Encounter for screening for human immunodeficiency virus [HIV]
* Z71.7, Human immunodeficiency virus [HIV] counseling
* Z72.51, High-risk heterosexual behavior

Furthermore, if the patient has been exposed to HIV, report code Z20.6, Contact with and (suspected) exposure to human immunodeficiency virus [HIV]. The exposure to HIV code should not be reported with codes for HIV positive status.

There are three possible outcomes from an HIV test:

* *The results are inconclusive.* If the results from this HIV test are inconclusive, then report code R75, Inconclusive laboratory evidence of human immunodeficiency virus [HIV].
* *The result is negative.* If the results are negative and the patient returns to discuss the findings, then report code Z71.7, Human immunodeficiency virus [HIV] counseling.

- *The result is positive.*
  - If the result is positive, and the patient is not experiencing any HIV-related symptoms, then report code Z21, Asymptomatic human immunodeficiency virus [HIV] infection status.
  - If the result is positive, and the patient is experiencing HIV-related symptoms, report code B20, Human immunodeficiency virus [HIV] disease. This code should be reported for all HIV or AIDS patients that have a positive HIV test and any HIV-related symptoms, ranging all the way to AIDS. Sequence B20 first, followed by any additional codes for HIV-related conditions. Note that even if the patient is not currently exhibiting any symptoms, it is still necessary to assign code B20, if they he or she has ever exhibited HIV-related symptoms. Once a patient has been assigned code B20, he or she can never go back to asymptomatic status.
  - If the result is positive and the patient is pregnant, report a code from category O98.7-, Human immunodeficiency virus [HIV] disease complicating pregnancy, childbirth and the puerperium, as well as code B20, followed by any additional code to identify HIV-related conditions, or Z21.7, for asymptomatic HIV status. See figure 14.5 for a graphic illustrating the coding process for HIV cases.

Figure 14.5. HIV coding

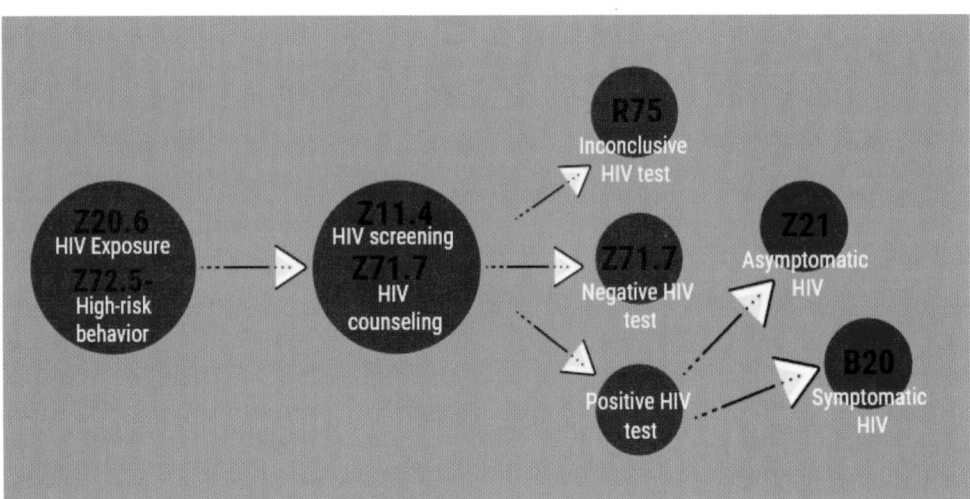

Once a patient receives an HIV-related diagnosis (either Z21 or B20), then either of these codes must be reported for every encounter with the patient, as this is a life-long condition that is not currently curable.

Sequencing of the HIV positive codes is also important (see figure 14.6 for the OGCR related to HIV coding).

- When a patient presents for an HIV-related condition, sequence B20 first, followed by any HIV-related condition(s). For example, an HIV positive patient presents for management of her pneumocystis carinii, which is related to her HIV status, the following codes would be reported in this order:
  - B20, Human immunodeficiency virus [HIV] disease
  - B59, Pneumocystosis

Figure 14.6. OGCR I.C.1.a

---

1. **Chapter 1: Certain Infectious and Parasitic Diseases (A00-B99)**

   a. **Human Immunodeficiency Virus (HIV) Infections**

      1) **Code only confirmed cases**

         Code only confirmed cases of HIV infection/illness. This is an exception to the hospital inpatient guideline Section II, H.

         In this context, "confirmation" does not require documentation of positive serology or culture for HIV; the provider's diagnostic statement that the patient is HIV positive, or has an HIV-related illness is sufficient.

      2) **Selection and sequencing of HIV codes**

         (a) **Patient admitted for HIV-related condition**

            If a patient is admitted for an HIV-related condition, the principal diagnosis should be B20, Human immunodeficiency virus [HIV] disease followed by additional diagnosis codes for all reported HIV-related conditions.

         (b) **Patient with HIV disease admitted for unrelated condition**

            If a patient with HIV disease is admitted for an unrelated condition (such as a traumatic injury), the code for the unrelated condition (e.g., the nature of injury code) should be the principal diagnosis. Other diagnoses would be B20 followed by additional diagnosis codes for all reported HIV-related conditions.

         (c) **Whether the patient is newly diagnosed**

            Whether the patient is newly diagnosed or has had previous admissions/encounters for HIV conditions is irrelevant to the sequencing decision.

         (d) **Asymptomatic human immunodeficiency virus**

            Z21, Asymptomatic human immunodeficiency virus [HIV] infection status, is to be applied when the patient without any documentation of symptoms is listed as being "HIV positive," "known HIV," "HIV test positive," or similar terminology. Do not use this code if the term "AIDS" is used or if the patient is treated for any HIV-related illness or is described as having any condition(s) resulting from his/her HIV positive status; use B20 in these cases.

         (e) **Patients with inconclusive HIV serology**

            Patients with inconclusive HIV serology, but no definitive diagnosis or manifestations of the illness, may be assigned code R75, Inconclusive laboratory evidence of human immunodeficiency virus [HIV].

         (f) **Previously diagnosed HIV-related illness**

            Patients with any known prior diagnosis of an HIV-related illness should be coded to B20. Once a patient has developed an HIV-related illness, the patient should always be assigned code B20 on every subsequent admission/encounter. Patients previously diagnosed with any HIV illness (B20) should never be assigned to R75 or Z21, Asymptomatic human immunodeficiency virus [HIV] infection status.

         (g) **HIV Infection in Pregnancy, Childbirth and the Puerperium**

            During pregnancy, childbirth or the puerperium, a patient admitted (or presenting for a health care encounter) because of an HIV-related illness should receive a principal diagnosis code of O98.7-, Human immunodeficiency [HIV] disease complicating pregnancy, childbirth and the puerperium, followed by B20 and the code(s) for the HIV-related illness(es). Codes from Chapter 15 always take sequencing priority.

            Patients with asymptomatic HIV infection status admitted (or presenting for a health care encounter) during pregnancy, childbirth, or the puerperium should receive codes of O98.7- and Z21.

         (h) **Encounters for testing for HIV**

            If a patient is being seen to determine his/her HIV status, use code Z11.4, Encounter for screening for human immunodeficiency virus [HIV]. Use additional codes for any associated high risk behavior.

            If a patient with signs or symptoms is being seen for HIV testing, code the signs and symptoms. An additional counseling code Z71.7, Human immunodeficiency virus [HIV] counseling, may be used if counseling is provided during the encounter for the test.

            When a patient returns to be informed of his/her HIV test results and the test result is negative, use code Z71.7, Human immunodeficiency virus [HIV] counseling.

            If the results are positive, see previous guidelines and assign codes as appropriate.

Source: CMS 2018.

- When a patient presents for a condition that is not related to HIV, sequence the unrelated condition first, followed by B20 and any codes for HIV-related condition(s). For example, if the HIV positive patient with pneumocystis carinii presented for a fracture of the right wrist, then the following codes would be reported in this order:
  - S62.101A, Fracture of unspecified carpal bone, right wrist, initial encounter for closed fracture
  - B20, Human immunodeficiency virus [HIV] disease
  - B59, Pneumocystosis

Coding for MRSA

Methicillin-resistant *Staphylococcus aureus* (MRSA) is a bacterium that can cause infections throughout the human body. It is resistant to certain antibiotics, making it especially hard to treat and cure. There are a handful of MRSA guidelines that are important to know when coding for this condition. See figure 14.7 for the official OGCR related to MRSA conditions.

Figure 14.7. OGCR I.C.1.e

---

e. Methicillin Resistant Staphylococcus aureus (MRSA) Conditions

 1) Selection and sequencing of MRSA codes

   (a) Combination codes for MRSA infection

   When a patient is diagnosed with an infection that is due to methicillin resistant Staphylococcus aureus (MRSA), and that infection has a combination code that includes the causal organism (e.g., sepsis, pneumonia) assign the appropriate combination code for the condition (e.g., code A41.02, Sepsis due to Methicillin resistant Staphylococcus aureus or code J15.212, Pneumonia due to Methicillin resistant Staphylococcus aureus). Do not assign code B95.62, Methicillin resistant Staphylococcus aureus infection as the cause of diseases classified elsewhere, as an additional code because the combination code includes the type of infection and the MRSA organism. Do not assign a code from subcategory Z16.11, Resistance to penicillins, as an additional diagnosis.

   See Section C.1. for instructions on coding and sequencing of sepsis and severe sepsis.

   (b) Other codes for MRSA infection

   When there is documentation of a current infection (e.g., wound infection, stitch abscess, urinary tract infection) due to MRSA, and that infection does not have a combination code that includes the causal organism, assign the appropriate code to identify the condition along with code B95.62, Methicillin resistant Staphylococcus aureus infection as the cause of diseases classified elsewhere for the MRSA infection. Do not assign a code from subcategory Z16.11, Resistance to penicillins.

   (c) Methicillin susceptible Staphylococcus aureus (MSSA) and MRSA colonization

   The condition or state of being colonized or carrying MSSA or MRSA is called colonization or carriage, while an individual person is described as being colonized or being a carrier. Colonization means that MSSA or MSRA is present on or in the body without necessarily causing illness. A positive MRSA colonization test might be documented by the provider as "MRSA screen positive" or "MRSA nasal swab positive".

   Assign code Z22.322, Carrier or suspected carrier of Methicillin resistant Staphylococcus aureus, for patients documented as having MRSA colonization. Assign code Z22.321, Carrier or suspected carrier of Methicillin susceptible Staphylococcus aureus, for patient documented as having MSSA colonization. Colonization is not necessarily indicative of a disease process or as the cause of a specific condition the patient may have unless documented as such by the provider.

   (d) MRSA colonization and infection

   If a patient is documented as having both MRSA colonization and infection during a hospital admission, code Z22.322, Carrier or suspected carrier of Methicillin resistant Staphylococcus aureus, and a code for the MRSA infection may both be assigned.

Source: CMS 2018.

- If the manifestation of the MRSA infection is not known or specified, code only for the organism with code A49.02, Methicillin-resistant *Staphylococcus aureus* infection, unspecified site. If the MRSA is the infectious agent causing sepsis, report code A41.02, Sepsis due to Methicillin-resistant *Staphylococcus aureus*.

- Use a combination code when available. There are several combination codes for MRSA as the infectious agent and the healthcare condition (the etiology and manifestation). When a combination code is present, it is only necessary to report the combination code. Do not report the combination code and the code for the infectious organism. One example of a MRSA combination code is J15.212, Pneumonia due to Methicillin-resistant *Staphylococcus aureus*. This code combines the etiology (MRSA) with the manifestation (pneumonia) into one code.

- When a combination code is not available, code for the condition and MRSA as the cause of the condition. When a combination code is not available, report one for the manifestation of the disease, along with B95.62, Methicillin-resistant *Staphylococcus aureus* infection as the cause of diseases classified elsewhere.

- If the patient is documented as an MRSA carrier or that he or she has an MRSA colonization, report code Z22.322, Carrier or suspected carrier of Methicillin-resistant *Staphylococcus aureus*. This code may be reported with the code for MRSA infection, if the patient has both conditions at the same time.

Key to Success

When reporting codes for MRSA, read the code descriptions carefully, as they are similar and in close proximity to MSSA codes. Methicillin-susceptible *Staphylococcus aureus* (MSSA) is a strain of the same bacteria that is susceptible to antibiotics, rather than resistant to them like MRSA. MSSA codes and MRSA codes read almost exactly alike, and only differ by one word, so they are easy to mistake for each other. For example, Z22.321, Carrier or suspected carrier of Methicillin-susceptible *Staphylococcus aureus*, and Z22.322, Carrier or suspected carrier of Methicillin-resistant *Staphylococcus aureus*.

HCC Coding Corner

HCC codes are scattered throughout chapter 1 of the ICD-10-CM code book, Certain Infectious and Parasitic Diseases. Most conditions that qualify as HCCs have a long-term impact on the patient's health. Additional categories of codes that all qualify as HCC codes include: Streptococcal sepsis (A40.-), Viral infections of the central nervous system (A81.-), Chronic viral hepatitis (B18.-), Human immunodeficiency virus disease (B20), Cytomegaloviral diseases (B25.-), Aspergillosis (B44.-), Cryptococcosus (B45.-), and Zygomycosis (B46.-). Codes that fit into an HCC should be documented carefully with all required components of HCC documentation.

For practice assigning diagnostic codes for laboratory procedures, complete the exercises in There's a Code for That 14.6.

14.6   Diagnostic coding for laboratory procedures

There's a Code for That

Read the following documentation of the laboratory or pathology service and identify the correct diagnosis code(s).

1. 23-year-old female with high-risk heterosexual behavior and exposure to HIV presents for HIV counseling and screening.

   ICD-10-CM codes: _____, _____, _____,

   _____

2. Lab culture positive for MRSA.

   ICD-10-CM code: _____

3. Group A streptococcal septicemia.

   ICD-10-CM code: _____

4. HIV positive patient is seen for management of AIDS-related Kaposi's sarcoma of the right lung.

   ICD-10-CM codes: _____, _____

5. Influenza due to novel influenza A/H5N1 virus.

   ICD-10-CM code: _____

6. Chlamydial epididymitis.

   ICD-10-CM code: _____

7. Salmonella gastroenteritis.

   ICD-10-CM code: _____

Putting It All Together: Coding for Laboratory and Pathology Services

Coding correctly for laboratory and pathology services requires an understanding of the various types of laboratory and pathology tests and the components of each test, as listed in the code descriptions.

Determination of the correct codes relies on the answers to the following questions.

- What type of laboratory or pathology procedure was performed?
  - For specific tests, what substance was tested?
  - For nonspecific tests, what type of specimen was tested?
  - What technique was used for the test?
- Was it qualitative or quantitative?
- How many tests were performed, and how many specimens were tested?
- How was the specimen collected?
  - Which facility collected the specimen? If it was the coder's facility, code for the collection technique (that is, venipuncture).

- o Did your facility test the specimen? If so, code for the laboratory procedure (for example, CBC).
- o Did your facility both collect and test the specimen? If so, code for both the collection and the testing.
- Is there an infectious organism present in the specimen?
  - o If so, code for the infectious agent.
    - ▫ If the manifestation of the infection is known, use either a combination code to identify both the manifestation and etiology of the infection, or separate codes to identify each.
  - o If no, then code for the signs, symptoms, or abnormal finding code.

Study the following vignette that demonstrates how to select the appropriate diagnosis and procedure codes. Then complete the following practice exercises in There's a Code for That 14.7.

Jessie has been working in healthcare billing and coding for a few years and most of her experience has been in primary care billing. She just moved to a new city and found a job as a coder for an independent laboratory clinic. The lab is large and employs numerous clinical and surgical pathologists, as well as several labs throughout the state that perform a wide range of tests. Jessie is studying some reference materials that she bought in order to prepare for her new job at the independent lab. She is currently coding from the following surgical pathology report.

SURGICAL PATHOLOGY

Specimen: 0.5 cm polyp of the ascending colon 0.2 cm polyp in the sigmoid colon

Clinical History: Patient presents for a screening colonoscopy. Family history significant for maternal history of adenocarcinoma of colon.

Gross Examination:
A. Cassette A labeled "ascending colon" contains a polypoid piece of tan mucosal tissue measuring 0.5 cm.
B. Cassette B labeled "sigmoid colon" contains one piece of light tan mucosal tissue 0.2.

Microscopic Examination:
Supportive of sessile serrated adenomatous polyp with low-grade adenomatous dysplasia in the ascending colon and tubular adenoma of the sigmoid colon.

Jessie knows from the report that the service performed was a surgical pathology test. She asks herself: What did the doctor do? In this case, the pathologist examined two polyps that were located in the colon. These were two separate tissue samples, so there should be one code assigned for each pathological examination. She searches the lists of tissues within each surgical pathology code, and locates Polyp, colorectal, *in the list of tissues for Level IV Surgical pathology. She assigns the following code:*

- *88305, Level IV Surgical pathology, gross and microscopic*

Now that Jessie has her procedure code, she asks herself: Why did the doctor do it? She notes that the patient has a family history of colon cancer, which should be reported with the appropriate family history code (chapter 8). Also, in the microscopic examination section of the report, she notes that the doctor wrote that the findings were "supportive of sessile serrated adenomatous polyp with low-grade adenomatous dysplasia in the ascending colon and tubular adenoma of the sigmoid colon."

She searches for the term Polyp *in the ICD-10-CM Index, and the subterm* Adenomatous, *which refers her to* see also Neoplasm, benign, by site. *She then refers to the Neoplasm Table, and locates the* colon *entry, with the cross-reference to* see also Neoplasm, intestine, large. *She refers to the entry* Intestine, intestinal, *and then the subterm* large *within the Table of Neoplasms. Here she finds multiple locations within the colon. The first polyp examined in the procedure was located in the ascending colon, and was determined to be a sessile serrated adenomatous polyp (benign neoplasm of the ascending colon), so she selects code D12.2. Now she locates the code for the second polyp, determined to be a tubular adenoma of the sigmoid colon (benign neoplasm of the sigmoid colon), so she selects code D12.5. She verifies each code within the Tabular List and reports the following diagnosis codes:*

- *D12.2, Benign neoplasm of the ascending colon*
- *D12.5, Benign neoplasm of the sigmoid colon*
- *Z80.0, Family history of malignant neoplasm of digestive organs*

She then rechecks the documentation to make sure she has coded everything for the encounter and reports the chosen codes.

14.7
There's a Code for That

Diagnostic and procedural coding for laboratory and pathology services

Read the following documentation and assign the appropriate CPT, HCPCS, and ICD-10-CM code(s) for the encounter.

1. Final cytopathology report reveals endocervical cell abnormalities on cervical/endocervical pap, thin layer preparation, collected in preservative fluid with automated and manual rescreening and review. Human Papilloma Virus HPV Assay by in-situ hybridization (16, 18, 31, 33, 35, 39, 45, 51, 52, 56, 58): none detected.

   CPT code: _____, _____

   ICD-10-CM codes: _____

2. Bacterial culture of wound exudate for MRSA aerobic isolate with susceptibility study via agar dilution method, confirms MRSA in skin abscess on right buttock.

   CPT code: _____, _____

   ICD-10-CM codes: _____, _____

End of Chapter Content

Instructions: Indicate whether the following statements are true or false (T or F). For false statements, rewrite the statement on the line below to make the statement true.

1. The patient must be present in order to run a laboratory test.

   _____

   _____

2. An independent laboratory is accredited to test and evaluate patient specimens free from a hospital or private practice.

_____

_____

3. Modifier -90 should be used when practicing pass-through billing.

_____

_____

4. Outside lab charges should be placed in box 24.B of the CMS-1500 claim form.

_____

_____

5. In laboratory coding, the modifier for the professional component is -PC.

_____

_____

6. Laboratories are prohibited from billing for the collection of lab samples via venipuncture.

_____

_____

7. Code selection for many laboratory and pathology codes depends on the type of the specimen tested.

_____

_____

8. A permanent block is embedded in ice so that it can be stored indefinitely.

_____

_____

9. The result of a quantitative examination is numerical.

_____

_____

10. A disease-oriented panel code may only be reported if more than half of the tests were performed.

_____

_____

Instructions: Choose the best answer.

1. What is the name of the billing practice in which a private practice bills for the laboratory service performed by an independent lab, and the lab bills the provider directly for the service?

   a. Fee for service billing
   b. Capitation
   c. Independent laboratory billing
   d. Pass-through billing

2. Which place of service code should be reported for services that were performed at an independent laboratory?

   a. 11
   b. 81
   c. 23
   d. 42

3. The professional component of a laboratory procedure is performed by which of the following?

   a. A pathologist
   b. A primary care physician
   c. A registered nurse
   d. An anesthesiologist

4. A doctor's office collected a patient blood sample and sent it to a lab for analysis. For what will the lab bill?

   a. The collection of the blood sample
   b. The testing of the blood
   c. Both the collection and the testing of the blood
   d. The lab handling fee only

5. A doctor's office collected a patient blood sample and sent it to a lab for analysis. For what will the doctor's office bill?

   a. The collection of the blood sample
   b. The testing of the blood
   c. Both the collection and the testing of the blood
   d. The lab handling fee only

6. A lab collected a blood sample from a patient and then tested the blood. For what will the lab bill?

   a. The collection and testing of the blood sample
   b. The preparation and testing of the blood
   c. The collection and preparation of the blood sample
   d. The lab handling fee only

7. An examination of the physical characteristics of a specimen is known as which of the following?

   a. Gross examination
   b. Microscopic examination
   c. Smear
   d. This type of exam is not included in lab services

8. The result from a specific test determined that it was contaminated with a substance. Which kind of test was it?

   a. Qualitative
   b. Quantitative
   c. A drug assay
   d. A chemistry study

9. Which type of laboratory procedure evaluates chromosomes for abnormalities?

   a. Cytogenetic studies
   b. Cytopathology
   c. Genomic sequencing procedures
   d. Multianalyte assays

10. Which code should be reported for a qualitative drug test read by instrument-assisted optical observation?

    a. 80305
    b. 80306
    c. 80307
    d. 80375

11. Which of the following codes is a nonspecific test?

    a. 81005
    b. 80047
    c. 82085
    d. 82017

12. Which code should be reported for a gross and microscopic full body autopsy, including the brain and spinal cord?

    a. 88007
    b. 88028
    c. 88027
    d. 88005

Instructions: Answer the following questions with the appropriate code(s) and modifier(s).

1. Therapeutic drug monitoring for quinidine in patient with atrial fibrillation.

   CPT code: _____

   ICD-10-CM code: _____

2. Hematocrit blood count for patient with polycythemia vera.

   CPT code: _____

   ICD-10-CM code: _____

3. Diphtheria immunoassay performed on patient recently returned from traveling abroad in Russia confirms presence of diphtheria.

   CPT code: _____

   ICD-10-CM code: _____

References

American Medical Association. 2017 (January). *Current Procedural Terminology (CPT)*. Chicago: AMA.

Centers for Medicare and Medicaid Services. 2018. ICD-10-CM Official Guidelines for Coding and Reporting FY 2018. https://www.cms.gov/Medicare/Coding/ICD10/Downloads/2018-ICD-10-CM-Coding-Guidelines.pdf.

Centers for Medicare and Medicaid Services. 2017. Details for title: CMS 1500. https://www.cms.gov/Medicare/CMS-Forms/CMS-Forms/CMS-Forms-Items/CMS1188854.html.

Rolls, G. 2017. An Introduction to Specimen Preparation. http://www.leicabiosystems.com/pathologyleaders/an-introduction-to-specimen-preparation/.

Tan, S.Y. and Y. Tatsumara. 2015 (October). George Papanicolaou (1883–1962): Discoverer of the Pap smear. *Singapore Med J* 56(10): 586–587. https://www.ncbi.nlm.nih.gov/pmc/articles/PMC4613936/.

Resources

American Society of Cytopathology. 2017. About Cytopathology. https://www.cytopathology.org/about-cytopathology/.

Cancer.Net. 2015 (April). After a Biopsy: Making the Diagnosis. http://www.cancer.net/navigating-cancer-care/diagnosing-cancer/reports-and-results/after-biopsy-making-diagnosis.

Centers for Medicare and Medicaid Services. 2017. CLIA Program and Medicare Laboratory Services. https://www.cms.gov/Outreach-and-Education/Medicare-Learning-Network-MLN/MLNProducts/downloads/CLIABrochure.pdf.

Johns Hopkins Medicine. 2017. Surgical Pathology. http://www.hopkinsmedicine.org/healthlibrary/conditions/pathology/surgical_pathology_85,P00967/.

CHAPTER

Orthopedic Services

Learning Objectives

- Understand the basics of billing and coding for orthopedic services.
- Examine procedural codes and guidelines for orthopedic services.

- Examine diagnosis coding and medical necessity for orthopedic services.
- Determine and apply ICD-10-CM, CPT, and HCPCS codes to orthopedic services.

Key Terms

Amputation
Arthritis
Arthrocentesis
Arthrodesis
Arthropathy
Arthroplasty
Arthroscopy
Closed fracture
Closed treatment
Comminuted fracture
Compound fracture
Compression fracture
Displaced fracture
Greenstick fracture
Gustilo-Anderson classification
Impacted fracture
Internal fixation device

Interspace
Kyphosis
Malunion
Manipulation
Monoarthritis
Musculoskeletal system
Non-displaced fracture
Nonunion
Oblique fracture
Open fracture
Open treatment
Orthopedic services
Orthopedist
Osteoarthritis
Pathological fracture
Percutaneous
Percutaneous skeletal fixation

Physeal fracture
Polyarthritis
Salter-Harris classification
Scoliosis
Segment
Segmental fracture
Skeletal traction
Skin traction
Spiral fracture
Sprain
Strain
Torus fracture
Traction
Transverse fracture
Traumatic fracture

Orthopedic services focus on the management and treatment of conditions affecting the musculoskeletal system—such as fractures, arthritis, joint sprains and strains, and osteoporosis. Orthopedics services may be performed in the outpatient office, inpatient hospital, or outpatient hospital setting, depending on the type of service and the needs of the patient. This chapter discusses the various orthopedic service procedure codes, as well as the diagnosis codes that identify the medical necessity for orthopedic services.

Orthopedics Basics

The **musculoskeletal system** is the body system comprised of all the bones, joints, muscles, cartilage, tendons, and ligaments in the human body. Comprehensively the musculoskeletal system works to provide movement, stability, and form to the human body. Due to the wide range of elements (like muscles, bones, or joints) within the musculoskeletal system, and the various medical conditions that can affect these elements, there are numerous subspecialties within the field of orthopedics. Orthopedic specialists focus on certain types of injuries, medical conditions, or treatment strategies.

Figure 15.1. Human skeleton

Source: ©AHIMA.

At the fundamental level, an orthopedist is a medical doctor who specializes in correcting congenital or acquired abnormalities of the bones and musculoskeletal system through the use of casting, bracing, and surgical techniques. Orthopedic specialists (also spelled orthopaedic specialists) may also treat and manage musculoskeletal conditions with physical therapy or medication. They may be referred to as "orthopods," or the specialty referred to as "ortho."

Additional orthopedic specialties include surgical specialties that focus solely on performing invasive surgeries on the orthopedic system, much like general surgeons focus on performing surgeries on the organ systems of the human body. Orthopedic surgeons are further subspecialized into specific musculoskeletal areas including hand, knee, foot and ankle, hip, shoulder, and spine. Each one of these orthopedic surgeons focuses on their respective body areas. Sports medicine is another type of orthopedic specialty, which focuses on sports injuries and the treatment (both surgical and nonsurgical) and management of injuries sustained in sports, with the goal of returning the patient to his or her pre-injury health.

Billing and coding of orthopedic services is similar to any other type of outpatient coding, and uses procedure codes from across the CPT code book. Diagnosis codes used for orthopedic coding are mainly located in chapter 13: Diseases of the Musculoskeletal System and Connective Tissue, as well as in chapter 19: Injury, Poisoning, and Certain Other Consequences of External Causes, although diagnosis codes for orthopedic services may be found throughout the ICD-10-CM code book.

Being an effective orthopedic coder requires strict attention to detail and a solid knowledge of the musculoskeletal system including muscles, bones, and tendons and ligaments that hold the body together. The coder must also assign codes from several different sections of the CPT code book, including evaluation and management (E/M) codes and codes from the Surgery and Radiology sections. See figure 15.1 for the front and back view of the human skeleton.

Procedural Coding for Orthopedic Services

Without a doubt, the most important subsection of procedure codes for orthopedics is the Musculoskeletal System subsection of the Surgery section. This subsection includes codes for fracture repair and manipulation, application of casts and strapping, joint injections, excision of both soft tissue and bone tumors, amputations, and arthrodesis. These procedures are stretched across the entirety of the Musculoskeletal System subsection, so coders will find themselves going back and forth within it. Therefore, it is important to review the table of contents at the beginning of the Musculoskeletal subsection closely before coding for these procedures.

The following sections discuss the format of the Musculoskeletal System subsection of the CPT code book, followed by specific procedures that include excision of bone and soft tissue tumors, arthrocentesis and joint injections, fracture repairs, application of casts and strapping, hip and knee replacements, arthrodesis and spinal instrumentation, amputations, and arthroscopies.

Format of the Musculoskeletal System Subsection

The Musculoskeletal System subsection is one of the most extensive subsections in the CPT code book because it contains codes for procedures for the largest list of body elements—including all of the bones, muscles, ligaments, and tendons in the human body. Because of its complexity, coders should first review and understand the format of the subsection and how codes are organized within it.

Figure 15.2. Organization of the Musculoskeletal System subsection

Source: AMA 2018, 133.

This subsection is organized by body area first, with categories for specific types of procedures in each subheading (see figure 15.2). The only exceptions to this are the sub-headings General, Application of Casts and Strapping, and Endoscopy/Arthroscopy. These subheadings are organized according to the type of procedure performed, rather than first organized by body area.

Within each subheading are the categories of procedures in each body area. Note that these are all similar: Incision; Excision; Manipulation; Introduction or Removal; Repair, Revision and/or Reconstruction; Fracture and/or Dislocation; Arthrodesis; Amputation; and Other Procedures. Note that all of these categories are also located throughout the Surgery section of the CPT code book (as discussed in chapter 11). In the Musculoskeletal System subsection, there are several categories specific to this sub-section, all of which are discussed in this chapter, including:

- Fracture and/or Dislocation. This category of codes identifies services performed specifically to treat fractures and dislocations.
- Arthrodesis. This category of codes includes all arthrodesis procedures only, performed to surgically fix a joint.
- Amputation. This category identifies procedures performed to amputate parts of the body.

The categories of codes listed beneath each subheading are specific to the procedures that can be performed on that particular body area or for that specific procedure. It is important to pay attention to these headings to ensure you are in the correct section of codes for the procedure being reported.

Musculoskeletal system coding requires an understanding of the basic components of these procedure categories, and the ability to apply this understanding to codes across all body areas. For example, once a coder knows the basics of coding for arthrodesis procedure, he or she can apply that knowledge to code for arthrodesis of the shoulder, humerus, or forearm or wrist.

Because the Musculoskeletal System subsection is so extensive, it is easy to get lost while searching for the correct code. Refer to the table of contents at the beginning of the subsection to find your bearings and get back on track. First, find the body area on which the procedure was performed, and then locate the category for the type of procedure performed. Go to this section of codes and search through the code descriptions until you find a code that looks correct. Then refer to the Index of the CPT code book to see if the code you chose in the Tabular matches the one in the Index. If they match, you have the right code. If not, find where you went wrong by referring to the Index and starting the process over again.

Key to Success

Learning how to maneuver through the CPT code book takes time, and every time you get lost, you learn something new—so do not get frustrated! It is all part of the learning process.

Remember that the Musculoskeletal System subsection is part of the Surgery section, which means that surgical guidelines and terminology are used in these codes. For a refresher on surgery basics, refer to chapter 11 (Surgical Services). Common procedural terminology in this section include the following:

- *-ectomy*, which means surgical removal; as in ostectomy, the removal of bone
- *-desis*, which means surgical fixation; as in arthrodesis, the surgical fixation of a joint
- *-otomy*, which means surgical incision; as in arthrotomy, the surgical incision of a joint
- *-plasty*, which means surgical repair; as in arthroplasty, the surgical repair of a joint
- *-centesis*, which means surgical puncture (often used to remove fluid); as in arthrocentesis, the removal of fluid from a joint
- *-oscopy*, which means an endoscopic examination or procedure; as in arthroscopy, an endoscopic-assisted procedure of the joint

Key to Success

Notice how the subheadings of the Musculoskeletal System subsection are generally organized from the head to the toes. This is common across the various subsections in the Surgery section of the CPT code book, as the subheadings are organized from one area of the body to another. As you become more accustomed to the ways in which the Surgery subsections are organized, you may find that locating codes is easier by accessing the specific body area or organ system, and then the type of procedure in each body area or organ system.

Excision of Bone and Soft Tissue Tumors

The Musculoskeletal System subsection of the CPT code book contains a number of codes for excision of both soft tissue and bone tumors, which may be either benign or malignant. It is highly probable that some of these excisions would be performed by a specialist other than an orthopedic surgeon, such as a general surgeon. However, they are discussed here in full as they are best understood in relation to each other.

Codes for the excision of tumors are based on the depth of the excision. Excisions of the skin, such as excisions of benign or malignant lesions, are identified with codes from the Integumentary System subsection. The excision codes found in the Musculo-skeletal System subsection are for deeper structures, such as the subcutaneous tissues, fascial and subfascial tissues, connective tissues within the subcutaneous and subfascial layers, and bone. Fascia is a sheet of connective tissue that encloses the structures of the muscles and other internal organs, and subfascial tissues are underneath the fascial layers, such as muscles. Procedures that are not performed on these deep structures are listed in the Integumentary System subsection of the CPT code book.

The tissue excised within any layer is only identified by the area from which it was excised, and does not depend on the type of tissue excised (that is, benign, malignant, or metastatic). Code selection is usually based on the location and the size of the tumor, with the exception of bone tumors. These procedures are on deeper structures of the body; procedures performed on the skin are coded from the Integumentary System subsection of the CPT code book. All of the following procedures listed are found in the Musculoskeletal System subsection of codes.

- *Excision of subcutaneous soft tissue tumors.* These tumors are below the skin, but above the deep fascia. Code selection depends on the location and the size of the tumor, which is based on the greatest diameter of the tumor plus the excisional margins (similar to the margins included within the excision of skin lesions). For example, code 22902, Excision, tumor, soft tissue of abdominal wall, subcutaneous; less than 3 cm.

- *Excision of fascial or subfascial soft tissue tumors.* These tumors are located within or below the deep fascia, but do not involve the bone. Code selection depends on the location and the size of the tumor, including excisional margins. For example, code 23076, Excision, tumor, soft tissue of shoulder area, subfascial (e.g., intramuscular); less than 5 cm.

- *Radical resection of soft connective tissue tumors.* These tumors have wide margins, and removal may involve excision of more than one layer of tissue. Code selection is based on the location and size of the tumor, including excisional margins. For example, 21557, Radical resection of tumor (e.g., sarcoma), soft tissue of neck or anterior thorax; less than 5 cm.

- *Excision of bone tumors.* These tumors are in the bone, and are typically very aggressive benign or malignant tumors. Code selection is based on the location of the tumor, and not on the size or type of tumor removed. For example, code 27360, Partial excision (craterization, saucerization, or diaphysectomy) bone, femur, proximal tibia and/or fibula (e.g., osteomyelitis or bone abscess).

To search for codes for the excision of tumors, look up the term *Excision* in the CPT Index, and refer to the subterm *Tumor*. There is a large section of subterms identifying codes for the removal of tumors. Note that many of these are within the code range 20005 to 29999, so they are musculoskeletal system procedure codes. An alternate method of locating the code for the tumor is to search for the subterm for the body area, organ, or bone under the Excision heading. For example, to find the code for the excision of a tumor in the humerus, search for the subterm *Humerus* under *Excision*, and note the subterm for *Tumor*, and the possible codes: 23150, 23155, 23156, 24110, 24115, 24116.

For practice assigning codes for excisions of bone and soft tissue, complete the exercises in There's a Code for That 15.1.

Excisions of bone and soft tissue

15.1

There's a Code for That

Read the following documentation of the procedure test and identify the correct excision of bone or soft tissue procedure code(s).

1. Excision of osteoid osteoma on right femur, with allograft and placement of internal fixation device.

   CPT code: _____, _____

2. Excision of 7 cm subfascial tumor of the left upper arm.

   CPT code: _____

3. Radical resection of squamous cell carcinoma of the mandible, with bone graft.

   CPT code: _____, _____

4. Excision of 2 cm benign soft tissue tumor in right foot.

   CPT code: _____

Arthrocentesis and Joint Injections

Arthrocentesis is the aspiration of a joint, a process that involves inserting a hollow needle into a joint or bursa to allow for the removal of fluid. Bursae are fluid-filled sacs beneath the skin that lie between tendons, ligaments, and bones, and assist in lubricating the joints. Inflammation of the bursa creates a condition called bursitis, which causes swelling and pain, and requires aspiration. Joint aspirations are performed for either diagnostic purposes—to obtain a sample of fluid from the joint and test it, or for therapeutic purposes by removing inflammation of effusive fluid from a joint, thereby relieving pressure and pain.

CPT codes for arthrocentesis (20600 to 20611) are based on the joint or bursa being aspirated, and whether or not imaging guidance is used during the procedure. For example, code 20610, Arthrocentesis, aspiration, and/or injection, major joint or bursa (e.g., shoulder, hip, knee, subacromial bursa); without ultrasound guidance identifies the joint involved (*major joint or bursa*) and if imaging guidance was used (*without ultrasound guidance*). Note the parenthetical guidance below the codes that identifies which codes should be used when imaging guidance is performed with the arthrocentesis.

Codes 20600 to 20611 include both the aspiration of fluid from a joint (arthrocentesis) and injection of a joint. As discussed in chapter 12 (Anesthesia and Pain Management), joint injections are performed for treatment of pain, to reduce inflammation, and to help lubricate the joint. Depending on the orthopedic specialty and the resources available to the provider, some orthopedic providers may choose to perform anesthetic joint injections for pain management, as described in chapter 12. Refer to figure 15.3 for an illustration of arthrocentesis techniques.

Key to Success

Do not confuse arthro*centesis* with arthro*desis*. Arthro*centesis* is the aspiration of a joint, while arthro*desis* is the surgical fixation of a joint—two completely different procedures. Arthrodesis procedures are discussed in depth later in this chapter.

Figure 15.3. Arthrocentesis techniques

Techniques for Aspiration of Joint Fluid

Knee. Needle inserted horizontally at medial or lateral margin of patella to pass beneath patella. 20-gauge needle used for most joints.

Ankle. Needle inserted just above and lateral to medial malleolus and medial to extensor hallucis longus tendon

Shoulder. Needle inserted at or just below coracoid process and medial to head of humerus

Elbow. With joint flexed 90°, needle inserted below lateral epicondyle and above olecranon

Finger joints. With joint partially flexed, 20- to 22-gauge needle inserted obliquely from dorsomedial or dorsolateral aspect

Wrist. With joint slightly flexed, needle inserted just distal to radius at ulnar margin of extensor pollicis longus tendon (demarcation of anatomic snuffbox)

Source: ©2010. Used with permission of Elsevier. All rights reserved.

For practice reporting arthrocentesis procedures, complete the exercises in There's a Code for That 15.2.

15.2

There's a Code for That

Arthrocentesis

Read the following documentation of the procedure test and identify the correct arthrodesis procedure code(s).

1. Arthrocentesis of bilateral elbow joints with ultrasound guidance.

   CPT code: _____ - _____

2. Cortisone injection of right hip, without ultrasound guidance.

   CPT code: _____ - _____

3. Aspiration of ganglion cyst of the left scapholunate and radioscaphoid joints.

   CPT code: _____, _____ - _____

Fracture Repair

Fracture repair and treatment is a large part of the job of an orthopedist. Coding for fracture repair correctly requires knowing the types of fractures as well as the various treatment techniques; this includes the differences in closed, open, and percutaneous skeletal fixation treatments for fractures.

Closed Treatment of Fractures

Closed treatment of a fracture means that the site of the fracture is not surgically opened to perform the repair. Closed treatment of a fracture is performed via four different methods:

- *With manipulation.* Manipulation is the attempt to return a fractured bone to its original location with manually applied forces. In other words, manipulation is the orthopedist applying forces by hand to put the bones back in place—pushing, pulling, or twisting the bone until it is in the original location (see figure 15.4).
- *Without manipulation.*
- *With traction.* Traction is the use of mechanical devices and mechanisms to straighten bones or relieve pressure. This is different than manipulation, which is done with hands. Traction employs the use of straps and sometimes mechanical devices such as pins or screws. There are two types of traction—skin traction and skeletal traction.
  - Skin traction uses straps, ropes, pulleys, and weights that are applied externally to the skin to slowly stretch and realign bones into place until they can be set and casted until fully healed (see figure 15.5).
  - Skeletal traction is an invasive form of traction in which a screw, pin, or wire is inserted into the bone, after which weights, ropes, and pulleys are used to pull the bone into the correct position.
- *Without traction.*

Figure 15.4. Closed treatment of Colles' fracture with manipulation

Reduction of Colles' fracture by manipulation method under local (infiltration) anesthesia:
1: Hyperextension and traction to break up impaction combined with direct thumb pressure; countertraction and fixation of forearm by assistant

2: With continued traction, counter-traction, ulnar deviation of the hand, and thumb pressure, the ends of the fragments are brought into apposition; the operator's index fingers press on the proximal fragment while the thumbs press on the distal one

3. The hand is now quickly flexed at the wrist, maintaining traction and pressure on the fragments to bring them into alignment.

A Colles' fracture is a common fracture of the distal radius, which often occurs as a result of a fall onto an outstretched hand.

Figure 15.5. Closed treatment of Colles' fracture with skin traction

Closed Reduction and Plaster Cast Immobilization of Colles Fracture

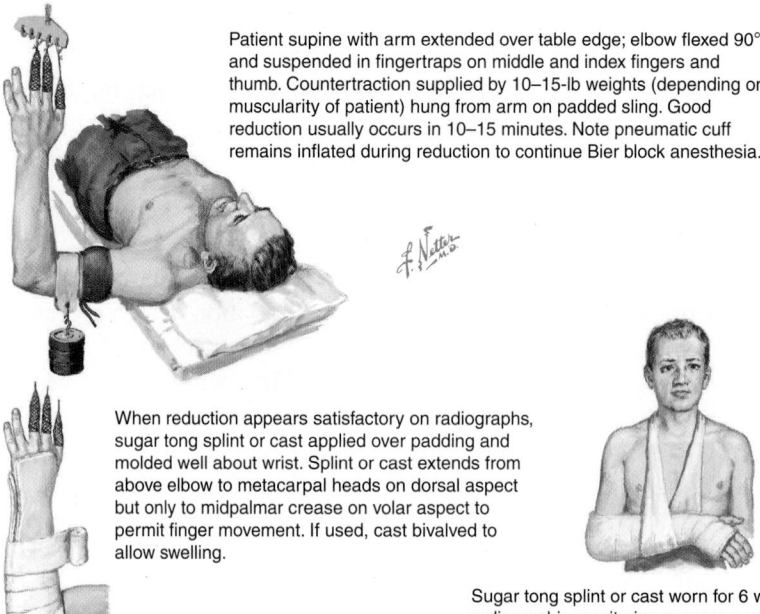

Patient supine with arm extended over table edge; elbow flexed 90° and suspended in fingertraps on middle and index fingers and thumb. Countertraction supplied by 10–15-lb weights (depending on muscularity of patient) hung from arm on padded sling. Good reduction usually occurs in 10–15 minutes. Note pneumatic cuff remains inflated during reduction to continue Bier block anesthesia.

When reduction appears satisfactory on radiographs, sugar tong splint or cast applied over padding and molded well about wrist. Splint or cast extends from above elbow to metacarpal heads on dorsal aspect but only to midpalmar crease on volar aspect to permit finger movement. If used, cast bivalved to allow swelling.

Sugar tong splint or cast worn for 6 weeks. Frequent radiographic monitoring necessary, especially during first 2 weeks. If slippage occurs, reduction repeated.

Open Treatment of Fractures

Open treatment of a fracture means that the fracture site has been surgically opened to see the fracture area or apply internal fixation devices. An internal fixation device is a device inserted into or across a bone or set of bones to fix it into place. Internal fixation devices are typically made from stainless steel or titanium and include plates, screws, nails, rods, wires, or pins (see figure 15.6).

Figure 15.6. Internal fixation device of the humerus

Source: Dilmen 2011.

Key to Success

Do not confuse open and closed *treatment* of fractures with open and closed *fractures*. Open and closed treatments refer to the way in which a fracture is treated. Open and closed fractures refer to the clinical presentation of the fracture (fracture types are discussed later in the chapter).

Percutaneous Skeletal Fixation

Percutaneous skeletal fixation is a type of fracture treatment in which fixation devices are placed across the fracture site, usually under x-ray imaging guidance. This procedure is neither closed (because it does break the skin), nor open (as the fracture site or bone is not surgically opened for visualization), but rather percutaneous. **Percutaneous** means through the skin, which is achieved by creating a small puncture in the skin and then inserting the medical instrument into the body through this opening. Percutaneous fixation is a process in which the fixation device(s) are placed through the skin and into the bone (see figure 15.7).

Figure 15.7. Percutaneous skeletal fixation of the tibia

Fractured tibia

External Fixation

Source: ©AHIMA.

Coding for Fracture Repair

Codes for fracture repair depend on the bone and the type of fracture treatment, including the elements discussed previously—with or without manipulation, open versus closed treatment, with or without traction (identify the type of traction, such as skin traction or skeletal traction), or with percutaneous skeletal fixation. To find the code for the fracture repair, search for the term *Fracture* in the CPT Index, followed by the subterm for the fracture site, and then the treatment type. If percutaneous skeletal fixation is provided along with fracture repair, report one code for each repair performed. For example, code 27517, Closed treatment of distal femoral epiphyseal separation; with manipulation, with or without skin or skeletal traction, identifies the manipulation (*with manipulation*), whether it was open or closed (*closed*), traction (*with or without skin or skeletal traction*). Note that skeletal fixation is not described in this code, which means that it was not an element in this fracture repair. See figure 15.8 for the elements of fracture repair coding.

Figure 15.8. Fracture repair coding

Application of Casts and Strapping

Typically after a fracture is repaired or set, a cast or strapping is applied to the body to immobilize the fracture site during the healing process. This initial application of casts or strapping is included in the procedure code for the procedure performed.

Codes for the Application of Casts or Strapping (29000 to 29799) should only be reported in the following instances:

- When the cast or application procedure is a replacement procedure performed during or after the period of follow-up care. For example, the initial cast was removed to gain access to the fracture site or due to damage, then the reapplication of the cast or strapping may be coded.

- When the application of cast or strapping is an initial service performed on a fracture, dislocation, or other injury that requires stabilization. For example, if the initial fracture did not require manipulation, fixation, or surgical repair, and only a cast was applied for mobilization. (AMA 2018)

Codes for the application of casts and strapping include removal of the cast or strapping, so when a patient presents for the removal of a cast it is not billable as a separate service.

Code selection depends on the site of the application of cast or strapping, and the type of cast or strapping used. When a separate brace, splint, or other permanent supply item is used, report the supply with the appropriate HCPCS code (as discussed in chapter 6, Supplies and Services). For example, HCPCS code A4580, Cast supplies (e.g., plaster), or A4590, Special casting material (e.g., fiberglass).

Complete the exercises in There's a Code for That 15.3 for practice reporting procedure codes for fracture repair, casts, and strapping procedures.

Fracture repair, casts, and strapping

15.3

There's a Code for That

Read the following documentation of the procedure test and identify the correct fracture repair, cast, and/or strapping procedure code(s).

1. Closed repair of right humeral fracture with manipulation and skeletal traction.

   CPT code: _____ - _____

2. Open treatment of fracture of displaced intraarticular calcaneous with internal fixation and primary iliac autograft.

   CPT code: _____

3. Closed treatment of fractures of the first, second, and third metacarpal bones, with manipulation.

   CPT code: _____, _____ - _____,

   _____ - _____

4. Closed reduction of fracture of the left fifth metacarpal base, with manipulation and percutaneous pinning.

   CPT code: _____, _____

5. Established patient with distal fracture of the left radius and ulna present for x-ray and evaluation of healing. She is one-month status post initial treatment, which involved a closed treatment of the fracture with skin traction and manipulation, and the insertion of pins. Complete x-ray of the left wrist completed today reveals a normally healing bone. Pins are stable and in original location. Fracture is re-casted with short-arm cast for immobility and patient is advised to return to office in two weeks for follow-up x-ray and evaluation.

   CPT code: _____, _____

Hip and Knee Replacements

Hip and knee replacements are commonly performed by orthopedic hip or knee surgeons. Known as **arthroplasty** procedures (surgical repair of a joint), they both replace the joint with a prosthetic device, with the goal of returning the joint to its previous functionality.

Coding for hip replacements depends on whether the replacement was a hemiarthroplasty (partial replacement), coded with 27125, Hemiarthroplasty, hip, partial (e.g., femoral stem prosthesis, bipolar arthroplasty), or if the procedure was a total hip replacement. A total hip replacement is coded with 27130, Arthroplasty, acetabular and proximal femoral prosthetic replacement (total hip arthroplasty), with or without autograft or allograft. Additional codes identify revision of previous hip replacement components and conversion from hip surgery to total hip arthroplasty (27132 to 27138). Hip prosthesis revisions are commonly performed to repair a hip prosthesis that has become damaged due to infection or due to regular wear and tear of the joint.

Codes for knee replacements, such as 27445, Arthroplasty, knee, hinge prosthesis (e.g., Walldius type), and knee prosthesis revisions, such as 27486, Revision of total knee arthroplasty, with or without allograft; 1 component, are dependent on the components included in the procedure. For example: 27446, Arthroplasty, knee, condyle and plateau; *medial OR lateral compartment,* or 27447, Arthroplasty, knee, condyle and plateau; *medial AND lateral compartments with or without patella resurfacing (total knee arthroplasty)* both describe different components included in the knee arthroplasty procedure. See figure 15.9 for an illustration of a total knee arthroplasty.

Figure 15.9. Total knee arthroplasty

Source: BruceBlaus 2015.

Arthrodesis and Spinal Instrumentation

Arthrodesis is the surgical fixation of a joint, performed to treat deformities of the bones and pain (see figure 15.10 for an image of arthrodesis of the spine). Codes for arthrodesis are based on the joint(s) involved, extent of the procedure, type of internal fixation (if applicable), and whether or not any grafts were used during the procedure. For example, an arthrodesis of the wrist could be reported with code 25820, Arthrodesis, wrist; limited, without bone graft (e.g., intercarpal or radiocarpal).

Arthrodesis of the spine is by far the most complex area for coding arthrodesis procedures. Arthrodesis of the spine codes first rely in the approach: lateral extracavitary (22532 to 22534); anterior or anterolateral (22548 to 22586); or posterior, posterolateral or lateral transverse process (22590 to 22634); or by spinal deformity, such as scoliosis

Figure 15.10. Arthrodesis of the spine

Source: BruceBlaus 2013.

or kyphosis (22800 to 22819). For example, 22800, Arthrodesis, posterior, for spinal deformity, with or without cast; up to 6 vertebral segments.

The approach technique, such as anterior or posterior, should be listed in the procedural description, and the coder should be able to discern this information to select the correct code. After the approach technique or medical condition is identified, codes depend on the site of the fusion, and may identify either the general vertebral area (cervical, thoracic, lumbar), or specific vertebrae involved in the procedure.

Because a vertebra cannot be fused to itself, it must be fused to another vertebra, either above or below it. The space between the two vertebrae is referred to as an **interspace** and the two vertebrae with the space between it is referred to as a **segment**. The CPT code book uses these two terms interchangeably when reporting the codes for the spaces between vertebrae. Some codes for arthrodesis procedures refer to the spaces between as segments, such as code 22802, Arthrodesis, posterior, for spinal deformity, with or without cast; 7 to 12 vertebral segments, while others refer to the spaces between as interspaces, such as 22585, Arthrodesis, anterior interbody technique, including minimal discectomy to prepare interspace (other than for decompression); each additional interspace.

When reporting arthrodesis for more interspaces than listed in the primary code, the coder should report the add-on code according the additional number of interspaces. For example, if a surgeon performed an arthrodesis of the thoracic vertebra T1 through T3, then this wound counts as two interspaces (or segments) (the space between T1 and T2, and T2 and T3), and would be coded as follows (count the spaces between the two vertebrae to total the correct number of procedures):

22532, Arthrodesis lateral extracavitary technique, including minimal discectomy to prepare interspace (other than for decompression); *thoracic*

22534, Arthrodesis lateral extracavitary technique, including minimal discectomy to prepare interspace (other than for decompression); thoracic or lumbar, *each additional vertebral segment*

Code 22532 identifies the surgical fixation of the first space, and code 22534 identifies the surgical fixation of the second space. 22534 is an add-on code, which is used to identify each additional vertebral segment involved in the procedure, and should be reported as many times as necessary to identify each segment. Count the spaces between the two vertebrae to count the correct number of procedures.

Amputation

An **amputation** is the complete removal of a body part, performed to remove dead, diseased, or damaged tissue, leaving only healthy and functional tissue behind. Depending on the site and cause of the amputation, it may be necessary to perform multiple amputations at the same site, moving from distal toward more proximal areas. Codes for amputations are based on the site of the amputation, any additional procedures, and whether the procedure is an initial (first) or a re-amputation (a subsequent amputation at the same body site, at a higher level).

To find the code for an amputation, search for the term *Amputation* in the CPT Index, and then the subterm for the area that was amputated. For example, the code for a single toe amputation would be 28810, Amputation, metatarsal, with toe, single.

Arthroscopy

An **arthroscopy** is an endoscopically-assisted procedure of a joint. Arthroscopies are less invasive than open surgeries and are used to perform repairs of a joint without

Figure 15.11. Arthroscopic surgery of the patella

Patellar Arthroscopic Surgery

Intraarticular shaver used to resect patellar area affected by severe chondromalacia

Arthroscopic appearance immediately after patellar shave

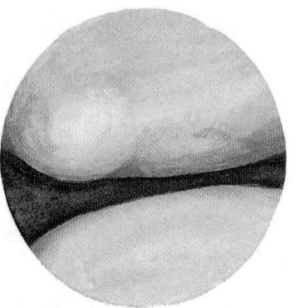

Fibrocartilaginous repair of articular surface of patella 15 months after shave

Preoperative "skyline" x-ray showing lateral subluxation of patella caused by imbalance of medial and lateral vastus muscles

Arthroscopic view of trans-cutaneous lateral release of patella by knife blade

Transcutaneous lateral release of patella guided by outside palpation and arthroscopic television monitoring

Postoperative x-ray showing reduction of patella in articular groove of femur

open surgery (see figure 15.11). Codes for arthroscopies are initially based on the joint involved, and then whether the procedure was diagnostic (with or without biopsy) or surgical. Codes for surgical arthroscopies are based on the type of surgery performed during the procedure. For example, code 29866, Arthroscopy, knee surgical; osteochondral autograft(s) (e.g., mosaicplasty) (includes harvesting of the autograft).

For practice reporting codes for orthopedic procedures, complete the exercises in There's a Code for That 15.4.

Orthopedic procedures

15.4

There's a Code for That

Read the following documentation of the procedure test and identify the procedure code(s).

1. Arthrodesis of T9 through T12, posterior approach.

   CPT code: _____, _____ X _____

2. Arthroscopic rotator cuff repair with partial acromioplasty, distal clavicle resection, and biceps tenodesis. (Hint: All these procedures were performed arthroscopically.)

   CPT code: _____, _____ - _____,

   _____ - _____, _____

Diagnostic Coding for Orthopedic Services

Diagnosis coding for orthopedic services requires an in-depth knowledge of two chapters in the ICD-10-CM code book—chapter 13: Diseases of the Musculoskeletal System and Connective Tissue, and chapter 19: Injury, Poisoning, and Certain Other Consequences of External Causes. Chapter 13 includes the myriad medical conditions that affect the musculoskeletal system, such as arthritis and osteoarthritis, gout, acquired joint disorders, joint pain and effusion, connective tissue disorders, spinal and vertebral conditions, and soft tissue disorders. Chapter 19 includes the myriad injuries to the musculoskeletal system, like fractures, sprains, and strains. Additional codes used by orthopedists may include those for congenital anomalies, nervous system disorders, and codes to identify underlying and comorbid conditions.

Coding for orthopedic diagnoses requires strict attention to detail, especially when it comes to fracture coding because fracture diagnosis codes are by far the most extensive set of diagnosis codes in the ICD-10-CM code book. Many codes require the following:

- *The specific identification of the site involved, including laterality.* Remember that if a condition presents bilaterally but no bilateral code exists, assign one code for each side (right and left).

- *Type of encounter.* The type of encounter is especially complicated for fracture codes, which can have up to 16 different encounter types.

- *External causes of injury.* If the patient has suffered any type of injury, the external cause codes for the injury need to be reported in addition to the primary code for the injury. (Refer to chapter 4 for instructions on how to use the Index to External Causes and chapter 10 for discussion of coding for external causes).

The following sections discuss diagnostic coding for fractures, arthropathies, spinal and vertebral conditions, sprains and strains, congenital and acquired deformities, and amputations.

Coding for Fractures

Fracture coding is detailed and includes many different components of the condition. When a patient has multiple fractures, sequence the worst or most severe fracture first. Code selection for fractures depends on the fracture type, fracture pattern, displacement of the bone, location of the fracture, the episode of care and healing status, and the external causes of the injury.

Key to Success

Remember, "worst comes first" when sequencing any injuries. This includes fractures. When multiple fractures are present, sequence the most severe fracture before less severe fractures.

Fracture Type

There are two main divisions in fracture coding—traumatic or pathological fractures. Pathological fractures are reported with codes from chapter 13 of the ICD-10-CM code book (the musculoskeletal system chapter), whereas traumatic fractures are reported with codes from chapter 19 of the ICD-10-CM code book (the injury chapter). See figure 15.12 for the OGCR related to coding for pathological fractures.

- A **pathological fracture** is one that occurs in a diseased bone, such as osteoporosis or neoplastic disease (bone cancer). These conditions are reported with codes from category M84, Disorder of continuity of bone. Pathological fractures that occur with osteoporosis are reported with the appropriate code from category

Figure 15.12. OGCR I.C.13.c and d

---

13. Chapter 13: Diseases of the Musculoskeletal System and Connective Tissue (M00-M99)

c. Coding of Pathologic Fractures

7th character A is for use as long as the patient is receiving active treatment for the fracture. While the patient may be seen by a new or different provider over the course of treatment for a pathological fracture, assignment of the 7th character is based on whether the patient is undergoing active treatment and not whether the provider is seeing the patient for the first time.

7th character, D is to be used for encounters after the patient has completed active treatment **for the fracture and is receiving routine care for the fracture during the healing or recovery phase**. The other 7th characters, listed under each subcategory in the Tabular List, are to be used for subsequent encounters for routine care of fractures during the healing and recovery phase as well as treatment of problems associated with the healing, such as malunions, nonunions, and sequelae.

Care for complications of surgical treatment for fracture repairs during the healing or recovery phase should be coded with the appropriate complication codes.

See Section I.C.19. Coding of traumatic fractures.

d. Osteoporosis

Osteoporosis is a systemic condition, meaning that all bones of the musculoskeletal system are affected. Therefore, site is not a component of the codes under category M81, Osteoporosis without current pathological fracture. The site codes under category M80, Osteoporosis with current pathological fracture, identify the site of the fracture, not the osteoporosis.

1) Osteoporosis without pathological fracture

Category M81, Osteoporosis without current pathological fracture, is for use for patients with osteoporosis who do not currently have a pathologic fracture due to the osteoporosis, even if they have had a fracture in the past. For patients with a history of osteoporosis fractures, status code Z87.310, Personal history of (healed) osteoporosis fracture, should follow the code from M81.

2) Osteoporosis with current pathological fracture

Category M80, Osteoporosis with current pathological fracture, is for patients who have a current pathologic fracture at the time of an encounter. The codes under M80 identify the site of the fracture. A code from category M80, not a traumatic fracture code, should be used for any patient with known osteoporosis who suffers a fracture, even if the patient had a minor fall or trauma, if that fall or trauma would not usually break a normal, healthy bone.

M80, Osteoporosis with current pathological fracture. Stress or fatigue fractures are also classified within category M84.

- A **traumatic fracture** is one that occurs as a result of some sort of traumatic injury. These conditions are reported with codes from chapter 19, to report the injury (fracture). Traumatic fractures can be either open or closed.
  - A **closed fracture** is one in which the broken bone does not penetrate the skin. If a fracture is not documented as either open or closed, report the code for the closed fracture (closed fracture is the default code).
  - An **open fracture**, also known as a **compound fracture**, is one in which the bone penetrates the skin. Open fractures can range from minor to complex, with vascular involvement. To classify the severity of an open fracture, the ICD-10-CM code book employs the Gustilo-Anderson classification system, discussed as follows.

Key to Success

If the documentation of the fracture does not specify if the fracture is open or closed, report the code for a closed fracture. If the fracture is not specified as open, report the closed fracture code.

Key to Success

When coding for fractures, it is important to distinguish between traumatic and non-traumatic fractures first, as each will lead you in two completely different directions. When searching for fractures in the Index of the ICD-10-CM code book, look up the term *Fracture*. (This is a large section.) The very first section of fracture entries is *Fracture, nontraumatic*, and then *Fracture, pathological*. All subsequent subterms are for pathological or non-traumatic fractures. Next, scan for the next fracture heading for *Fracture, traumatic*; all of these subterms are for traumatic fractures. If necessary, draw a line in the Index of your ICD-10-CM code book to make this difference more obvious.

- *Gustilo-Anderson classification* is used to identify the type of open fracture, which is included as part of the code description for open fractures. The classification system is as follows (see figure 15.13):
  - Type I. This is an open fracture with a clean wound less than 1 cm long.
  - Type II. This is an open fracture with an open wound greater than 1 cm long, which does not have extensive soft tissue damage, flaps, or avulsions of tissue.
  - Type IIIA. This is an open fracture with soft tissue coverage of the wound measuring more than 10 cm, with extensive soft tissue lacerations or flaps, or one due to high-energy trauma.
  - Type IIIB. This is an open fracture with extensive soft tissue injury and bone exposure, usually highly contaminated with foreign material.
  - Type IIIC. This is an open fracture that involves a large wound with arterial injury. (Kim 2012)

Figure 15.13. Gustilo-Anderson classification

Gustilo and Anderson classification of open fracture

Type I. Wound <1 cm long

Type II. Wound 1 to 10 cm long but without significant soft tissue stripping, gross contamination, or high-energy fracture patterns

Type IIIA. Wound >10 cm long or lesser skin lesions with gross contamination and/or high-energy fracture patterns. Bone coverage adequate

Type IIIB. Extensive soft tissue stripping that typically needs some type of soft tissue flap for coverage

Type IIIC. Large wound with major arterial injury

Fracture Pattern

The pattern of the fracture identifies the way in which the bone broke, and this is an important consideration in the way the fracture is treated. The treatment performed for each of these fractures depends on the severity and location of the fracture. For example, a mild transverse fracture may be treated without manipulation and a simple cast, whereas a severe transverse fracture of a long bone of the upper extremity may require open treatment or skeletal fixation. The following fracture types impact code selection for certain bones, when applicable (see figure 15.14):

- **Greenstick fractures** occur when a bone bends and cracks on one side (similar to a green branch, which may bend and only break one side). This fracture type occurs most often in children, as their bones are less brittle and more flexible, which results in incomplete fractures.
- **Transverse fractures** travel horizontally across the bone.
- **Spiral fractures** spiral around and extend down the length of the bone.
- **Oblique fractures** travel diagonally across the bone.
- **Comminuted fractures** have more than two parts, usually with multiple broken pieces.
- **Segmental fractures** are made up of at least two fracture lines, which isolate a larger section of bone.
- **Torus fractures** occur in children, when only one part of the bone buckles. This is also referred to as an incomplete fracture.
- **Impacted fracture** are ones in which the ends of a bone are pushed into each other. This is also referred to as a buckle fracture.
- **Compression fractures** are found in the spine, and occur when one or more vertebrae collapse under their own pressure.

Figure 15.14. Fracture patterns

Source: OpenStax College 2013.

Displacement

Fractures are identified as either displaced or non-displaced. A displaced fracture is one in which the bone moves so the two ends of the bones are misaligned (see figure 15.15). A non-displaced fracture is one in which the bone itself is fractured, but the bone has not moved and is still properly aligned. If a fracture is not documented as either displaced or non-displaced, report the code for the displaced fracture (displaced fracture is the default code).

Location

Fracture codes often identify the exact location of the fracture—both the involved in the fracture and the precise site of the fracture, such as the shaft, head, neck, distal,

Figure 15.15. Types of fracture displacement

Valgus angulation   Varus angulation   Anterior angulation   Posterior angulation

Shortening   Translation

proximal, styloid process, epiphysis, and such. The laterality is also indicated as left or right. There are no bilateral fracture codes; if the condition presents bilaterally, assign one code for each side. **Physeal fractures**, fractures of the growth plate in long bones in children, are identified using the **Salter-Harris classification** system (see figure 15.16). This classification identifies the type of physeal fracture, according to the following:

Figure 15.16. Salter-Harris classification

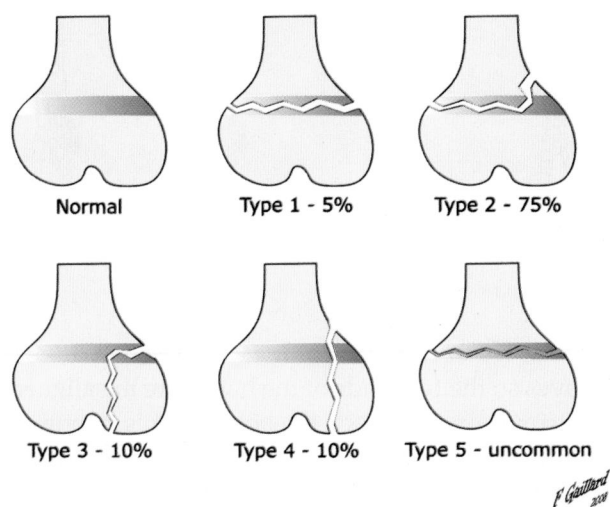

Normal   Type 1 - 5%   Type 2 - 75%

Type 3 - 10%   Type 4 - 10%   Type 5 - uncommon

Source: Gaillard 2012.

- Type I fractures pass all the way through the growth plate, completely missing the bone.

- Type II fractures pass through most of the growth plate and upward through the metaphysis of the bone.

- Type III fractures pass through the growth plate and down through the epiphysis.

- Type IV fractures pass through the entire growth plate, including the metaphysis and the epiphysis.

- Type V are a crushing type injury, which do not displace the growth plate but cause direct damage to it (Cepela 2016).

Figure 15.17 lists additional OGCR related to coding for traumatic fractures.

Figure 15.17. OGCR I.C.19.c.1 and OGCR I.C.19.c.2

---

c. Coding of Traumatic Fractures

The principles of multiple coding of injuries should be followed in coding fractures. Fractures of specified sites are coded individually by site in accordance with both the provisions within categories S02, S12, S22, S32, S42, S49, S52, S59, S62, S72, S79, S82, S89, S92 and the level of detail furnished by medical record content.

A fracture not indicated as open or closed should be coded to closed. A fracture not indicated whether displaced or not displaced should be coded to displaced.

More specific guidelines are as follows:

1) Initial vs. Subsequent Encounter for Fractures

Traumatic fractures are coded using the appropriate 7th character for initial encounter (A, B, C) for each encounter where the patient is receiving active treatment for the fracture. The appropriate 7th character for initial encounter should also be assigned for a patient who delayed seeking treatment for the fracture or nonunion.

Fractures are coded using the appropriate 7th character for subsequent care for encounters after the patient has completed active treatment of the fracture and is receiving routine care for the fracture during the healing or recovery phase.

Care for complications of surgical treatment for fracture repairs during the healing or recovery phase should be coded with the appropriate complication codes.

Care of complications of fractures, such as malunion and nonunion, should be reported with the appropriate 7th character for subsequent care with nonunion (K, M, N,) or subsequent care with malunion (P, Q, R).

Malunion/nonunion: The appropriate 7th character for initial encounter should also be assigned for a patient who delayed seeking treatment for the fracture or nonunion.

The open fracture designations in the assignment of the 7th character for fractures of the forearm, femur and lower leg, including ankle are based on the Gustilo open fracture classification. When the Gustilo classification type is not specified for an open fracture, the 7th character for open fracture type I or II should be assigned (B, E, H, M, Q).

A code from category M80, not a traumatic fracture code, should be used for any patient with known osteoporosis who suffers a fracture, even if the patient had a minor fall or trauma, if that fall or trauma would not usually break a normal, healthy bone.

See Section I.C.13. Osteoporosis.

The aftercare Z codes should not be used for aftercare for traumatic fractures. For aftercare of a traumatic fracture, assign the acute fracture code with the appropriate 7th character.

2) Multiple fractures sequencing

Multiple fractures are sequenced in accordance with the severity of the fracture.

Source: CMS 2018.

Episode of Care and Healing Status

Identifying the episode of care for fracture codes is complicated, and for some fracture types there are as many as 16 different classifications (see figure 15.18 for a list of the 16 seventh-character encounter types). Follow these steps to identify the correct encounter of care:

Figure 15.18. Encounters of care for fracture codes*

	The appropriate seventhcharacter is to be added to all codes form category S52
A	initial encounter for closed fracture
B	initial encounter for open fracture type I or II initial encounter for open fracture NOS
C	initial encounter for open fracture type IIIA, IIIB, or IIIC
D	subsequent encounter for closed fracture with routine healing
E	subsequent encounter for open fracture type I or II with routine healing
F	subsequent encounter for open fracture type IIIA, IIIB, or IIIC with routine healing
G	subsequent encounter for closed fracture with delayed healing
H	subsequent encounter for open fracture type I or II with delayed healing
J	subsequent encounter for open fracture type IIIA, IIIB, or IIIC with delayed healing
K	subsequent encounter for closed fracture with nonunion
M	subsequent encounter for open fracture type I or II with nonunion
N	subsequent encounter for open fracture type IIIA, IIIB, or IIIC with nonunion
P	subsequent encounter for closed fracture with malunion
Q	subsequent encounter for open fracture type I or II with malunion
R	subsequent encounter for open fracture type IIIA, IIIB, or IIIC with malunion
S	sequela

⇧ **Encounter**　⇧ **Open or closed fracture**　⇧ **Gustilo classification**　⇧ **Healing status**

*Not all 16 episodes of care are options for all fracture codes.

- The episode of care should be identified as either initial, subsequent, or sequela.
- For open fracture, identify the Gustilo classification for the fracture, in terms of type I or II, or type IIIA, IIIB, or IIIC.
- For subsequent encounters, identify the healing status of the fracture, in terms of:
  - Routine healing
  - Delayed healing
  - Nonunion of fracture (when the bones have not fused back together)
  - Malunion of fracture (when the bones have fused back together in the wrong position)

External Causes of the Injury

Codes for the external cause of the injury identify the injury mechanism (how the patient was injured), place of occurrence when the injury happened, activity in which the patient was engaged when the injury occurred, and patient status at the time of injury.

Review figures 15.19 and 15.20, which illustrate the components of fracture codes and a decision process for fracture coding, then complete the exercises in There's a Code for That 15.5 for practice reporting fracture diagnosis codes.

Figure 15.19. Fracture code components

S52.342M, Displaced spiral fracture of shaft of radius, left arm, subsequent encounter for open fracture type I or II with nonunion

Fracture type: open
Gustilo classification: type I or II
Pattern: spiral
Displacement: displaced
Location: shaft of radius
Laterality: left
Encounter: subsequent
Healing status: nonunion

Figure 15.20. Fracture coding

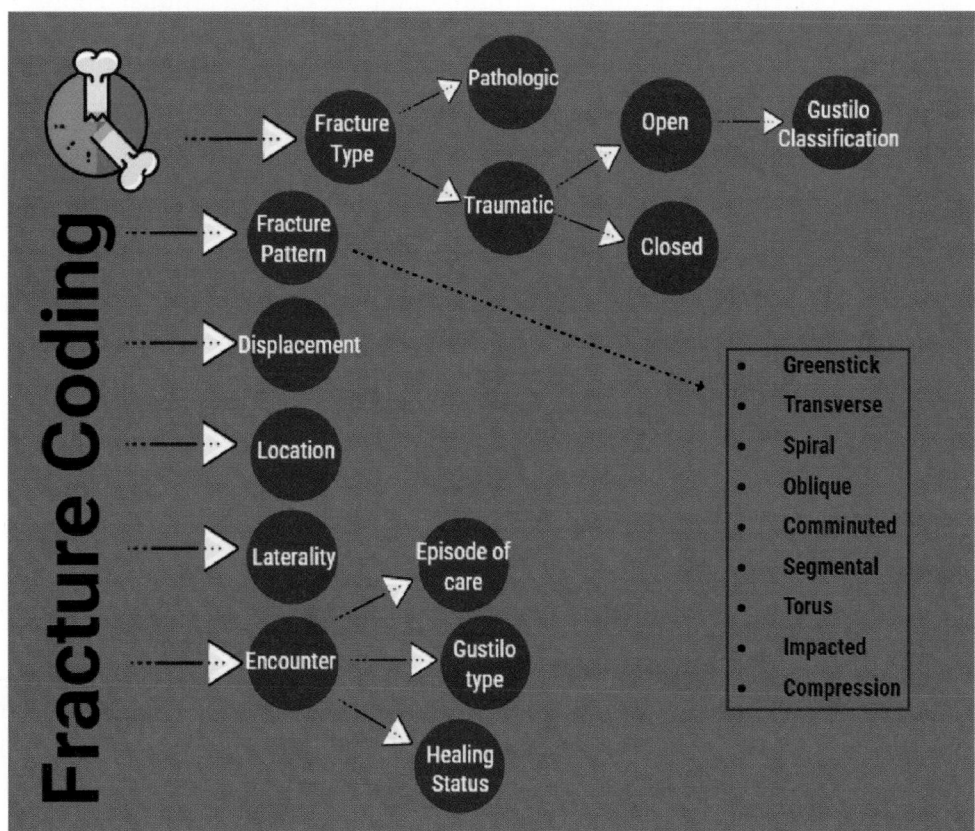

(Continued on next page)

Fracture coding

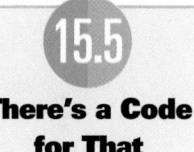

There's a Code for That

Read the following documentation of and assign the appropriate diagnosis code(s) for the fracture and any additional conditions.

1. 27-year-old male presents for initial treatment of his closed trimalleolar fracture of the left ankle.

   ICD-10-CM code: _____

2. 27-year-old male presents for removal of cast and subsequent x-ray of his trimalleolar fracture of the left ankle. X-ray reveals nonunion of the fracture.

   ICD-10-CM code: _____

3. X-ray results reveal an open, type II, displaced compound comminuted fracture of the right radial shaft.

   ICD-10-CM code: _____

4. Frontal skull fracture with subsequent subdural hemorrhage.

   ICD-10-CM codes: _____, _____

5. Sports-related injuries resulting in fractures of three right ribs, fractured right wrist, and contusion of right chest over rib fractures.

   ICD-10-CM codes: _____, _____

Continued

6. 60-year-old female presents with arthritis of the left hip as a residual of hip fracture five years ago.

ICD-10-CM codes: _____, _____

7. Traumatic lateral epicondyle fracture of the left elbow, subsequent encounter with routine healing.

ICD-10-CM codes: _____

8. Stress fracture of right foot, subsequent encounter with delayed healing.

ICD-10-CM codes: _____

9. Pathological fracture of right humerus due to secondary neoplasm of bone. Secondary encounter for evaluation of nonunion of fracture.

ICD-10-CM codes: _____, _____

 ## Arthropathies

An **arthropathy** is any disease of the joints, the most common of which is **arthritis**, an inflammation of the joints. There are numerous types of arthritis including infectious arthritis (as a response to an infectious organism), rheumatoid arthritis (RA), and juvenile arthritis. Most forms of arthritis (not osteoarthritis) are also included in HCC coding, so documentation of these conditions is especially important. **Osteoarthritis** is a type of arthritis that results from wear and tear on the joints over a period of time, and often occurs in the hips and knees.

Coding for arthritis thus requires identification of the type of arthritis. It further requires identification of the location and the specific joint(s) involved. Arthritis that occurs in many different areas is referred to as **polyarthritis** or polyosteoarthritis, while arthritis in a localized joint is referred to as **monoarthritis**. It is also important to identify any underlying or comorbid conditions. For example, M08.261, Juvenile rheumatoid arthritis with systemic onset, right knee, identifies the type of arthritis (*juvenile RA with systemic onset*), the location and joint involved (*right knee*).

Spinal and Vertebral Conditions

Many of the spinal and vertebral conditions discussed in chapter 12 (Anesthesia and Pain Management) may also be treated by orthopedic spinal surgeons for definitive repair and treatment. These conditions include intervertebral disc disorders, spinal stenosis, neck and back pain, and radiculopathy. Remember that most of these conditions require specific identification on where exactly the condition occurs: occipito-atlanto-axial, cervical, cervicothoracic, thoracic, thoracolumbar, lumbar, lumbosacral, sacral, and sacrococcygeal sites.

Sprains and Strains

Sprains and strains are common joint injuries and are usually managed by sports medicine providers, especially for patients involved in sports. Though sprain and strain sound alike, do not get them confused—they are two separate conditions and are coded separately. A **sprain** is the stretching or tearing of a ligament (see figure 15.21). A **strain** is an injury to a muscle or tendon, which ranges from a simple stretching of the muscle or tendon to complete tear of the muscle and tendon (see figure 15.22).

Figure 15.21. Sprain

A sprain stretches the ligaments in the ankle and lower leg.
Source: Scientificanimations.com 2016.

Figure 15.22. Strain

Hamstring
Tendon Tear

A severe hamstring strain in which the tendon has been torn from the bone.
Source: Reprinted by permission from AAOS 2015.

Codes for sprains and strains identify the specific joint involved and the ligament, tendon, or muscle, if known. Furthermore, since these are all classified as injury codes, they all require the identification of the episode of care for the encounter. To look up the code for a sprain, search for the main term *Sprain* in the ICD-10-CM Index, and then search for the specific area of sprain. For example: S93.411A, Sprain of calcaneo-fibular ligament of right ankle, initial encounter. To search for a strain in the Index of the ICD-10-CM code book, search for either the main term *Strain*, or if the strain is of a muscle, search for the main term *Injury*, followed by *muscle*, then search for the specific muscle strained. For example: S76.311A, Strain of muscle, fascia and tendon of the posterior muscle group at thigh level, right thigh, initial encounter.

Congenital and Acquired Deformities

Both congenital and acquired deformities are treated by orthopedists and orthopedic surgeons to correct and return the body area to its original function, improve function, or to reduce pain. Congenital deformities are ones present at birth, whereas acquired conditions develop over a period of time or later in life because of a traumatic event or disease state.

Scoliosis, a condition in which the spine curves sideways (see figure 15.23), and kyphosis, a condition in which the back rounds forward, are two examples of musculoskeletal deformities that can be either congenital or acquired. When looking up a code for a musculoskeletal deformity, search for the specific term for the type of deformity, such as *Scoliosis*, and then either *acquired, congenital,* or the specified type of the deformity. Congenital disorders are all coded from chapter 17: Congenital Malformations, Deformations and Chromosomal Abnormalities of the ICD-10-CM code book.

Figure 15.23. Scoliosis

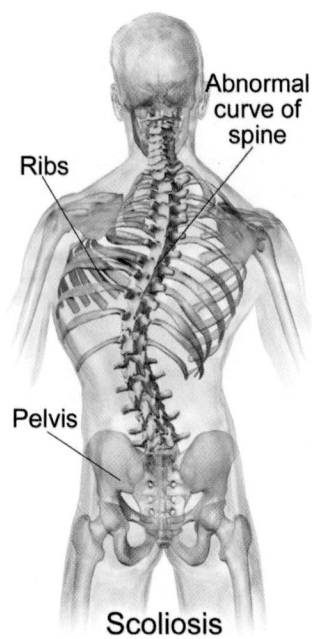

Ribs

Abnormal curve of spine

Pelvis

Scoliosis

Source: Blausen.com staff 2013.

Amputation

When coding for an amputation, search for the term *Amputation* in the ICD-10-CM Index, and then locate the code for the site of the amputation. Codes for amputations of the extremities may also identify the level of amputation, such as amputation of the lower leg (S88), which can be reported as at the knee level (S88.0-) or at level between knee and ankle (S88.1-). They further identify the amputation as either complete, in that the entire extremity has been amputated, or if the patient has suffered only a partial amputation of the extremity (in which some of the soft tissue, vascular structures, or bone remains).

If the documentation does not identify the amputation as either partial or complete, code it as a complete amputation. Because an amputation is a life-long medical condition that may require medical services for the rest of the patient's life, diagnosis codes for amputations do impact HCC coding and thus require complete documentation and careful code selection.

Orthopedic Aftercare

Aftercare is the healthcare provided to patients after the healing phase of an injury or illness has completed. Orthopedic aftercare is the care provided to patients that have sustained fractures, joint replacements, or other orthopedic services. These aftercare encounters are reported with E/M codes to identify the encounter with the patient; and medical necessity for the services is identified with the appropriate code from category Z47, Orthopedic aftercare. These aftercare services include:

- Z47.1, Aftercare following joint replacement surgery
- Z47.2, Encounter for removal of internal fixation device
- Z47.31, Aftercare following explantation of shoulder joint prosthesis
- Z47.32, Aftercare following explantation of hip joint prosthesis
- Z47.33, Aftercare following explantation of knee joint prosthesis
- Z47.81, Encounter for orthopedic aftercare following surgical amputation
- Z47.82, Encounter for orthopedic aftercare following scoliosis surgery
- Z47.89, Encounter for other orthopedic aftercare

These aftercare codes should not be used to identify care for an acute injury, but they may be used with additional codes to describe the patient's condition. For example, if a patient received a hip joint prosthesis two months ago, and presents to his or her orthopod's office for an aftercare appointment and complains of difficulty walking, then the coder would assign the Z code for the aftercare (Z47.32), and the code for difficulty walking (R26.2, Difficulty in walking, not elsewhere classified).

Pay close attention to the Tabular instructions in this range of codes to ensure that all codes are reported. For example, under code Z47.81, Encounter for orthopedic aftercare following surgical amputation, there is a note to use an additional code to identify the limb that was amputated. For practice reporting diagnosis codes for orthopedic conditions, complete the exercises in There's a Code for That 15.6.

15.6

There's a Code for That

Orthopedic diagnosis coding

Read the following documentation of and assign the appropriate diagnosis code(s) for the patient's condition(s).

1. 54-year-old male presents with instability of the right knee due to old complex tear of lateral meniscus of the right side.

   ICD-10-CM code: _____ , _____

2. 25-year-old athlete presents with peripheral tear of the medial meniscus of the left knee. She was seen at urgent care last night after sustaining the injury.

   ICD-10-CM code: _____

(Continued on next page)

15.6

Continued

3. Strain of right Achilles tendon, initial encounter.

ICD-10-CM code: _____

4. Left ACL sprain, initial encounter.

ICD-10-CM code: _____

Putting It All Together: Coding for Orthopedic Services

Coding correctly for orthopedic services requires an in-depth understanding of the Musculoskeletal System subsection of the CPT code book, as well as the ability to code for E/M and Radiology procedures, when necessary.

Determination of the correct codes relies on the answers to the following questions.

- What type of orthopedic procedure was performed?
  - Fracture repair, excision of tumor, arthrodesis, arthrocentesis, or such.
  - What technique was used for the procedure? How large was it? What components were included? Were any additional procedures performed?
- Are there any applicable modifiers for the procedure?
  - Remember to add modifiers for bilateral procedures, distinct procedural services, repeat services, and multiple procedures.
- Is there a definitive diagnosis for the procedure? If so, then code for the definitive diagnosis. If not, then code for the signs and symptoms, such as joint pain.

Study the following vignette that demonstrates how to select the appropriate diagnosis and procedure codes. Then complete the practice exercises in There's a Code for That 15.7.

It is Towana's first day on the job in the orthopedics office, and her office manager has given her a handful of easy coding cases to work on while she is still in training. She is coding the following: Two-view x-ray of the fingers of the left hand reveal closed displaced fracture of medial phalanx of left middle finger. Closed reduction with manipulation of the phalangeal shaft of the middle phalanx with application of static finger splint.

She asks herself: What did the doctor? In this case, the doctor performed an x-ray of the fingers, then reduced the fracture with manipulation, and applied a static finger splint. Since her office owns the radiology equipment and employs the orthopedist, she knows that she will bill the global fee for the x-ray. She will also need to bill for the fracture treatment as well as the cast. Because the application of the cast is included in the initial fracture treatment service, she only needs to code for the cast itself, and not the application of the cast. She selects the following codes:

- *26720, Closed treatment of phalangeal shaft fracture, proximal or middle phalanx, finger or thumb; without manipulation, each.*
- *73140, Radiologic examination, finger(s), minimum of 2 views*
- *Q4049, Finger splint, static*

Now that Towana has her procedure codes, she asks herself: Why did the doctor do it? The patient was diagnosed with a closed displaced fracture of medial phalanx of left middle finger. This was an initial encounter for the fracture because the patient is receiving active treatment for the injury. She searched the ICD-10-CM Index for Fracture, traumatic, *selects the location, laterality, and type of fracture, and adds the seventh-character extension to the end of the code for initial encounter for closed fracture. She reports the following diagnosis code:*

- *S62.623A, Displaced fracture of medial phalanx of left middle finger, initial encounter for closed fracture*

She then rechecks the documentation to make sure she has coded everything for the encounter, and reports the chosen codes.

Diagnostic and procedural coding for orthopedic services

15.7

There's a Code for That

Read the following documentation and assign the appropriate CPT, HCPCS, and ICD-10-CM code(s) for the encounter.

1. 40-year-old morbidly obese (due to excess calories) male with fever and chills presents with swelling, pain, and redness of his right knee, which has progressed over the last two days. He is a type 2 diabetic and currently dependent on chewing tobacco. Three-view x-ray of right knee are negative for fracture but are indicative of effusion. Joint aspirated of effusive fluid in office. Impression: infective tenosynovitis of the right knee.

   CPT code: _____ -_____, _____ -_____

   ICD-10-CM codes: _____, _____, _____,

   _____

2. 82-year-old otherwise healthy female slipped in the kitchen of her single-family home and fell on her left hip. AP x-ray performed in the hospital facility ED revealed displaced oblique fracture of the center of the femoral neck. Midcervical fracture of the right femur treated via open treatment of femoral fracture with placement of internal fixation device. (Tip: In this case, do not code for the x-ray, as it is performed in the emergency department setting of a hospital facility.)

   CPT code: _____ -_____

   ICD-10-CM codes: _____, _____,

   _____

HCC

End of Chapter Content

Instructions: Indicate whether the following statements are true or false (T or F). For false statements, rewrite the statement on the line below to make the statement true.

1. An orthopedic surgeon is an orthopedic doctor that specializes in surgeries of the musculoskeletal system.

   _____

   _____

2. Orthopedic services may only be performed in the surgical suite of an outpatient hospital.

   _____

   _____

3. Arthrodesis procedures aspirate fluid from a joint.

   _____

   _____

4. The Musculoskeletal System subsection in the CPT code book is organized by body area first.

   _____

   _____

5. To search for the code for an excision of a soft tissue tumor in the CPT Index, first look up the term *soft tissue.*

   _____

   _____

6. When coding for arthrodesis, vertebral segments and interspaces are measured in the same manner.

   _____

   _____

7. Manipulation of a fracture is the attempt to return the bone to its original location.

   _____

   _____

8. There are three types of traction for fracture treatments.

   _____

   _____

9. The application of a cast or strapping is included in the initial fracture repair code.

_____

_____

10. Codes for the excision of a soft tissue tumor rely on the location of the tumor, but not the size.

_____

_____

Instructions: Choose the best answer.

1. Which type of orthopedic specialist would perform a surgery of the metacarpals?

a. Orthopedic spine surgeon
b. Orthopedic hand surgeon
c. Orthopedic foot and ankle surgeon
d. Orthopedic shoulder surgeon

2. Which chapter of the ICD-10-CM code book includes the codes for fractures?

a. Diseases of the Musculoskeletal System
b. Injury, Poisoning, and Certain Other Consequences of External Causes
c. External Causes of Morbidity
d. Congenital Malformations, Deformations, and Chromosomal Abnormalities

3. Which of the following suffixes means surgical incision?

a. _-desis_
b. _-centesis_
c. _-ectomy_
d. _-otomy_

4. Which type of tumor excision includes the removal of a tumor below the skin but above the deep fascia?

a. Excision of subcutaneous soft tissue tumors
b. Excision of fascial or subfascial soft tissue tumors
c. Excision of soft connective tissue tumors
d. Excision of bone tumors

5. Which of the following arthrocentesis codes would be assigned for the finger joint?

a. 20600
b. 20605
c. 20610
d. 20612

6. Which type of fracture treatment employs the use of straps, ropes, pulleys, and weights applied externally to the body?

a. Skin traction
b. Skeletal traction
c. Percutaneous skeletal fixation
d. Internal fixation

7. Which type of fracture repair surgically opens the body to visualize the fracture site?

a. Open
b. Closed
c. Internal fixation
d. Percutaneous skeletal fixation

8. Which of the following codes would be reported for a total hip arthroplasty?

a. 27438
b. 27138
c. 27130
d. 27447

9. Which of the following ICD-10 categories would be used for a pathological fracture in osteoporosis?

a. S52
b. M80
c. M84
d. M85

10. An open fracture is also known as which of the following?

a. Closed
b. Comminuted
c. Gustilo
d. Compound

11. Which classification system is used to classify physeal fractures?

a. Gustilo-Anderson

b. Salter-Harris

c. ICD-10-CM codes

d. Rule of Nines

12. Which of the following types of fractures results in two or more fracture lines that isolate a large section of bone?

a. Comminuted

b. Compound

c. Torus

d. Segmental

13. Which of the following injuries identifies a strain?

a. The stretching of ligaments in the ankle

b. The stretching of ligaments in the shoulder

c. The tearing of muscle in the groin

d. The tearing of a ligament in the groin

Instructions: Answer the following questions with the appropriate code(s) and modifier(s).

1. Fracture of shaft of right femur, subsequent encounter for open type IIIA fracture with delayed healing. AP x-ray performed in office confirms slow healing. Long-leg cast reapplied in office and patient will follow up in three weeks.

CPT codes: _____-____,

_____-____

ICD-10-CM code: _____

2. 30-year-old male was playing basketball when he felt a snap in his left ankle and intense calf pain. This is a healthy man with unremarkable medical history. Does not smoke or drink. Physical examination revealed passive range of motion and inability to plantarflex the left foot. Two-view radiography of the left ankle is negative for fracture. Clinical impression: spontaneous rupture of Achilles tendon. Definitive procedure performed was a surgical repair and reattachment of Achilles tendon, without graft.

CPT codes: _____-____,

_____-____

ICD-10-CM code: _____, _____

3. Trigger finger of the left index, middle, and ring fingers.

ICD-10-CM code: _____, _____,

_____

4. Radial styloid tenosynovitis.

ICD-10-CM code: _____

5. Ganglion cyst of left wrist and right hip.

ICD-10-CM code: _____

6. Complete tear of the rotator cuff of the right shoulder.

ICD-10-CM code: _____

7. 43-year-old male presents with pain in the right leg and knee joint. He plays tag football on the weekend and reports falling on his knee this past weekend. X-rays negative for fracture.

ICD-10-CM code: _____

References

American Academy of Orthopaedic Surgeons. 2015. Hamstring Tendon Tear. Digital Image. American Academy of Orthopedic Surgeons. Accessed December, 2017. https://orthoinfo.aaos.org/en/diseases --conditions/sprains-strains-and-other-soft-tissue-injuries.

American Medical Association. 2018. *CPT© 2018 Professional Edition.* Chicago: AMA.

BruceBlaus. 2015. "Knee Replacement.png." Digital image. Wikimedia Commons. Accessed December, 2017. https://commons.wikimedia.org/wiki/File:Knee _Replacement.png.

BruceBlaus. 2013. "Blausen 0446 HarringtonRods. png." Digital image. Wikimedia Commons. Accessed December, 2017. https://commons.wikimedia.org/wiki /File:Blausen_0446_HarringtonRods.png.

Blausen.com staff. 2013. "Blausen 0785 Scoliosis 01.png." Digital image. Wikimedia Commons. Accessed December, 2017.

https://en.wikipedia.org/wiki/Scoliosis#/media /File:Blausen_0785_Scoliosis_01.png.

Centers for Medicare and Medicaid Services. 2018. ICD-10-CM Official Guidelines for Coding and Reporting FY 2018. https://www.cms.gov/Medicare /Coding/ICD10/Downloads/2018-ICD-10-CM-Coding-Guidelines.pdf.

Cepela, D.J., Tartaglione, J.P., and T.P. Dooley. 2016 (November). Classifications in Brief: Salter-Harris Classification of Pediatric Physeal Fractures. https://doi .org/10.1007/s11999-016-4891-3.

Dilmen, N. 2011. "Medical X-Ray imaging LHH05 nevit. jpg." Digital image. Wikimedia Commons. Accessed

December, 2017. https://commons.wikimedia.org /wiki/Category:X-rays_of_internal_fixation#/media /File:Medical_X-Ray_imaging_LHH05_nevit.jpg.

Gaillard, F. 2012. "SalterHarris.svg." Digital image. Wikimedia Commons. Accessed December, 2017. https://commons.wikimedia.org/wiki/File:SalterHarris. svg.

Kim, P.H. and S.S. Leopold. 2012 (May 9). Gustilo-Anderson Classification. *Clin Orthop Relat Res* (11): 3270–3274. https://www.ncbi.nlm.nih.gov/pmc/articles /PMC3462875/#CR17.

OpenStax College. 2013. "612 Types of Fractures.jpg." Digital Image. Wikimedia Commons. Accessed December, 2017. https://en.wikipedia.org/wiki/Bone _fracture#/media/File:612_Types_of_Fractures.jpg.

Scientificanimations.com. 2016. "Sprain SAG.jpg." Digital image. Wikimedia Commons. Accessed December, 2017. https://commons.wikimedia.org/wiki/File:Sprain _SAG.jpg.

Beach, W., and J.B. Samora. 2017. Coding and Billing: A Global Perspective. http://www.aaos.org /CustomTemplates/Content.aspx?id=22436.

Centers for Medicare and Medicaid Services. ICD-10 Clinical Concepts for Orthopedics. https://www .cms.gov/medicare/coding/icd10/downloads /icd10clinicalconceptsorthopedics1.pdf.

Haralson III, R.H.and M.S. Vaught. 2004 (August). Coding spinal procedures; Avoid confusion by following these tips. http://www2.aaos.org/bulletin/aug04/code.htm.

Jones, L. Lesion / Tumor Excision & Would Repair CPT Guidelines. https://newsletters.ahima.org /Newsletters/Code_Write/2016/November/CW1116 _LesiontumorTool.pdf.

Lohr, K.M., A. Gonsalves, L. Root, and J.K. Talbot-Stern. 2016 (September 26). Bursitis. http://emedicine .medscape.com/article/2145588-overview.

Resources

American Academy of Orthopaedic Surgeons. 2017. Sprains, Strains and Other Soft-Tissue Injuries. http://orthoinfo .aaos.org/topic.cfm?topic=a00111.

American Medical Association. 2013. *Advanced Anatomy and Physiology for ICD-10-CM/PCS*. Salt Lake City, UT: Contexo Media.

CHAPTER 16

Physical, Occupational, and Speech Therapy Services

Learning Objectives

- Understand the basics of billing and coding for physical, occupational, and speech therapy services.
- Examine procedural codes and guidelines for physical, speech, and occupational therapy services.

- Examine diagnosis coding and medical necessity for physical, speech, and occupational therapy services.
- Determine and apply ICD-10-CM, CPT, and HCPCS codes to physical, speech, and occupational therapy services.

Key Terms

8-minute rule
Amputation
Amputee
Amyotrophic lateral sclerosis (ALS)
Aphonia
Augmentative and alternative
   communication (AAC)
Cognitive communication disorder
Constant attendance code
Dentofacial anomaly
Dominant side

Dyslexia
Dysphagia
Electrical stimulation
Hubbard tank
Hypernasality
Iontophoresis
Language disorder
Multiple sclerosis (MS)
Occupational therapist (OT)
Occupational therapy services
Physical therapist (PT)

Physical therapy services
Service-based code
Social communication disorder
Speech-language pathologist
   (SLP)
Speech therapy services
Therapy services
Time-based code
Traumatic brain injury (TBI)
Treatment modality
Vasopneumatic device

Therapy services are treatments aimed at rehabilitating the patient to optimal bodily function. These services are uniquely tailored to the needs of individual patients, so that patients can receive the best possible rehabilitation or functional training to live their lives without outside support. Discussed in this chapter are physical, occupational, and speech therapy services, all of which are designed to help patients reduce pain, improve function, and live their lives as independently as possible.

Physical therapy services are noninvasive procedures and treatments that alleviate pain and improve and restore mobility to limbs and areas of the body. Occupational therapy services are noninvasive procedures aimed at improving fine motor skills and functions (such as brushing teeth or writing with a pencil). Speech therapy services, also referred to as speech language pathology, help adults and children improve their speech, advance social and cognitive communication skills, and treat swallowing disorders. Some speech therapy services may also be performed by otorhinolaryngologists, otherwise known as ear, nose, and throat doctors (ENTs), who may treat or study the medical causes of speech and swallowing disorders.

Procedural codes for therapy services make up a small slice of CPT codes, so coding for physical, occupational, or speech therapy services is not as complicated as some other specialties. This chapter discusses the basics of coding for therapy services, as well as procedural coding for therapy services and common therapy diagnosis codes.

Therapy Basics

Physical, speech, and occupational therapy services are often combined so that several providers of multiple therapy types can work together to help patients with multiple needs, such as a patient who might need physical and occupational training after receiving a lower arm prosthesis. Individual therapists may also work with medical specialists to help improve patient function and outcomes. For example, a physical therapist may work with an orthopedist or sports medicine doctor to help patients recover from sports injuries. Physical, speech, and occupational therapists must be licensed to practice in their state, and may not determine patient medical diagnoses. All of the services they perform must be requested by an authorized provider who has determined the patient's diagnosis and the need for therapy services.

When coding for therapy services, coders focus on the relatively small selection of therapy codes for physical, occupational, and speech therapy services located in the Medicine section of the CPT code book, and base diagnosis code selection on the documentation provided by the patient's requesting provider. The healthcare provider diagnoses the patient and then requests a specific therapy service from either a physical, occupational, or speech therapist to help treat a deficit (discussed in full later in this chapter). Coders must also keep in mind the basics of billing for all three types of therapy services.

Speech, physical, and occupational therapists also develop a plan of care that is individualized for each patient, which includes an evaluation of the patient and his or her speech, physical, or occupational functioning, and a plan of interventions to help the patient reach his or her goals.

This chapter discusses three types of therapy—physical, occupational, and speech—and their providers and services performed. It also identifies the settings in which services are provided, the basics of billing and coding for therapy services, and also physician orders, authorizations for therapy services, and advanced beneficiary notices (ABNs).

Physical Therapy

A **physical therapist (PT)** is a licensed healthcare professional who focuses on non-invasive procedures that alleviate pain and improve and restore mobility. Unlike surgeons who perform invasive restorative procedures, physical therapists perform an in-depth functional evaluation of each individual patient (upon physician orders) to develop a plan of care that includes multiple methods or procedures (modalities) to help improve movement, reduce pain, restore body functionality, and prevent patient disability. These services are typically provided in one or more individual treatment periods, or rehabilitative sessions, in which the therapist focuses on gross motor skills, range of motion for large joints, and body movement. PTs teach patients how to manage their own condition to achieve long-term health benefits and bodily function, often without the use of prescription medications.

PT services are usually performed immediately after an injury, surgery, or other medical condition, which may result in loss of function or disability. For example, a patient who has just received a total hip arthroplasty may receive physical therapy services after surgery to retrain the body to use the new hip joint and ensure total functionality of the hip prosthesis. This would include training in coordination, endurance, muscle function, and range of motion. PT services in this case not only help restore function but also help to regain strength, balance, prevent patient falls, and decrease pain.

Physical therapists may perform their services in various settings, including inpatient and outpatient hospitals, private practices, home healthcare agencies, nursing homes, schools, and sports and fitness facilities. For example, they may see patients in a sports facility on the weekends, at a private practice during the week, and in the outpatient hospital setting on occasion. Therefore, when coding for PT services it is important to verify the place of service code for each service performed.

Occupational Therapy

An **occupational therapist (OT)** is a healthcare professional who uses constructive activities to help restore a patient's ability to perform essential activities of daily living (occupations) and improve or maintain functional ability. Unlike physical therapists, occupational therapists focus more on fine motor skills that allow individuals to perform activities of daily living, such as brushing teeth, eating with a fork, or holding a pencil.

Occupational therapy interventions include helping children and adults with disabilities to participate in school and social settings, assisting patients with recovery from illness or injury, and restoring full function of abilities to adult patients who have suffered physical or cognitive problems, such as a stroke.

Just as physical therapists may perform their services in a number of different settings, occupational therapists also provide services across settings such as inpatient and outpatient hospitals, private practices, nursing homes, and schools. Again, always select the appropriate place of service code that corresponds to the location in which services were rendered.

Speech Therapy

A healthcare professional who provides speech therapy services is referred to as a **speech-language pathologist (SLP)**. SLPs perform a number of different procedures in the form of therapeutic services that help adults and children improve speech and social and cognitive communication skills; they also treat swallowing disorders. Speech therapy may include treatment of speaking problems (such as fluency), problems with voice resonance, and difficulties with pronunciation.

SLPs provide a wide range of services depending on the needs of the patient and include rehabilitation for patients with hearing problems, development of communication systems for patients with expressive or language comprehension problems, strengthening oral muscle function for patients with swallowing disorders, and even treatment of cognitive status such as orientation, memory, and reasoning skills.

Note that SLPs, just like PTs and OTs, may perform services across a wide range of settings including inpatient and outpatient hospitals, private practices, home healthcare agencies, nursing homes, and schools. Thus, the place of service for SLP services should always be verified when reporting codes.

Physician Orders, Authorizations, and Advanced Beneficiary Notices

When a PT, OT, or SLP provides services to a patient, is it upon the order of a healthcare provider or PCP who has either diagnosed the patient with the medical condition, disorder, or disability, r the surgeon who performed the surgery. In either case, the healthcare professional has identified that the patient needs a certain therapeutic service (PT, OT, or SLP) and referred the patient to the therapist for services. The patient's diagnosis (or signs and symptoms) are usually included on the orders for the therapy service. Because they are not medical doctors, PTs, OTs, and SLPs are not authorized to diagnose patients—they must rely on the diagnosis code(s) included on the orders for services.

Understanding the billing process for therapy claims is essential, as it may impact the way in which the claim for therapy services is coded and the amount or frequency of therapy services the patient is allowed to receive. For example, if the insurance requires that a referral is on file before the therapy services are provided, then it will not pay for any services rendered until the referral is authorized and on file.

Certain insurance companies may have a specific dollar amount capped annually for therapy services; for example, Medicare only permits a specific dollar amount for therapy services per year (CMS 2017). Anything over this amount must be specifically documented as reasonable and medically necessary or it will not be paid. This determination is made by the therapy provider, patient, and the patient's requesting healthcare provider. Ultimately, the patient's insurance can decide to approve or deny additional services (unless the patient chooses to pay for the services out-of-pocket).

If a service is provided to a Medicare patient and it is expected that Medicare will not reimburse for the service (and the patient will be responsible for payment), the patient must be given an advanced beneficiary notice (ABN) of noncoverage (discussed in chapter 2). This document notifies the patient that Medicare may not pay for the service, and that the patient may have to assume full financial responsibility for the services provided (CMS 2017).

When an ABN is given to the patient, to the coder must append a modifier to the procedure code indicating to Medicare that the ABN was provided. These include the following:

- GA, Waiver of liability statement issued as required by payer policy, individual case. This modifier indicates that the ABN was signed and is on file at the provider's office, which allows the provider to bill the patient for the service, if the service is denied by Medicare.
- GX, Notice of liability issued, voluntary under payer policy. This modifier is used to indicate that an ABN was signed for a noncovered service that will not be paid by Medicare. This service will be billed to the patient.

- GY, Item or service statutorily excluded, does not meet the definition of any Medicare benefit or, for non-Medicare insurers, is not a contract benefit. This modifier is used to notify Medicare that the provider understands that this is a noncovered service and will not be reimbursed.
- GZ, Item or service expected to be denied as not reasonable or necessary. This modifier is used to identify instances in which an ABN may have been required but was not obtained from the patient. (CMS 2015)

Other insurance payers may set a limit of services rather than a dollar amount. For example, a commercial insurance company may authorize five rehabilitation sessions for a physical therapy patient. If additional services are needed after those five services have been provided, then the insurance company must approve a new request. If it is not approved, then the patient will be responsible for the services.

The services provided by each individual therapy provider are distinct and intended to treat a specific functionality or disability with a particular modality. Procedure codes for PT, OT, and SLP services are found in the Medicine section of the CPT code book.

Key to Success

Therapy providers are not typically classified as healthcare professionals according to CMS or CPT guidelines, and are therefore unable to provide any type of medical service other than the therapy services they are qualified to perform. In other words, physical and occupational therapists and speech language pathologists are not qualified to provide evaluation and management (E/M) encounters, surgical procedures, or medical procedures other than therapy services. Qualification for therapy services depends on state licensing regulations and insurance regulations, so the exact services allowed may differ from state to state or by insurance company.

Procedural Coding for Therapy Services

Procedure codes for physical and occupational therapy, and speech language pathology services are all included in the Medicine section of the CPT code book. Physical and occupational therapy use similar modalities, whereas speech language services use a different set of modalities and procedures. A small selection of HCPCS codes are employed for both in addition to CPT codes.

Physical and Occupational Therapy Procedures

Physical and occupational therapy codes are found in the Medicine section of the CPT code book in the Physical Medicine and Rehabilitation (97010 to 97799) subsection. Codes in this section identify physical and occupational therapy evaluation and re-evaluations, treatment modalities, therapeutic procedures, tests and measurements, and orthotic and prosthetic management. The services identified in this section may be reported for some physical or occupational therapists, but may not be reported for others; this depends on the types of services for which each individual therapy provider is qualified, trained, and has the resources to perform. For example, a physical therapist with the necessary equipment to perform Hubbard tank treatments may do so, and report the service with the code 97036, Application of a modality to 1 or more areas; Hubbard tank, each 15 minutes.

Physical and Occupational Therapy Evaluations

Both physical and occupational therapy services are initiated with an evaluation service, which includes a patient history, examination or assessment, and the development of a plan of treatment used to deliver the physical or occupational therapy services to the patient.

Physical therapy evaluations (97161 to 97164) include a patient history and examination, and the development of a plan of care. They are similar in nature to E/M codes, as they include the three key components of history, examination, and clinical decision making in addition to the development of a plan of care. There are three levels of physical therapy evaluations—low complexity, moderate complexity, and high complexity, which depend on the level of difficulty for each of the key components in the code description. Note that the levels of complexity listed in these codes are not the same as the levels of complexity for E/M codes. The exact components within each level of complexity are included in the full code description for each respective therapy evaluation service. For example, codes 97161, Physical therapy evaluation: low complexity through 97163, Physical therapy evaluation: high complexity, identify the initial evaluation service, whereas code 97164, Re-evaluation of physical therapy established plan of care is reported for a re-evaluation of the established physical therapy plan of care.

Occupational therapy evaluations (97165 to 97168) are also similar to E/M codes, except the key component of the codes differ slightly from physical therapy evaluation codes. The key components for occupational therapy evaluations include an occupational profile and client medical and therapy history, an assessment of occupational performance, clinical decision making, and the development of a plan of care. There are three levels of codes for occupational therapy evaluations—low complexity, moderate complexity, and high complexity—that depend on the levels of the four key components. Codes 97165, Occupational therapy evaluation, low complexity through 97167, Occupational therapy evaluation, high complexity, identify initial evaluations, whereas code 97168, Re-evaluation of occupational therapy established plan of care, is reported for a re-evaluation of an established occupational therapy plan of care. See figure 16.1 for the key components of physical and occupational therapy evaluations.

Evaluations for either physical or occupational therapy are performed as an initial service, and the plan of care is developed for the remaining therapy services that will be provided to the patient. A re-evaluation is used to perform an additional assessment of the patient and make any necessary changes to the plan of care. Neither of these services are performed at every visit. Rather, once the evaluation is completed and the plan of care is developed, only the specific therapeutic modalities or procedures will be performed. The only exception to this is if the patient needs a re-evaluation,

Figure 16.1. Key components of therapy evaluations

Key Components of Evaluations

Physical Therapy
- History
- Examination
- Clinical decision making
- Development of plan of care

Occupational Therapy
- Occupational profile and client history
- Assessment of occupational performance
- Clinical decision making
- Development of plan of care

in which case a new plan of care will determine the services the patient will receive. For example, after an initial evaluation, a physical therapist may create a plan of care including the gross motor function of a lower-limb amputee, and include 10 treatments over the course of three months. After the three-month period, the physical therapist notes that the patient has not made as much progress as anticipated by the original plan of care, and so performs a re-evaluation and the development of a new plan of care that includes additional treatments (Jannenga 2014).

Physical and Occupational Therapy Modalities and Procedures

Physical and occupational treatment services employ a range of **treatment modalities**—methods of therapeutic treatment designed to treat or rehabilitate a specific patient condition. Codes for therapy services identify the specific modality employed during the service, which is either service-based or time-based.

Treatment Modalities

Treatment modalities for physical therapy services help to strengthen, relax, or heal a specific muscle or group of muscles. Modalities for occupational therapy services help to improve circulation, decrease pain, improve elasticity of muscles and body movement, improve joint mobility, as well as reduce inflammation and swelling. The codes for the specific modality do not change depending on if they were employed for occupational or therapeutic services. Coders should select the appropriate code according to the modality used, without regard to the type of healthcare provider who performed the service.

Therapeutic modalities include the use of specialized equipment or devices, and may include massage, application of tape, and exercises. Additional therapeutic modalities are as follows:

- *Hot and/or cold packs.* Coded with 97010, Application of a modality to 1 or more areas; hot or cold packs, hot packs are used to help relax tight muscles and decrease pain and muscle spasms, and are typically applied before a treatment session. Cold packs are used after a treatment session to reduce pain and inflammation.

- *Electrical stimulation.* **Electrical stimulation** causes one muscle or a group of muscles to contract, which helps to increase muscle strength and blood supply to the muscle, and decrease pain. Codes for electrical stimulation identify the type of stimulation performed and differ depending on whether the code selected is service-based or time-based (discussed later in this chapter). Code 97014, Application of modality to 1 or more areas; *electrical stimulation (unattended)*, should be reported for electrical stimulation treatment for a patient when the therapist is not in constant physical attendance. Alternatively, code 97032, Application of modality to 1 or more areas; *electrical stimulation (manual), each 15 minutes*, should be reported when the therapist is in constant physical attendance. **Iontophoresis** (97033) is a form of electrical stimulation used to push medication through the skin to the affected body area, muscle, tendon, or ligament (see figure 16.2). Note that the medication administered during the iontophoresis must be prescribed by the patient's healthcare provider.

- *Ultrasound.* The high or low frequency sound waves from an ultrasound machine are used by therapists to penetrate muscle tissues to warm them and help in relaxation techniques, as well as increase circulation and reduce inflammation. This is coded with 97035, Application of a modality to 1 or more areas; *ultrasound, each 15 minutes*.

Figure 16.2. Iontophoresis

Source: ©2017. Used with permission by Perimed.

- *Paraffin bath.* Paraffin is a wax heated together with mineral oil and used as a treatment for patients with arthritis or joint conditions. The procedure is performed by coating the hand with multiple coats of the wax mixture, letting it to dry between coats, and allowing it to heat the hand for a small amount of time. It is reported with code 97018, Application of a modality to 1 or more areas; *paraffin bath.*
- *Ultraviolet therapy.* This procedure is used to help improve circulation and bring oxygen to body tissues, by employing ultraviolet rays. It is coded with 97028, Application of a modality to 1 or more areas; *ultraviolet.*
- *Diathermy and infrared therapy.* These two therapeutic procedures produce a warming sensation directed at a specific body area or muscle. They are reported with 97024, Application of a modality to 1 or more areas; diathermy (e.g., microwave), and 97026, Application of a modality to 1 or more areas; infrared.
- *Whirlpool and immersion.* A whirlpool is a large tank or tub filled with warm water that uses water jets and bubbles to help clean wounds or improve flexibility of muscles. Whirlpool treatments are reported with code 97022, Application of a modality to 1 or more areas; whirlpool. A Hubbard tank (reported with code 97036, Application of a modality to 1 or more areas; Hubbard tank, each 15 minutes), is a large tub in which the patient can be fully immersed, allowing patients to perform exercises while in the water.
- *Vasopneumatic device.* A vasopneumatic device is used on the external extremities, like the arms and legs, applying external pressure to the soft tissues and decreasing swelling. Use of a vasopneumatic device is reported with code 97016, Application of a modality to 1 or more areas; vasopneumatic devices.

Figure 16.3 illustrates a physical therapist providing care to a patient.

Medicare may require the submission of HCPCS codes for certain services, when HCPCS codes are available. HCPCS codes for therapy services can be found in the HCPCS code book by searching under the term *Therapy*, and then selecting the subterm for the specific type of therapy service provided, or by searching the Index for the specific type of therapy service provided. Most, but not all, therapy services in the HCPCS code book are found in Temporary Procedures/Professional Services (G0000 to G9999). For example, code G0129, Occupational therapy services requiring the skills of a qualified occupational therapist, furnished as a component of a partial hospitalization treatment program, per session (45 minutes or more).

Figure 16.3. Physical therapy

Source: Airman First Class Danielle Grannan 2009.

Modifiers Used in Therapy Services
New modifiers -96 and -97 were added to the 2018 CPT code set specifically for therapy services. For more information, please see the student workbook.

Service-Based and Time-Based Codes
Physical and occupational therapy services are divided into two types of codes: service-based and time-based. A **service-based code** is one that describes a full service, such as a physical therapy evaluation (97161 to 97163), application of hot or cold packs (97010), or the performance of electrical stimulation (97014). Service-based codes are untimed, and one code should be reported no matter how long the provider spent performing the service.

Time-based codes, also known as **constant attendance codes**, are reported according to the length of time the provider spent performing the service. These are easily distinguished from service-based codes, as the code description identifies the amount of time per code. For example, code 97110, Therapeutic procedure, 1 or more areas, each 15 minutes; therapeutic exercises to develop strength and endurance, range of motion and flexibility. This code describes the amount of time during which the provider must be in constant attendance in order to report the code. In this case, the therapy provider must be face-to-face with the patient, constantly attending the patient's side, for the amount of time described in the code.

Reporting time-based codes becomes a bit more complicated when the healthcare practitioner does not provide the full 15 minutes of the therapy service, as identified in the code. In order to bill for the full code, the provider must perform at least 8 minutes of the service. For example, if the provider was in constant attendance for 10 minutes, then he or she would be able to bill for the service. For any time *over* 15 minutes, the additional time must be at least 8 minutes over the 15-minute unit to report an additional unit of the service. This is known as the **8-minute rule**. For example, a provider performed 23 minutes of electrical stimulation to a patient with atrophy of leg muscles. The code for the service is 97032, Application of a modality to 1 or more areas; electrical stimulation (manual), each 15 minutes, and would be reported with two units, for example 97032 × 2 (the first unit would account for the initial 15 minutes of the service, and the second unit would account for the additional 8 minutes of the service). Each additional 8 minutes over the last 15-minute mark equals one additional unit. If less than 8 additional minutes are spent (over the last 15-minute mark), do not report an additional unit (see figure 16.4).

Figure 16.4. The 8-minute rule

97032	15 (1 unit)
97032	8 (1 unit)
Code(s) reported: **97032 X 2**	**Total time spent:** **23 minutes**

97032	15 (1 unit)
97032	15 (1 unit)
97032	5 (not reported)
Code(s) reported: **97032 X 2**	**Total time spent:** **35 minutes**

It is important to note that Medicare follows the 8-minute rule, but not all third-party payers follow suit. When reporting time-based codes for insurance plans other than Medicare, be sure to follow the specific guidelines for each insurance for reporting time-based services. For practice reporting physical and occupational therapy procedures, complete the exercises in There's a Code for That 16.1.

16.1

There's a Code for That

Physical and occupational therapy procedures

Read the following documentation of the service and identify the procedure code(s).

1. Application of hot packs to right ankle and knee joints.

   CPT code: _____

2. Patient received paraffin bath treatment on both hands.

   CPT code: _____

3. 30 minutes of therapeutic exercise including activities to increase R shoulder ROM and strengthening of R side.

   CPT code: _____ × _____

4. Gait training with comprehensive motion analysis by 3D kinematics, with dynamic plantar pressure measurements during walking.

   CPT code: _____

5. 45 minutes of myofascial release therapeutic massage.

CPT code: _____ × _____

6. High complexity occupational therapy evaluation with subsequent 20 minutes of training on activities of daily living, including training in adaptive equipment.

CPT codes: _____, _____

Speech Therapy Procedures

Codes for speech therapy and speech language pathology services are found in the Medicine section of the CPT code book in the Special Otorhinolaryngologic Services (92502 to 92700) subsection. This section includes a variety of codes that may be performed by speech language pathologists or ENTs. Additional codes from the Surgery section, such as endoscopic examination of the esophagus, may also be reported as necessary, depending on the services provided by the SLP.

Treatments provided by speech language pathologists are designed to rehabilitate and improve swallowing function and communication ability, as well as oral speaking and language ability. They include:

- *Swallowing function.* Swallowing disorders are common conditions, especially in the elderly population, and can cause a range of additional health problems such as weight loss, dehydration, aspiration pneumonia, and obstruction of the airway. Swallowing studies help to diagnose the cause of the patient's dysphagia (difficulty swallowing) and improve swallowing ability. Codes for swallowing function studies (92610 to 92617) identify the method of the test, and whether the SLP provided the full procedure or only the interpretation and report of the test. For example, code 92613, Flexible endoscopic evaluation of swallowing by cine or video recording; interpretation and report only, identifies the type of swallowing study (flexible endoscopic by cine or video recording) and that the therapist only provided the interpretation and report of the study (and did not perform the actual endoscopy). Treatment of a swallowing disorder is coded with 92526, Treatment of swallowing dysfunction and/or oral function for feeding.

- *Augmentative and alternative communication.* Augmentative and alternative communication (AAC) is used to communicate with other people and does not include oral communication. For example, an augmentative form of communication includes hand gestures or facial expressions when speaking. These gestures augment and add meaning to the oral words that are spoken. Patients with speech problems rely on AAC to help them communicate with others and may use special devices to further augment their communication and provide alternative communication. Codes for AAC services (92597, 92605 to 92609) identify the type of service (evaluation or therapeutic service), as well as the type of AAC device. Codes 92605, 92618, 92607, and 92608 are time-based codes that identify the amount of time spent on the evaluation. HCPCS code V5336, Repair/modification of augmentative communicative system or device (excludes adaptive hearing aid), should be reported when the SLP performs either a repair or modification of the AAC device. See figure 16.5 for an example of a speech-generating AAC device.

Figure 16.5. Speech generating AAC device

This AAC device allows the user to press the image for the idea or phrase they would like to communicate.

Source: Poule 2009.

- *Speech and language services.* Speech and language services are provided to patients with a range of communication disorders. **Language disorders** are difficulties with understanding or producing oral speech. They include receptive language disorders (when a patient has trouble understanding others) and expressive language disorders (when a patient has trouble sharing his or her thoughts and feelings with others), and may be in either oral or written form. **Social communication disorders** occur when a patient has difficulty understanding social cues in verbal and nonverbal communication, such as sitting down for a formal meal or telling a story from start to finish. **Cognitive communication disorders** include difficulties for patients when organizing thoughts, remembering, paying attention, planning, and problem-solving (ASLHA 2017). The way in which an SLP treats a speech and language disorder depends on the type of disorder the patient has. Furthermore, services range from noninvasive evaluations of voice and resonance to minimally invasive procedures, such as a nasopharyngoscopy (an endoscopic examination of the nose and throat). Procedures to treat speech and language disorders include:

  o 92507, Treatment of speech, language, voice, communication, and/or auditory processing disorder; *individual,* or 92508, Treatment of speech, language, voice, communication, and/or auditory processing disorder; *group, 2 or more individuals.*

  o Endoscopic examinations and function studies (92511 to 92516).

  o Evaluations of hearing loss and rehabilitation status (92626 to 92633).

  o Assessments and testing of aphasia and cognitive development (96105 to 96111, 96125).

  o Techniques to improve sensory and cognitive ability (97127 and 97533).

  o Telephone and online assessments and management services (98966 to 98969) and medical team conferences with primary care and other practitioners (99366 to 99368) (note that the codes for medical team conferences are in the E/M section of the CPT code book).

The diagnostic codes used to identify the medical necessity for therapy services are not assigned by therapy providers, as PTs, OTs, and SLPs are not authorized to assign medical diagnoses to patients. However, this does not mean that therapy services do not need ICD-10-CM codes. Rather, the ICD-10-CM codes assigned for therapy services rely on the documentation of the patient's condition by the primary care or referring provider. Complete the exercises in There's a Code for That 16.2 for practice reporting codes for speech therapy procedures.

Speech therapy procedures

16.2

There's a Code for That

Read the following documentation of the service and identify the procedure code(s).

1. Treatment of language processing disorder, individual.
   CPT code: _____

2. Evaluation of receptive/expressive language on 5-year-old male patient.
   CPT code: _____

3. 30 minutes of direct patient development of cognitive skills (attention, memory, and problem-solving).
   CPT code: _____ × _____

4. Programming and modification of non-speech generating device.
   CPT code: _____

5. Modification of AAC device.
   CPT code: _____

Diagnostic Coding for Therapy Services

Therapy services treat a vast range of conditions throughout the human body, from congenital malformations to acquired deformities, traumatic injuries, musculoskeletal conditions, and neurological impairments. Patients undergoing therapy receive a diagnosis from a primary care physician or other treating physician, who has determined that the patient needs some sort of therapeutic treatment to help the patient either return to original function or improve function after an injury or other medical condition.

ICD-10-CM codes are used to identify the medical necessity for physical and occupational therapy services, which includes musculoskeletal conditions, injuries, and problems with patient's fine and gross motor functioning. This medical necessity also includes neurological conditions, such as sequela from a stroke or cerebrovascular accident, or multiple sclerosis (MS). Medical necessity for occupational therapy services also includes behavioral and mental disorders, which may impair a patient's ability to function in a social setting.

Medical necessity for speech language pathology services includes disorders that impair or inhibit communication and affect the ability to swallow or hear. This includes physical conditions such as malignant neoplasm of the throat or dentofacial anomalies, as well as psychological and behavioral disorders that affect social communication and speaking difficulties.

Ultimately, reporting diagnosis codes for any type of therapy service requires a general knowledge of the ICD-10–CM code book, the ability to assign codes from across many chapters of the ICD-10-CM code book, and interpreting guidelines to ensure correct code selection.

Physical and Occupational Therapy Conditions

Many of the medical conditions treated by physical and occupational therapists result from injuries and musculoskeletal conditions, congenital malformations and anomalies, mental and developmental disorders, and neurological conditions.

Injuries and Musculoskeletal Conditions

Traumatic injuries range from simple fractures that heal without any side effects or necessary treatment or surgical interventions, to severe disfiguring injuries that require surgical interventions, medical treatments, and rehabilitative therapy services. Therefore, coding for injuries and related conditions of the musculoskeletal system (such as joint pain) can also range from reporting symptoms to reporting complex combinations of injuries, musculoskeletal conditions, and side effects.

Injuries are coded from chapter 19: Injury, Poisoning and Certain Other Consequences of External Causes, and musculoskeletal conditions are coded from chapter 13: Diseases of the Musculoskeletal System and Connective Tissue. Medical conditions from these chapters treated by occupational and physical therapists include:

- *Joint pain.* Joint pain (such as back, neck, arm, shoulder, leg, knee, ankle, and foot pain) is a common symptom treated by physical and occupational therapists. It may be a result of a past injury, medical condition, or side effect of surgical treatment. Rehabilitative therapy treatments of joint pain are aimed at reducing the amount of pain and restoring full range of motion of the joint. When searching for a joint pain code, refer to the term *Pain* in the Main Index of the ICD-10-CM code book, then refer to the subterm *joint*, and then the specific joint. Codes for joint pain also identify the laterality of the condition, such as right or left, the codes for which are found in the Tabular List of the codes. For example, M25.561, Pain in right knee.

- *Arthritis and degenerative joint diseases.* The numerous different types of arthritis may also require therapeutic services to reduce pain and restore functionality. Coding for any type of arthritis requires the identification of the specific type of arthritis—such as osteoarthritis, rheumatoid, juvenile, or infective arthritis—and the specific site involved. Remember that if a definitive diagnosis is identified, then it is not necessary to report the signs or symptoms included in the definitive diagnosis. For example, if the definitive diagnosis is arthritis, then it would not be necessary to report any associated swelling, pain, or reduced range of motion in the arthritic joints. If a patient was treated for severe bilateral osteoarthritis of the hips that caused pain, swelling, and lack of range of motion and caused her to ambulate with a walker, the only diagnosis code reported would be M16.0, Bilateral primary osteoarthritis of hip.

HCC Coding Corner

Note that some, but not all, arthropathies are included in HCC coding, such as pyogenic arthritis, infectious arthritis, reactive arthropathies, inflammatory arthritis (including rheumatoid), and juvenile arthritis.

- *Sports injuries.* Sports injuries occur from either a single instance of a motion or movement resulting in an injury, such as a torn ligament or muscle strain; or an injury resulting from repetitive movements, such as tendinitis of the elbow from playing tennis (tennis elbow). Physical therapists may further specialize in rehabilitative sports therapy to help restore function to the affected area and make it possible for the patient to resume athletic activities. Some of the more common conditions treated for sports injuries include tears of the anterior cruciate ligament (ACL) in the knee, rotator cuff strains, tendinitis, and various strains and sprains. When searching for a sport-related injury, identifying the external causes surrounding the injury, including the patient's activity, place of occurrence, injury mechanism, and the patient status at the time of the injury is necessary. For example, code S43.422A, Sprain of left rotator cuff capsule, initial encounter.

- *Amputation.* An **amputation** is the surgical removal of all or a portion of a body part. Often an amputation is performed surgically on an extremity due to a medical condition, such as gangrene, or from a traumatic injury that has either removed the body part or caused so much damage to the body part that it must be removed. Physical and occupational therapy services focus on helping the **amputee**, the patient who has undergone an amputation, learn how to function with a prosthetic device. For example, a lower leg amputee may receive physical therapy services to learn to walk again with the use of a prosthetic leg. Refer to chapter 15 for the discussion on amputation ICD-10-CM codes.

- *Head injury.* Head injuries can range from a concussion that requires little more than observation, to severe and debilitating **traumatic brain injuries (TBI)** requiring invasive surgery and a lifetime of medical treatment and rehabilitative services. Physical and occupational therapists can help patients regain function after a TBI by helping the patient relearn both fine and gross movements. TBI patients may also require the services of a speech therapist as well, depending on the type of injury. TBIs are coded from category S06, Intracranial Injury, and identify the type of injury (such as cerebral edema, diffuse traumatic brain injury, focal traumatic brain injury, contusion and laceration of cerebrum) and the duration of any loss of consciousness suffered by the patient—also if the patient returned to pre-injury level of consciousness, if the patient did not return to pre-existing level of consciousness, or if the patient died (either due to the brain injury or another injury) before regaining consciousness. As with amputation codes, almost all TBI codes are included in HCC coding, so care should be taken to ensure the correct documentation and code selection for these conditions.

- *Spinal cord injuries and paralytic syndromes.* Spinal cord injuries may range in neurological symptoms from tingling and weakness to full paralysis. When coding for a spinal cord injury, identify the specific type of injury, level of the injury (such as cervical or lumbar), and then the specific vertebra(e) involved in the injury. If multiple spinal cord injuries are present, code to the highest level of the injury (for example, code to the cervical level rather than the lumbar level). Paralytic syndromes are coded from category G81, Hemiplegia and hemiparesis, G82, Paraplegia (paraparesis) and quadriplegia (quadriparesis), and G83, Other paralytic syndromes. Codes from these categories should be reported when the condition is documented without further specification, or if the condition is old or longstanding and the cause is unspecified. These codes may also be used in addition to the code for the original injury, such as spinal cord injury. For example, if the documentation only states that the patient is paraplegic, but does not specify the cause of the paraplegia, then report a code from category G82. When coding for paralytic syndromes, codes identify the condition as affecting either the dominant or nondominant side of the body. The **dominant side** is the side that the patient prefers when performing daily functions—writing with the right hand would mean that a person is right-handed. When the dominant side is not identified in the provider's documentation, then code as the following:

- For ambidextrous patients, report the right side as dominant.
- If the left side is affected, report the condition as affecting the nondominant side.
- If the right side is affected, report the condition as affecting the dominant side.

In other words, the right side is the default dominant side. Note that both spinal cord injuries as well as paralytic syndromes are included in HCC coding (see figure 16.6 for the OGCR related to coding for the dominant versus nondominant sides).

Figure 16.6. OGCR I.C.6.a

---

6. Chapter 6: Diseases of the Nervous System (G00-G99)

a. Dominant/nondominant side

Codes from category G81, Hemiplegia and hemiparesis, and subcategories, G83.1, Monoplegia of lower limb, G83.2, Monoplegia of upper limb, and G83.3, Monoplegia, unspecified, identify whether the dominant or nondominant side is affected. Should the affected side be documented, but not specified as dominant or nondominant, and the classification system does not indicate a default, code selection is as follows:

- For ambidextrous patients, the default should be dominant.
- If the left side is affected, the default is non-dominant.
- If the right side is affected, the default is dominant.

Source: CMS 2018.

Congenital Malformations and Anomalies

A congenital malformation or anomaly is one with which a patient is born. Some congenital malformations may result in musculoskeletal disfigurement to such an extent that the patient requires either physical or occupational therapy (or both) in order to learn how to function.

Congenital malformations are reported from chapter 17: Congenital Malformations, Deformations and Chromosomal Abnormalities. These codes may be reported throughout the life of the patient. When searching for a congenital malformation in the ICD-10-CM Index, find the main term to identify the specific type of malformation, and then the subterm for the congenital version of the condition.

Also included in chapter 17 are codes for chromosomal abnormalities, such as Down Syndrome. These are reported with codes from Chromosomal abnormalities, not elsewhere classified (Q90 to Q99). Code selection depends on the identification of the specific type of chromosomal abnormality, such as Q95.1, Chromosome inversion in normal individual. Some abnormalities may also be identified by their resulting syndromes, such as Q93.3, Deletion of short arm of chromosome 4 (Wolff-Hirschhorn syndrome). Note that almost all chromosomal abnormalities are included in HCC coding.

Mental and Developmental Disorders

There are a host of mental and developmental disorders that may require therapeutic services to help patients function in a social environment. For example, patients with autism spectrum disorder (ASD) (F84.0, Autistic disorder) may need help learning how to perform everyday tasks without becoming overwhelmed by external influences, such as loud noises or changes in lighting and other environmental factors. Patients with emotional disturbances or mental disorders, such as disruptive mood dysregulation disorder (F34.81, Disruptive mood dysregulation disorder) or excoriation (skin-picking) disorder (F42.4, Excoriation (skin-picking) disorder) may also need therapeutic services in order to function in a social setting or to remove unwanted behaviors.

Codes for mental and developmental disorders may be found in chapter 5: Mental, Behavioral and Neurodevelopmental Disorders, and chapter 6: Diseases of the Nervous System of the ICD-10-CM code book. If the mental disorder is due to a known physiological condition, report the code for the underlying physiological condition in addition to the code for the mental disorder.

Neurological Conditions

Both physical and occupational therapists may treat patients with neurological conditions. These include degenerative neurological conditions such as multiple sclerosis (MS), a disease that affects the central nervous system and causes nerve deterioration and damage, and amyotrophic lateral sclerosis (ALS), also known as Lou Gehrig's Disease, a degenerative disease in which motor neurons slowly die causing muscle weakness, stiffness, and twitching, and for which there is no cure.

Stroke and intracerebral incidents may also result in a range of physical or neurological conditions, such as paralysis and dysphasia. Coding for strokes and intracerebral incidents, such as intracranial hemorrhage and cerebral infarction is a bit complicated. It is important to understand the difference between a service that is provided to a patient who is currently experiencing a cerebrovascular incident (patient is receiving acute care for the incident), and one that is receiving services for the sequela (late effects) of the incident. Cerebrovascular diseases (I60 to I69) are identified as either the current cerebrovascular disease (I60 to I66) (the acute incident), or a specific sequela following the cerebrovascular disease (I69) (the late effect of the incident).

For example, if a patient is admitted to the hospital for a cerebral infarction due to an embolism of the basilar artery, then the code reported would be I63.12, Cerebral infarction due to embolism of basilar artery. This diagnosis code would be reported for all services provided to treat the cerebral infarction, such as imaging or surgical services. However, therapists only treat the sequela that arise from a stroke—difficulty swallowing or speaking, paralysis, or deficits in cognitive functioning—so it would be incorrect to code for the actual cerebrovascular disease. Instead, report the code for the sequela(e) of the disease, such as cognitive or speech deficits (from category I69). For example, if the patient with the cerebral infarction of the basilar artery suffered hemiplegia due to the infarction, and the patient is receiving physical or occupational therapy to treat the hemiplegia, then the code reported would be I69.351, Hemiplegia and hemiparesis following cerebral infarction affecting right dominant side.

Note that many neurological conditions, because they are life-long and sometimes degenerative diseases, are included in HCC coding and should be coded to the highest specificity possible with complete documentation.

Key to Success

All codes for sequelae of cerebrovascular diseases are found in category I69 of the ICD-10-CM code book. These codes should not be used to identify the specific type of cerebrovascular disease, but rather the effect resulting from the cerebrovascular disease, like cognitive or speech deficits or paralysis. Pay attention to the guidelines in the Tabular, as reporting codes for additional or specific types of sequelae may be necessary. If the effects of the cerebrovascular disease are unknown or undocumented, or if there are no sequelae, assign a code from category I60 to I66.

Speech Therapy Conditions

Speech therapy and speech language pathology services are provided to patients who have problems swallowing, speaking, and hearing, as well as patients who need rehabilitation because of a communication disorder. As in diagnosis coding for physical and occupational therapy services, codes that identify the medical necessity for SLP services are found throughout the ICD-10-CM code book. SLPs also treat patients that are experiencing sequela of a stroke or cerebrovascular incident and paralytic syndromes, in addition to those with congenital anomalies and malformations, such as cleft lip or palate. Additional conditions include the following.

- *Neoplasms.* Benign and malignant neoplasms may affect a patient's ability to speak, hear, swallow, or otherwise communicate. They include neoplasms of the lip, tongue, parts of the mouth, tonsil, oropharynx, and esophagus, as well as nasal cavity, middle ear, larynx, and trachea. When coding for neoplasms, remember the basics of neoplasm code selection (refer to chapter 4 for the basics on how to code from the Table of Neoplasms):
  - If the histologic type of the neoplasm is known, search for the histologic type of neoplasm in the ICD-10-CM Index. If not, then search the Table of Neoplasms for the site of the neoplasm.
  - Once the site of the neoplasm is located, find the code in the Table of Neoplasms that identifies the type of neoplasm—either malignant, benign, uncertain, or unspecified. Malignant neoplasms are identified as either primary, secondary, or carcinoma in situ (ca in situ).
  - Verify the code for the neoplasm in the Tabular List.
  - If the patient has a history of neoplasm and is no longer undergoing treatment for the condition, then report the code for history of neoplasm. If the neoplasm has been removed but the patient is still undergoing treatment for the neoplasm (such as chemotherapy), then report the code for the neoplasm as if it still exists. For example, if a patient had undergone a partial glossectomy (removal of the tongue) due to primary malignancy of the tongue, and is now receiving chemotherapy for the treatment of the neoplasm, in addition to SLP services for rehabilitation of speech, then the coder would report the code for the neoplasm (because the patient is still undergoing treatment for the neoplasm, even though it was already excised) and the code(s) for any speech deficits or other problems requiring treatment.
- *Developmental Disorders.* Developmental disorders related to speech and language (F80, Specific developmental disorders of speech and language), scholastic skills (F81, Specific developmental disorders of scholastic skills), motor

function (F82, Specific developmental disorder of motor function), and pervasive developmental disorders (F84, Pervasive developmental disorders) may require SLP services to help the patient communicate effectively with others. For example, a patient with F80.0, Phonological disorder, may require SLP services to help with functional speech, remove a lisp, or improve articulation of specific sounds. Report any additional codes for associated hearing loss, medical or neurological condition, or intellectual disability. Note that pervasive developmental disorders (category F84) are included in HCC coding and should be assigned with care.

- *Dentofacial anomalies*. Dentofacial anomalies (M26) are malformations of the jaw and face, resulting from abnormal dental or facial growth. Although they are musculoskeletal in origin, these anomalies can affect the patient's ability to speak or form words, and may require speech therapy services.

- *Signs and symptoms*. Speech therapy services may also be required to treat the signs and symptoms of other or undiagnosed disorders. These include category R47, Speech disturbances, not elsewhere classified, which includes codes for dysphasia (difficulty speaking) and other speech disturbances. If an underlying condition is causing the speech disturbance, it should be reported in addition to the fluency or speech disorder. Category R48, Dyslexia and other symbolic dysfunctions, not elsewhere classified, includes the codes for dyslexia (difficulty reading) and other symbolic dysfunctions. Category R49, Voice and resonance disorders, includes codes for aphonia (loss of voice) and hypernasality (excessive nasal tone to the voice). Swallowing disorders are reported with codes from category R13, Aphagia and dysphagia. Dysphagia codes identify the specific phase of dysphagia. When a patient suffers dysphagia due to a stroke or cerebrovascular incident, report the sequela of stroke code and the dysphagia code.

Key to Success

Be particularly careful when assigning codes for either dysphasia or dysphagia. They are pronounced essentially the same way, and the spelling of the words only differ by one letter. Dysphasia with an "s" is for difficulty speaking, while dysphagia with a "g" is for difficulty swallowing. Think "s" for speaking (difficulty speaking) and "g" for gulping (difficulty gulping).

For practice reporting diagnosis codes for physical, occupational, and speech therapy services, complete the exercises in There's a Code for That 16.3.

PT, OT, and ST diagnosis coding

16.3

There's a Code for That

Read the following documentation and assign the appropriate diagnosis code(s) for the patient's condition(s).

1. 12-year-old male with cerebral palsy and spastic diplegia.

   ICD-10-CM code: _____

(Continued on next page)

Continued

2. Late stage Huntington's disease.

ICD-10-CM code: _____

3. 70-year-old female with primary osteoarthritis of the right knee with knee stiffness following total right knee arthroplasty presents for physical therapy including range of motion exercises.

ICD-10-CM codes: _____ , _____ ,

_____

4. 50-year-old male with chronic posterior cervicalgia, increasing over the last 6 weeks.

ICD-10-CM codes: _____ , _____

Putting It All Together: Coding for Therapy Services

Coding correctly for therapy services requires an understanding of the services provided by physical, occupational, and speech therapists, the specific selection of CPT codes they use, and the ability to assign diagnosis codes from various chapters of the ICD-10-CM code book.

Determination of the correct codes relies on the answers to the following questions.

- What type of therapy procedure was performed? If the service was an evaluation, was it an initial or re-evaluation, and what level of service was provided?
- For physical and occupational therapy services, is the service represented by a time-based code or a service-based code? If the code is time based, how much time was spent providing the service?
- Were any additional procedures performed?
- Are there any applicable modifiers for the procedure?
- Is there a definitive diagnosis for the procedure? If so, then code for the definitive diagnosis. If not, then code for the signs and symptoms.
  - If multiple therapeutic services were provided, each service must be linked with the appropriate ICD-10-CM codes to identify the medical necessity for the service provided.
- Are there any additional or underlying conditions that need to be reported, such as an underlying mental or neurological disability or intellectual disability?

Study the following vignette that demonstrates how to select the appropriate diagnosis and procedure codes. Then complete the following practice exercises in There's a Code for That 16.4.

Juan has been working in medical billing and coding for a few years now, and has just moved to a new city where he got a job as a coder in a therapy practice. His new workplace employs about 30 different therapy providers, each of whom performs services at multiple different locations around the city. The therapists that work for his practice include physical, occupational, and speech therapists. Juan is coding for the services provided by the therapists at the therapy group. Right now he is working on coding the following physical therapy note: 72-year-old female patient was seen at the clinic for the first time after a subarachnoid hemorrhage (CVA). Sequela from the CVA includes monoplegia of right arm (patient is left-handed), resulting in inability to perform functional ADLs (activities of daily living) and lack of normal mobility. Her healthcare history is also significant for essential hypertension, type II diabetes, and urge incontinence. A high complexity physical therapy evaluation concluded that the patient's plan of care will include therapeutic exercises to increase the range of motion of the right arm and shoulder, with strengthening exercises of the right side. Functional training to assist in overall mobility and balance, posture, and gait training.

Juan asks himself: What did the therapist do? In this case, the therapist performed a high complexity physical therapy evaluation and developed a plan of care, including therapeutic exercises and functional training. Only the evaluation was performed at this point and no actual therapeutic services were performed. He selects the following code for the physical therapy evaluation:

- *97163, Physical therapy evaluation: high complexity*

Now that Juan has the procedure code, he asks himself: Why did the therapist do it? In this case, the patient has monoplegia of the upper right (nondominant) arm (because the patient is left-handed), due to a subarachnoid hemorrhage, as well as three other significant conditions: essential hypertension, type II diabetes, and urge incontinence. He knows that to code for the sequela of subarachnoid hemorrhage, he needs to use a combination code from category I69 to identify both the hemiplegia as well as the CVA. He selects the following codes for the patient's conditions:

- *I69.033, Monoplegia of upper limb following nontraumatic subarachnoid hemorrhage affecting right nondominant side*
- *I10, Essential (primary) hypertension*
- *E11.9, Type 2 diabetes mellitus without complications*
- *N39.41, Urge incontinence*

He then rechecks the documentation to make sure he has coded everything for the encounter and reports the chosen codes.

Diagnostic and procedural coding for therapy services

16.4

There's a Code for That

Read the following documentation and assign the appropriate CPT, HCPCS, and ICD-10-CM code(s) for the encounter.

1. 16-year-old male is admitted to inpatient rehab; status post complete spinal cord injury at the T12 level resulting in complete paraplegia below the T12 level. Plan of care was developed at the last encounter and today patient received 40 minutes of wheelchair training including rolling, posture changes, transfers, and wheelchair mobility of different surfaces.

   CPT code: _____ × _____

   ICD-10-CM codes: _____, _____

(Continued on next page)

16.4

Continued

2. An 85-year-old male sustained a subarachnoid hemorrhage in his home three weeks ago. He now suffers from right-sided hemiparesis, difficulty swallowing, and expressive aphasia. SLP completed an evaluation of oral and pharyngeal swallowing function and diagnosed the patient with oropharyngeal dysphagia.

CPT code: _____

ICD-10-CM codes: _____, _____

3. 25-year-old female with Down Syndrome received 1 hour of work training, including money management and work task analysis.

CPT code: _____

ICD-10-CM codes: _____

End of Chapter Content

Instructions: Indicate whether the following statements are true or false (T or F). For false statements, rewrite the statement on the line below to make the statement true.

1. A physical therapist specializes in procedures on activities of daily living that require fine motor skills.

_____

_____

2. SLPs treat speaking problems such a fluency, problems with voice resonance, and problems with pronunciation.

_____

_____

3. Therapy providers never need a request from a healthcare provider to begin therapy services.

_____

_____

4. Medicare has no limit to the amount of therapy services that can be billed within a calendar year.

_____

_____

5. A treatment modality for physical therapy services is a method of therapeutic treatment.

_____

_____

6. Iontophoresis is a type of electrical stimulation.

_____

_____

7. The 8-minute rule is used for service-based codes.

_____

_____

8. Some of the codes for occupational therapy services can be found in the Special Otorhinolaryngologic Services subsection of the CPT code book.

_____

_____

9. Augmentative and alternative communication (AAC) does not include oral communication.

_____

_____

10. Joint pain is a condition commonly treated by physical therapists.

_____

_____

Instructions: Choose the best answer.

1. Which of the following therapists would perform therapeutic exercises on a patient to help them with swallowing function?
   a. Speech language pathologist
   b. Physical therapist
   c. Occupational therapist
   d. Oral-maxillofacial surgeon

2. Which of the following activities would a physical therapist assist a patient in performing?
   a. Brushing teeth
   b. Speaking
   c. Walking
   d. Eating with a fork

3. Which of the following activities would an occupational therapist help a patient in performing?
   a. Balancing while standing up
   b. Understanding directions
   c. Debriding a wound
   d. Writing with a pencil

4. Which modifier should be used when an ABN may have been required but was not obtained from the patient?
   a. GA
   b. GX
   c. GY
   d. GZ

5. Which of the following is a key component of physical therapy evaluations?
   a. Development of plan of care
   b. Medical evaluation and management
   c. Pharmaceutical management
   d. Prescription of medications

6. Which of the following codes identifies a re-evaluation for occupational therapy services?
   a. 97165
   b. 97164
   c. 97163
   d. 97168

7. Which type of device applies external pressure to the soft tissues and is used to decrease swelling?

   a. Vasopneumatic
   b. Iontophoresis
   c. Diathermy
   d. Whirlpool

8. Using the 8-minute rule, how many units would you report for a therapeutic service that took 43 minutes to complete?

   a. 3
   b. 4
   c. 5
   d. 6

9. Which of the following codes identifies an evaluation for the use of an AAC device to supplement oral speaking?

   a. 92597
   b. 92605
   c. 92609
   d. 92607

10. Which of the following includes problems with understanding or producing oral speech?

    a. Cognitive communication disorders
    b. Social communication disorders
    c. Language disorders
    d. All of the above

11. When searching the ICD-10-CM Index for joint pain of the right hip, which term do you search for first?

    a. Joint
    b. Pain
    c. Right
    d. Hip

12. Which of the following types of anomalies are malformations of the jaw and face?

    a. Oropharyngeal
    b. Dentofacial
    c. Congenital
    d. Hypernasal

Instructions: Answer the following questions with the appropriate code(s) and modifier(s) when necessary.

1. 65-year-old male with adhesive capsulitis of the shoulder receives 30 minutes of aquatic therapy with therapeutic exercises. Before therapy begins, PT places hot packs on the affected area for 15 minutes.

   CPT codes: _____ × _____, _____

   ICD-10 code: _____

2. 7-year-old male is referred to SLP by his PCP. He was recently begun stuttering in his elementary class and he presents today for evaluation of speech fluency.

   CPT codes: _____

   ICD-10 code: _____

References

American Speech-Language-Hearing Association. *Speech-Language Pathologists.* http://www.asha.org/Students/Speech-Language-Pathologists/.

Centers for Medicare and Medicaid Services. 2018. ICD-10-CM Official Guidelines for Coding and Reporting FY 2018. https://www.cms.gov/Medicare/Coding/ICD10/Downloads/2018-ICD-10-CM-Coding-Guidelines.pdf.

Centers for Medicare and Medicaid Services. January 2017 (January). Medicare Limits on Therapy Services. https://www.medicare.gov/Pubs/pdf/10988-Medicare-Limits-Therapy-Services.pdf.

Centers for Medicare and Medicaid Services. 2015 (October). Medicare Advance Beneficiary Notices. https://www.cms.gov/Outreach-and-Education/Medicare-Learning-Network-MLN/MLNProducts/downloads/abn_booklet_icn006266.pdf.

Jannenga, H. 2014 (June 3). Founder Letter: 97002 and 97004 (Re-Evaluation) Myths Debunked. https://www.webpt.com/blog/post/founder-letter-97002-and-97004-re-evaluation-myths-debunked.

Poule. 2009. "Minimo.jpg. Digital image." Wikimedia Commons. Accessed December, 2017. https://commons.wikimedia.org/wiki/File:Minimo.jpg.

Resources

American Occupational Therapy Association. 2017. What is Occupational Therapy? https://www.aota.org/Conference-Events/OTMonth/what-is-OT.aspx.

American Physical Therapy Association. 2015 (November 24). Identifying the Correct Codes for ICD-10 (ICD-10-CM). http://www.apta.org/ICD10/IdentifyingCodes/.

American Physical Therapy Association. 2015 (November 24). Who Are Physical Therapists? http://www.apta.org/AboutPTs/.

American Physical Therapy Association. 2015 (July 22). Coding Interpretations: Group Therapy Patient Scenarios. http://www.apta.org/Payment/Coding/GroupTherapyScenarios/.

American Speech-Language-Hearing Association. 2017. Model Superbill for Speech-Language Pathology. http://www.asha.org/uploadedFiles/ModelSuperbillSLP.pdf.

Jannenga, H. 2016 (March 17). Physical Therapists' Guide to Billing. https://www.webpt.com/physical-therapists-guide-to-billing.

Jannenga, H. 2016 (February 2). Physical Therapists' Guide to the 8-Minute Rule. WebPThttps://www.webpt.com/8-minute-rule.

Jannenga, H. 2016 (January 25). Physical Therapists' Guide to CPT Codes. https://www.webpt.com/cpt-codes.

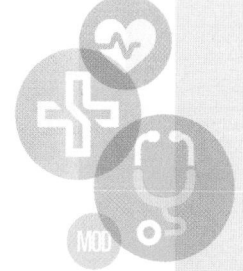

Obstetrics and Gynecology Services

Learning Objectives

- Understand the basics of billing and coding for obstetrics and gynecology services.
- Examine procedural codes and guidelines for obstetrics and gynecology services.

- Examine diagnosis coding and medical necessity for obstetrics and gynecology services.
- Determine and apply ICD-10-CM, CPT, and HCPCS codes to obstetrics and gynecology services.

Key Terms

Abortion
Antepartum
Bartholin's glands
Birthing center
Cerclage
Certified nurse midwife (CNM)
Cervix uteri
Conization
Corpus uteri
Diaphragm
Endocervical curettage (ECC)
External os
Fallopian tubes
Gestation
Gestational condition
Gravida
Gynecologists
Incidental pregnancy
Internal os
Intrauterine device (IUD)

Introitus
Labia majora
Labia minora
Last menstrual period (LMP)
Loop electrosurgical excision procedure (LEEP)
Marsupialization
Maternal fetal medicine (MFM) specialist
Maternity services
Non-obstetric
Nuchal cord
Nulligravida
Nulliparous
Obstetric
Obstetrics and gynecology services
Obstetricians
Outcome of delivery code
Ovaries
Oviducts

Parity (or para)
Perinatal
Perinatologist
Perineum
Peripartum
Pessary
Postpartum
Puerperium
Products of conception (POC)
Reproductive endocrinology and infertility (REI) specialist
Reproductive surgery
Sequencing priority
Trimesters
Uterus
Vagina
Vaginectomy
Vulva

Obstetrics and gynecology services (OB/GYN) are focused on the gynecological and reproductive health of female patients, as well as providing services for pregnant patients and performing deliveries. Obstetrics services are provided to pregnant patients and focus on the reproductive health of the patient, including managing the patient's pregnancy and delivering the fetus at childbirth. Gynecological services focus on the genital and reproductive health of female patients and include services to monitor, diagnose, and treat female patients. Gynecological services may also treat genitourinary conditions of female patients, which include conditions of the female genital and urinary systems, such as urinary tract infection or urinary incontinence.

Obstetrics and gynecology coding includes both gynecological and urinary system treatments and procedures on non-pregnant females, as well as maternity-related procedures on pregnant females. Coding for obstetric and gynecologic services requires an understanding of the medical terminology used and the services included in the global package for maternity care. This chapter discusses the basics of billing and coding for both gynecology and obstetrics, the medical terminology used and procedural and diagnostic coding for obstetrics and gynecology services.

Obstetrics and Gynecology Basics

Obstetrics and gynecology are times combined into one specialty, called OB/GYN (OB for obstetrics and GYN for gynecology) or OBGYNE. Although they are technically two different healthcare specialties, both obstetricians and gynecologists often combine into small or large group practices that both treat female patients throughout their life cycles including during pregnancy.

Proper coding for OB/GYN services requires an understanding of the special services performed by each type of healthcare provider, and the unique terminology used in the OB/GYN field.

OB/GYN Providers

Gynecologists are healthcare providers who specialize in the female reproductive system including the vagina, uterus, and ovaries, as well as the breasts. Gynecologists also help diagnose and treat conditions that affect the urinary system, such as urinary tract infections, sexually transmitted diseases, and urinary incontinence. Obstetricians are healthcare providers who specialize in the health of a patient during pregnancy, childbirth, and the postpartum period. This includes managing the health, growth, and development of the pregnant mother and fetus, performing the delivery at childbirth, and necessary follow-up care for the mother after delivery. Obstetricians and gynecologists may also specialize in surgical treatments of the female genital and reproductive system, as well as the urinary system, such as surgery to correct urinary incontinence or hysterectomy.

Note that gynecologists and other primary care physicians or healthcare providers may see patients during pregnancy for non-pregnancy-related conditions (such as an injury), but these visits are to manage a health condition suffered by the pregnant female, and not to manage the pregnancy itself. Coders must interpret when the services treat or manage the patient's pregnancy, or if the pregnancy is incidental to the patient's treatment (more on incidental pregnancy coding is discussed later in this chapter).

As gynecologists and obstetricians specialize in reproductive health of female patients, some healthcare providers are qualified to perform both OB and GYN procedures. However, a major distinction in OB/GYN coding is the difference between obstetric and non-obstetric procedures and conditions. Obstetric refers to a procedure performed on a pregnant woman or condition related to a woman's pregnancy, such as a delivery or complication of pregnancy. These services are also referred to as **maternity services**. Non-obstetric refers to a procedure performed to treat or manage signs and symptoms, or other encounter for gynecological or genitourinary services, such as reproductive, urinary, and breast health. OB/GYN services are closely related and when coding for OB/GYN services, procedures and diagnosis codes are differentiated based on whether or not the patient in question is pregnant, and if the services were related to the patient's pregnancy. Non-obstetric procedures and treatments are usually performed by a gynecologist, and obstetric procedures are performed by an obstetrician.

Because of the range of OB/GYN services provided, there are additional provider types of which coders should be aware, as well as the different healthcare settings in which OB/GYN services are provided.

Additional OB/GYN Specialties and Subspecialties

There are a handful of additional healthcare specialists who perform OB/GYN services. Fortunately for the coder, these different specialties do not impact codes selected for the services performed.

- Certified nurse midwife (CNM). A CNM is a mid-level practitioner (as discussed in chapter 1) with an advanced degree as a registered nurse in midwifery, the study of assisting pregnant females in obstetric care and childbirth, including the postpartum period, female care, and birth control. Remember that as a mid-level provider, CNMs must practice under a licensed physician. CNMs may or may not be licensed to perform deliveries, depending on the state in which they practice.

- Maternal fetal medicine (MFM) specialist. An MFM specialist, also known as a perinatologist, is a medical doctor who specializes in high-risk pregnancies and focuses on the health of the mother and fetus before, during, and after pregnancy. MFM doctors are obstetricians with additional training in managing the health of both the fetus and the mother during risky pregnancies, including additional testing, imaging services, and management of the pregnancy.

- Reproductive endocrinology and infertility (REI) specialist. Otherwise known as a fertility specialist, an REI is a medical doctor with additional training and expertise in human reproduction, including the function of hormones in reproduction. A related specialty is reproductive surgery, which focuses on surgical treatments to treat infertility. Reproductive surgery services are reported with codes from the Reproductive Medicine Procedures (89250 to 89398) subsection of the Laboratory and Pathology section of the CPT code book (refer to chapter 14).

Place of Service for OB/GYN Services

Depending on the service performed, both gynecologists and obstetricians may perform services in the outpatient office setting or surgeries and deliveries in the inpatient hospital setting. Deliveries may also be performed at a certified birthing center, a facility that specializes in providing a comfortable setting for labor, delivery, postpartum care, and immediate newborn care. Birthing centers are not hospitals, but they do have specialized equipment and trained staff to assist with healthcare needs. If a medical emergency occurs during the labor and delivery process, or with the newborn after childbirth, the patient may have to be transported to an inpatient hospital facility for evaluation and treatment. If an obstetrician performs any services at a birthing center, use POS code 24, for a "facility, other than a hospital's maternity facilities or a physician's office, which provides a setting for labor, delivery, and immediate postpartum care as well as immediate care of newborns" (AMA 2017).

Pregnancy Timeline and Terminology

When it comes to OB/GYN coding, especially coding for maternity services, it is important to understand the timeline of pregnancy, services involved, and terminology used to discuss pregnancy, childbirth, and the postpartum period. This terminology is used in both CPT and ICD-10-CM coding, and is essential in reporting procedural codes for maternity services and diagnosis codes for pregnancy, childbirth, and the puerperium.

Pregnancy Timeline

Pregnancy-related services are reported along a continuum of care (that is, the pregnancy timeline), which begins at the patient's last menstrual period and ends six weeks after childbirth. The **last menstrual period (LMP)** is the first day of the patient's last period; this date is used to estimate the date of conception, and subsequently the estimated date of delivery, 40 weeks after the LMP. The period of pregnancy before childbirth is known as the **antepartum,** or pre-partum, period, and lasts 40 weeks (or until childbirth). The **postpartum** period extends after childbirth to six weeks post-delivery. The postpartum period is also referred to as the **puerperium** (from birth to six weeks after birth). The **peripartum** period pertains to the mother's health and healthcare services, and extends from about one month before childbirth to up to five months after childbirth. The **perinatal** period also extends before and after childbirth, but pertains to the health and healthcare services for the fetus (and later newborn). The perinatal period extends from 20 to 28 weeks before childbirth to up to 6 weeks post-delivery. See figure 17.1 for a visual representation of the pregnancy timeline.

Figure 17.1. Pregnancy timeline

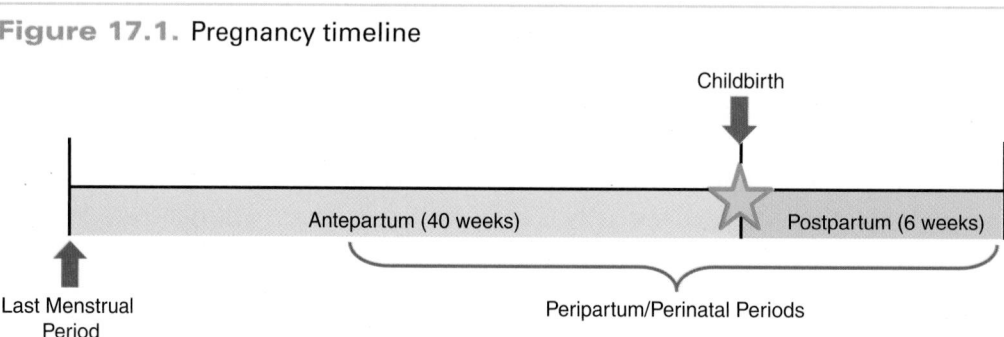

This timeline becomes more important later in this chapter when discussing maternity services and the global maternity package.

Pregnancy Terminology

There are several important terms regarding OB/GYN conditions, and this small section is by no means a full list of the medical terms a coder must know in order to report procedure and diagnosis codes for OB/GYN services. When coding for OB/GYN services, remember to use a medical dictionary and any other available resources when confronted with an unfamiliar term or phrase.

Pregnant women are often referred to by their gravida status, such as G3P2. The "G" refers to gravida, which means pregnant female. The "P" means parity (or para), the number of previous pregnancies. The numbers between refer to the number of times the patient has been pregnant (after the G) and the number of times the patient has carried to full-term (after the P). For example, a G3P2 patient is currently pregnant, and has been pregnant three times (G3), and carried to full-term two times (P2). This number and letter combination is used as a shorthand to refer to patients when they present for OB/GYN services. However, keep in mind that the gravida and parity status of a patient only impacts code selection for patients who are elderly, or if the patient has had multiple miscarriages or abortions (this is discussed later in this chapter). A nulligravida female is one who has never been pregnant, and a nulliparous female is one who has never carried a pregnancy longer than 20 weeks.

Trimesters of pregnancy are an additional concept that should be fully understood when coding for OB/GYN services. The 40 weeks of pregnancy are divided into three trimesters, which are roughly three-month periods of time into which the 40 weeks of pregnancy are grouped (see figure 17.2). The three trimesters are based upon the following timeframes:

- First trimester: conception to 13 weeks, 6 days
- Second trimester: 14 weeks to 27 weeks, 6 days
- Third trimester: 28 weeks to delivery

Figure 17.2. Trimesters of pregnancy

Many codes identify the specific trimester of pregnancy. Also important to understand is the estimated weeks of gestation, which is identified with an additional code. Gestation is the time between conception (the moment at which the egg is fertilized) and birth (when the fetus is delivered). There are approximately 40 weeks of gestation for a pregnant human female, divided into three trimesters.

Key to Success

When reporting codes for any type of obstetric or maternity service, keep in mind the difference between the pregnant woman (mother) and the fetus (child). Many terms are similar but refer to either the mother or the baby. For example, the peripartum period refers to the mother's health, while the perinatal period refers to the growth and development of the fetus and eventually the newborn. This is also important to keep in mind when reporting diagnosis codes for the mom versus the baby, as sometimes the codes are similar and difficult to distinguish from one another. Remember, all

OB/GYN services are provided on the pregnant female patient. Any services provided to the infant, once born, are provided by a pediatrician or neonatal specialist. A neonatal specialist is a medical doctor who typically works in a Neonatal Intensive Care Unit (NICU) of a hospital to provide intensive care to severely ill or premature infants.

Just as with OB/GYN terminology, there is a difference between OB/GYN services provided to patients who are not pregnant (non-obstetric services) and services provided to pregnant patients. Diagnosis codes also differ based on whether or not the patient is pregnant, and if that pregnancy is related to the service(s) performed or if it is incidental to the services performed.

Procedural Coding for OB/GYN Services

Procedural coding for OB/GYN services depends on whether or not the service was maternity related. Non-obstetric surgical services are coded from the Female Genital subsection of the CPT code book, and obstetric services are coded from the Maternity subsection of the CPT code book. Evaluation and management (E/M) codes are also commonly reported in the outpatient office setting for gynecological services, as most office visits are reported with an E/M code, using additional codes to identify either procedures performed in the office or surgical procedures performed in the hospital setting.

Key to Success

Many healthcare specialties like OB/GYN report a great deal of E/M codes, as these codes identify outpatient office visits. If the decision for surgery or other medical treatment or diagnostic service is made during an office visit, then additional codes from throughout the CPT code book are used to identify the subsequent services performed.

Gynecology Services

Most gynecology services use evaluation and management (E/M) codes for outpatient office visits. If a patient is seen and no surgical, medicine, imaging, or laboratory procedures are performed, the encounter should be reported with the appropriate E/M code. For example, if a patient presents to the office of her gynecologist for an annual female examination, this service is reported with the appropriate E/M code. For a reminder of how to correctly select and report and evaluation and management services, refer to chapter 8 (Primary Care).

If, at the E/M encounter, a decision for surgery is made, or if a procedure is performed in addition to the E/M encounter (such as the insertion of an intrauterine device), then that service is reported with the appropriate code from the Female Genital subsection of the CPT code book. Note, however, that it is not appropriate to always report an E/M code with the minor surgical procedure code (like the insertion of an IUD). The E/M service must be a significant, separately identifiable service from the minor surgical procedure, as the minor surgical procedure already includes payment for the pre-procedure, intra-procedure, and post-procedure work (refer to chapter 11 for the components of the surgical package).

The Female Genital subsection is organized according to the anatomy of the female genital system, beginning with the vulva, perineum, and introitus; followed by the vagina, cervix uteri, corpus uteri, oviducts; and then the ovaries.

Vulva, Perineum, and Introitus

The external female genitalia are comprised of the vulva, perineum, and introitus (see figure 17.3). The perineum is the area between the vagina and the anus. The vulva consists of the labia (both labia majora and labia minora), the bulb of the vestibule, vestibule of the vagina, the greater vestibular glands (known as Bartholin's glands, which/- secrete mucus to lubricate the vagina), the lesser vestibular gland, and the vagina orifice, also known as the introitus. The labia majora is the tissue that surrounds the labia minora and the clitoris. The labia minora surrounds the vaginal vestibule and the external urethra.

Figure 17.3. External female genitalia

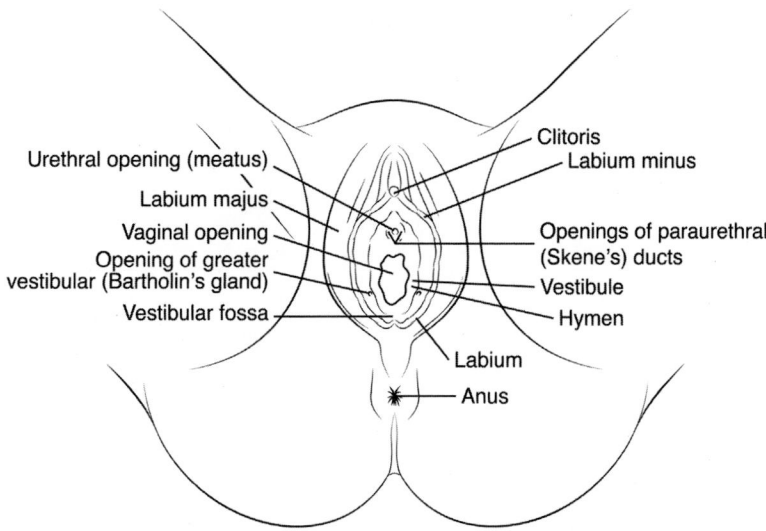

Source: ©AHIMA.

Procedures on the external female genitalia include incision and drainage of abscesses, and marsupialization of Bartholin's gland cysts. Marsupialization is a procedure in which a cyst is incised along one edge to form an open pouch, and then sutured open to allow for continuous drainage (see figure 17.4). This procedure is coded with 56440, Marsupialization of Bartholin's gland cyst.

Vulvar lesions may be biopsied, destroyed, or removed. Destruction of vulvar lesions is categorized based on whether the destruction was simple (56501) or extensive (56515), and includes destruction by any method (laser surgery, electrosurgery, cryosurgery, or chemosurgery). Remember that destruction of a lesion is different than excision of a lesion. In lesion excision, the tissue or lesion is removed via a scalpel or sharp edge, whereas with destruction, the tissue is destroyed and there is nothing left. There is one code for biopsy of vulvar or perineal lesion, 56605, Biopsy of vulva or perineum (separate procedure); *1 lesion*, with an add-on code for each additional lesion: 56606, Biopsy of vulva or perineum (separate procedure); *each separate additional lesion.*

Excision of vulvar lesions are based on two different principles—the depth of the removal and the extent of the removal. These definitions apply to vulvectomy codes found in codes 56620 through 56640. The depth of a vulvectomy is referred to as either simple or radical:

- A *simple* vulvectomy is the removal of the skin and superficial tissues.
- A *radical* vulvectomy is the removal of the skin and deep subcutaneous tissues.

Figure 17.4. Marsupialization of Bartholin's gland cyst

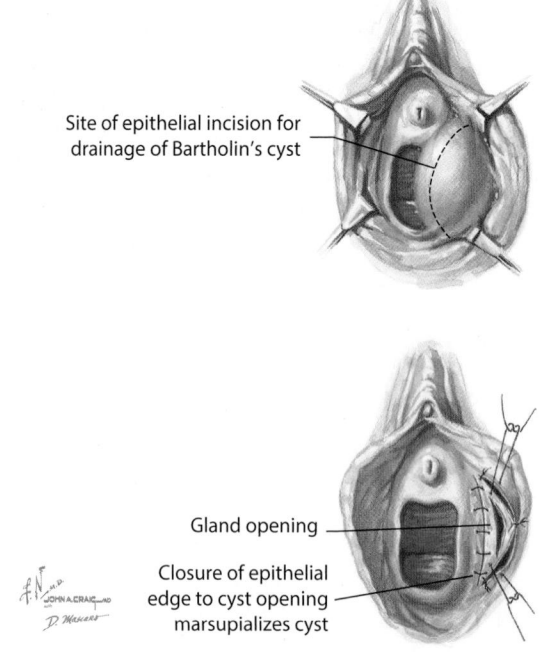

Source: ©2008. Used with permission of Elsevier. All rights reserved.

Vulvectomies are also described according to the extent of the tissue removal, or how large of a surface area of tissue was removed. These are either partial or complete:

- A *partial* vulvectomy is the removal of less than 80 percent of the vulvar area.
- A *complete* vulvectomy is the removal of more than 80 percent of the vulvar area.

When coding for a vulvectomy, both the depth and the extent of the removal must be identified. For example, code 56620, Vulvectomy simple; partial. This code reports a simple, partial vulvectomy—the removal of only skin and subcutaneous tissues of less than 80 percent of the vulvar area.

Vagina

The **vagina** is the lower portion of the birth canal, which serves as the conduit for the birth of a fetus, uterine secretions and menstrual flow, and the receptacle for semen from a male during intercourse. The medical prefix for vagina is *colpo-*, and many of the procedural terms in this subheading use this prefix. For example, a *colposcopy* is an endoscopic examination of the vagina, and a *colporrhaphy* is the surgical repair of the vagina.

Procedures on the vagina are more varied in nature, and include incision, destruction, excision, introduction, repair, and endoscopy. Incision (57000 to 57023) procedures performed for drainage of abscesses and hematomas. Note that code 57022, Incision and drainage of vaginal hematoma; *obstetrical/postpartum*, reports the drainage of a hematoma (blood-filled sac) that was related to an obstetric or postpartum condition. However, code 57023, Incision and drainage of vaginal hematoma; *non-obstetrical (e.g., post-trauma, spontaneous bleeding)*, is for the same procedure but due to a non-obstetric condition. Always remember this difference when reporting codes for female genital procedures, as it often results in the selection of a different code.

Additional procedures on the vagina include destruction of vaginal lesions and excisions. Excision codes are divided based on whether the procedure was a biopsy, either simple or extensive (57100, 57105), or a **vaginectomy** (removal of all or part of the vagina). Vaginectomy codes (57106 to 57135) are categorized based on whether the removal is a partial removal of the vaginal wall (the selective removal of the upper or lower portion of the vagina), or if it was a complete removal of the vaginal wall. Both partial and complete removals have additional codes to identify the removal of paravaginal tissue (radical vaginectomy) with or without bilateral total pelvic lymphadenectomy and para-aortic lymph node sampling (biopsy). Vaginectomy procedures may or may not be followed with plastic repairs of the vagina.

Introduction procedures of the vagina include irrigation or application of therapeutic substances for bacterial, parasitic, or fungoid diseases (57150), as well as the insertion of brachytherapy elements. Brachytherapy is a type of radiation treatment for cancer, which is discussed in chapter 18 (Medical Specialist Services). Note that many of the body systems throughout the CPT surgical section include the insertion of brachytherapy elements, including female genital, male genital, and urinary systems.

Also within the introduction category is code 57160, Fitting and insertion of a pessary or other intravaginal support device. A **pessary** is a small device placed inside the vagina to support the internal structures of the female reproductive system such as the uterus, vagina, bladder, or rectum (see figure 17.5). They can be used to help treat pelvic organ prolapse or stress incontinence, for example. Code 57170, Diaphragm or cervical cap fitting with instructions, is for the manual fitting of a diaphragm. A **diaphragm** is a barrier birth control method in which a small, cup-like device is placed over the cervix during intercourse, along with spermicide that is later removed (see figure 17.6). Note that when the procedure for either a pessary or a diaphragm is performed, the pessary or diaphragm is also supplied to the patient. The supply of the actual device is reported with the appropriate HCPCS code, such as A4561, Pessary, rubber, any type, A4562, Pessary, non-rubber, any type, or A4261, Cervical cap for contraceptive use.

Vaginal repairs are reported with codes 57200 through 57335. Codes depend on the specific type of repair, whether the procedure is obstetric or non-obstetric, and the approach to the procedure.

Figure 17.5. Pessary

Uterus — Rectum

Bladder

Vagina

Pessary

Figure 17.6. Insertion of diaphragm

Also included in these codes are procedures for stress incontinence—when physical movement or stress, such as a sneeze or jumping up and down, causes a leakage of urine. Code 57288 Sling operation for stress incontinence (e.g., fascia or synthetic), reports an open approach to the procedure. Note that the procedure for stress incontinence performed via a laparoscopic approach is reported with code 51992, Laparoscopy, surgical; sling operation for stress incontinence (e.g., fascia or synthetic), which is in the urinary system section of codes.

Endoscopic examinations and procedures of the vagina are reported with codes 57420 through 57426. However, it is important to pay attention to the notes in this section, as they identify additional or more appropriate codes when more than just the vagina is visualized or accessed during the procedure. For example, under code 57421, Colposcopy of the entire vagina, with cervix if present; with biopsy(s) of vagina/cervix, are parenthetical notes including: *For colposcopic visualization of cervix and adjacent upper vagina, use 57452.* Note that this section of codes also includes three laparoscopic procedures of the vagina, 57423 through 57426.

Cervix Uteri

The cervix uteri, also known as the cervix, is the lowest part of the uterus, about two to three centimeters long and round in shape, and forms a canal from the upper portion of the vagina to the uterus (see figure 17.7). The lower end of the cervix is called the external os, and the upper end, which opens into the uterus, is called the internal os. The cervical canal allows sperm to travel from the vagina to the uterus, and flattens and dilates during vaginal childbirth to open and allow for the passage of the fetus from the uterus through the birth canal.

Procedures on the cervix include biopsies performed to check for malignant cells and removal of cervical tissue (Endoscopy codes located in 57452 to 57461; Excision codes located in 57500 to 57558). When coding for an excision of cervical tissue, it is necessary to identify the manner in which the procedure was performed—either via endoscope or excision. Also identify whether the excision of tissue was for a biopsy,

Figure 17.7. Cervix uteri, corpus uteri, oviducts, and ovaries

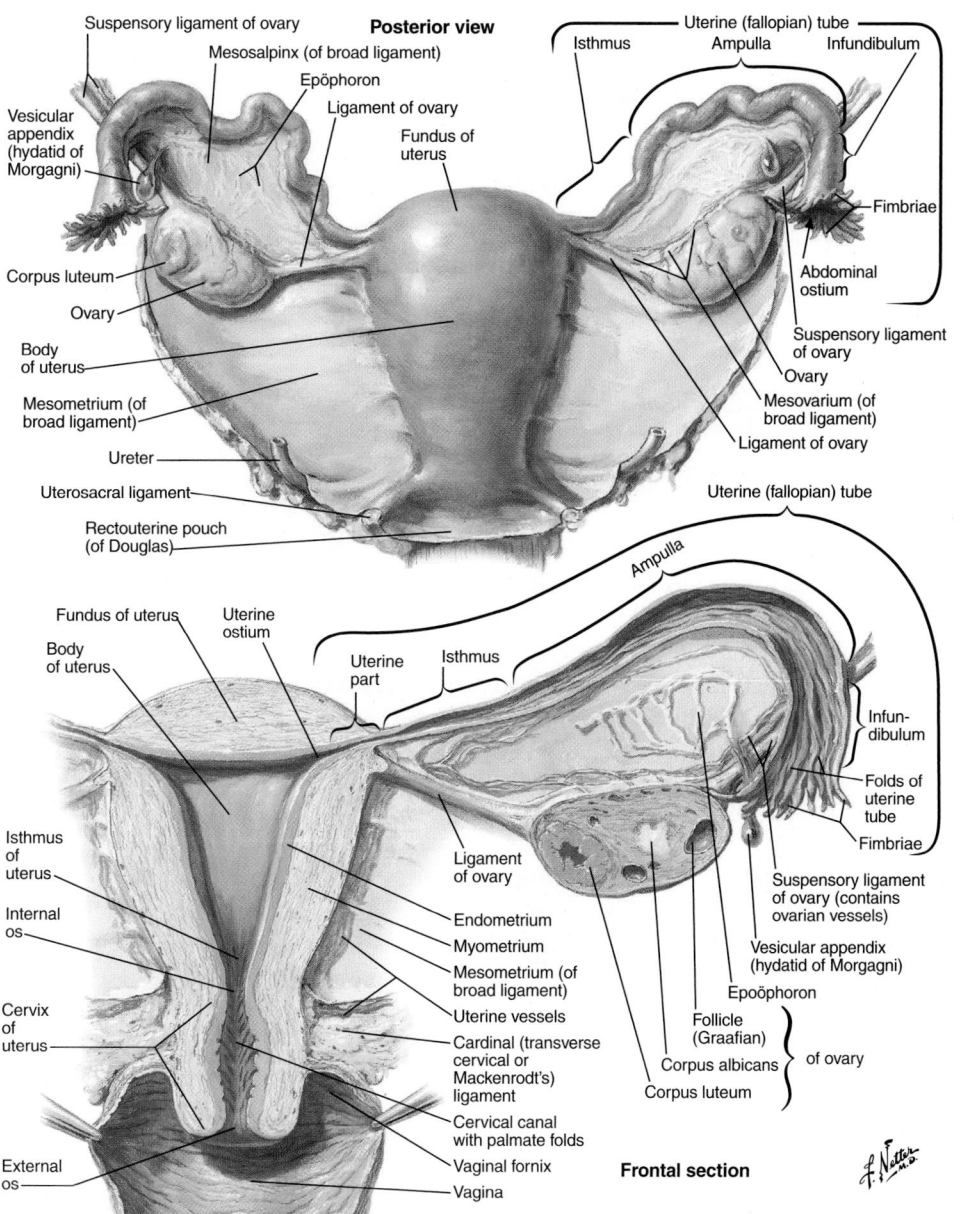

and the manner in which the tissue was removed. Cervical tissue removals are performed via the following procedures.

- **Endocervical curettage (ECC).** Procedure in which a curette is used to scrape cells off the cervical canal. For example, code 57505, Endocervical curettage (not done as part of a dilation and curettage).

- **Loop electrosurgical excision procedure (LEEP).** Procedure in which a fine wire with an electrical charge is used to remove cervical tissue. An LEEP may be performed for biopsy or excisional purposes. For example, code 57522, Conization of cervix, with or without fulguration, with or without dilation and curettage, with or without repair; loop electrode excision.

- **Conization.** A procedure that uses either an electrical wire (LEEP), cold knife, or laser to remove a cone of tissue from the cervix, either for diagnostic purposes

Figure 17.8. Conization of the cervix with cold knife

(biopsy) or to remove cancerous or pre-cancerous cells (see figure 17.8). For example, code 57461, Colposcopy of the cervix including upper/adjacent vagina; with loop electrode conization of the cervix.

Additional procedures performed on the cervix uteri include repair, including cerclage of the cervix. A **cerclage** of the cervix is a stitch or band device that helps the cervix remain closed at the external os. It can be done either for cervical incompetence in a non-obstetric case, or during pregnancy in women with history of cervical incompetence or miscarriage. Note that the codes for cerclage reflect whether or not the patient is obstetric: 57700, Cerclage of uterine cervix, nonobstetrical, versus 59320, Cerclage of cervix, during pregnancy; vaginal, or 59325, Cerclage of cervix, during pregnancy; abdominal.

Corpus Uteri

The **corpus uteri**, also known as the uterus, is the body of the uterus above the internal os of the cervix and connects to the fallopian tubes at the fundus at the top of the uterus (refer to figure 17.7). Lined with endometrial cells, the **uterus** is where the fetus develops during gestation.

Procedures on the uterus include excisions, which range from biopsy of endometrial cells in the lining of the uterus to the complete removal of the uterus, cervix, ovaries, and fallopian tubes. When reporting codes for any type of removal procedure, it is important to first determine the components included in the procedure. For example, was the procedure a biopsy and, if so, what tissue was biopsied? If the procedure was an excision of the uterus, what additional components were removed (uterus, cervix, fallopian tubes, or ovaries)? Furthermore, how was the procedure performed? Open excisions of the uterus are reported with codes 58100 through 58294, whereas laparoscopic procedures are reported with codes 58541 through 58579. Total hysterectomy codes depend on the weight of the excised organ—250 g or less, or 250 g or more.

There are also introduction procedures in the uterus; for example, the introduction or removal of **intrauterine device (IUD)** (58300, Insertion of intrauterine device (IUD), or 58301, Removal of intrauterine device (IUD)). An IUD is a small, T-shaped device inserted into the uterus for birth control purposes (see figure 17.9). Like coding for the

Figure 17.9. Intrauterine device

Source: ©AHIMA.

fitting or insertion of a pessary or diaphragm, the HCPCS code for the IUD itself is needed when reporting the insertion of an IUD. For example, J7300, Intrauterine copper contraceptive.

Oviducts and Ovaries

The **oviducts**, also known as the **fallopian tubes**, are the ducts through which eggs released from the ovaries travel. The fallopian tubes are attached to the fundus of the uterus and resemble long tubes, ending with small finger-like fimbriae. The **ovaries** are the glands found on either side of the uterus, below and behind the fallopian tubes, anchored to the uterus with suspensory ligaments. The ovaries form eggs that are released at regular intervals and travel through the fallopian tubes into the uterus where they are either fertilized by sperm or shed by the body (refer to figure 17.7).

Procedures on the oviducts include ligation, transection, or occlusion of the fallopian tubes for birth control purposes (Incision, 58600 to 58615) and laparoscopic procedures on the fallopian tubes (Laparoscopy 58660 to 58679). When coding for the excision of fallopian tubes, it is necessary to identify the procedure as either the removal of just the fallopian tubes (58700, Salpingectomy, complete or partial, unilateral or bilateral) or removal of both the fallopian tubes and the ovaries (58720, Salpingo-oophorectomy, complete or partial, unilateral or bilateral).

Codes for the removal of ovaries identify the type of removal (biopsy, wedge resection or bisection, cystectomy, or total removal), and identify additional components included in the excision procedure, such as lymphadenectomy or omentectomy.

Key to Success

When coding for procedures on the fallopian tubes or ovaries, remember that these are paired organs, meaning that procedures may be performed either unilaterally or bilaterally. Sometimes codes differ depending on whether the procedure was performed on either one or both sides, so look for this when reporting codes for the fallopian tubes and ovaries.

For practice assigning codes for OB/GYN services, complete the exercises in There's a Code for That 17.1.

17.1

There's a Code for That

Coding for OB/GYN services

Read the following documentation from OB/GYN encounters and services and assign the appropriate CPT and HCPCS codes. (Note that some of these encounters may require E/M codes, surgical codes, or both).

1. 23-year-old established patient presents to the office of her gynecologist complaining of fatigue, nausea, and two missed periods. She took a pregnancy test at home, which was positive, and presents today to get a confirmation pregnancy test. E/M service provided includes problem-focused history and examination, and straightforward medial decision making. Urine pregnancy test performed in office is positive.

   CPT codes: _____, _____

2. Code for the complete radical vulvectomy with inguinofemoral lymphadenectomy of the left nodes.

   CPT code: _____

3. Perineoplasty to repair traumatic laceration of the perineum.

   CPT code: _____

4. Laparoscopic supracervical hysterectomy with bilateral salpingo-oophorectomy for uterus weighing 278 grams.

   CPT code: _____

5. 26-year-old female multigravida presents for contraceptive counseling and the insertion of IUD. After 20 minutes spent counseling the patient, Mirena IUD contraceptive (52 mg levonogestrel-releasing) was inserted into cervix without incident.

   CPT codes: _____, _____, _____

6. Endoscopic biopsy of the cervix with endometrial sampling.

   CPT codes: _____, _____

7. Patient with pelvic pain and discomfort for 3 weeks presents for examination. During a detailed history she admits that during her last menstrual period she lost a tampon after insertion. Detailed pelvic examination reveals impacted tampon, near cervical opening. Tampon removed without incident, patient tolerated the procedure well.

   CPT code: _____

Maternity and Obstetric Services

Maternity services are reported from the Maternity Care and Delivery (59000 to 59899) subsection of the CPT code book. This section includes codes for services unrelated to childbirth and delivery, but still related to the fetus and care of the mother, as well as services related to routine antenatal, delivery, and postpartum care of the mother.

Maternity Care

Maternity care procedures include Antepartum and Fetal Invasive Services (59000 to 59076), Excision (59100 to 59160), Introduction (59200), Repair (59300 to 59350), Abortion (59812 to 59857), and Other Procedures (59866 to 59899).

- Antepartum and fetal invasive services are related to the growth and development of both the mother and the fetus, and include both diagnostic procedures designed to test the health of the fetus, such as 59025, Fetal non-stress test, as well as therapeutic procedures designed to treat the health of the mother or the fetus, such as 59001, Amniocentesis; therapeutic amniotic fluid reduction (includes ultrasound guidance).

- Excision procedures include surgical treatment of ectopic pregnancies. An ectopic pregnancy is one in which the fertilized egg has implanted outside of the uterus. Codes for the surgical removal of an ectopic pregnancy depend on the site of the implantation, such as 59130, Surgical treatment of ectopic pregnancy; abdominal pregnancy, or 59140, Surgical treatment of ectopic pregnancy; cervical, with evacuation.

- Introduction. There is only one code in the introduction category, which is 59200, Insertion of cervical dilator (e.g., luminaria, prostaglandin). A cervical dilator is a small tampon-like device with a small amount of labor-inducing hormones placed against the cervix to help it soften and thin out before inducing labor.

- Repair codes include an episiotomy repair by a healthcare provider other than the one who performed the episiotomy during the delivery (59300), as well as obstetric cerclage (59320 to 59325) and repair of ruptured uterus (59350).

- Abortion procedures are performed to evacuate the uterus of the products of conception (POC). Products of conception are the remaining fetal and placental tissues after either a spontaneous miscarriage or elective pregnancy termination.

- Other procedures include multifetal pregnancy reductions, uterine evacuation and curettage for hydatidiform mole, removal of cerclage sutures under anesthesia, and unlisted maternity care and delivery procedures.

Delivery

Correctly reporting codes for delivery procedures depends on an understanding of the global maternity package. Just like a surgical package, the global delivery package includes several services, ranging from antepartum care to delivery and postpartum care; noted as follows.

- Antepartum services:
  - Initial and subsequent prenatal history and physical examinations
  - Recording of maternal weight, blood pressure, fetal heart tones
  - Routine chemical urinalysis
  - Monthly visits up to 28 weeks of gestation
  - Biweekly visits up to 36 weeks of gestation
  - Weekly visits at week 37 until delivery
- Delivery services:
  - Admission to the hospital, including admission history and physical examination
  - Management of uncomplicated labor
  - Delivery (vaginal or cesarean), including episiotomy and use of forceps
- Postpartum services:
  - Office or other outpatient visits following delivery

When a single provider (or if the patient saw multiple providers from the same group) performed all of the antepartum, delivery, and postpartum services, then only one single code identifying the services is reported. For example, if a doctor performed all the antepartum visits, a vaginal delivery, and then the postpartum checkup, then he or she would report code 59400, Routine obstetric care including antepartum care, vaginal delivery (with or without episiotomy, and/or forceps) and postpartum care

Figure 17.10. The global maternity package

59400, Routine obstetric care including **antepartum** care, vaginal **delivery** (with or without episiotomy, and/or forceps) and **postpartum** care

(see figure 17.10). This one code reports the entire package related to the patient's routine antepartum care, delivery, and routine postpartum care.

However, there are several services not included in routine care. These services should be reported separately, outside of the global maternity package, and include the following:

- Pregnancy confirmation during a problem-oriented or preventive visit. This should be coded with the appropriate E/M code.
- Any visits during the antepartum period that are not routine care related to the patient's pregnancy. For example, a sick visit would not be included in the global maternity package. This would be coded with the appropriate E/M code.
- Medical complications of the pregnancy, such as cardiac problems, neurological problems, diabetes, hypertension, toxemia, hyperemesis (excessive vomiting), preterm labor, premature rupture of membranes, or trauma.
- Medical problems complicating labor and delivery that require additional resources.
- Surgical complications of pregnancy, such as appendectomy, hernia, ovarian cyst, or Bartholin's cyst, that require care during the pregnancy or delivery. These services would be reported with the appropriate surgery codes.

When a healthcare provider only performs a portion of the global maternity service—for example, only the delivery or a portion of the antepartum visits—then those specific services would be reported according to the exact service the provider performed. For example, if the provider only performed the vaginal delivery because the original doctor was unavailable, then he or she would report code 59409, Vaginal delivery only (with or without episiotomy and/or forceps).

Key to Success

Remember when breaking up the global maternity package to code only for the service that your provider performed. For example, if your provider only performed a portion of the antepartum appointments, then code only for those services. The remaining services provided by other practitioners will be reported by those practitioners.

Coding for maternity services is further complicated by different types of deliveries as well as multiple births.

Types of Deliveries

The CPT code book identifies four different types of births, each of which are coded with a different range of CPT codes (for individual components and for the global maternity package).

- Vaginal delivery (59400 to 59414).
- Cesarean delivery (59510 to 59525).
- Vaginal birth after cesarean (VBAC) (59610 to 59614). A VBAC is when a woman who has previously given birth via cesarean section successfully gives birth vaginally.
- Cesarean delivery after attempted VBAC (59618 to 59622). This type of delivery is reported when a VBAC is attempted, but for medical reasons must be converted to a cesarean delivery.

When coding for deliveries, first determine the type of delivery (as listed previously) and then the specific service provided (either the global maternity package or a part thereof). Note that codes 59425 to 59430 identify either antepartum care (depending on the number of visits) or postpartum care, and do not identify the type of delivery. For these codes, the type of delivery is not relevant because the provider did not perform any of the delivery service.

Figure 17.11. Multiple births

Multiple Births

Reporting the delivery services for multiple births depends on the type of deliveries and the third-party payer. Unless the insurance has specific reporting requirements, report multiple (twin or more) births as follows (see figure 17.11):

- Multiple birth, all born vaginally. Report code 59400 for the global maternity package with vaginal delivery, in addition to 59409, Vaginal delivery only, appended with modifier -59 to identify the additional procedure as a distinct service.

- Multiple birth, all born via cesarean. Report code 59510 for the global maternity package with cesarean delivery. This code should be reported only once. However, if there was a significant amount of additional work involved, modifier -22 should be reported to identify the increased procedural service.

- Multiple births in which one twin is vaginal and the other is born via cesarean, report 59510 for the global maternity package for the cesarean delivery (the work involved in the cesarean delivery is higher, so it should be reported as the primary service). Also report code 59409, Vaginal delivery only, appended with modifier -51 for the multiple procedures.

Key to Success

Again, note that these multiple birth delivery guidelines are likely to change. One insurance provider might require modifier -59, Distinct procedural service, while another insurance provider might require modifier -51, Multiple procedures. One insurance provider may allow you to bill the routine delivery code with two or more units, whereas another requires the use of modifier -22, Increased procedural services. Ultimately, report the delivery of multiples according to the guidelines set forth by the payer that is covering the service.

Complete the exercises in There's a Code for That 17.2 for practice reporting maternity and obstetric services.

17.2 Coding for maternity and obstetric services

There's a Code for That

Read the following documentation from maternity encounters and services and assign the appropriate CPT codes.

1. Vaginal cerclage on a pregnant 34-year-old G5P1 with history of incompetent cervix.

   CPT code: _____

2. Cesarean delivery only.

   CPT code: _____

3. 30-year-old pregnant female received five antepartum visits from Dr. A, and then moved across the state, where Dr. B completed the remaining antepartum care, a cesarean delivery, and the postpartum check.

   Identify the CPT code for Dr. A's services: _____

   Identify the CPT code for Dr. B's services: _____

4. Routine vaginal delivery with episiotomy, including antepartum and postpartum care.

   CPT code: _____

5. Amniocentesis with imaging guidance for fluid reduction.

CPT code: _____

6. Surgical treatment of septic abortion.

CPT code: _____

Diagnosis Coding for OB/GYN Services

Diagnosis coding for OB/GYN services generally falls into two broad categories: diseases of the genitourinary system for gynecological services, and codes for pregnancy, childbirth, and the puerperium for obstetric services. A handful of Z-codes for routine examinations, screenings, and additional information for patient encounters are also important to report for OB/GYN services (refer to chapter 8 for a discussion of Z-codes). Codes for abnormal findings and encounters for examinations are also important to understand in OB/GYN coding.

Diseases of the Genitourinary System

Gynecological services are reported primarily with codes from chapter 14: Diseases of the Genitourinary System, of the ICD-10-CM code book. However, additional codes may be used to identify specific signs and symptoms, such as dysuria or abnormal lab findings. Z-codes may also be reported for medical examinations, screenings, personal or family history, or additional pertinent patient information related to the encounter. This chapter includes codes for both the urinary and genital systems for both males and females, and is first organized by urinary conditions, such as Glomerular diseases (N00 to N08), Renal tubulo-interstitial diseases (N10 to N16), Acute kidney failure and chronic kidney disease (N17 to N19), Urolithiasis (N20 to N23), Other diseases of the kidney and ureter (N25 to N29), and Other diseases of the urinary system (N30 to N39). Note that when coding for these categories, there are several valid three-character codes and a handful of notes to report additional code(s) for underlying conditions, an infectious or toxic agent, or a causal condition, when necessary.

Codes in these categories are also applicable to both males and females, as they affect the urinary system. The next category of codes in the chapter, Diseases of male genital organs (N40 to N53) pertain specifically to male patients. As with other codes for urinary conditions, pay attention to the notes in the Tabular that indicate when to include additional codes to identify underlying condition(s), infectious agent, or causal condition. Notice that the codes in this category all have a small male symbol next to them in the Tabular List (♂), which indicates that these diagnosis codes may only be used for male patients. Additional diagnosis and procedure codes for male genital and urinary systems are discussed in chapter 18.

Remaining categories of codes in this chapter are for Disorders of breast (N60 to N65), which may be applicable for either male or female patients, followed by Inflammatory diseases of female pelvic organs (N70 to N77) and Noninflammatory diseases of the female genital tract (N80 to N98). Note that these last two categories pertain to only female patients. As such, they all each have a small female symbol (♀). (The presence or absence of the male or female symbols depends on the publisher of the ICD-10-CM code book. Note that these symbols may not be present in all code books.)

Abnormal Findings and Encounters for Examinations

OB/GYN providers may also see patients for signs, symptoms, and abnormal findings of the genitourinary system, which are reported with codes from chapter 19: Symptoms, Signs, and Abnormal Clinical and Laboratory Findings, Not Elsewhere Classified. Abnormal findings are reported with codes from category R87, Abnormal findings in specimens from female genital organs. These include abnormal findings from pap smears and cellular changes, which may indicate cancer, among other findings.

Encounters for examinations and screenings identify that the patient presented for a gynecological examination and are reported with codes from category Z01.4, Encounter for gynecological examination. A code from this category should be reported when a woman presents for a routine gynecological examination. If an abnormal finding is encountered at the examination, such as a genitourinary condition, abnormal laboratory finding, or sign or symptom, report the code for the abnormal finding in addition to the code for the routine screening (with abnormal findings).

Encounter codes may also be necessary in identifying when a patient receives a contraceptive (Z30, Encounter for contraceptive management) or procreative encounter (Z31, Encounter for procreative management), such as counseling provided to a patient considering a specific type of birth control or regarding fertility. Codes for contraceptive management may also be used when a patient returns for a refill or evaluation and management of a current birth control method, to begin a new birth control method, or to cease a birth control method (such as the removal of an IUD). When coding for contraceptive management, identify the specific type of contraceptive used and the specific contraceptive management service provided. For example, Z30.46, Encounter for surveillance of implantable subdermal contraceptive, identifies the service provided (*surveillance*) and the type of contraceptive (*implantable subdermal*).

Complete the exercises in There's a Code for That 17.3 for practice assigning OB/GYN diagnosis codes.

17.3

There's a Code for That

Coding for OB/GYN services

Read the following documentation from OB/GYN encounters and services and assign the appropriate ICD-10-CM codes.

1. 13-year-old female presents complaining of heavy periods. She started her period two months ago and her mother is bringing her in today for examination. Impression: pubertal menorrhagia.

   ICD-10-CM code: _____

2. Infertility counseling for a 27-year-old G1P2 with polycystic ovarian syndrome (PCOS).

   ICD-10-CM codes: _____, _____

3. Abnormal pap smear.

   ICD-10-CM code: _____

4. 55-year-old female with menopause (started approximately 6 months ago) presents complaining of hot flashes, sleeplessness, and headaches.

   ICD-10-CM codes: _____, _____. _____

5. Acute vulvovaginitis.

   ICD-10-CM code: _____

Pregnancy, Childbirth, and the Puerperium

Conditions related to pregnancy, childbirth, and the puerperium are reported with codes from chapter 15: Pregnancy, Childbirth, and the Puerperium of the ICD-10-CM code book, as well as from chapter 21: Factors Influencing Health Status and Contact with Health Services (Z-codes).

Codes from chapter 15 begin with the letter O making it easy to remember that O codes are for obstetric services. However, keep in mind that obstetric coding can be a bit more complicated than other types of coding, as the codes in this chapter tend to be longer as they require more characters. More codes are also needed to fully identify all of the medical conditions present, as well as the estimated weeks of gestation of the pregnancy. A good rule to follow when assigning codes for obstetric patients is to code until you can code no longer. Review the diagnostic statement and ensure that a diagnosis code is assigned for every healthcare condition affecting the patient.

There are also several important guidelines that govern how and when to assign codes for pregnancy, childbirth, and the puerperium. These useful guidelines help coders assign the correct codes and also refer to additional codes, including Z-codes, when necessary. Remember that many obstetric cases will contain codes from both chapter 15 as well as Z-codes from chapter 21. See figure 17.12 for the OGCR related to obstetrical and reproductive services.

Figure 17.12. OGCR I.C.21.c.11

---

11) Encounters for Obstetrical and Reproductive Services

See Section I.C.15. Pregnancy, Childbirth, and the Puerperium, for further instruction on the use of these codes.

Z codes for pregnancy are for use in those circumstances when none of the problems or complications included in the codes from the Obstetrics chapter exist (a routine prenatal visit or postpartum care). Codes in category Z34, Encounter for supervision of normal pregnancy, are always first-listed and are not to be used with any other code from the OB chapter.

Codes in category Z3A, Weeks of gestation, may be assigned to provide additional information about the pregnancy. Category Z3A codes should not be assigned for pregnancies with abortive outcomes (categories O00-O08), elective termination of pregnancy (code **Z33.2**), nor for postpartum conditions, as category Z3A is not applicable to these conditions. The date of the admission should be used to determine weeks of gestation for inpatient admissions that encompass more than one gestational week.

The outcome of delivery, category Z37, should be included on all maternal delivery records. It is always a secondary code. Codes in category Z37 should not be used on the newborn record.

Z codes for family planning (contraceptive) or procreative management and counseling should be included on an obstetric record either during the pregnancy or the postpartum stage, if applicable.

Z codes/categories for obstetrical and reproductive services:

Z30	Encounter for contraceptive management
Z31	Encounter for procreative management
Z32.2	Encounter for childbirth instruction
Z32.3	Encounter for childcare instruction
Z33	Pregnant state
Z34	Encounter for supervision of normal pregnancy
Z36	Encounter for antenatal screening of mother
Z3A	Weeks of gestation
Z37	Outcome of delivery
Z39	Encounter for maternal postpartum care and examination
Z76.81	Expectant mother prebirth pediatrician visit

Guidelines for Coding Obstetric Diagnoses

Guidelines for coding obstetric (OB) cases require an understanding of the numerous components and additional codes that should be reported when a patient presents for obstetric services. These include guidelines for sequencing of pregnancy conditions and incidental pregnancy, estimated weeks of gestation, encounters for pregnancy-related services, identification of the fetus in multiple pregnancies, delivery guidelines, and pre-existing versus gestational conditions. Figure 17.13 lists the OGCR related to coding for OB conditions. As you read the following sections, return to this figure to identify the individual OGCR for coding for these conditions.

Sequencing and Incidental Pregnancy

Codes from chapter 15 have sequencing priority over codes from other chapters. Sequencing priority means that these codes should be assigned *before* codes from other chapters.

Codes from chapter 15 are commonly assigned with codes from other chapters of the ICD-10-CM code book. In these instances, it is necessary to sequence the O-code before the additional codes for the encounter. This guideline overrules other sequencing priority guidelines from other chapters. For example, HIV guidelines state that the code B20 for symptomatic HIV should be sequenced as the first-listed diagnosis on a claim. However, if the HIV-positive patient is pregnant, then code O98.7-, Human immunodeficiency virus [HIV] disease complicating pregnancy, childbirth and the puerperium should be sequenced before the code to identify the type of HIV. In this case, the fact that the patient is pregnant and has HIV is more important than simply the diagnosis of HIV.

However, there is one exception to this rule. When a patient presents for an encounter that is completely unrelated to the pregnancy such as a finger laceration, then the pregnancy should be coded as incidental to the encounter. An **incidental pregnancy** is one that in no way complicates the reason for the healthcare encounter. When a pregnancy is incidental to the encounter, the coder must assign a code for the reason for the encounter, such as finger laceration, and the code for incidental pregnancy to indicate that the patient is pregnant, but the pregnancy does not impact, nor is it impacted by, the reason for the encounter: Z33.1, Pregnant state, incidental.

Estimated Weeks of Gestation

Whenever a pregnant patient presents for any type of obstetric service or childbirth, it is necessary to report a code from category Z3A, Weeks of gestation. For example, if a patient reported to the office of her obstetrician for a routine prenatal examination and she was 30 weeks pregnant, then code Z3A.30, 30 weeks gestation of pregnancy, should be reported in addition to any other codes assigned at that visit. According to ICD-10-CM guidelines, category Z3A codes should not be assigned:

* For pregnancies with abortive outcomes (categories O00 to O08)
* For elective termination of pregnancy (Z33.32)
* For postpartum conditions (and the patient is no longer pregnant)

Weeks of gestation codes are organized in such a way that they are relatively easy to assign, as the last two digits identify the number of weeks. For example, a patient at 20 weeks gestation is assigned code Z3A.20. A patient at 24 weeks gestation is assigned code Z3A.24. A patient at 32 weeks gestation is assigned code Z3A.32. And so on. The last two digits identify the number of weeks. (Note that this rule does not apply before 8 weeks gestation or after 42 weeks gestation.)

Figure 17.13. OGCR I.C.15

15. Chapter 15: Pregnancy, Childbirth and the Puerperium (O00-O9A)

a. General Rules for Obstetric Cases

1) Codes from chapter 15 and sequencing priority

Obstetric cases require codes from chapter 15, codes in the range O00-O9A, Pregnancy, Childbirth, and the Puerperium. Chapter 15 codes have sequencing priority over codes from other chapters. Additional codes from other chapters may be used in conjunction with chapter 15 codes to further specify conditions. Should the provider document that the pregnancy is incidental to the encounter, then code Z33.1, Pregnant state, incidental, should be used in place of any chapter 15 codes. It is the provider's responsibility to state that the condition being treated is not affecting the pregnancy.

2) Chapter 15 codes used only on the maternal record

Chapter 15 codes are to be used only on the maternal record, never on the record of the newborn.

3) Final character for trimester

The majority of codes in Chapter 15 have a final character indicating the trimester of pregnancy. The timeframes for the trimesters are indicated at the beginning of the chapter. If trimester is not a component of a code it is because the condition always occurs in a specific trimester, or the concept of trimester of pregnancy is not applicable. Certain codes have characters for only certain trimesters because the condition does not occur in all trimesters, but it may occur in more than just one.

Assignment of the final character for trimester should be based on the provider's documentation of the trimester (or number of weeks) for the current admission/encounter. This applies to the assignment of trimester for pre-existing conditions as well as those that develop during or are due to the pregnancy. The provider's documentation of the number of weeks may be used to assign the appropriate code identifying the trimester.

Whenever delivery occurs during the current admission, and there is an "in childbirth" option for the obstetric complication being coded, the "in childbirth" code should be assigned.

4) Selection of trimester for inpatient admissions that encompass more than one trimester

In instances when a patient is admitted to a hospital for complications of pregnancy during one trimester and remains in the hospital into a subsequent trimester, the trimester character for the antepartum complication code should be assigned on the basis of the trimester when the complication developed, not the trimester of the discharge. If the condition developed prior to the current admission/encounter or represents a pre-existing condition, the trimester character for the trimester at the time of the admission/encounter should be assigned.

5) Unspecified trimester

Each category that includes codes for trimester has a code for "unspecified trimester." The "unspecified trimester" code should rarely be used, such as when the documentation in the record is insufficient to determine the trimester and it is not possible to obtain clarification.

6) 7ᵗʰ character for Fetus Identification

Where applicable, a 7ᵗʰ character is to be assigned for certain categories (O31, O32, O33.3 - O33.6, O35, O36, O40, O41, O60.1, O60.2, O64, and O69) to identify the fetus for which the complication code applies.

Assign 7ᵗʰ character "0":

- For single gestations
- When the documentation in the record is insufficient to determine the fetus affected and it is not possible to obtain clarification.
- When it is not possible to clinically determine which fetus is affected.

b. Selection of OB Principal or First-listed Diagnosis

1) Routine outpatient prenatal visits

For routine outpatient prenatal visits when no complications are present, a code from category Z34, Encounter for supervision of normal pregnancy, should be used as the first-listed diagnosis. These codes should not be used in conjunction with chapter 15 codes.

2) Supervision of High-Risk Pregnancy

Codes from category O09, Supervision of high-risk pregnancy, are intended for use only during the prenatal period. For complications during the labor or delivery episode as a result of a high-risk pregnancy, assign the applicable complication codes from Chapter 15. If there are no complications during the labor or delivery episode, assign code O80, Encounter for full-term uncomplicated delivery.

For routine prenatal outpatient visits for patients with high-risk pregnancies, a code from category O09, Supervision of high-risk pregnancy, should be used as the first-listed diagnosis. Secondary chapter 15 codes may be used in conjunction with these codes if appropriate.

(Continued on next page)

Figure 17.13. *(Continued)*

b. Selection of OB Principal or First-listed Diagnosis

1) Routine outpatient prenatal visits

For routine outpatient prenatal visits when no complications are present, a code from category Z34, Encounter for supervision of normal pregnancy, should be used as the first-listed diagnosis. These codes should not be used in conjunction with chapter 15 codes.

2) Supervision of High-Risk Pregnancy

Codes from category O09, Supervision of high-risk pregnancy, are intended for use only during the prenatal period. For complications during the labor or delivery episode as a result of a high-risk pregnancy, assign the applicable complication codes from Chapter 15. If there are no complications during the labor or delivery episode, assign code O80, Encounter for full-term uncomplicated delivery.

For routine prenatal outpatient visits for patients with high-risk pregnancies, a code from category O09, Supervision of high-risk pregnancy, should be used as the first-listed diagnosis. Secondary chapter 15 codes may be used in conjunction with these codes if appropriate.

3) Episodes when no delivery occurs

In episodes when no delivery occurs, the principal diagnosis should correspond to the principal complication of the pregnancy which necessitated the encounter. Should more than one complication exist, all of which are treated or monitored, any of the complications codes may be sequenced first.

4) When a delivery occurs

When an obstetric patient is admitted and delivers during that admission, the condition that prompted the admission should be sequenced as the principal diagnosis. If multiple conditions prompted the admission, sequence the one most related to the delivery as the principal diagnosis. A code for any complication of the delivery should be assigned as an additional diagnosis. In cases of cesarean delivery, if the patient was admitted with a condition that resulted in the performance of a cesarean procedure, that condition should be selected as the principal diagnosis. If the reason for the admission was unrelated to the condition resulting in the cesarean delivery, the condition related to the reason for the admission should be selected as the principal diagnosis.

5) Outcome of delivery

A code from category Z37, Outcome of delivery, should be included on every maternal record when a delivery has occurred. These codes are not to be used on subsequent records or on the newborn record.

c. Pre-existing conditions versus conditions due to the pregnancy

Certain categories in Chapter 15 distinguish between conditions of the mother that existed prior to pregnancy (pre-existing) and those that are a direct result of pregnancy. When assigning codes from Chapter 15, it is important to assess if a condition was pre-existing prior to pregnancy or developed during or due to the pregnancy in order to assign the correct code.

Categories that do not distinguish between pre-existing and pregnancy- related conditions may be used for either. It is acceptable to use codes specifically for the puerperium with codes complicating pregnancy and childbirth if a condition arises postpartum during the delivery encounter.

d. Pre-existing hypertension in pregnancy

Category O10, Pre-existing hypertension complicating pregnancy, childbirth and the puerperium, includes codes for hypertensive heart and hypertensive chronic kidney disease. When assigning one of the O10 codes that includes hypertensive heart disease or hypertensive chronic kidney disease, it is necessary to add a secondary code from the appropriate hypertension category to specify the type of heart failure or chronic kidney disease.

See Section I.C.9. Hypertension.

e. Fetal Conditions Affecting the Management of the Mother

1) Codes from categories O35 and O36

Codes from categories O35, Maternal care for known or suspected fetal abnormality and damage, and O36, Maternal care for other fetal problems, are assigned only when the fetal condition is actually responsible for modifying the management of the mother, i.e., by requiring diagnostic studies, additional observation, special care, or termination of pregnancy. The fact that the fetal condition exists does not justify assigning a code from this series to the mother's record.

2) In utero surgery

In cases when surgery is performed on the fetus, a diagnosis code from category O35, Maternal care for known or suspected fetal abnormality and damage, should be assigned identifying the fetal condition. Assign the appropriate procedure code for the procedure performed.

No code from Chapter 16, the perinatal codes, should be used on the mother's record to identify fetal conditions. Surgery performed in utero on a fetus is still to be coded as an obstetric encounter.

f. HIV Infection in Pregnancy, Childbirth and the Puerperium

During pregnancy, childbirth or the puerperium, a patient admitted because of an HIV-related illness should receive a principal diagnosis from subcategory O98.7-, Human immunodeficiency [HIV] disease complicating pregnancy, childbirth and the puerperium, followed by the code(s) for the HIV-related illness(es).

Patients with asymptomatic HIV infection status admitted during pregnancy, childbirth, or the puerperium should receive codes of O98.7- and Z21, Asymptomatic human immunodeficiency virus [HIV] infection status.

g. Diabetes mellitus in pregnancy

Diabetes mellitus is a significant complicating factor in pregnancy. Pregnant women who are diabetic should be assigned a code from category O24, Diabetes mellitus in pregnancy, childbirth, and the puerperium, first, followed by the appropriate diabetes code(s) (E08- E13) from Chapter 4.

h. Long term use of insulin and oral hypoglycemics

See section I.C.4.a.3 for information on the long term use of insulin and oral hypoglycemic.

i. Gestational (pregnancy induced) diabetes

Gestational (pregnancy induced) diabetes can occur during the second and third trimester of pregnancy in women who were not diabetic prior to pregnancy. Gestational diabetes can cause complications in the pregnancy similar to those of pre-existing diabetes mellitus. It also puts the woman at greater risk of developing diabetes after the pregnancy. Codes for gestational diabetes are in subcategory O24.4, Gestational diabetes mellitus. No other code from category O24, Diabetes mellitus in pregnancy, childbirth, and the puerperium, should be used with a code from O24.4

The codes under subcategory O24.4 include diet controlled, insulin controlled, and controlled by oral hypoglycemic drugs. If a patient with gestational diabetes is treated with both diet and insulin, only the code for insulin-controlled is required. If a patient with gestational diabetes is treated with both diet and oral hypoglycemic medications, only the code for "controlled by oral hypoglycemic drugs" is required.

Code Z79.4, Long-term (current) use of insulin or code Z79.84, Long-term (current) use of oral hypoglycemic drugs, should not be assigned with codes from subcategory O24.4.

An abnormal glucose tolerance in pregnancy is assigned a code from subcategory O99.81, Abnormal glucose complicating pregnancy, childbirth, and the puerperium.

j. Sepsis and septic shock complicating abortion, pregnancy, childbirth and the puerperium

When assigning a chapter 15 code for sepsis complicating abortion, pregnancy, childbirth, and the puerperium, a code for the specific type of infection should be assigned as an additional diagnosis. If severe sepsis is present, a code from subcategory R65.2, Severe sepsis, and code(s) for associated organ dysfunction(s) should also be assigned as additional diagnoses.

k. Puerperal sepsis

Code O85, Puerperal sepsis, should be assigned with a secondary code to identify the causal organism (e.g., for a bacterial infection, assign a code from category B95-B96, Bacterial infections in conditions classified elsewhere). A code from category A40, Streptococcal sepsis, or A41, Other sepsis, should not be used for puerperal sepsis. If applicable, use additional codes to identify severe sepsis (R65.2-) and any associated acute organ dysfunction.

l. Alcohol and tobacco use during pregnancy, childbirth and the puerperium

1) Alcohol use during pregnancy, childbirth and the puerperium

Codes under subcategory O99.31, Alcohol use complicating pregnancy, childbirth, and the puerperium, should be assigned for any pregnancy case when a mother uses alcohol during the pregnancy or postpartum. A secondary code from category F10, Alcohol related disorders, should also be assigned to identify manifestations of the alcohol use.

2) Tobacco use during pregnancy, childbirth and the puerperium

Codes under subcategory O99.33, Smoking (tobacco) complicating pregnancy, childbirth, and the puerperium, should be assigned for any pregnancy case when a mother uses any type of tobacco product during the pregnancy or postpartum. A secondary code from category F17, Nicotine dependence, should also be assigned to identify the type of nicotine dependence.

m. Poisoning, toxic effects, adverse effects and underdosing in a pregnant patient

A code from subcategory O9A.2, Injury, poisoning and certain other consequences of external causes complicating pregnancy, childbirth, and the puerperium, should be sequenced first, followed by the appropriate injury, poisoning,

(Continued on next page)

Figure 17.13. *(Continued)*

toxic effect, adverse effect or underdosing code, and then the additional code(s) that specifies the condition caused by the poisoning, toxic effect, adverse effect or underdosing.

See Section I.C.19. Adverse effects, poisoning, underdosing and toxic effects.

n. Normal Delivery, Code O80

1) Encounter for full term uncomplicated delivery

Code O80 should be assigned when a woman is admitted for a full-term normal delivery and delivers a single, healthy infant without any complications antepartum, during the delivery, or postpartum during the delivery episode. Code O80 is always a principal diagnosis. It is not to be used if any other code from chapter 15 is needed to describe a current complication of the antenatal, delivery, or perinatal period. Additional codes from other chapters may be used with code O80 if they are not related to or are in any way complicating the pregnancy.

2) Uncomplicated delivery with resolved antepartum complication

Code O80 may be used if the patient had a complication at some point during the pregnancy, but the complication is not present at the time of the admission for delivery.

3) Outcome of delivery for O80

Z37.0, Single live birth, is the only outcome of delivery code appropriate for use with O80.

o. The Peripartum and Postpartum Periods

1) Peripartum and Postpartum periods

The postpartum period begins immediately after delivery and continues for six weeks following delivery. The peripartum period is defined as the last month of pregnancy to five months postpartum.

2) Peripartum and postpartum complication

A postpartum complication is any complication occurring within the six-week period.

3) Pregnancy-related complications after 6 week period

Chapter 15 codes may also be used to describe pregnancy-related complications after the peripartum or postpartum period if the provider documents that a condition is pregnancy related.

4) Admission for routine postpartum care following delivery outside hospital

When the mother delivers outside the hospital prior to admission and is admitted for routine postpartum care and no complications are noted, code Z39.0, Encounter for care and examination of mother immediately after delivery, should be assigned as the principal diagnosis.

5) Pregnancy associated cardiomyopathy

Pregnancy associated cardiomyopathy, code O90.3, is unique in that it may be diagnosed in the third trimester of pregnancy but may continue to progress months after delivery. For this reason, it is referred to as peripartum cardiomyopathy. Code O90.3 is only for use when the cardiomyopathy develops as a result of pregnancy in a woman who did not have pre-existing heart disease.

p. Code O94, Sequelae of complication of pregnancy, childbirth, and the puerperium

1) Code O94

Code O94, Sequelae of complication of pregnancy, childbirth, and the puerperium, is for use in those cases when an initial complication of a pregnancy develops a sequelae requiring care or treatment at a future date.

2) After the initial postpartum period

This code may be used at any time after the initial postpartum period.

3) Sequencing of Code O94

This code, like all sequela codes, is to be sequenced following the code describing the sequelae of the complication.

q. Termination of Pregnancy and Spontaneous abortions

1) Abortion with Liveborn Fetus

When an attempted termination of pregnancy results in a liveborn fetus, assign code Z33.2, Encounter for elective termination of pregnancy and a code from category Z37, Outcome of Delivery.

2) Retained Products of Conception following an abortion

Subsequent encounters for retained products of conception following a spontaneous abortion or elective termination of pregnancy, **without complications** are assigned O03.**4, Incomplete spontaneous,** abortion **without complication,** or codes O07.4, Failed attempted termination of pregnancy without complication. This advice is appropriate even when the patient was discharged previously with a discharge diagnosis of complete abortion. **If the patient has a specific complication associated with the spontaneous abortion or elective termination of pregnancy in addition to retained products of conception, assign the appropriate complication in category O03 or O07 instead of code O03.4 or O07.4.**

3) **Complications leading to abortion**

   Codes from Chapter 15 may be used as additional codes to identify any documented complications of the pregnancy in conjunction with codes in categories in **O04**, O07 and O08.

r. **Abuse in a pregnant patient**

   For suspected or confirmed cases of abuse of a pregnant patient, a code(s) from subcategories O9A.3, Physical abuse complicating pregnancy, childbirth, and the puerperium, O9A.4, Sexual abuse complicating pregnancy, childbirth, and the puerperium, and O9A.5, Psychological abuse complicating pregnancy, childbirth, and the puerperium, should be sequenced first, followed by the appropriate codes (if applicable) to identify any associated current injury due to physical abuse, sexual abuse, and the perpetrator of abuse.

   See Section I.C.19. Adult and child abuse, neglect and other maltreatment.

Source: CMS 2018.

Key to Success

Keep the weeks of gestation guideline in mind when coding for pregnancy-related services. Unless the patient is in the postpartum period or the pregnancy is aborted or terminated, then every obstetric case should have at least two codes—one for the reason for the encounter (primary diagnosis) and another from category Z3A to identify the weeks of gestation. If the weeks of gestation are not identified in the documentation, then do not assign a weeks of gestation code.

Encounter for Pregnancy Services

Just like in injury codes, the encounter should be identified for a pregnant patient when she receives pregnancy-related services. However, the encounters do not identify if the service is initial, subsequent, or sequela, but rather where the patient is on the pregnancy timeline.

These encounters include the antepartum, childbirth, or puerperal (postpartum) periods. If the patient is in the antepartum period, then identify the specific trimester of the pregnancy. Remember that the first trimester is from conception to less than 14 weeks, 0 days; the second trimester is from 14 weeks, 0 days to less than 28 weeks, 0 days; and the third trimester is from 28 weeks, 0 days until delivery (see figure 17.14).

Figure 17.14. Encounters for pregnancy-related services

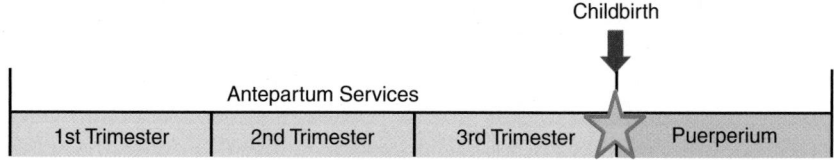

Note that not all codes identify the encounter for pregnancy-related services. If the condition reported is a condition that always occurs in a specific trimester, then the component of trimester is not included in the code. Some codes have only certain trimesters applicable, because said condition can only occur in specific trimesters. Ultimately, it is important to read the code description thoroughly, and always check to see if an additional character is required to identify the trimester of pregnancy, childbirth, or the puerperium.

If the specific trimester is not included in the documentation, but the number of weeks is included, it is the coder's responsibility to assign the correct trimester of pregnancy code. If neither the trimester nor the number of weeks of gestation are documented, assign the code for unspecified trimester.

Identification of Fetus in Multiple Pregnancies

When a patient with a multiple pregnancy (twins, triplets) presents for services, and a specific complication exists for one of the fetuses, it is necessary to assign a complication of pregnancy (O-code) to identify the complication for that specific fetus. For example, if fetus 1 in a twin birth is born with a nuchal cord (umbilical cord around the neck) without compression, and fetus 2 has no complications, then to the coder must assign code O69.81X1, Labor and delivery complicated by cord around neck, without compression, fetus 1. The seventh character "1" identifies that fetus 1 was affected by the nuchal cord.

The seventh-character "0" for "not applicable" should be used in the following circumstances:

- The pregnancy is a single gestation.
- The documentation does not specify which fetus was affected by the complication.
- When it is not clinically possible to identify which fetus is affected by the complication.

Delivery Guidelines

When coding for pregnancy-related services, coders should identify whether or not a delivery has occurred. The following guidelines apply:

- When no delivery occurs the first-listed diagnosis should be the primary complication that necessitated the patient encounter. If more than one complication is present, assign one code for each complication.

- When a delivery occurs at a patient admission, the condition that prompted the admission should be sequenced as the first diagnosis. If the patient has multiple conditions, the one that is most related to the patient delivery should be sequenced first. Any additional complication of pregnancy codes should be sequenced after the first-listed code.

- When a delivery occurs, an outcome of delivery code should be assigned. The outcome of delivery code identifies the number of births and if they were live or stillborn. The outcome of delivery is reported with the appropriate code from category Z37, Outcome of delivery. Note that this code is to be used only on the maternal record, and never on the newborn's record.

- When a delivery occurs, if it is a normal delivery, then code O80, Encounter for full-term uncomplicated delivery, should be assigned. A normal delivery is one that: requires minimal or no assistance; occurs with or without episiotomy; occurs without fetal manipulation (such as rotation version); occurs without instrumentation (such as forceps); is a spontaneous, vaginal delivery, single birth of a full-term, liveborn infant.

  Code O80 may not be used with any other code from chapter 15 (O-code). The only additional code that may be reported with O80 is the additional code to identify the outcome of delivery (Z37) and weeks of gestation (Z3A).

Category Z37, Outcome of delivery, is used to identify that a pregnant patient presented for delivery and code Z37 identifies the outcome of that delivery, such as a single liveborn. This is similar to the code assigned on the record for a liveborn infant, category Z38, Liveborn infants according to place of birth and type of delivery. A code from category Z38 should be assigned only on the newborn's record to identify the newborn's place of birth, type of delivery, and multiple-birth status. The Z37 code is assigned on the mother's record when she delivers. The Z38 code is assigned on the newborn's record when he or she is born and receives healthcare services. When in doubt regarding which code to assign, look at the notation in the Tabular that identifies the code as either being applicable to a maternity case or to a newborn case.

Key to Success

Do not confuse the outcome of delivery code (Z37.-), which is used on a maternal record, with the code for liveborn infants according to place of birth and type of delivery (Z38.-), which is assigned on the newborn's record. To help differentiate between these two categories of codes, remember to keep an eye out for the indicators in the Tabular List that identify whether the code should be used on a maternal or a newborn record (such as the little "M" or the little "N").

Pre-existing versus Gestational Conditions

A pre-existing condition is a known condition of the patient before she became pregnant, such as hypertension or type 2 diabetes. On the other hand, a gestational condition is one that is a direct result from pregnancy, such as gestational hypertension or gestational diabetes. Gestational conditions are also referred to as pregnancy-induced conditions.

Codes differ based on whether the condition was pre-existing or gestational. For example, category O10, Pre-existing hypertension complicating pregnancy, childbirth, and the puerperium, should be assigned for a patient who had hypertension prior to becoming pregnant. However, category O13, Gestational [pregnancy-induced] hypertension without significant proteinuria, should be assigned for a patient that did not have hypertension before becoming pregnant, and but now has hypertension due to her pregnancy.

It is important to pay attention to the guidelines in the Tabular for pre-existing conditions, as many guidelines alert the coder that an additional code should be reported to identify the underlying or pre-existing condition. In these cases, the additional condition would not be a complication of pregnancy code, but the code for the specific complication (such as I10, Essential (primary) hypertension).

For practice reporting diagnosis codes for maternity and obstetric services, complete the exercises in There's a Code for That 17.4.

Coding for maternity and obstetric services

17.4

Read the following documentation from maternity encounters and services and assign the appropriate ICD-10-CM codes.

There's a Code for That

1. Supervision of normal third pregnancy, 16 weeks of gestation.

   ICD-10-CM codes: _____ , _____

(Continued on next page)

17.4

Continued

2. 32 weeks pregnant G2P1 female presents with 2nd degree burn of her left forearm due to a kitchen injury.

   ICD-10-CM codes: _____, _____, _____

3. 22-week pregnant HIV-positive female presents for evaluation. She tested positive for HIV three years ago and has not shown any symptoms yet.

   ICD-10-CM codes: _____, _____, _____

4. 26-year-old female presents with gestational diabetes. She has it under control with the use of oral hypoglycemics.

   ICD-10-CM codes: _____, _____

5. 23-year-old patient presents for tobacco cessation counseling. She is currently 20 weeks pregnant, and smokes approximately 10 cigarettes per day.

   ICD-10-CM codes: _____, _____, _____,
   _____

Putting It All Together: Coding for OB/GYN Services

Coding correctly for OB/GYN services requires an understanding of the differences between gynecological and obstetric services, as well as the guidelines for reporting obstetric diagnosis codes. Determination of the correct codes relies on the answers to the following questions.

- What type of service or procedure was performed, and did the encounter include an E/M service?
  - If so, report the code for the E/M service and any codes for additional procedures (such as the removal of an IUD).
  - If not, report only the code(s) for the service(s) or procedure(s) that were performed.
- Is the service obstetric or non-obstetric?
- Are there any applicable modifiers for the procedure(s)?
- For gynecological services, is there a definitive diagnosis for the encounter? If so, then code for the definitive diagnosis. If not, then report the code for the sign, symptom, or abnormal finding.
- Is the patient presenting for an examination, screening, counseling, or management service? If so, report the Z-code for the encounter type.
- For pregnant patients:
  - Is the pregnancy incidental to the service being provided?
  - Why is the patient presenting to the encounter?
    - Is it a routine examination? If yes, then report the appropriate Z-code.
    - Are there complications of the pregnancy? If yes, assign one code per complication.
    - Where is the patient on the pregnancy timeline?
    - Did a delivery occur?

- ▫ Is it a multiple pregnancy, and which fetus is affected by the complication?
- ▫ What is the estimated week of gestation for the pregnancy?
- Are there any additional conditions that need to be reported, such as pre-existing or underlying conditions?

Study the following vignette that demonstrates how to select the appropriate diagnosis and procedure codes. Then complete the following practice exercises in There's a Code for That 17.5.

Melissa is working as a healthcare coder at a local OB/GYN group practice as she completes her health information management program online. Today she is coding for the deliveries that her OB provided at the hospital over the weekend. She is currently coding the following record: "32-year-old G5P3 high-risk female with history of Factor V deficiency blood clotting disorder presented for induction. Patient is at 36 weeks of gestation. Pitocin was administered at approx. 8am. I checked patient at 12:30 to assess her progress and decided that she was progressing nicely, with 4 cm dilation and 20 percent effacement. Epidural anesthesia was administered by anesthesiologist at approx. 3:30, and labor progressed over the next two hours. At 5:30 I prepped patient for delivery and at 5:47 a male infant with noncompressed triple nuchal cord was delivered vaginally without the use of episiotomy or forceps. I managed this patient throughout her antepartum period (12 visits total) but patient states that she is moving in two weeks. Antepartum hospital and delivery records will be forwarded to her new doctor before the postpartum check with the new doctor."

Melissa asks herself: What did the doctor do? In this case, the doctor performed the vaginal delivery of an infant in the hospital. The note also mentions that the same doctor also performed the antepartum care, but that the patient will be moving soon and will receive the postpartum check from a different doctor. In this case, Melissa needs to report the antepartum care as well as the vaginal delivery. She cannot report code 59400, Routine obstetric care including antepartum care, vaginal delivery (with or without episiotomy, and/or forceps) and postpartum care because the doctor will not be providing the postpartum care. So she reports one code for the antepartum care (for 12 visits), as well as the vaginal delivery:

- *59426, Antepartum care only, 7 or more visits*
- *59409, Vaginal delivery only (with or without episiotomy and/or forceps)*

Melissa does not have to report any of the other services that were performed, because she is only coding for the services that her doctor performed. The anesthesiologist will bill for the epidural, and the hospital will bill for the remaining services.

Now that Melissa has the procedure codes, she asks herself: Why did the doctor do it? In this case, there are several different diagnosis codes that need to be reported to identify the medical necessity for the services performed. Furthermore, she needs to pay attention to how she will link the procedure codes and diagnosis codes.

She decides to report the codes for the delivery first. Melissa remembers that a good measurement for diagnosis coding in OB services is to code until she can code no longer code. Looking at the report, the patient is presenting for delivery, so she knows that she will select the diagnosis codes and identify "delivery" as the encounter for the services. First, the doctor notes that the patient is a high-risk pregnancy due to a Factor V deficiency blood clotting disorder, so she searches the ICD-10-CM Index for Pregnancy, complicated by, *and then* Diseases, *and then* diseases of the blood. *She goes to the Tabular and verified her code selection with childbirth as the encounter, and selects the code: O99.12,*

Other diseases of the blood and blood-forming organs and certain disorders involving the immune mechanism complicating childbirth. She now needs to identify the code for the delivery of the infant with noncompressed triple nuchal cord, and finds the code O69.81X0, Labor and delivery complicated by cord around neck, without compression, not applicable or unspecified. She selected "0" as the seventh character because this was as single pregnancy, and so the seventh characters used to identify the fetus in multiple pregnancies is not applicable. The only other code she needs for this visit at this point is to identify the outcome of the delivery (a single live birth), and the weeks of gestation. She reports the following codes for the maternity record:

- *O99.12, Other diseases of the blood and blood-forming organs and certain disorders involving the immune mechanism complicating childbirth*
- *O69.81X0, Labor and delivery complicated by cord around neck, without compression, not applicable or unspecified.*
- *Z37.0, Single live birth*
- *Z3A.36, 36 weeks gestation of pregnancy*

She then rechecks the documentation to make sure she has coded everything for the encounter and reports the chosen codes. Note that the O-codes (obstetric codes) are sequenced first in this scenario, followed by the two Z-codes to identify the outcome of the delivery and the weeks of gestation of the pregnancy. Remember that O-codes have sequencing priority, so they should be sequenced before any other codes reported on the claim. The Z-codes for the outcome of delivery and weeks of gestation should be sequenced after all other codes that may also be included on the claim.

17.5 Diagnostic and procedural coding for OB/GYN services

There's a Code for That

Read the following documentation and assign the appropriate CPT, HCPCS, and ICD-10 CM code(s) for the encounter.

1. Dilation and curettage of patient with moderate uterine endometriosis.

   CPT code: _____

   ICD-10-CM code: _____

2. VBAC delivery of a single female infant, born at 38 weeks of gestation. Patient suffered second degree perineal laceration during delivery.

   CPT code: _____

   ICD-10-CM codes: _____, _____, _____,

   _____

3. 17-year-old sexually active female presents with severe abdominal pain and cramping during menstruation. Pelvic examination performed in office revealed numerous ovarian cysts bilaterally. Detailed history and examination with MDM of moderate complexity.

   CPT code: _____

   ICD-10-CM code: _____, _____

End of Chapter Content

Instructions: Indicate whether the following statements are true or false (T or F). For false statements, rewrite the statement on the line below to make the statement true.

1. A gynecologist is more likely to treat non-obstetric conditions.

_____

_____

2. An obstetric procedure may also be referred to as a maternity procedure.

_____

_____

3. The place of service code for an infant born in a birthing center is 21.

_____

_____

4. The date used to estimate the patient's date of delivery of a fetus is the last menstrual period.

_____

_____

5. A nulliparous female has had multiple pregnancies that were carried to full term.

_____

_____

6. The organization of the female genital subsection of the CPT book begins with the ovaries and ends with the vulva, perineum, and introitus.

_____

_____

7. A conization procedure removes a portion of tissue from the cervix.

_____

_____

8. A pessary is a stitch that helps the cervix remain closed at the external os.

_____

_____

(Continued on next page)

(Continued)

9. A VBAC is a type of delivery in which the pregnant female has had a previous cesarean and is attempting to deliver vaginally.

_____

_____

10. Contraceptive management diagnosis codes should be used when a patient comes in for a refill of her contraceptive prescription.

_____

_____

Instructions: Choose the best answer.

1. Which of the following services would more likely be performed by an obstetrician?

a. Delivery of a fetus

b. Treatment of urinary tract infection

c. Urinary sling procedure for incontinence

d. Treatment of a sexually transmitted infection

2. Which of the following healthcare providers specializes in fertility?

a. Certified nurse midwife (CNM)

b. Reproductive endocrinology and infertility (REI) specialist

c. Maternal fetal medicine (MFM) specialist

d. Gynecologist

3. Which of the following periods extends from the date of delivery to the six weeks following delivery?

a. Antepartum

b. Perinatal

c. Postpartum

d. Peripartum

4. A G4P2 female has carried a pregnancy to full term how many times?

a. 4

b. 6

c. 2

d. You cannot tell from this gravida/para status

5. Which of the following trimesters encompasses the time between 14 weeks to 27 weeks, 6 days of pregnancy?

a. First trimester

b. Second trimester

c. Third trimester

6. "The incision along the edge of a cyst to form an open pouch for drainage" is which type of procedure?

a. Centesis

b. Incision and drainage

c. Excision

d. Marsupialization

7. Which of the following vulvectomies involves the removal of skin and deep subcutaneous tissues?

a. Radical

b. Simple

c. Complete

d. Partial

8. Which of the following devices is used as a cervical cap to cover the cervix for birth control purposes?

a. Diaphragm

b. Pessary

c. IUD

d. Cerclage

9. Which of the following are included in antepartum services when coding for the global routine delivery package?

   a. Management of labor

   b. Monthly visits with the OB provider

   c. Admission to the hospital

   d. Delivery of the fetus

10. The global delivery package includes which of the following?

    a. Antepartum services

    b. Delivery

    c. Postpartum checkup

    d. Antepartum, delivery, and postpartum services

11. Which of the following best describes the concept of an "incidental pregnancy"?

    a. A pregnancy that was not intended

    b. A pregnancy that occurred out of wedlock

    c. A pregnancy that impacts the medical decision making of the provider

    d. A pregnancy that does not impact the medical decision making of the pregnancy

12. Category Z3A codes identify which of the following?

    a. Trimester

    b. Fetus

    c. Weeks of gestation

    d. BMI

13. Which of the following codes would be reported to identify the outcome of delivery on the maternal record?

    a. Z37.1

    b. O80

    c. Z38.00

    d. O82

Instructions: Answer the following questions with the appropriate code(s) and modifier(s).

1. 40-week pregnant female presents for spontaneous delivery of normal full-term liveborn female infant, delivered vaginally without assistance, no episiotomy, fetal manipulation, or instrumentation used.

   CPT codes: _____

   ICD-10 code: _____, _____,

   _____

2. Total laparoscopic hysterectomy of uterus (307 grams) for intramural uterine fibroids.

   CPT codes: _____

   ICD-10 code: _____

3. Laparoscopic colpopexy for incomplete uterovaginal prolapse.

   CPT codes: _____

   ICD-10 code: _____

References

American Medical Association. 2017. *CPT 2017 Professional Edition*. Chicago: AMA.

Centers for Medicare and Medicaid Services. 2018. ICD-10-CM Official Guidelines for Coding and Reporting FY 2018. https://www.cms.gov/Medicare/Coding/ICD10/Downloads/2018-ICD-10-CM-Coding-Guidelines.pdf.

Resources

American Congress of Obstetricians and Gynecologists. 2017. Coding Question of the Month. https://www.acog.org/About-ACOG/ACOG-Departments/Coding/Coding-Question-of-the-Month?IsMobileSet=falsehttps://www.acog.org/About-ACOG/ACOG-Departments/Coding/Coding-Question-of-the-Month?IsMobileSet=false.

American Medical Association. 2013. *Advanced Anatomy and Physiology for ICD-10-CM/PCS*. Salt Lake City, UT: Contexo Media.

Centers for Medicare and Medicaid Services. 2017. ICD-10 Clinical Concepts for OB/GYN. https://www.cms.gov/Medicare/Coding/ICD10/Downloads/ICD10ClinicalConceptsOBGYN1.pdf.

United Healthcare Oxford. 2017 (October 1). Obstetrical Policy. https://www.oxhp.com/secure/policy/obstetrical_policy.pdf.

CHAPTER 18

Healthcare Specialist Services, Part I

Learning Objectives

- Understand the basics of billing and coding for healthcare specialist services, including consultations, hematology and oncology, neurology, and urology and nephrology services.
- Examine procedural codes and guidelines, diagnosis coding, and medical necessity for

hematology and oncology, neurology, and urology and nephrology services.
- Determine and apply ICD-10-CM, CPT, and HCPCS codes to hematology and oncology, neurology, and urology and nephrology services.

Key Terms

Alzheimer's disease
Anemia
Benign prostatic hyperplasia (BPH)
Brachytherapy
Catheterizations
Cerebrospinal fluid (CSF) shunt
Chemodenervation
Chemotherapy
Circumcision
Consultation
Corpora cavernosa
Corpora spongiosum
Craniectomy
Craniotomy
Dementia
Dialysis
Dosimetry
Electroencephalogram (EEG)
Electronic brachytherapy
Epididymis
Epilepsy
Extracorporeal shock wave
    lithotripsy (ESWL)
Hematologist

Hemodialysis
Hydration
Hydrocele
Infusion
Injection
Intensity Modulated Radiation
    Treatment Delivery (IMRT)
Interstitial brachytherapy
Intracavitary brachytherapy
Intractable condition
Kidney
Lower urinary tract symptoms
    (LUTS)
Nephrolithiasis
Nephrolithotomy
Nephrologist
Neurologist
Neuropsychiatry
Neurosurgery
Oncologist
Orchiopexy
Parkinson's disease
Penis
Peritoneal dialysis

Prostate
Push
Radiation oncologist
Scrotum
Seminal vesicles
Spermatic cord
Staghorn calculus
Status epilepticus
Stereotactic body radiation
    treatment (SBRT)
Stereotactic radiosurgery (SRS)
Testes
Transurethral resection of the
    prostate (TURP)
Tunica vaginalis
Ureters
Urethra
Urinary bladder
Urodynamics
Urologist
Vas deferens
Vasectomy

There are dozens of different medical specialties—from general practitioners who care for the entire health of a patient, like a primary care provider (PCP), to subspecialists who only treat and manage a small number of medical conditions, such as a pediatric endocrinologist. Healthcare specialists all focus on a specific type of body system, medical condition, or treatment type (refer to chapter 1 for a list of healthcare specialties).

Various types of healthcare specialist services have been discussed in this text, including obstetrics and gynecology, therapy providers, primary care practitioners, eye and vision services, and behavioral health services. This chapter discusses three additional specialties: hematology and oncology, neurology, and urology and nephrology. Chapter 19 discusses gastroenterology and cardiology. However, this text does not address every healthcare specialty in which a coder may practice. It is important to keep in mind that a professional entering the world of coding must be flexible, pay close attention to detail, and follow coding guidelines, all while using a solid understanding of both human anatomy and physiology and medical terminology.

Healthcare Specialist Basics

When coding for services provided by a healthcare specialist, remember that a referral or prior authorization may be required before services can be provided to the patient. Healthcare specialists also provide consultations, which are evaluation and management (E/M) services that have a different set of coding guidelines. Finally, it is important to understand the specific types of services provided by hematologists and oncologists, neurologists, and urologists and nephrologists.

Referrals for Specialist Services

When coding for any type of healthcare specialty, it is important to remember that a healthcare specialist usually does not accept patients that have not been specifically referred to his or her office (see chapter 2 for more information on referrals, including how they function). Patients who see a healthcare specialist most likely have been seen first by a primary care or other provider who has determined that the patient needs specialized care, evaluation, or treatment. For example, a patient is not able to determine that he or she has cancer and therefore must see an oncologist. Rather, this patient would be diagnosed first by his PCP, after consulting with a pathologist or radiologist, and then sent to an oncologist for evaluation and treatment.

Remember that a referral depends on the patient's third-party payer (chapter 2), as some policies do not require a referral nor prior authorization before services are provided to the patient. If a referral is required but not obtained prior to service being rendered, and the referral (or authorization) number is not clearly identified on the CMS-1500 form, then the insurance company may deny payment for the claim.

Consultations

A consultation is an E/M encounter that is provided by one healthcare professional, often a specialist, at the request of another healthcare professional such as a primary care practitioner. The consultant healthcare professional provides an evaluation and management service, which may consist of all of the components of a typical E/M encounter including a history, examination, and medical decision making, and then provides recommendations regarding the care of the patient. In this way, a consultation is similar to an outpatient office visit, for example, but with the additional element of the service being specifically requested by another provider so that the consulting provider can suggest treatment options or provide recommendations or advice regarding the patient's condition and its management.

A consultation differs from a referral, which is a request for care from one healthcare provider to another. A consultation is requested so that the consulting physician (specialist) can either recommend care for a specific condition or decide if he or she will take over the care of the patient and the specified condition. For example, a patient with an anal fissure may be sent to consult with a general surgeon to see if surgical treatment of the fissure is an option, and to discuss pros, cons, and risks of the surgery. The general surgeon may then render any necessary service, including the surgical treatment.

In order to qualify as a consultation service for billing purposes, it must be formally requested by a healthcare provider (not by the patient or his family), the request must be in writing, and it must be documented in the patient's health record. Furthermore, the consultant's findings must be documented in a written report that is given to the requesting provider once the service is rendered and the consultation is complete. This leads to the three Rs of consultations: request, render, and report (see figure 18.1).

Figure 18.1. Three Rs of consultations

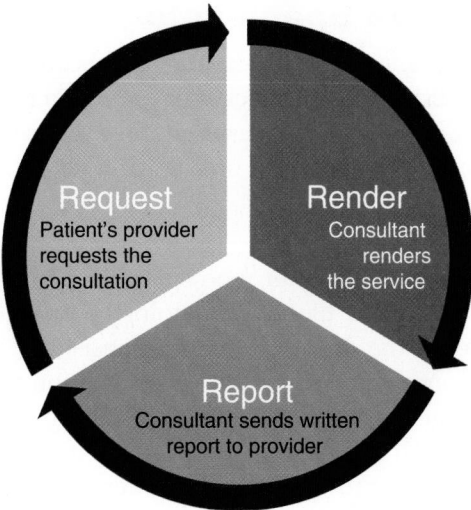

In order to report the code for a consultation service, the consultation must have been formally requested by the patient's healthcare provider. This is the *request*. Then the consultant (such as the healthcare specialist) provides the service to the patient. If additional procedures or services are necessary to treat, diagnose, or manage the patient, these services may be performed in addition to the consultation and will be coded separately. This is the *rendering* of the service. After the service is rendered, the consultant must create a written report of the findings from the service and send this to the requesting provider. This is the *report*.

If the three components of the consultation are not met, then the service may not be billed as a consultation. It is important to understand the necessary components of a consultation and when it is possible to bill for them, as Medicare does not pay for consultation codes (CMS 2009). Other third-party payers may or may not pay for consultations, so it is important to understand the guidelines for each patient's third-party payer to ensure the claim is coded correctly. If the patient's insurance does not pay for consultations, the service provided should be reported using the appropriate inpatient or outpatient office evaluation and management code. For example, if a surgical consultation is performed in the office setting for a patient requesting a bunionectomy (including the request from the patient's PCP, the rendering of the evaluation and consultation by the surgeon, and the report from the surgeon to the PCP), but the patient's insurance does not cover consultation codes, then the coder would need to report the appropriate outpatient office E/M code (99201 through 99215) to identify the encounter with the patient, rather than the consultation E/M code.

Key to Success

Note again that Medicare does not pay for consultation services. Other third-party payers may also follow Medicare policy and deny payment for consultation codes. When you are reporting consultation E/M codes, verify with the patient's third-party payer to determine which codes to use. If the third-party payer does not pay for consultation codes (99241 to 99255), then report the service with the appropriate E/M code from the outpatient/office (99201 to 99215) or inpatient (99221 to 99239) E/M encounter codes.

Types of Healthcare Specialists

As mentioned previously, there are dozens of healthcare specialists. As medicine evolves, even more specialties and subspecialties grow as a result of new technologies and healthcare advances. This chapter focuses on three different healthcare specialties: hematology and oncology, neurology, and urology and nephrology.

Hematology and Oncology

A **hematologist** is a healthcare provider who specializes in the diagnosis, treatment, and prevention of diseases of the blood (hematology). An **oncologist** is a healthcare provider who specializes in the development, diagnosis, and treatment of malignant neoplasms and tumors (oncology). These two specialization areas are often combined into one specialty called hematology/oncology, which provides study and treatment for medical conditions of both the blood and tumors. This dual specialty may also be referred to as hem/onc. Similar to OB/GYN providers, providers may choose to specialize in hematology only, or oncology only, but often combine into group practices, as the two specialties are so closely related. Other specialists and subspecialists that work in hematology and oncology include medical or clinical oncologists, who treat cancer with treatments such as chemotherapy; surgical oncologists, who surgically remove tumors; and **radiation oncologists**, also known as interventional radiologists, who specialize in the treatment of cancers via radiation treatments (Cancer.net 2015).

Most of the services rendered by hematology and oncology providers are E/M services to evaluate and manage patients, as well as provide and manage cancer treatments such as chemotherapy, radiation therapy (radiation oncology), and surgical removals. Most of the conditions managed by hematologists and oncologists involve neoplasms and disorders of the blood.

Neurology

A **neurologist** is a medical doctor who specializes in the diagnosis and treatment of neurological disorders, including disorders of the nerves and the nervous system. Neurologists may further specialize in **neuropsychiatry**, treatment of mental or behavioral disturbances as a result of neurological conditions, or **neurosurgery**, surgical treatment of disorders of the nerves and nervous system.

Neurologists treat patients with neurological disorders of both the central nervous system, such as brain or spinal cord injuries, and the peripheral nervous system, such as peripheral neuropathies. Many of the surgical codes for neurological procedures are located in the Nervous system subsection of the CPT code book.

Urology and Nephrology

A medical doctor who specializes in the diagnosis and treatment of conditions of the urinary system and the male and female genital systems is a **urologist** (AUA 2017). A **nephrologist** is a medical doctor who focuses on the diagnosis and treatment of conditions of the kidneys, such as chronic kidney disease. Urologists may also treat specific disorders of the kidneys, but nephrologists focus solely on the kidneys.

Because urologists and nephrologists perform numerous surgery-based procedures, the majority of codes for urology and nephrology services are reported from the Urinary and Male Genital System subsections of the CPT code book. Additional codes may be reported from the Female Genital subsection of the CPT code book, when these services are performed by a urologist or nephrologist rather than an OB/GYN provider. Most diagnosis codes reported for medical necessity identify diseases of the genitourinary system.

Consultation Coding for Healthcare Specialist Services

As noted in the previous section, procedure codes for any type of healthcare specialist services depend on the type of specialty and the services provided. This section discusses consultation coding, which may be used by any type of healthcare provider.

To report a code for an office or other outpatient consultation, the service may be provided in any of the following settings:

- Outpatient or other ambulatory facility (like an ASC), including outpatient office
- Hospital observation area
- Home
- Domiciliary or rest home
- Emergency department

Office or other outpatient consultations are reported with codes 99241, Office consultation for a new or established patient, which requires these 3 key components: a problem focused history; a problem focused examination; and straightforward medical decision making through 99245, Office consultation for a new or established patient, which requires these 3 key components: a comprehensive history; a comprehensive examination; and medical decision making of high complexity. As long as there is always a request in writing and the service is medically necessary, as many outpatient consultations as necessary may be reported per patient per provider,

Consultations may also be provided in the inpatient setting, to the following patients:

- Hospital inpatients
- Residents of nursing facilities
- Patients in a partial hospital setting (as discussed in chapter 7)

In the inpatient setting, only one consultation service may be reported per patient per admission. For example, if a consultation was billed by Dr. A for Patient B, then Dr. A cannot bill for another consultation with the same patient unless Patient B has a new admission to the hospital. For example, if a consultation was provided for a gastrointestinal problem, and the patient was treated and discharged but returned the next day and was admitted again, and the same doctor provided another consultation for the same gastrointestinal problem, then the doctor can report each consultation as they occurred during separate admissions. Inpatient consultations are reported with codes 99251, Inpatient consultation for a new or established patient, which requires these 3 key components: a problem-focused history, a problem-focused examination; and straightforward medical decision making through 99255, Office consultation for a new or established patient, which requires these 3 key components: a comprehensive history; a comprehensive examination; and medical decision making of high complexity.

Key to Success

Consultation codes are located in the E/M section of the CPT code book, after Hospital Inpatient Services (99221 to 99239).

Codes for consultations are much like the codes for outpatient office or inpatient encounters because they rely on determining the levels of the three key components (history, examination, and medical decision making) to then determine the level of consultation service provided (as discussed in chapters 7 and 8). However, unlike outpatient office visit encounters, consultation codes do not differ based on whether the service was provided to a new or established patient. Both inpatient and outpatient consultations require all three key components to be at the level described in the code or higher.

Procedural and Diagnostic Coding for Hematology and Oncology

Procedures for hematology and oncology services are found throughout the CPT code book. For example, surgical removal of neoplastic organs and insertion of brachytherapy elements are found in the Surgery section, in each respective subsection; radiation oncology procedures are found in the Radiology section; and infusion procedures for chemotherapy are found in the Medicine section.

Surgical treatment of neoplasms (both benign and malignant) may involve surgical removal. Surgical removal codes are included in the Surgery section of the CPT code book, in their respective body system subsections. For example, the code for the removal of an osteosarcoma (cancer of the bone) would be located in the Musculoskeletal System subsection. To search for the removal of a lesion, organ, or part of an organ, search the CPT Index for the term *Excision* or *Resection* and then search for either the lesion or the type of body tissue or organ that was removed. Using the same example, search for the code for an osteosarcoma of the humerus, then for the term *Resection* in the Index, then *Tumor*, and then find *Humerus*. Next to the term *Humerus*, the coder will find the code for the radical resection of a tumor of the humerus, code 23220, Radical resection of tumor, proximal humerus.

Together with surgical removal of neoplastic tumors, cancers may also be treated in several different ways, and often combine one or more treatment methods. For example, a patient with a malignant neoplasm of the breast might undergo a mastectomy procedure to remove the neoplastic tissue and undergo chemotherapy.

Coding for hematology and oncology requires a strict attention to detail, and an in-depth knowledge of the types of treatments for neoplasms—including brachytherapy, radiation therapy, and chemotherapy. It also requires an in-depth knowledge of diagnosis coding guidelines for neoplasms and the services associated with neoplastic conditions.

Brachytherapy

Brachytherapy is a cancer treatment method in which small radioactive seeds, capsules, or elements are surgically placed in or near a cancer or cancerous organ (USNLM 2016a). These seeds may also be referred to as brachytherapy sources, and are specifically designed to treat the neoplasm as best as possible. These small seeds emit radiation to the cancerous tissue, while reducing radiation exposure to the remaining tissues at the same time, resulting in a precise treatment directed at the malignant neoplasm. Brachytherapy treatments include several different components including simulation and planning, which are components of radiation oncology codes (discussed in the following section). Simulation and planning services include the virtual delivery of the brachytherapy treatment to the patient, planning of how the procedure will be performed, and how and where the brachytherapy sources will be implanted into the patient.

Surgical codes for brachytherapy report the actual implantation of the seeds or capsules into the specific organ. These codes are found in the Introduction categories (see chapter 11) in each respective body system because the brachytherapy elements are directly introduced into the body tissues. The placement of brachytherapy elements may be interstitial or intracavitary. Interstitial brachytherapy involves placing the radioactive elements directly into the tumor or organ. Intracavitary brachytherapy involves placing the radioactive elements into a body cavity, such as the vagina or the bladder.

There are two further distinctions in brachytherapy treatment—clinical and electronic brachytherapy. Clinical brachytherapy is the use of radioactive elements, as described previously. Electronic brachytherapy is the use of a small, high-dose x-ray source, applied directly to the malignancy. It is used as an emerging treatment for skin cancer and, as such, codes for electronic brachytherapy treatments are Category III codes.

Key to Success

Do not forget about Category III codes. These codes report new and emerging services and procedures, and all end with the letter T. Codes for electronic brachytherapy, for example, include 0394T, High dose rate electronic brachytherapy, skin surface application, per fraction, includes basic dosimetry, when performed.

Codes for the surgical placement of brachytherapy elements differ based on the body area or organ being treated and the method of brachytherapy used (namely, interstitial or intracavitary). For example, code 49411, Placement of interstitial device(s) for radiation therapy guidance (e.g., fiducial markers, dosimeter), percutaneous, intra-abdominal, intra-pelvic (except prostate), and/or retroperitoneum, single or multiple, identifies the brachytherapy device placement as in the *intra-abdominal, intra-pelvic, or retroperitoneal* space and the device as *interstitial*. To find the codes for brachytherapy element placement search for the term *Brachytherapy* in the CPT Index, and then the specific service related to the brachytherapy treatment, such as *interstitial application, intracavitary application,* or *planning*.

Because the surgeon is placing a medical device into the patient, it is necessary to report the HCPCS code for the brachytherapy source(s) (the device) in addition to the code for the surgical placement (reported with a CPT code). To search for brachytherapy sources in the HCPCS Index, search under the term *Brachytherapy radioelements,* or *Radioelements for brachytherapy.* However, the exact phrase for the radioelement source may differ depending on the publisher of the HCPCS code book. Brachytherapy source HCPCS codes identify the type of source and are per source codes, in that one source is reported per code. So, if 10 sources are used, then the HCPCS code should be reported times 10. For example, code C2638, Brachytherapy source, stranded, iodine-125, per source, reports a stranded iodine-125 brachytherapy source. If 10 of these sources are implanted into the patient, then the code for the sources would be C2638 × 10.

In addition to the brachytherapy source insertion and the code for the brachytherapy itself, codes from the radiation oncology subsection of the CPT code book must be reported to identify the brachytherapy planning, simulation, and treatment. Clinical Brachytherapy (77750 to 77799) codes identify the actual brachytherapy treatment and application of the radioactive elements, solution, or source. For example, code 77761, Intracavitary radiation source application; simple. They are grouped based on the complexity of the service (simple: 1 to 4 sources, intermediate: 5 to 10 sources, or complex: greater than 10 sources) and the type of brachytherapy treatment performed.

When a brachytherapy service is performed, it is carefully planned and simulated to ensure that the method of treatment and dose are appropriate to treat the cancer while maintaining the surrounding healthy tissues. These services are included in the Radiation Oncology subsection of the CPT code book.

Radiation Oncology

The Radiation Oncology (77261 to 77799) subsection of the CPT code book reports services that use radioactive treatments for malignant neoplasms. Antineoplastic radiation therapy is a complex, carefully planned, designed, simulated, and delivered treatment that contains numerous components. The first stage of radiation treatment is a clinical consultation with a hematologist or oncologist who determines the need for radiation treatment and begins the radiation oncology service(s). This consultation and any other E/M services are reported with codes from the E/M section.

After the decision to treat the patient via radiation therapy, the radiation oncology services begin, of which the first step is clinical treatment planning and simulation of the treatment. Clinical treatment planning involves:

- Interpreting special tests
- Locating tumors
- Determining treatment volume
- Determining treatment time and dosage
- Choosing the treatment modality
- Determining the number and size of treatment ports
- Selecting treatment devices (AMA 2017)

Simulation is the process of targeting the anatomy to be treated during the procedure and determining the optimal process of radiation treatment for the patient (AMA 2017). These procedures are reported with codes 77261, Therapeutic radiology treatment planning; simple, through 77299, Unlisted procedure, therapeutic radiology clinical treatment planning. Planning and simulation codes are categorized based on whether the service is simple, intermediate, or complex, as defined in the guidelines for each category of codes.

Key to Success

One way to help ensure you are coding from the correct section in the Radiation Oncology subsection is to pay attention to the subheadings within the subsection of codes. Subheadings include Clinical Treatment Planning, Medical Radiation Physics, Dosimetry, Treatment Devices and Special Services, Stereotactic Radiation Delivery, Other Procedures, Radiation Treatment Delivery, and Radiation Treatment Management (among others). Before assigning codes for radiation oncology codes, be sure to review these headings and see how each selection of codes is organized. This will help you keep in track when searching for radiation oncology codes.

After the radiation treatment is planned and simulated, a process called dosimetry is performed to calculate the exact dose amount. In order to give the patient the dose of medication determined by the dosimetry calculation, treatment devices—such as patient immobilization devices or radiation-beam modification devices—are designed and created to administer the radiation. Additional consultations are also performed to inform the patient of the dosage and treatment plan. These services are reported with codes 77295, 3-dimensional radiotherapy plan, including dose-volume histograms, through 77370, Special medical radiation physics consultation.

After coding for the planning, simulation, dosimetry, and creation of device, then code for the delivery of different types of radiation treatments. The codes for delivery types are as follows.

- Stereotactic Radiation Treatment Delivery (77371 to 77373). Stereotactic radiosurgery (SRS) is a type of radiation treatment used for intracranial lesions that delivers a precision dose of radiation. SRS services are reported with codes 77371 and 77372. Whole-body SRS treatment, referred to as stereotactic body radiation treatment (SBRT), is a developing type of stereotactic treatment used on body tumors. SBRT is reported with code 77373.

- Radiation Treatment Delivery (77401 to 77417, 77385 to 77387, 77424, 77425). Radiation treatment delivery codes depend on the type of radiation treatment delivered and the complexity of the service (simple, intermediate, or complex). Some codes also identify the treatment session for the radiation delivery. Radiation treatment delivery codes in this section include Intensity Modulated Radiation Treatment Delivery (IMRT), a radiation treatment method that uses computer-based mapping to create dosing distributions delivered by a radiotherapy treatment machine.

- Neutron Beam Treatment Delivery (77423). Neutron beam radiation therapy codes identify neutron beam radiation treatments.

- Proton Beam Treatment Delivery (77520 to 77525). These codes identify radiation therapy services performed with proton beam radiation treatments.

Management of radiation treatments is reported with codes from the Radiation Treatment Management (77427 to 77499) subsection. These codes identify the management services provided by the physician to the patient during the radiation treatment phase. This includes a minimum of one examination (including assessment of the patient's response to the radiation treatments), coordination of the care and treatment of the patient, and review of each imaging or lab service. All of these services are included in the one radiation treatment management code, as defined by the CPT guidelines before the selection of codes for radiation treatment management.

In sum, radiation oncology coding is a complex subspecialty of coding that requires a comprehensive understanding of the types of treatments and delivery methods, including planning, simulating, and designing the process of radiation treatments for each individual patient.

Infusions

Infusion services for cancer patients are for the delivery of chemotherapy for patients with malignant neoplasms. **Chemotherapy** in general terms is the use of a drug to treat a medical condition. For hematology and oncology, chemotherapy is used to treat patients with malignant neoplasms by administering an infusion of antineoplastic chemotherapeutic agents.

Chemotherapy infusion codes are reported from the Hydration, Therapeutic, Prophylactic, Diagnostic Injections and Infusions, and Chemotherapy and Other Highly Complex Drug or Highly Complex Biologic Agent Administration (96360 to 96549) subsections of codes. Coding for chemotherapy requires the identification of both the infusion service and the drug that was administered during the infusion. The ability to accurately code for infusion services relies on the understanding of a number of important concepts related to infusion services. Note that not all of the following are infusions, but are interrelated types of procedures that entail administering therapeutic, chemotherapeutic, or other substances directly into the patient's blood stream.

- *Hydration*. A **hydration** service is the administration of fluids or electrolytes without the presence of drugs. A hydration line may be started and then later used to administer drugs through the same intravenous (IV) insertion site. According to CPT guidelines, if a hydration line is started in order to keep the vein open before or after a therapeutic or chemotherapy infusion, then the hydration service is not reported.

- *Injection*. An **injection** is given intramuscularly (into the muscle) to administer a therapeutic substance. Injections in this section of codes are *not* used to report the injection of vaccines, but rather a therapeutic, prophylactic, or diagnostic substance. Unlike a hydration or infusion service, an injection is given in a quick "shot" dose.

- *Infusion*. An **infusion** is the administration of a diagnostic, prophylactic, or therapeutic fluid or drug, given over a period of time longer than 15 minutes. This is the same as a hydration saline drip, except that the substance being administered is therapeutic rather than hydrating.

- *Push*. A **push** is the administration of a therapeutic, prophylactic, or diagnostic substance via an IV line (not an injection). A push can be administered together with an infusion or hydration. The difference between a push and an infusion is the timeframe. A push is an infusion of 15 minutes or less.

When coding for chemotherapy infusion codes, first identify the service as the administration of hydration, a therapeutic substance, or chemotherapy.

Another important component of infusion coding is the identification of the service as initial, sequential, or concurrent, as the code reported for the infusion service will differ. Note that these guidelines differ depending on whether the service was performed in the inpatient setting or the outpatient setting. An initial infusion is the primary reason for the encounter and includes the administration of the first or initial substance. A sequential infusion is the infusion or push of a new therapeutic substance after the initial infusion service. In order to qualify as a sequential infusion service, a new substance or drug must be administered through the same injection site.

A concurrent infusion is the infusion of a new therapeutic substance at the same time as an existing infusion. A concurrent infusion is administered simultaneously with the initial infusion. When coding for multiple infusions, read the infusion guidelines in the CPT code book to help identify which infusion should be reported as initial, sequential, or concurrent, and to ensure correct code selection.

Key to Success

When coding for multiple infusions, carefully read the guidelines for these services in the CPT code book to ensure you report the infusion services appropriately. This is a long section of guidelines that includes a lot of detailed information. Remember to highlight and make notes in your CPT book to make sure you understand these guidelines and select the correct CPT codes.

Hydrations

Hydration services are reported with codes 96360, Intravenous infusion, hydration; *initial, 31 minutes to 1 hour*, and 96361, Intravenous infusion, hydration; *each additional hour*. Note that these codes identify the amount of time spent providing the hydration service. The first hour should be reported with 96360, with code 96361 added for each additional hour of service provided. For example, if a patient received six hours of hydration therapy, then the coder should report 96360 for the first hour, and then 96361 × 5 for the additional five hours, equaling six hours total (96360, 96361 × 5).

The parenthetical note under 96361 in the CPT code book specifies to report 96361 for hydration of greater than 30 minutes, up to one hour. What this means is that to report the add-on code 96361, the additional time must be *at least* 30 minutes over the hour. For example, if the hydration service lasted for 5 hours 20 minutes, then the codes reported would be as follows: 96360, 96361 × 4, equaling five total hours. The last 20 minutes are not counted, as they must add up to an additional 30 minutes to report the add-on code 96361 again.

Therapeutic, Prophylactic, and Diagnostic Injections and Infusions

Injections and infusions of therapeutic, prophylactic, and diagnostic substances are reported with codes 96365 to 96379. Note that these codes do not report the injection or infusion of chemotherapy agents; these codes specifically exclude chemotherapeutic substances. When selecting codes from this section, the coder must identify the service as an injection, an infusion, or a push, the type of administration (namely, subcutaneous, intramuscular, intra-arterial, intravenous), and the amount of time it took to perform the service. As with hydration codes, the initial hour is reported with the initial code and an add-on code to identify each additional hour (30 minutes or more).

Chemotherapy Injections and Infusions

Chemotherapy administration codes are located in the Chemotherapy and Other Highly Complex Drug or Highly Complex Biologic Agent Administration subsection (96401 to 96549). This subsection is divided into three sections: Injections and Intravenous Infusions, Intra-arterial Administrations, and Other Injection and Infusion Services.

- Injections and Intravenous Infusions report the administration of chemotherapy via an injection or intravenous infusion. Codes differ based on the type of administration (intramuscular, subcutaneous, intralesional, or intravenous), the type of antineoplastic substance, and the time it took to administer the service. Just as with hydration and therapeutic infusions, report the first hour with the code for initial service and then the add-on code for each additional hour (30 minutes or more).

- Intra-arterial Administrations report the administration of a chemotherapeutic agent directly into an arterial structure. Codes identify the time it took to administer the service and the technique used.

Other Injection and Infusion Services codes report the administration of chemotherapeutic substances into other body structures, such as the pleural or peritoneal cavity, as well as additional services related to the delivery of chemotherapy. For example, code 96440, Chemotherapy administration into pleural cavity, requiring and including thoracentesis. Complete the exercises in There's a Code for That 18.1 for practice reporting hematology and oncology procedure codes.

18.1

There's a Code for That

Hematology and oncology procedures

Read the following documentation of the service and identify the CPT procedure code(s).

1. Insertion of vaginal brachytherapy device for female patient with endometrial cancer, with design and construction of simple treatment device.

   CPT codes: _____, _____

2. Complex simulated field setting for therapeutic radiation treatment.

   CPT code: _____

3. Application of intermediate intracavitary radiation source.

   CPT code: _____

4. Simple radiology treatment planning.

   CPT code: _____

5. Complex radiation treatment delivery.

   CPT code: _____

6. Two hours of IV hydration therapy.

   CPT codes: _____, _____

7. Intramuscular administration of hormonal anti-neoplastic chemotherapy.

   CPT codes: _____

8. Spinal puncture with intrathecal administration of chemotherapy.

   CPT codes: _____

Hematology and Oncology Diagnoses

Hematologists and oncologists treat both disorders of the blood and neoplasms. When reporting diagnosis codes for neoplasms, there are a number of guidelines that impact code selection and sequencing of which the coder should be aware.

Blood Disorders

Disorders of the blood are reported with codes from chapter 3: Diseases of the Blood and Blood-Forming Organs of the ICD-10–CM code book. Note that there are no chapter-specific coding guidelines for reporting the conditions in this chapter, so the coder must pay attention to specific instructions in the Tabular and rely on provider documentation for correct code selection.

Perhaps one of the most common conditions in this chapter is anemia. Anemia occurs when a person has abnormally low red blood cells or hemoglobin in the blood. There are several different types of anemia that can be caused by a number of underlying conditions, or it may be idiopathic. Anemic conditions are reported with codes from categories D50 to D53, Nutritional anemias, D55 to D59, Hemolytic anemias, and D60 to D64, Aplastic and other anemias and other bone marrow failure syndromes. When coding for anemias, pay attention to the specific type of anemia, as well as any additional or underlying conditions or external causes. Note also that many anemia codes are important in risk adjustment and HCC coding.

Category D63, Anemia in chronic disease classified elsewhere, is a special category of anemia manifestation codes. These codes identify anemia that is a manifestation of a specific disease, which is classified elsewhere in the ICD-10-CM code book. For example, code D63.0, Anemia in neoplastic disease, should be reported for a patient who has a neoplastic disease (such as cancer) that has resulted in anemia. Manifestation codes can *never* be reported by themselves, they must always follow the code for the primary condition (that caused the manifestation).

Neoplasms

Neoplasms are all reported with codes from chapter 2: Neoplasms of the ICD-10-CM code book. For a refresher on neoplasm coding refer to chapter 4 of this text for a description of the different types of neoplasms and how to locate neoplasms on the ICD-10-CM Index.

Neoplasm coding guidelines define the sequencing of neoplasms when a patient has more than one neoplasm, as well as the coding and sequencing of complications, administration of antineoplastic therapies, and current versus personal history of malignancies (see figure 18.2).

Neoplasm Sequencing

According to ICD-10-CM guidelines, when a patient has more than one malignancy the sequencing depends on the reason for the encounter. Primary malignancies are the originating site of the neoplasm, and secondary malignancies are places to where the cancer has spread. If the patient is being seen for treatment of the primary malignancy, sequence the primary malignancy first, followed by the secondary malignancy. If the patient is being seen for the secondary malignancy, sequence the secondary malignancy first, followed by the code for the primary malignancy.

Coding and Sequencing of Complications

Pay attention to sequencing guidelines when reporting malignancies with complications such as anemia, dehydration, or other complications resulting from the neoplasm, antineoplastic therapy, or surgical procedure.

When a patient presents for treatment of anemia due to a neoplasm, sequence the code for the neoplasm before the code for the anemia. If the anemia is a direct result of antineoplastic therapy—such as chemotherapy or radiation therapy—and the patient is being treated for the anemia, then sequence the code for the anemia first, followed by the code for the malignancy and the adverse effect of antineoplastic therapy code (T45.1X5-, Adverse effect of antineoplastic and immunosuppressive drugs), or the abnormal reaction from radiation therapy code (Y84.2, Radiological procedure and radiotherapy as the cause of abnormal reaction of the patient, or of later complication, without mention of misadventure at the time of the procedure).

Figure 18.2. OGCR I.C.2

2. Chapter 2: Neoplasms (C00-D49)

General guidelines

Chapter 2 of the ICD-10-CM contains the codes for most benign and all malignant neoplasms. Certain benign neoplasms, such as prostatic adenomas, may be found in the specific body system chapters. To properly code a neoplasm it is necessary to determine from the record if the neoplasm is benign, in-situ, malignant, or of uncertain histologic behavior. If malignant, any secondary (metastatic) sites should also be determined.

Primary malignant neoplasms overlapping site boundaries

A primary malignant neoplasm that overlaps two or more contiguous (next to each other) sites should be classified to the subcategory/code .8 ('overlapping lesion'), unless the combination is specifically indexed elsewhere. For multiple neoplasms of the same site that are not contiguous such as tumors in different quadrants of the same breast, codes for each site should be assigned.

Malignant neoplasm of ectopic tissue

Malignant neoplasms of ectopic tissue are to be coded to the site of origin mentioned, e.g., ectopic pancreatic malignant neoplasms involving the stomach are coded to **malignant neoplasm of** pancreas, unspecified (C25.9).

The neoplasm table in the Alphabetic Index should be referenced first. However, if the histological term is documented, that term should be referenced first, rather than going immediately to the Neoplasm Table, in order to determine which column in the Neoplasm Table is appropriate. For example, if the documentation indicates "adenoma," refer to the term in the Alphabetic Index to review the entries under this term and the instructional note to "see also neoplasm, by site, benign." The table provides the proper code based on the type of neoplasm and the site. It is important to select the proper column in the table that corresponds to the type of neoplasm. The Tabular List should then be referenced to verify that the correct code has been selected from the table and that a more specific site code does not exist.

See Section I.C.21. Factors influencing health status and contact with health services, Status, for information regarding Z15.0, codes for genetic susceptibility to cancer.

a. Treatment directed at the malignancy

If the treatment is directed at the malignancy, designate the malignancy as the principal diagnosis.

The only exception to this guideline is if a patient admission/encounter is solely for the administration of chemotherapy, immunotherapy or **external beam** radiation therapy, assign the appropriate Z51.-- code as the first-listed or principal diagnosis, and the diagnosis or problem for which the service is being performed as a secondary diagnosis.

b. Treatment of secondary site

When a patient is admitted because of a primary neoplasm with metastasis and treatment is directed toward the secondary site only, the secondary neoplasm is designated as the principal diagnosis even though the primary malignancy is still present.

c. Coding and sequencing of complications

Coding and sequencing of complications associated with the malignancies or with the therapy thereof are subject to the following guidelines:

1) Anemia associated with malignancy

When admission/encounter is for management of an anemia associated with the malignancy, and the treatment is only for anemia, the appropriate code for the malignancy is sequenced as the principal or first-listed diagnosis followed by the appropriate code for the anemia (such as code D63.0, Anemia in neoplastic disease).

2) Anemia associated with chemotherapy, immunotherapy and radiation therapy

When the admission/encounter is for management of an anemia associated with an adverse effect of the administration of chemotherapy or immunotherapy and the only treatment is for the anemia, the anemia code is sequenced first followed by the appropriate codes for the neoplasm and the adverse effect (T45.1X5, Adverse effect of antineoplastic and immunosuppressive drugs).

When the admission/encounter is for management of an anemia associated with an adverse effect of radiotherapy, the anemia code should be sequenced first, followed by the appropriate neoplasm code and code Y84.2, Radiological procedure and radiotherapy as the cause of abnormal reaction of the patient, or of later complication, without mention of misadventure at the time of the procedure.

3) Management of dehydration due to the malignancy

When the admission/encounter is for management of dehydration due to the malignancy and only the dehydration is being treated (intravenous rehydration), the dehydration is sequenced first, followed by the code(s) for the malignancy.

4) Treatment of a complication resulting from a surgical procedure

When the admission/encounter is for treatment of a complication resulting from a surgical procedure, designate the complication as the principal or first-listed diagnosis if treatment is directed at resolving the complication.

d. Primary malignancy previously excised

When a primary malignancy has been previously excised or eradicated from its site and there is no further treatment directed to that site and there is no evidence of any existing primary malignancy, a code from category Z85, Personal history of malignant neoplasm, should be used to indicate the former site of the malignancy. Any mention of extension, invasion, or metastasis to another site is coded as a secondary malignant neoplasm to that site. The secondary site may be the principal or first-listed with the Z85 code used as a secondary code.

e. Admissions/Encounters involving chemotherapy, immunotherapy and radiation therapy

1) Episode of care involves surgical removal of neoplasm

When an episode of care involves the surgical removal of a neoplasm, primary or secondary site, followed by adjunct chemotherapy or radiation treatment during the same episode of care, the code for the neoplasm should be assigned as principal or first-listed diagnosis.

2) Patient admission/encounter solely for administration of chemotherapy, immunotherapy and radiation therapy

If a patient admission/encounter is solely for the administration of chemotherapy, immunotherapy or **external beam** radiation therapy assign code Z51.0, Encounter for antineoplastic radiation therapy, or Z51.11, Encounter for antineoplastic chemotherapy, or Z51.12, Encounter for antineoplastic immunotherapy as the first-listed or principal diagnosis. If a patient receives more than one of these therapies during the same admission more than one of these codes may be assigned, in any sequence.

The malignancy for which the therapy is being administered should be assigned as a secondary diagnosis.

If a patient admission/encounter is for the insertion or implantation of radioactive elements (e.g., brachytherapy) the appropriate code for the malignancy is sequenced as the principal or first-listed diagnosis. Code Z51.0 should not be assigned.

3) Patient admitted for radiation therapy, chemotherapy or immunotherapy and develops complications

When a patient is admitted for the purpose of **external beam** radiotherapy, immunotherapy or chemotherapy and develops complications such as uncontrolled nausea and vomiting or dehydration, the principal or first-listed diagnosis is Z51.0, Encounter for antineoplastic radiation therapy, or Z51.11, Encounter for antineoplastic chemotherapy, or Z51.12, Encounter for antineoplastic immunotherapy followed by any codes for the complications.

When a patient is admitted for the purpose of insertion or implantation of radioactive elements (e.g., brachytherapy) and develops complications such as uncontrolled nausea and vomiting or dehydration, the principal or first-listed diagnosis is the appropriate code for the malignancy followed by any codes for the complications.

f. Admission/encounter to determine extent of malignancy

When the reason for admission/encounter is to determine the extent of the malignancy, or for a procedure such as paracentesis or thoracentesis, the primary malignancy or appropriate metastatic site is designated as the principal or first-listed diagnosis, even though chemotherapy or radiotherapy is administered.

g. Symptoms, signs, and abnormal findings listed in Chapter 18 associated with neoplasms

Symptoms, signs, and ill-defined conditions listed in Chapter 18 characteristic of, or associated with, an existing primary or secondary site malignancy cannot be used to replace the malignancy as principal or first-listed diagnosis, regardless of the number of admissions or encounters for treatment and care of the neoplasm.

See section I.C.21. Factors influencing health status and contact with health services, Encounter for prophylactic organ removal.

h. Admission/encounter for pain control/management

See Section I.C.6. for information on coding admission/encounter for pain control/management.

i. Malignancy in two or more noncontiguous sites

A patient may have more than one malignant tumor in the same organ. These tumors may represent different primaries or metastatic disease, depending on the site. Should the documentation be unclear, the provider should be queried as to the status of each tumor so that the correct codes can be assigned.

j. Disseminated malignant neoplasm, unspecified

Code C80.0, Disseminated malignant neoplasm, unspecified, is for use only in those cases where the patient has advanced metastatic disease and no known primary or secondary sites are specified. It should not be used in place of assigning codes for the primary site and all known secondary sites.

(Continued on next page)

Figure 18.2. *(Continued)*

k. Malignant neoplasm without specification of site

Code C80.1, Malignant (primary) neoplasm, unspecified, equates to Cancer, unspecified. This code should only be used when no determination can be made as to the primary site of a malignancy. This code should rarely be used in the inpatient setting.

l. Sequencing of neoplasm codes

1) Encounter for treatment of primary malignancy

If the reason for the encounter is for treatment of a primary malignancy, assign the malignancy as the principal/first-listed diagnosis. The primary site is to be sequenced first, followed by any metastatic sites.

2) Encounter for treatment of secondary malignancy

When an encounter is for a primary malignancy with metastasis and treatment is directed toward the metastatic (secondary) site(s) only, the metastatic site(s) is designated as the principal/first-listed diagnosis. The primary malignancy is coded as an additional code.

3) Malignant neoplasm in a pregnant patient

When a pregnant woman has a malignant neoplasm, a code from subcategory O9A.1-, Malignant neoplasm complicating pregnancy, childbirth, and the puerperium, should be sequenced first, followed by the appropriate code from Chapter 2 to indicate the type of neoplasm.

4) Encounter for complication associated with a neoplasm

When an encounter is for management of a complication associated with a neoplasm, such as dehydration, and the treatment is only for the complication, the complication is coded first, followed by the appropriate code(s) for the neoplasm.

The exception to this guideline is anemia. When the admission/encounter is for management of an anemia associated with the malignancy, and the treatment is only for anemia, the appropriate code for the malignancy is sequenced as the principal or first-listed diagnosis followed by code D63.0, Anemia in neoplastic disease.

5) Complication from surgical procedure for treatment of a neoplasm

When an encounter is for treatment of a complication resulting from a surgical procedure performed for the treatment of the neoplasm, designate the complication as the principal/first- listed diagnosis. See guideline regarding the coding of a current malignancy versus personal history to determine if the code for the neoplasm should also be assigned.

6) Pathologic fracture due to a neoplasm

When an encounter is for a pathological fracture due to a neoplasm, and the focus of treatment is the fracture, a code from subcategory M84.5, Pathological fracture in neoplastic disease, should be sequenced first, followed by the code for the neoplasm.

If the focus of treatment is the neoplasm with an associated pathological fracture, the neoplasm code should be sequenced first, followed by a code from M84.5 for the pathological fracture.

m. Current malignancy versus personal history of malignancy

When a primary malignancy has been excised but further treatment, such as an additional surgery for the malignancy, radiation therapy or chemotherapy is directed to that site, the primary malignancy code should be used until treatment is completed.

When a primary malignancy has been previously excised or eradicated from its site, there is no further treatment (of the malignancy) directed to that site, and there is no evidence of any existing primary malignancy, a code from category Z85, Personal history of malignant neoplasm, should be used to indicate the former site of the malignancy.

See Section I.C.21. Factors influencing health status and contact with health services, History (of)

n. Leukemia, Multiple Myeloma, and Malignant Plasma Cell Neoplasms in remission versus personal history

The categories for leukemia, and category C90, Multiple myeloma and malignant plasma cell neoplasms, have codes indicating whether or not the leukemia has achieved remission. There are also codes Z85.6, Personal history of leukemia, and Z85.79, Personal history of other malignant neoplasms of lymphoid, hematopoietic and related tissues. If the documentation is unclear, as to whether the leukemia has achieved remission, the provider should be queried.

See Section I.C.21. Factors influencing health status and contact with health services, History (of)

> **o. Aftercare following surgery for neoplasm**
>
> See Section I.C.21. Factors influencing health status and contact with health services, Aftercare
>
> **p. Follow-up care for completed treatment of a malignancy**
>
> See Section I.C.21. Factors influencing health status and contact with health services, Follow-up
>
> **q. Prophylactic organ removal for prevention of malignancy**
>
> See Section I.C. 21, Factors influencing health status and contact with health services, Prophylactic organ removal
>
> **r. Malignant neoplasm associated with transplanted organ**
>
> A malignant neoplasm of a transplanted organ should be coded as a transplant complication. Assign first the appropriate code from category T86.-, Complications of transplanted organs and tissue, followed by code C80.2, Malignant neoplasm associated with transplanted organ. Use an additional code for the specific malignancy.

Source: CMS 2018.

If a patient presents for treatment of either dehydration as a result of a malignancy or a complication from a surgical procedure, sequence either the dehydration or the complication first, followed by the code for the malignancy.

Administration of Antineoplastic Therapy

If the patient presents for the administration of antineoplastic chemotherapy, immunotherapy, or radiation therapy, then sequence one of the following Z-codes first, followed by the code for the malignancy. If the patient received more than one type of antineoplastic therapy, report one of each of the following Z-codes for each type of antineoplastic therapy performed. These Z-codes are:

- Z51.0, Encounter for antineoplastic radiation therapy
- Z51.11, Encounter for antineoplastic chemotherapy
- Z51.12, Encounter for antineoplastic immunotherapy

If a patient develops complications like nausea or vomiting as a result of the antineoplastic therapy during the encounter, then report the Z-code first, followed by the codes for the complications and the adverse effect of antineoplastic therapy or abnormal reaction to radiation therapy code.

Current versus Personal History of Neoplasm

Neoplasms should be reported as current until the patient is no longer undergoing any type of treatment toward that specific neoplasm (even if that neoplasm has been surgically removed). Report the current malignancy code until the patient is no longer receiving any type of treatment for that malignancy.

Once the malignancy has been excised or successfully treated, there is no longer any treatment directed at the site, and there is no evidence of existing malignancy, then report the code for personal history of malignant neoplasm (from category Z85). For example, if a patient with breast cancer has a mastectomy, but is still undergoing chemotherapy treatments, then the coder should report the code for the breast cancer even though the patient has received a mastectomy. Once the patient completes the chemotherapy regimen and is no longer receiving any type of treatment for that breast cancer, then the coder should report the history of breast cancer code.

For practice reporting diagnosis codes for hematology and oncology services, complete the exercises in There's a Code for That 18.2.

18.2 Hematology and oncology diagnosis coding

There's a Code for That

Read the following documentation and assign the appropriate diagnosis code(s) for the patient's condition(s).

1. Iron deficiency anemia, NOS.

   ICD-10-CM code: _____

2. Anemia due to cancer of the pancreas.

   ICD-10-CM codes: _____, _____

3. Primary malignant neoplasm of the tongue, frenulum linguae.

   ICD-10-CM code: _____

4. 36-year-old female with family history of breast cancer is BRCA1 gene mutation positive, presents today for biopsy of lump in the upper outer quadrant of the right breast.

   ICD-10-CM codes: _____, _____, _____

5. Metastatic cancer of the left lung.

   ICD-10-CM code: _____

6. 42-year-old patient presents for antineoplastic chemotherapy for angiosarcoma of the liver.

   ICD-10-CM codes: _____, _____

Procedural and Diagnostic Coding for Neurology

Codes for nervous system procedures are found in two sections of the CPT code book: the Surgery section and the Medicine section. Codes in the Nervous System subsection of the Surgery section identify invasive surgical procedures like placement of a cerebrospinal fluid shunt, whereas codes in the Medicine section identify mostly noninvasive procedures and studies of the neurological system, such as routine electroencephalography (EEG). Diagnoses commonly seen by neurologists and neurosurgeons include mental and behavioral disorders, as well as medical conditions of the nervous system.

Nervous System Surgical Procedures

The nervous system surgery codes are divided into two main divisions, which correspond with the two main divisions in the human nervous system—the central nervous system (CNS) and the peripheral nervous system (PNS). The central nervous system is comprised of all of the nerves of the brain and the spinal cord. The peripheral nervous system is comprised of all the other nerves throughout the body (USNLM, 2016b). Procedures on the central nervous system are reported with codes from the Skull, Meninges, and Brain (61000 to 62258) and Spine and Spinal Cord (62263 to 63746) subsections, and procedures on the peripheral nervous system are reported with codes from the Extracranial Nerves, Peripheral Nerves, and Autonomic Nervous System (64400 to 64999).

Skull, Meninges, and Brain

Procedures on the skull, meninges, and brain include the creation of an access point into the skull, such as a subdural tap through a fontanelle (the soft spot on the head of an infant), a twist drill hole, burr hole, trephine, or craniectomy or craniotomy (see figure 18.3). Twist drill, burr hole, and trephine procedures are all used to create a small opening into the skull, either for diagnostic or therapeutic purposes. Code selection depends on the type of opening created and the purpose of the procedure. For example, code 61105, Twist drill hole for subdural or ventricular puncture.

Figure 18.3. Craniotomy

Source: Cancer Research UK 2014a.

Craniectomy and Craniotomy codes (61304 to 61576) are more numerous and identify the specific type of procedure (craniectomy or craniotomy), area of the procedure, and purpose of the procedure or any additional services performed. For example, code 61510, Craniectomy, trephination, bone flap craniotomy; for excision of brain tumor, supratentorial, except meningioma. Craniectomies are performed to remove a portion of skull for an indicated reason, such as a lesion of the skull or damaged area, or to allow for a therapeutic procedure. Craniotomies are performed to remove a portion of the skull to allow access into the cranium or for therapeutic reasons, such as to relieve pressure or allow for drainage.

Key to Success

Do not get confused between craniectomies and craniotomies. A **craniectomy** is the removal of a portion of the skull. A **craniotomy** is an incision into the skull. The difference between the two is that in a craniotomy, the piece of skull is removed for therapeutic or diagnostic reasons, then placed back in its original location, whereas in a craniectomy, the fragment of bone is not replaced.

Surgeries of the skull base (61580 to 61619) are detailed procedures that require a number of qualified surgeons working as a team to complete the surgery. There are three different components to a surgery of the skull base: the approach procedure, the definitive procedure, and the repair/reconstructive procedure. The approach and the definitive procedures are always coded separately, with different CPT codes. The approach procedure describes the way in which the skull base is dissected open to reveal the lesion, as well as any additional procedures performed to gain access to the lesion, such as removal of sinuses or removal of facial bones. The definitive procedure describes the service that was performed on the lesion once access was gained, such as resection or excision of the lesion. The repair or reconstruction procedure is only coded if the repair required extensive dural grafting, cranioplasty, local or regional myocutaneous pedicle flaps, or extensive skin grafts. Figure 18.4 provides an overview of the anatomy of the skull.

Figure 18.4. Anatomy of the skull

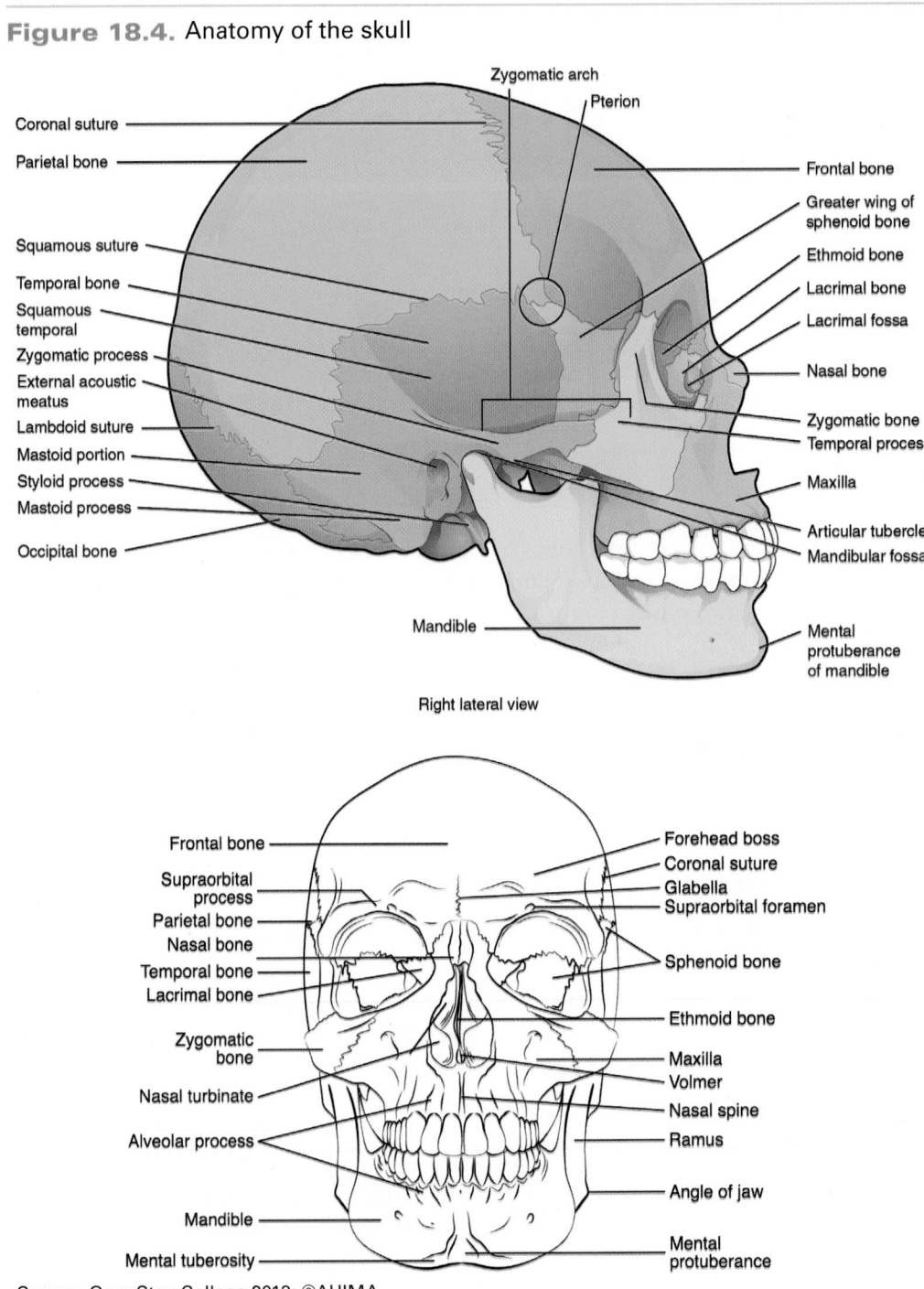

Source: OpenStax College 2013; ©AHIMA.

Additional procedures on the skull, meninges, and brain include surgical repairs of intracranial aneurysms, arteriovenous malformations, and vascular diseases (61680 to 61711), as well as insertion of intracranial neurostimulators (61850 to 61888), which may be used as a part of interventional pain management service.

Services to create, repair, and remove cerebrospinal fluid shunts are reported with codes from the Cerebrospinal Fluid (CSF) Shunt (62180 to 62258) subheading. A **cerebrospinal fluid (CSF) shunt** is a small one-way valve that is inserted within the ventricles of a patient's brain to allow for the drainage of cerebrospinal fluid from the brain and into the peritoneal cavity (see figure 18.5). This is a common treatment for hydrocephalus, in which the ventricles of the brain do not drain cerebrospinal fluid, causing a buildup of fluid in the skull. Coding for CSF shunts depends on the type of device, area being accessed, and definitive service, such as creation of shunt, replacement or revision of shunt, reprogramming, or removal of the complete CSF shunt device. For example, code 62230, Replacement or revision of cerebrospinal fluid shunt, obstructed valve, or distal catheter in shunt system.

Figure 18.5. CSF shunt

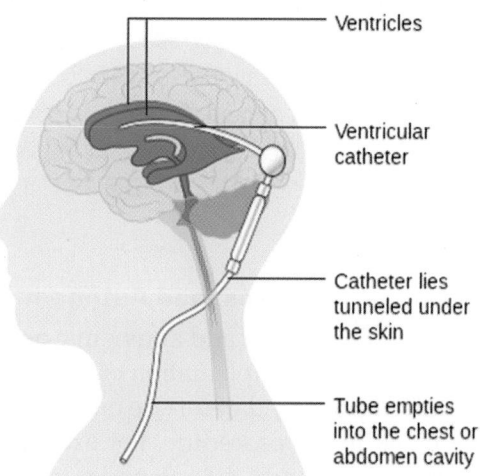

Ventricles

Ventricular catheter

Catheter lies tunneled under the skin

Tube empties into the chest or abdomen cavity

Source: Cancer Research UK 2014b.

Key to Success

Do not get confused between a *shunt* and a *stent*. A shunt is a tube placed inside the body to help remove fluid, such as cerebrospinal fluid, from one area to another. A stent is a device placed within a tubular body to keep it open. Shunts are often used in cardiovascular procedures, which are described in chapter 19, to keep blood vessels open and to increase blood flow.

Spine and Spinal Cord

Procedures on the spine and spinal cord include procedures like epidural injections, as well as procedures on the spine and vertebral column, such as laminectomies. Many of these procedures are performed by anesthesiologists and interventional pain management specialists, such as therapeutic or anesthetic injections and implantations of neurostimulators for pain relief. Orthopedic spinal surgeons may also perform many of the procedures on the spine itself, such as excision of herniated discs and decompression of neural elements.

When reporting codes for procedures on the spine, a good rule of thumb is to always check for the spinal area in the code description (for instance, lumbar or thoracic), and remember that vertebrae have two sides. If a procedure is performed on both sides of the vertebra, it should be reported as a bilateral service (modifier -50). Read code descriptions thoroughly to ensure correct code selection and the application of any necessary modifiers. For example, code 63020, Laminotomy (hemilaminectomy), with decompression of nerve root(s), including partial facetectomy, foraminotomy and/or excision of herniated intervertebral disc; 1 interspace, cervical describes the spinal area (*cervical*), and describes a unilateral procedure. In the parenthetical notes under the code description, it states: For bilateral procedure, report 63020 with modifier 50. This means that code 63020 describes a unilateral procedure, so if the procedure was performed on both sides, it should be reported with modifier -50.

Key to Success

Remember that when coding for procedures on the vertebrae or spinal column, some codes describe the number of interspaces or vertebral segments involved in the procedure. For more than one interspace or vertebral segment, check for the add-on code that is used to identify each additional interspace or segment. For example, if the provider performed the procedure described by code 63020 on three interspaces in the cervical region, then the coder should report code 63020 once for the first segment, and then the add-on code 63035, Each additional interspace, cervical or lumbar, twice for the additional two segments: 63020, 63035 × 2.

Extracranial Nerves, Peripheral Nerves, and Autonomic Nervous System

Procedures on the extracranial, peripheral, and autonomic nerves include injections of anesthetic and therapeutic substances, implantation of neurostimulators, and destruction of nerves. When performing any kind of service on a nerve, it is necessary to identify the specific nerve involved in the procedure. For example, code 64402, Injection, anesthetic agent; facial nerve. In many of the categories, nerves are grouped by their type, such as somatic nerves, paravertebral spinal nerves and branches, autonomic nerves, and sympathetic nerves.

Codes 64600 through 64681 report destruction by neurolytic agent (for example, chemical, thermal, electrical, or radiofrequency), and chemodenervation procedures. Chemodenervation is the injection of botulinum toxin, a potent neurotoxin, to an affected nerve for various reasons including pain management and reduction of muscle spasticity. Like nerve injection procedures, chemodenervation codes identify the specific nerve or muscle being treated. Check for add-on codes in this section to fully report each injection performed.

Additional procedures in this section include:

- Neuroplasty (Exploration, Neurolysis or Nerve Decompression) (64702 to 64727) codes, which report plastic surgical decompression or freeing of intact nerves from scar tissue.
- Transection or Avulsion (64732 to 64772) codes, which report the actual transection (cutting of the nerve) or avulsion (tearing away) of nerves for therapeutic purposes.
- Excision (64774 to 64823) codes report the surgical removal of either nerves or tumors on specific nerves.

- Neurorrhaphy (64831 to 64876) codes report the surgical repair of nerves via suture or anastomosis.
- Neurorrhaphy With Nerve Graft, Vein Graft, or Conduit (64885 to 64913) codes report surgical repair of nerves using a graft for the repair.

Neurology Medicine Procedures

There are also several neurology procedures in the Medicine section of the CPT code book. These include specialized tests and treatments to help diagnose, treat, and assist with surgical procedures. These procedures include:

- Sleep Medicine (95803 to 95811).
- Routine Electroencephalography (EEG) (95812 to 95830). An **electroencephalogram (EEG)** is a diagnostic study of the electrical impulses of the brain. EEGs are useful in diagnosing neurological conditions such as epilepsy, brain tumors, encephalitis, encephalopathy, strokes, sleep disorders, and dementia.
- Muscle and Range of Motion Testing (95831 to 95857).
- Electromyography (95860 to 95887).
- Muscle Testing and Guidance (95873 to 95875).
- Nerve Conduction Studies (95905 to 95913).
- Intraoperative Neurophysiology (95940 and 95941).
- Autonomic Function Tests (95921 to 95924, 95943).
- Evoked Potentials and Reflex Tests (95925 to 95937).
- Special EEG Tests (95950 to 95967). Like routine EEGs, special EEGs are recordings of the brain's electrical impulses. However, these EEGs are extended or performed in a different manner than routine EEGs.
- Neurostimulators, Analysis-Programming (95970 to 95982).
- Motion Analysis (96000 to 96004).
- Functional Brain Mapping (96020).

As with coding for all CPT codes, reporting neurology medicine procedures described by the codes in this list requires a strict attention to detail and understanding of how to report CPT codes properly.

Complete the exercises in There's a Code for That 18.3 for practice reporting neurology procedure codes.

Neurology procedures

18.3

There's a Code for That

Read the following documentation of the service and identify the CPT procedure code(s).

1. Infratentorial trephine.

   CPT code: _____

2. Craniectomy of the posterior fossa of the skull for excision of meningioma.

   CPT code: _____

(Continued on next page)

18.3

Continued

3. Simple dural repair of intracranial arteriovenous malformation.

   CPT code: _____

4. Creation of subdural-pleural CSF shunt.

   CPT code: _____

5. Cervical laminectomy with exploration and decompression of spinal cord without discectomy, of three vertebral segments.

   CPT code: _____

6. Thoracic discectomy and decompression of spinal cord and nerve roots, T3 to T6.

   CPT code: _____ , _____

Neurology Diagnoses

The majority of diagnosis codes reported by neurologists are located in chapter 5: Mental, Behavioral, and Neurodevelopmental Disorders, and chapter 6: Diseases of the Nervous System, of the ICD-10-CM code book. However, keep in mind that neurology conditions may present with additional comorbidities or complications that would be coded from other chapters of the ICD-10-CM code book. Also, neurologists will see patients who have suffered traumatic brain injuries or stroke victims. Refer to chapter 16 on how to report strokes and cerebrovascular incidents, as well as traumatic brain injuries.

Mental, Behavioral, and Neurodevelopmental Disorders

The only coding guidelines that pertain to coding for conditions from the Mental, Behavioral, and Neurodevelopmental Disorders chapter are for the reporting of pain disorders due to psychological factors and mental disorders due to psychoactive substance use.

One commonly seen condition coded from this chapter is dementia. Dementia is the term for loss of memory and mental abilities due to an underlying physical change in the brain. Codes for dementia are located in categories F01, Vascular dementia, F02, Dementia in diseases classified elsewhere, and F03, Unspecified dementia. For both vascular and dementia in diseases classified elsewhere, there is a note in the Tabular to code first for the underling physiological condition, such as cerebrovascular incident (stroke) or Alzheimer's disease. Note that dementia codes are included in HCC and special attention should be paid to the documentation and reporting of the most specified dementia codes.

Chapter 5 also includes codes for mental disorders such as schizophrenia, mood disorders, and depression. Many of these conditions are discussed in chapter 7 regarding behavioral health services. As a rule of thumb, neurologists treat mental diagnoses that are a result of an underlying physiological condition, such as vascular dementia—dementia caused by a vascular disease of the brain. However, these conditions do sometimes present in conjunction with mental disorders often treated by a behavioral health practitioner.

Diseases of the Nervous System

Neurologists treat a wide range of neurological conditions, most of which are included in chapter 6: Diseases of the Nervous System, of the ICD-10-CM code book. Note that the guidelines for this chapter pertain to dominant and nondominant sides and pain, discussed in chapters 16 and 12 of this text, respectively. Conditions treated by neurologists in this chapter of the ICD-10-CM book include the following (note that many of these conditions are also classified as HCC codes, so it is important to ensure that these codes are documented fully and coded to the highest level of specificity).

- Extrapyramidal and movement disorders (G20 to G26), including Parkinson's disease (G20). **Parkinson's disease** is a progressive disorder of the central nervous system that causes tremors rigidity, and postural problems.

- Other degenerative diseases of the nervous system (G30 to G32), including Alzheimer's disease (G30.-). **Alzheimer's disease** is a progressive form of dementia that causes loss of memories and cognitive abilities that interfere with activities of daily living. Codes for Alzheimer's disease specify whether the condition is early-onset (before the age of 65), late onset, or other form. Note the guidelines in the Tabular to use an additional code to identify Alzheimer's dementia with or without behavioral disturbance (F02.80, Dementia in other diseases classified elsewhere without behavioral disturbance, or F02.81, Dementia in other diseases classified elsewhere with behavioral disturbance). According to ICD-10-CM Tabular notes, the appropriate code for dementia or delirium should always accompany the code for Alzheimer's disease. When sequencing Alzheimer's disease and dementia, sequence the Alzheimer's code first, followed by the code for the dementia (either with or without behavioral disturbance) or delirium.

- Episodic and Paroxysmal Disorders (G40-G47), including Epilepsy and recurrent seizures (G40). **Epilepsy** is a neurological condition that manifests in sensory disturbances, loss of consciousness, and seizures (convulsions) as a result of abnormal electrical activity in the brain. Codes for epilepsy identify various components, which make them some of the more complex codes in ICD-10-CM. These include:
    - *The type of epilepsy*. For example, localization-related (focal) (partial) symptomatic epilepsy, generalized idiopathic epilepsy, or juvenile myoclonic epilepsy.
    - *The type of seizures*. For example, seizures of localized onset, simple partial seizures, or complex partial seizures.
    - *Intractability status*. An **intractable condition** is one that does not respond to medical treatment. For example, an intractable migraine is one that does not respond to migraine pain medication. Intractable epilepsy is difficult or impossible to control with treatment. Codes for epilepsy identify whether the condition is intractable or not.
    - *Status epilepticus*. **Status epilepticus** is a type of epilepsy in which the seizures occur too close together for the patient to fully recover in-between seizures, or when a seizure lasts for a long period of time. Codes for epilepsy also identify whether the condition presents with status epilepticus or not.

  For example, code G40.019, Localization-related (focal) (partial) idiopathic epilepsy and epileptic syndromes, with seizures of localized onset, intractable, without status epilepticus, identifies the type of epilepsy (*localization-related*), type of seizures (*localized onset*), intractability status (*intractable*), and with or without status epilepticus (*without status epilepticus*).

- Additional conditions in this chapter include migraines, nerve disorders, neuropathies, and paralytic syndromes.

Complete the exercises in There's a Code for That 18.4 for practice reporting neurology diagnosis codes.

18.4 Neurology diagnosis coding

There's a Code for That

Read the following documentation and assign the appropriate diagnosis code(s) for the patient's condition(s).

1. Parkinson's disease with dementia with aggressive and combative behavior.

   ICD-10-CM code: _____, _____

2. Congenital nonprogressive ataxia.

   ICD-10-CM code: _____

3. Parkinsonism due to vascular malformation.

   ICD-10-CM code: _____

4. Lewy body dementia without behavioral disturbance.

   ICD-10-CM code: _____, _____

5. Multiple sclerosis.

   ICD-10-CM code: _____

6. Intractable absence epileptic syndrome, without status epilepticus.

   ICD-10-CM code: _____

Procedural and Diagnostic Coding for Urology and Nephrology

Coding for urology and nephrology services requires an understanding of at least two subsections of the CPT code book: the Urinary System and Male Genital System. Remember that urologists may also perform some procedures on the female urinary system, which are located in the Female Genital System subsection as well (such as a sling operation for stress incontinence). Dialysis is performed for patients with chronic kidney disease and end-stage renal disease, and codes for dialysis and end-stage renal disease services are found in the Medicine section of the CPT code book.

Urinary System Procedures

Surgical procedures on the urinary system are all located in the Urinary System subsection of the CPT code book. This subsection is organized into four main sections, according to the four main organs in the urinary system: kidneys, ureters, bladder, and urethra.

The kidneys are two bean-shaped organs that function to filter waste products from the blood and to control electrolyte balance and the body's balance of fluid. In this process, the kidneys create urine, which passes through the urinary system through the ureters—two thin tubes that connect the kidneys to the urinary bladder. The urinary bladder, also known as the bladder, is a hollow muscular organ that holds urine until it is emptied from the body through the urethra. The urethra is the last part of the urinary system, through which urine passes during elimination from the bladder. In females, the urethra is about 1 to 1.5 inches long, ending directly in front of the vaginal opening and located between the labia. In males, the urethra is about 7 to 8 inches long, beginning at the bladder and ending at the urethral orifice at the tip of the penis. The prostate is a gland only found in males that stores and assists in making seminal fluid, and sits under the urinary bladder surrounding part of the urethra. See figure 18.6 for an overview of urinary system anatomy.

Figure 18.6. Urinary system anatomy

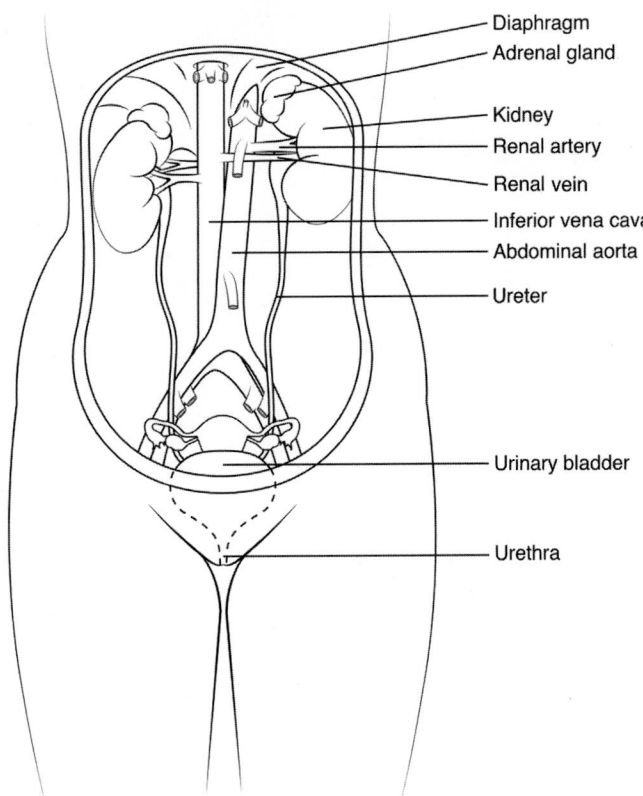

- Diaphragm
- Adrenal gland
- Kidney
- Renal artery
- Renal vein
- Inferior vena cava
- Abdominal aorta
- Ureter
- Urinary bladder
- Urethra

Source: ©AHIMA.

Kidney

Surgical procedures on the kidneys are reported with codes from the Kidney section (50010 to 50593). Note that nephrologists, as specialists in the diagnosis and treatment of kidney disorders, are more likely to perform procedures on the kidneys, although some minor procedures may be performed by urologists as well. This depends on the resources, training, and availability of the healthcare specialists.

Many of the surgical procedures on the kidneys are for the treatment of nephrolithiasis, or kidney stones. Kidney stones—also known as renal calculi—are usually small, condensed deposits of minerals and other solids that form in the kidneys (see figure 18.7). To expel the stone from the urinary tract, it passes through the urinary system, down the ureters, through the bladder, and out through the urethra. This is a painful and sometimes lengthy process. However, if the stone is too large to pass naturally through the urinary tract, or if it becomes obstructed (stuck), it must be treated surgically. Large nephrolithiasis, known as staghorn calculus, completely fill the renal pelvis (the area within the kidney), and are too big to pass naturally through the urinary system and may require surgical treatment.

Codes for the open incision of the kidneys are located in the Incision category (50010 to 50135), and include codes for the incision and drainage of renal abscesses, as well as nephrolithotomy—incision into the kidney for the removal of a kidney stone.

Figure 18.7. Renal calculi

Renal Calculi

Multiple small calculi

Plain film: multiple renal calculi

Bilateral staghorn calculi

Staghorn calculus plus smaller stone

Nephrolithotomy codes identify the type of operation and the type of calculus. For example, code 50075, Nephrolithotomy; removal of large staghorn calculus filling renal pelvis and calyces (including anatomic pyelolithotomy), reports an incisional procedure to remove a staghorn calculus from the kidney.

MOD Because kidneys are bilateral organs, the coder must identify the laterality of the procedure by appending modifier -RT or -LT, for right or left side. Unless there are specific notations in the Tabular, if the procedure was performed bilaterally, append modifier -50 to report the bilateral service. Note that the way unilateral or bilateral codes are reported may depend on the third-party payer; always check the payer requirements to ensure correct modifier selection.

Excision (50200 to 50290) codes identify excisional procedures performed in the kidneys, such as renal biopsies and excision of kidneys. If the excision of the kidney is part of a kidney transplantation procedure, it is coded from the Renal Transplantation (50300 to 50380) subsection. Remember that there are three main components to any major organ transplant—organ removal, backbench work, and recipient transplantation (refer to chapter 11, Surgical Services). Note that a donated kidney may come from either a living or cadaver donor, and kidney transplants may be performed with or without the removal of the recipient's kidney. Both of these components impact code selection. For example, code 50365, Renal allotransplantation, implantation of graft; with recipient nephrectomy.

Kidney Introduction (50382 to 50435) procedures include the placement and removal of catheters (both internally dwelling as well as externally accessible) in the renal pelvis, and the creation of nephrostomies and injection procedures.

Laparoscopic procedures of the kidney are reported with codes 50541 to 50549. Many of these procedures are also located in other procedural categories, with the exception that codes in this section all identify laparoscopic procedures. For example, code 50547, Laparoscopy, surgical; donor nephrectomy (including cold preservation), from living donor, is the same procedure as code 50320, Donor nephrectomy (including cold preservation); open, from living donor with the exception that code 50547 is performed via the laparoscopic approach, and code 50320 is performed via the open approach.

Codes for Endoscopy (50551 to 50580) of the kidneys differ depending on the approach to the endoscopic procedure (through nephrostomy or nephrotomy), and the definitive procedure performed during the endoscopy (such as removal of calculus).

The Other Procedures (50590 to 50593) category of codes contain the code 50590, Lithotripsy, extracorporeal shock wave. **Extracorporeal shock wave lithotripsy (ESWL)** is a procedure in which shock waves are sent through the patient's body to break up a nephrolithiasis into tiny fragments. Once the stone is broken up it naturally passes through the urinary system (see figure 18.8).

Figure 18.8. Extracorporeal shockwave lithotripsy (ESWL)

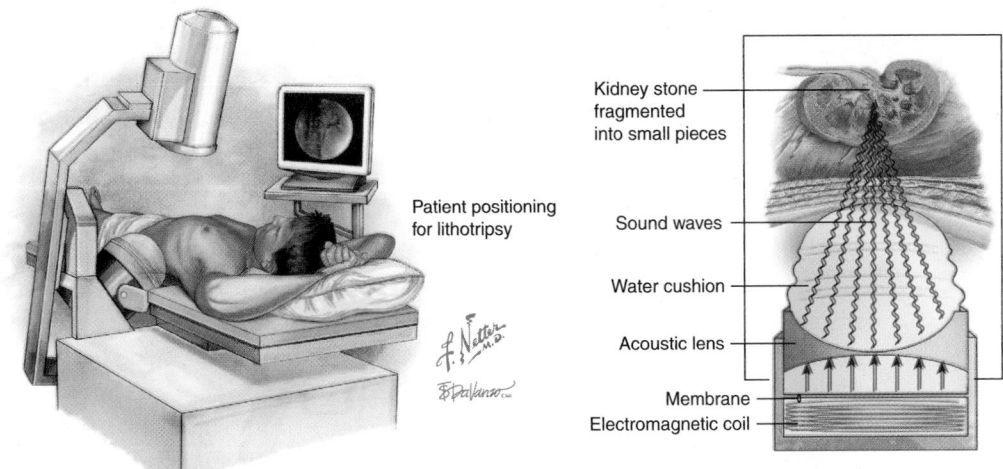

Kidney stone fragmented into small pieces

Patient positioning for lithotripsy

Sound waves

Water cushion

Acoustic lens

Membrane

Electromagnetic coil

Ureter

Procedures on the ureters include Incision (50600 to 50630), Excision (50650 to 50660), Introduction (50684 to 50695), Repair (50700 to 50940), Laparoscopy (50945 to 50980), and Endoscopy (50951 to 50980). When coding for ureteral procedures, identify the procedure as being performed on the right or left side, or if the procedure was performed bilaterally. Note that these components are not included in the code descriptions. For example, code 50605, Ureterotomy for insertion of indwelling stent, all types, does not identify the procedure as either unilateral or bilateral. In this case, the documentation should identify the laterality of the procedure, and the coder should append modifier -50 if the procedure was performed bilaterally, or modifier -LT or -RT to identify the laterality of the procedure.

Bladder

There are more procedures on the bladder than for any other organ in the urinary system. These include procedures for the removal of calculi, destruction and removal of lesions and tissue, introduction procedures, and repair procedures.

Key to Success

The medical prefix for the bladder is *cyst/o-*, so numerous procedures in this subheading refer to *cystotomy, cystectomy, cystotomy,* and such. If you think of a cyst as a fluid-filled sac, it is easy to remember that *cyst/o-* refers to the bladder— a sac that holds urine.

Procedures on the bladder include:

- Incision (51020 to 51080) codes identify surgical incisions into the bladder to remove calculi, insert radioactive material as a treatment for cancer, or drainage.
- Removal (51100 to 51102) codes report the surgical aspiration of bladder contents via needle, trocar or intracatheter, or with insertion of suprapubic catheter.
- Excision (51500 to 51597) codes identify the removal of the bladder or additional urinary components. When coding for cystectomies, identify the components removed and any additional procedures performed.
- Introduction (51600 to 51720) codes report the introduction of a catheter, injected substance, or cystostomy tube. This subheading includes codes for urinary catheterizations. **Catheterizations** are common procedures that involve the insertion of a catheter tube in through the urethra and into the bladder to drain urine. There are two types of catheterizations—straight and indwelling:
  - Straight catheterization, coded with 51701, Insertion of non-indwelling bladder catheter (e.g., straight catheterization for residual urine) is performed by inserting a catheter through the urethra and into the bladder to drain urine from the bladder. This procedure is performed to either completely drain the bladder or to collect a urine sample. Once the urine is drained, the catheter is removed.
  - Indwelling catheterization, coded with 51702, Insertion of temporary indwelling bladder catheter; simple (e.g., Foley), or 51703, Insertion of temporary indwelling bladder catheter; complicated (e.g., altered anatomy, fractured catheter/balloon) is performed by inserting a catheter with a small balloon at the tip through the urethra and into the bladder, where the balloon is inflated so that it stays in place (see figure 18.9). This allows the urine to drain from the bladder for a longer period of time, into a collection bag. Indwelling catheters are used for continuous drainage for patients who are undergoing surgery, bedridden, or are otherwise unable to mobilize themselves to the toilet. Indwelling catheters may stay in place for

several days, depending on the patient's medical condition and the safety implications of a long-term bladder catheterization.

- Urodynamics (51725 to 51798) codes report a variety of procedures. Urodynamics is the study of the motion and flow of urine. These codes identify procedures designed to study urinary flow and pressure, as well as additional studies on the nerve conduction of the anal or urethral sphincter, and measurement of urinary post-voiding.

- Repair (51800 to 51980) codes report the surgical repair of the bladder and associated components, as well as closure of fistulas. Some of these procedures include repair of components located in the female genital system, so it is important to pay attention to the parenthetical notes in the Tabular list to ensure correct code selection.

- Laparoscopy (51990 to 51999) codes report two different types of sling operations for stress incontinence in which sutures are placed near the bladder to support the neck of the urethra. If this procedure is performed via the open approach, it is reported with the appropriate code from the female vaginal system. When performed via the open approach, urinary incontinence surgeries for males are coded from the Urethra subheading of codes in the Repair category. Again, it is important to pay attention to the parenthetical notes in the Tabular List to ensure correct code selection.

- Endoscopy—Cystoscopy, Urethroscopy, Cystourethroscopy (52000 to 52010) codes identify endoscopic procedures of the urinary system. This subsection includes Transurethral Surgery of the Urethra and Bladder (52204 to 52318) and of the Ureter and Pelvis (52320 to 52356), as well as endoscopic procedures of the Vesical Neck and Prostate (52400 to 52700). Procedures on the vesical neck and prostate include transurethral procedures on the prostate. One of the most common medical conditions of the prostate is benign prostatic hyperplasia (BPH), a condition in which the prostate gland is enlarged, causing urinary frequency and urgency, nocturia (urinating at night), and urinary retention (among other symptoms). As a treatment for BPH and the lower urinary tract symptoms, prostatic tissue can be surgically removed to reduce obstruction and pressure on the bladder and

Figure 18.9. Indwelling catheterization

urethra. One of the ways in which this tissue is removed is via a procedure called a **transurethral resection of the prostate (TURP)** (see figure 18.10). Coded with 52601, Transurethral electrosurgical resection of the prostate, including control of postoperative bleeding, complete (vasectomy, meatotomy, cystourethroscopy, urethral calibration and/or dilation, and internal urethrotomy are included), this procedure involves the insertion of a resectoscope through the male urethra, which is threaded to the area of the prostate tissue to be removed. An electrocautery knife is then used to cut away at the enlarged prostatic tissue. Transurethral excision or destruction of prostatic tissue may also be performed via laser coagulation of the prostate (52647), laser vaporization of the prostate (52648), and laser enucleation of the prostate (52649). Open procedures of the prostate are reported with codes from the Male Genital System subsection under the heading Prostate (55700 through 55899).

Figure 18.10. Transurethral resection of the prostate (TURP)

Source: ©2009. Used with permission of Elsevier. All rights reserved.

Key to Success

Do not get confused between a *cystoscopy* and a *cystourethroscopy*, though these two procedures are similar. A cystourethroscopy is the endoscopic examination of both the urethra and the bladder, whereas a cystoscopy is the examination of just the bladder. However, because an imaging procedure of the bladder typically passes through the urethra (to gain access to the bladder), endoscopic examinations of the bladder may be referred to as cystourethroscopies (including the urethra and the bladder). Thus, endoscopic examinations of the bladder are listed in the section of codes for cystourethroscopies in the CPT code book. If you read the parent code for each procedure in the endoscopy section of the bladder, you will see that all these procedures are described as cystourethroscopies. When the documentation of a healthcare procedure identifies the procedure as a *cystoscopy*, you should select the appropriate *cystourethroscopy* code. Although these two procedures are technically different, the terms are used interchangeably in the CPT book.

Key to Success

Transurethral excisions of prostatic tissue are technically prostatectomies, as they remove the tissue of the prostate. This is confusing, as prostatectomy codes are also included in the Male Genital System subsection. The difference between the two is that prostatectomies in the Urinary System subsection are all performed through the transurethral approach, whereas prostatectomies in the Male Genital System are all performed via an open excisional approach.

Urethra

Procedures on the urethra include Incision (53000 to 53085), Excision (53200 to 53275), Repair (53400 to 53520), Manipulation (53600 to 53665), and Other Procedures (53850 to 53899). Some of these procedures indicate patient gender, as the male and female urethra differ. Note that three of the procedures in the Other Procedures category (53850 to 53855) are additional procedures that may be performed to remove prostatic tissue (via microwave or radiofrequency thermotherapy) and to insert an indwelling prostatic urethral stent.

Male Genital Procedures

Surgical procedures on the male genital system are all located in the Male Genital System subsection of the CPT code book. This subsection is divided based on the specific anatomy of the male genital system including the penis, testis, epididymis, tunica vaginalis, scrotum, vas deferens, spermatic cord, seminal vesicles, and prostate.

The penis is the main male reproductive organ and is made up of two types of tissue: corpora cavernosa, which is made up of erectile tissue, and corpora spongiosum, which lies under the corpora cavernosa and forms the internal shape of the penis with a bulbous shape at the end of the penis and helps to prevent urethral compression during erection. The testes, glands of the reproductive and endocrine systems, produce and store sperm and male sex hormones. In healthy males, there are two testes (or testicles) located behind the penis in a pouch of skin called the scrotum. The tunica vaginalis is a layer of tissue covering the testes in the shape of a pouch. The epididymis is a duct behind the testes, in which newly created sperm cells mature and then move into the vas deferens. The vas deferens (also referred to as the vas or ductus deferens) are made of smooth muscle and are located within the spermatic cord, a cord-like structure made up of the vas deferens and surrounding tissues. The vas deferens transport sperm from the epididymis to the urethra, which is later ejaculated through the urethral orifice. The seminal vesicles are small male accessory sex glands that help to form the lubricating fluid of semen. The prostate is a gland, located under the urinary bladder and in front of the rectum, helps in making and storing seminal fluid. See figures 18.11 and 18.12 for an overview of the male genital and reproductive systems.

Key to Success

The male genital system is made up of numerous anatomical components. However, the number of procedures that can be performed on those components is relatively small. If you are having problems finding codes in the Male Genital System subsection, locate the subheading for the anatomical area on which the procedure is being performed (such as the tunica vaginalis), and then try searching the available codes for the procedure that was performed.

Figure 18.11. Male genital system

Source: ©AHIMA.

Figure 18.12. Cross-section of male genital system

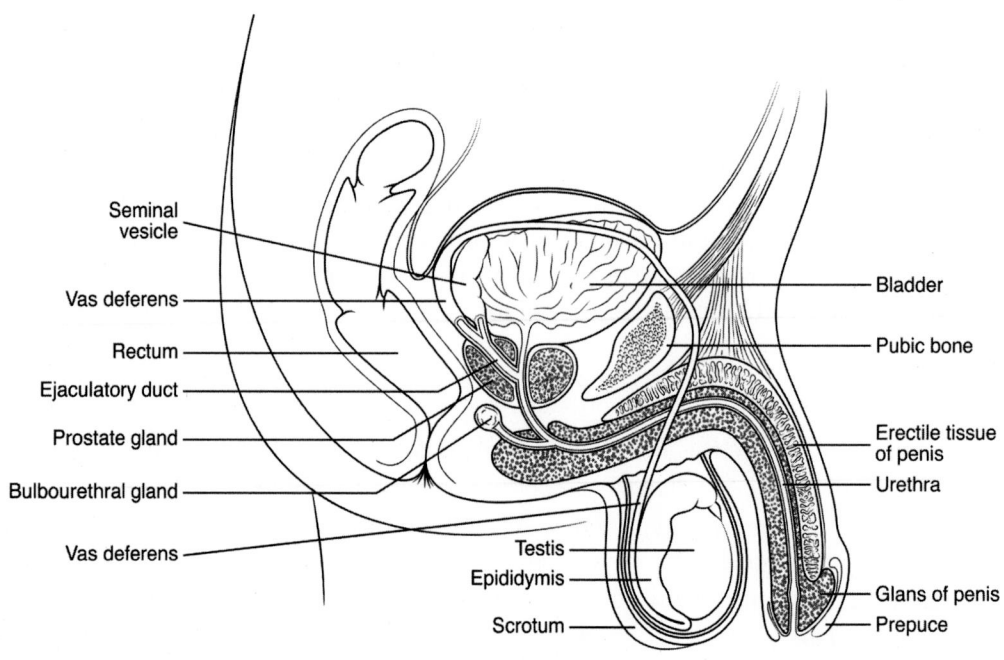

Source: ©AHIMA.

Penis

The Penis (54000 to 54450) subheading contains the largest amount of codes in the Male Genital System subsection. These procedures include incision, destruction, and excision procedures. Keep in mind that when performing a procedure on the penis, the surgeon is not working on the skin of the penis, but rather the deep tissues of the penis. For example, instead of the destruction of a lesion on the skin of the penis, code 54050, Destruction of lesion(s), penis (e.g., condyloma, papilloma, molluscum contagiosum, herpetic vesicle), simple; chemical, should be reported for the destruction of a lesion of the penile tissue under the subcutaneous layer of skin. This is a common distinction in surgical coding—if the procedure was performed on the skin of an organ or on the deeper structures.

A common excision procedure performed on the penis is a circumcision, coded with 54150, Circumcision, using clamp or other device with regional dorsal penile or ring block, through 54161, Circumcision, surgical excision other than clamp, device, or dorsal slit; older than 28 days of age. A circumcision is the surgical removal of the foreskin at the tip of the penis. When coding for circumcisions, identify the method of circumcision (clamp or device) and whether a penile ring block was used for anesthesia. If a penile ring block was not used, then identify the age of the patient (a neonate 28 days or less, or older than 28 days of age).

Additional procedures on the penis include Introduction (54200 to 54250), Repair (54300 to 54400), and Manipulation (54450).

Testis

Testis (54500 to 54699) report procedures for the biopsy and excision of testis (both via open approach and laparoscopically), exploration, and repair. Exploration (54550 to 54560) codes are reported for the exploration of undescended testes. Undescended testes may need to be surgically fixated in the scrotal sac in a procedure known as an orchiopexy. Orchiopexy codes are located in both the Repair (54600 to 54680) and Laparoscopy (54690 to 54699) categories, depending on the approach to the procedure.

Epididymis

Epididymis (54700 to 54901) codes identify procedures to incise and drain abscess or hematoma of the epididymis, biopsy or excision of lesion of the epididymis, exploration, and repair.

Tunica Vaginalis

Tunica Vaginalis (55000 to 55060) codes identify the treatment of hydrocele of the tunica vaginalis, a fluid-filled sac that can cause pain and discomfort. Treatment includes puncture aspiration, excision, or repair of a tunica vaginalis hydrocele.

Scrotum

Scrotum (55100 to 55180) codes identify procedures performed on the scrotal sac (not the skin of the scrotum), such as removal of foreign bodies, drainage of abscess, resection, and repair.

Vas Deferens

The most common procedure performed within the Vas Deferens (55200 to 55450) subheading of codes is a vasectomy, coded with 55250, Vasectomy, unilateral or bilateral (separate procedure), including postoperative semen examination(s). This is an outpatient procedure that is performed commonly for elective sterilization. In the procedure, a small section of the vas deferens are cut and removed, so that semen does not flow through the vas to the urethra during ejaculation. This is a procedure that can be reversed through a vasovasostomy or vasovasorrhaphy, connecting the vas back together again.

Spermatic Cord

Spermatic Cord (55500 to 55559) codes report procedures on the spermatic cord, including excision of lesions, hydroceles, or varicocele. Note that these procedures can be performed either via open incision or laparoscopically.

Seminal Vesicles

Seminal Vesicles (55600 to 55680) procedures include either incision or excision procedures, with a specific code for the excision of a Mullerian duct cyst, which can cause urinary urgency, frequency, dysuria, and urinary obstruction, among other symptoms. The code for the excision of the Mullerian duct cyst is 55680, Excision of Mullerian duct cyst.

Prostate

Prostate (55700 to 55899) procedures include biopsy of the prostate, and drainage of prostatic abscesses, as well as excision of the prostate via open or laparoscopic approaches. Prostatectomy codes located in this section include the removal of the entire prostate, rather than a small section of prostatic tissue (as in transurethral resection of the prostate). Open prostatectomy codes differ depending on the approach to the procedure (open, laparoscopic, perineal, suprapubic, retropubic), and the elements included in the excision procedure.

Dialysis

Dialysis is the process of filtering waste products from the blood, which replaces the function of the kidneys for patients with end-stage renal disease or renal failure. There are two types of dialysis—hemodialysis and peritoneal dialysis. Hemodialysis is the process of filtering the blood of waste products using a dialyzer machine, which removes the waste products from the blood. Peritoneal dialysis involves the placement of a dialyzing solution into the peritoneal cavity in the abdomen, where it removes waste products from the body and is then drained, removing extra fluid and waste products.

Codes for dialysis are found in the Medicine section of the CPT code book, in the Dialysis (90935 to 90999) subsection. There are four subheadings of codes.

- Hemodialysis (90935 to 90940). Hemodialysis procedure codes identify the actual dialysis service performed per date of service.
- Miscellaneous Dialysis Procedures (90945 to 90947). Miscellaneous dialysis procedure codes are used for dialysis procedures other than hemodialysis, such as peritoneal dialysis.
- End-Stage Renal Disease Services (90951 to 90970). End-stage renal disease (ESRD) service codes are reported once per month to identify the services provided to the patient in relation to the patient's ESRD. These services include the establishment of a dialyzing cycle, outpatient E/M of the dialysis visits, telephone calls and other patient management reported on a monthly basis.

Codes 90951 through 90966 report a full month of services, whereas codes 90967 through 90970 report ESRD-related services per day. Code selection for ESRD-related services requires identification of the age of the patient, and the number of face-to-face visits between the patient and healthcare provider per month. For example, code 90961, End-stage renal disease (ESRD) related services monthly, for patients 20 years of age and older; with 2-3 face-to-face visits by a physician or other qualified health care professional per month identifies the age of the patient (*20 years of age or older*) as well as the number of face-to-face visits with the healthcare provider (2-3).

- Other Dialysis Procedures (90989 and 90999). Other dialysis procedure codes include patient training on use of dialysis equipment as well as an unlisted dialysis services code.

Complete the exercises in There's a Code for That 18.5 for practice reporting codes for urology and nephrology procedures.

Urology and nephrology procedures

18.5

There's a Code for That

Read the following documentation of the service and identify the CPT procedure code(s).

1. Nephrolithotomy with removal of calculus, complicated by congenital kidney malformation.

   CPT code: _____

2. Simple Foley Y-pyeloplasty with pyelostomy and ureteral splinting.

   CPT code: _____

3. ESWL.

   CPT code: _____

4. Complex cystometrogram with voiding pressure studies and simple uroflowmetry.

   CPT code: _____ - _____, _____

5. Removal of plastic implant from penile tissue.

   CPT code: _____

6. Bilateral vesiculectomy.

   CPT code: _____ - _____

7. Retropubic radical prostatectomy performed with nerve sparing and laparoscopic robotic assistance.

   CPT code: _____

8. ESRD related services for 25-year-old female, including two face-to-face visits per month.

   CPT code: _____

9. Peritoneal dialysis with single evaluation and management encounter with healthcare provider.

   CPT code: _____

Urology and Nephrology Diagnosis Codes

Diagnosis codes reported by urologists and nephrologists are located in chapter 14: Diseases of the Genitourinary System, of the ICD-10-CM code book. Coding guidelines for this chapter discuss coding situations for chronic kidney disease, a common nephrology diagnosis. Additional, important diagnoses for urology and nephrology include nephrolithiasis and benign prostatic hyperplasia.

Chronic Kidney Disease

Chronic kidney disease (CKD) and acute kidney failure are all coded from the section Acute Kidney Failure and Chronic Kidney Disease (N17 to N19). Codes for CKD, located in category N18, identify the stage of the CKD and if the patient is in end-stage renal disease. All codes in category N18 for chronic kidney disease are classified as HCC codes, so pay special attention when selecting these codes to ensure they are coded to the highest level of specificity. According to ICD-10-CM coding guidelines, when coding for CKD, use an additional code to identify either diabetic or hypertensive CKD, whether the patient has previously received a kidney transplant (Z94.0, Kidney transplant status), or if the patient is currently on dialysis (Z99.2, Dependence on renal dialysis). See figure 18.13 for the guidelines related to CKD coding. For example, if a patient with hypertensive stage 5 CKD and hypertensive heart failure who is currently dependent on renal dialysis presented for treatment, the codes reported would be as follows:

- I13.2, Hypertensive heart and chronic kidney disease with heart failure and with stage 5 chronic kidney disease, or end-stage renal disease
- I50.9, Heart failure, unspecified
- N18.5, Chronic kidney disease, stage 5
- Z99.2, Dependence on renal dialysis

Figure 18.13. OGCR I.C.14

---

14. **Chapter 14: Diseases of the Genitourinary System (N00-N99)**

a. **Chronic kidney disease**

1) **Stages of chronic kidney disease (CKD)**

The ICD-10-CM classifies CKD based on severity. The severity of CKD is designated by stages 1-5. Stage 2, code N18.2, equates to mild CKD; stage 3, code N18.3, equates to moderate CKD; and stage 4, code N18.4, equates to severe CKD. Code N18.6, End stage renal disease (ESRD), is assigned when the provider has documented end-stage-renal disease (ESRD).

If both a stage of CKD and ESRD are documented, assign code N18.6 only.

2) **Chronic kidney disease and kidney transplant status**

Patients who have undergone kidney transplant may still have some form of chronic kidney disease (CKD) because the kidney transplant may not fully restore kidney function. Therefore, the presence of CKD alone does not constitute a transplant complication. Assign the appropriate N18 code for the patient's stage of CKD and code Z94.0, Kidney transplant status. If a transplant complication such as failure or rejection or other transplant complication is documented, see section I.C.19.g for information on coding complications of a kidney transplant. If the documentation is unclear as to whether the patient has a complication of the transplant, query the provider.

3) **Chronic kidney disease with other conditions**

Patients with CKD may also suffer from other serious conditions, most commonly diabetes mellitus and hypertension. The sequencing of the CKD code in relationship to codes for other contributing conditions is based on the conventions in the Tabular List.

See I.C.9. Hypertensive chronic kidney disease.

See I.C.19. Chronic kidney disease and kidney transplant complications.

Nephrolithiasis

Nephrolithiasis and urinary calculi are all reported with codes from section Urolithiasis (N20 to N23). These codes identify the location of the stone—in kidney, ureter, kidney with ureter, or such. If the calculus is due to an underlying condition, report the code for the underlying condition first.

Benign Prostatic Hyperplasia

As mentioned previously, benign prostatic hyperplasia (BPH) is one of the most common conditions affecting the prostate. BPH is reported with the appropriate code from category N40, Benign prostatic hyperplasia, and code selection depends on whether the condition is BPH or nodular prostate, and if it presents with or without lower urinary tract symptoms. **Lower urinary tract symptoms (LUTS)** include the various symptoms that can present with BPH, such as urinary frequency, urinary retention, or urinary urgency. Note that these symptoms can also present without BPH, but when they are present with BPH, then add one code per symptom. For example, if a 60-year-old male patient with BPH presented with the LUTS of urinary obstruction and a weak urinary system, the codes reported would be as follows:

- N40.1, Benign prostatic hyperplasia with lower urinary tract symptoms
- N13.8, Other obstructive and reflux uropathy
- R39.12, Poor urinary stream

Key to Success

Coding for BPH is one instance in which you code for both the definitive diagnosis and the symptoms of the disease. In this case, when a patient presents with BPH with LUTS, it is not only acceptable but required to code for *both* the definitive diagnosis and the symptoms.

For practice reporting diagnosis codes for urology and nephrology conditions, complete the exercises in There's a Code for That 18.6.

Urology and nephrology diagnosis coding

18.6

There's a Code for That

Read the following documentation and assign the appropriate diagnosis code(s) for the patient's condition(s).

1. Patient with ESRD is on daily dialyzing schedule and kidney transplant list.

   ICD-10-CM codes: _____, _____

2. Overactive bladder.

   ICD-10-CM code: _____

3. Erectile dysfunction due to hypogonadism.

   ICD-10-CM codes: _____, _____

4. BPH with straining upon urination.

   ICD-10-CM codes: _____, _____

(Continued on next page)

Continued

5. Prostate cancer.

   ICD-10-CM code: _____

6. 35-year-old multigravida presents with both urge and stress incontinence.

   ICD-10-CM code: _____

Putting It All Together: Coding for Healthcare Specialist Services, Part I

Coding for healthcare specialist services requires carefully reading the documentation of the service provided, then accessing each code book to find the procedure or service provided and the corresponding diagnosis or diagnoses to support the medical necessity for the service. Procedural and supply codes are found in the CPT and HCPCS code books, and diagnosis codes are found in the ICD-10-CM code book.

Determination of the correct codes relies on the answers to the following questions.

- What services were provided to the patient?
    - Was an E/M service provided?
        - If the service provided was a consultation, determine if the consultation code may be reported, based on the patient's third-party payer. If the third-party payer does not reimburse for consultation codes, report the appropriate E/M code for the service provided.
    - Were any additional procedures performed, such as labs, x-rays or other imaging services, or any additional medical or surgical procedures?
- Are there any applicable modifiers or add-on codes?
- Is there a definitive diagnosis for the encounter? If yes, this should be the first-listed diagnosis code. If not, then use the code for the signs or symptoms.
- Include any additional diagnosis codes for comorbidities or complications, if necessary.

Study the following vignette that demonstrates how to select the appropriate diagnosis and procedure codes. Then complete the practice exercises in There's a Code for That 18.7.

Maria is studying for her coding examination and she is currently coding the case for a 67-year-old male patient. This patient went to his primary care physician complaining of urinary urgency and frequency. The PCP performed a digital rectal examination and found that the patient's prostate was significantly enlarged, and sent the patient to a urologist for a consultation. Maria is now coding for the services performed by the urologist: After a detailed history and examination and moderate complexity MDM consultation, the urologist performed a total prostate-specific antigen test, which revealed an abnormally high PSA. He then performed a needle biopsy of the prostate, which revealed malignant cells. The urologist diagnosed the patient with malignant neoplasm of the prostate, and referred the patient to an oncologist to discuss antineoplastic treatment, including surgery. The urologist then compiled his findings and prepared a report for the PCP regarding the findings from the encounter and suggested treatment.

First, Maria asks herself: What did the healthcare provider do? The physician performed a consultation service, as well as a total PSA and then needle biopsy of the prostate. After the urologist performed the E/M service (the consultation), he decided to perform a biopsy (a surgical procedure), and so she knows that modifier -57, Decision for surgery, should be appended to the E/M code. Maria also knows that many payers do not reimburse for consultation services, so after verifying that the patient's insurance will pay for the consultation code, she reports the following procedure codes:

- 99243-57, Office consultation for a new or established patient, which requires these 3 key components: a detailed history; a detailed examination; and medical decision making of low complexity
- 84153, Prostate specific antigen (PSA); total
- 55700, Biopsy, prostate; needle or punch, single or multiple, any approach

Now that she has the procedure codes, Maria asks herself: Why did the healthcare provider do it? The patient was referred to the urologist because the PCP found an enlarged prostate and the patient was complaining of urinary symptoms. The urologist performed the PSA test and found an abnormally high PSA level and after the biopsy confirmed the diagnosis of malignant neoplasm of the prostate. Maria needs to report two diagnosis codes—one for the prostate cancer and one for the high PSA levels. She refers to the Table of Neoplasms and selects the code for primary malignant neoplasm of the prostate (because the neoplasm is not specified as secondary or carcinoma in situ, she uses the default code for primary malignant cancer). She then finds the code for elevated PSA, and verifies both codes in the Tabular List. She then reports the following codes:

- C61, Malignant neoplasm of prostate
- R97.20, Elevated prostate specific antigen [PSA]

She then rechecks the documentation to make sure she has coded everything for the encounter and reports the chosen codes on the claim for the service.

Diagnostic and procedural coding for medical specialist services

18.6

There's a Code for That

Read the following documentation and assign the appropriate CPT, HCPCS, and ICD-10 CM code(s) for the encounter.

1. Outpatient office consultation for 45-year-old female patient with estrogen-receptor positive (ER+) cancer of the upper-outer quadrant of left female breast. Comprehensive history and examination with high complexity MDM. Patient medical history is also significant for a significant family history of breast cancer and has elected for a radical double mastectomy.

   CPT code: _____

   ICD-10-CM code: _____, _____, _____

(Continued on next page)

18.6

Continued

2. Surgical oncologist treated osteosarcoma of the femur of the left leg via surgical resection.

CPT code: _____

ICD-10-CM code: _____

3. Suture of sciatic nerve for injury of the sciatic nerve at the left hip.

CPT code: _____

ICD-10-CM code: _____

4. Inpatient neuro consultation for a 42-year-old male with epilepsy (approx. 20 years). He suffers daily from generalized convulsive (idiopathic) epilepsy, not intractable, with status epilepticus. Provider performed a comprehensive history, detailed examination, and MDM of moderate complexity.

CPT code: _____

ICD-10-CM code: _____

HCC

End of Chapter Content

Instructions: Indicate whether the following statements are true or false (T or F). For false statements, rewrite the statement on the line below to make the statement true.

1. Once a consultation is complete, the consulting provider must provide the requesting provider with a report of his or her findings.

_____

_____

2. If the patient's insurance does not reimburse for consultation codes, then E/M codes should be used in their place.

_____

_____

3. A neurologist treats conditions of the urinary tract, including the kidneys.

_____

_____

4. A push is given in a period of time under 15 minutes.

_____

_____

5. A personal history of neoplasm code should be used when the patient is undergoing treatment for a neoplasm.

_____

_____

6. Chemodenervation is the injection of a therapeutic substance to a nerve.

_____

_____

7. Status epilepticus occurs when the patient is unresponsive to treatment.

_____

_____

8. The prostate gland is only found in males.

_____

_____

9. Codes in the Penis (54000 to 54450) subheading include procedures on the skin of the penis.

_____

_____

10. Dialysis is often performed on patients with little or no liver function.

_____

_____

Instructions: Choose the best answer.

1. Which of the following parties may request a consultation for a patient?

 a. The patient's healthcare provider
 b. The patient's family
 c. The surgeon
 d. The patient's employer

2. Which of the following describes the rendering of a consultation service?

 a. The healthcare provider requesting the service from the consultation
 b. The consultation providing the healthcare service to the patient
 c. The consultant providing a written report of findings form the consultation
 d. The referral request sent to the insurance company

3. Which of the following types of providers would provide a brachytherapy service?

 a. Urologist
 b. OB/GYN
 c. Oncologist
 d. Nephrologist

4. Which of the following types of healthcare providers would perform a renal transplant?

 a. Neurologist
 b. Hematologist
 c. Urologist
 d. Nephrologist

5. Which of the following is a surgical treatment for a neoplasm?

a. Chemotherapy infusions
b. Brachytherapy
c. Excision
d. Radiation treatment

6. Which of the following is the intravenous administration of diagnostic, therapeutic, or prophylactic substance, given over a period of time longer than 15 minutes?

a. Infusion
b. Push
c. Drip
d. Injection

7. Which of the following codes would be used when a patient presents for antineoplastic chemotherapy?

a. Z99.2
b. Z51.0
c. Z51.11
d. Z51.12

8. Which of the following procedures removes a piece of skull without replacing it?

a. Trephine
b. Craniotomy
c. Craniectomy
d. Incision

9. When reporting codes for procedures on the spine, what should the coder always check for?

a. The type of excision performed
b. The area of the spine and whether it was unilateral or bilateral
c. The spinal instrumentation used in the procedure
d. Whether or not there was a neurostimulator placed

10. Which type of procedure is the repair of a nerve via suture or anastomosis?

a. Excision
b. Avulsion
c. Neuroplasty
d. Neurorrhaphy

11. Which of the following is an organ that filters waste products from the blood?

a. Ureter
b. Bladder
c. Urethra
d. Kidney

12. Which type of calculus completely fills the renal pelvis?

a. Nephrolithiasis
b. Staghorn calculus
c. Cholelithiasis
d. Choledocholithiasis

13. Which of the following codes would be reported for the transurethral coagulation of the prostate?

a. 52601
b. 52648
c. 52647
d. 52649

14. Codes for male circumcisions are found in which of the following subheadings in the Male Genital System subsection?

a. Penis
b. Integumentary
c. Scrotum
d. Vas deferens

Instructions: Answer the following questions with the appropriate code(s) and modifier(s).

1. Extradural resection of metastatic lesion of the left temporal lobe, using infratemporal pre-auricular approach to middle cranial fossa, including disarticulation of the mandible and parotidectomy.

CPT codes: _____-_____, _____

ICD-10 code: _____

2. Suture of kidney laceration performed on patient who suffered a moderate laceration to the right kidney.

CPT codes: _____

ICD-10 code: _____

3. Patient with sepsis without septic shock and with acute kidney failure is undergoing hemodialysis, requiring multiple evaluations by the healthcare provider and revision of the dialyzing schedule.

CPT codes: _____

ICD-10 code: _____, _____,
_____, _____

4. Initial dilation of urethral stricture by passage of urethral dilator, in a male with post-traumatic anterior urethral stricture.

CPT codes: _____

ICD-10 code: _____

References

American Medical Association. 2017 (January). *Current Procedural Terminology (CPT)*. Chicago: AMA.

American Urological Association. 2017. Definition of a Urologist. http://www.auanet.org/guidelines /definition-of-a-urologist.

Cancer.net. 2015 (November). Types of Oncologists. https://www.cancer.net/navigating-cancer-care /cancer-basics/cancer-care-team/types-oncologists.

Cancer Research UK. 2014a. "Diagram showing a craniotomy CRUK 063.svg." Digital image. Wikimedia Commons. Accessed December, 2017. https:// en.wikipedia.org/wiki/Craniotomy#/media/File: Diagram_showing_a_craniotomy_CRUK_063.svg.

Cancer Research UK. 2014b. "Diagram showing a brain shunt CRUK 052.svg." Digital image. Wikimedia Commons. Accessed December, 2017. https:// en.wikipedia.org/wiki/Cerebral_shunt#/media /File:Diagram_showing_a_brain_shunt_CRUK_052.svg.

Centers for Medicare and Medicaid Services. 2009 (December 14). Revisions to Consultation Services Payment Policy. https://www.cms.gov/Outreach -and-Education/Medicare-Learning-Network-MLN /MLNMattersArticles/downloads/mm6740.pdf.

OpenStax College. 2013. 705 Lateral View of Skull-01. jpg." Digital image. Wikimedia Commons. Accessed December, 2017. https://commons.wikimedia.org /wiki/Category:Anatomical_plates_and_drawings_of _the_human_skull#/media/File:705_Lateral_View_of _Skull-01.jpg.

US National Library of Medicine. 2016a (December 30). Brachytherapy. https://www.ncbi.nlm.nih.gov/pub medhealth/PMH0072483/.

US National Library of Medicine. 2016b (August 16). How Does the Nervous System Work? https://www.ncbi.nlm .nih.gov/pubmedhealth/PMH0072574/.

Resources

Alzheimer's Association. 2017. Types of Dementia. http:// www.alz.org/dementia/types-of-dementia.asp.

Alzheimer's Association. 2017. What Is Alzheimer's? http://www.alz.org/alzheimers_disease_what_is _alzheimers.asp.

American Association of Medical Dosimetrists. 2016 (June 15). Deciphering Brachytherapy Coding and Documentation. http://atlanta2016.medicaldosimetry .org/2016AnnualConference/assets/File/Wednesday /Brown.pdf.

American Medical Association. 2013. *Advanced Anatomy and Physiology for ICD-10-CM/PCS*. Salt Lake City, UT: Contexo Media.

Devaraju, S., R. Nerli, and M Hiremath. 2012 (Autumn). A large Mullerian duct cyst presenting as an abdominal mass with ipsilateral renal agenesis: An unusual presentation. *Nephrourol Mon* 4(4):640–643. https:// www.ncbi.nlm.nih.gov/pmc/articles/PMC3614304/.

Endicott, M. 2012 (November). Taking the sting out of injection and infusion coding. *Journal of AHIMA* 83/911):74–76. http://bok.ahima.org/doc?oid=105755# .WVKPvmgrI2w.

Flewelling, C.2015 (June). Injection and infusion coding offers high stakes: Outpatient coders must play their cards right. *Journal of AHIMA* 86(6): extended online version. http://bok.ahima.org/doc?oid=107707# .WVKP0GgrI2w.

Mayo Clinic. 2014 (May 20). EEG (electroencephalogram). http://www.mayoclinic.org/tests-procedures/eeg /basics/definition/prc-20014093.

Parkinson's Disease Foundation. 2017. What is Parkinson's Disease? http://www.pdf.org/about_pd.

RadiologyInfo.org. 2017 (February 17). Stereotactic Radiosurgery (SRS) and Stereotactic Body Radiotherapy (SBRT). https://www.radiologyinfo.org/en/info .cfm?pg=stereotactic.

US National Library of Medicine. 2017. Dialysis. https:// www.ncbi.nlm.nih.gov/pubmedhealth/PMHT0022165/.

US National Library of Medicine. 2017. Hemodialysis. https://www.ncbi.nlm.nih.gov/pubmedhealth /PMHT0022166/.

US National Library of Medicine. 2017. Peritoneal Dialysis. https://www.ncbi.nlm.nih.gov/pubmedhealth /PMHT0022170/.

US National Library of Medicine. 2017. Status Epilepticus. https://meshb.nlm.nih.gov/record/ui?ui=D013226.

Wheeler, A. 2017 (May 5). Therapeutic Injections for Pain Management. http://emedicine.medscape.com /article/1143675-overview#a9.

CHAPTER 19

Healthcare Specialist Services, Part II

Learning Objectives

- Examine procedural codes and guidelines, diagnosis coding, and medical necessity for gastroenterology and cardiology services.

- Determine and apply ICD-10-CM, CPT, and HCPCS codes to gastroenterology and cardiology services.

Key Terms

Abdominal aortic aneurysm (AAA)
Angiography
Aneurysm
Atherosclerosis
Bariatric surgery
Cardiac electrophysiology
Cardiologist
Cardiopulmonary bypass (CPB)
Cardiothoracic surgery
Central venous access devices (CVAD)
Colonoscopy
Colorectal surgery
Coronary artery bypass grafts (CABG)

Coronary artery disease
Deep vein thrombosis (DVT)
Dissecting aneurysm
Diverticulitis
Diverticulosis
Embolus
Endovascular procedure
Esophagogastroduodenoscopy (EGD)
Gastric bypass
Gastroenterologist
Gastro-esophageal reflux disease (GERD)
Implantable cardiac defibrillator (ICD)

Non-ruptured aneurysms
Pacemaker
Patient-activated cardiac event recorder
Percutaneous transluminal coronary angioplasty (PTCA)
Pericardium
Proctosigmoidoscopy
Pulmonary embolism
Ruptured aneurysm
Sigmoidoscopy
Thrombosis
Transluminal procedure
Varicose vein

This chapter discusses two additional healthcare specialties—gastroenterology and cardiology services. Coders must pay close attention to detail, follow coding guidelines, and use their understanding of medical terminology, and human anatomy and physiology when coding for these specialties.

Procedural and Diagnostic Coding for Gastroenterology

A **gastroenterologist** is a healthcare provider who specializes in the diagnosis and treatment of disorders of the digestive system, including but not limited to disorders of the esophagus, stomach, intestines, colon, and rectum and anus. Gastroenterologists can further specialize in surgical gastroenterology, or **bariatric surgery** (surgery performed on the stomach or intestines to induce weight loss), or **colorectal surgery** (surgery of the colon, rectum, and anus).

The majority of the surgical codes reported by gastroenterologists are located in the Digestive System subsection of the CPT code book, with a small selection of codes located in the Medicine section. Diagnosis codes for gastroenterology services are located mainly in the chapter for diseases of the digestive system—chapter 11 of the ICD-10-CM code book. The following sections discuss procedural and diagnostic coding for gastroenterology procedures.

Key to Success

Note that gastroenterologists are commonly referred to as "GI" doctors, as they treat the gastrointestinal system (gastro=G, intestinal=I).

Gastroenterology Procedures

Gastroenterology procedures range from medical studies of the function of the gastrointestinal system to invasive surgical procedures. Gastroenterology (91010 to 91133) procedures, such as acid perfusion tests for esophageal reflux, are found in the Medicine section of the CPT code book. Gastroenterology surgical procedures are located in the Digestive System subsection of the Surgery section of the CPT code book. This section includes codes for all components of the digestive system, beginning with the lips and vestibule of the mouth, through the alimentary tract to the rectum and anus (see figure 19.1). It also includes procedures on organs that assist in the digestive process, such as the liver, biliary tract, and pancreas, as well as the abdomen, peritoneum, and omentum. These sections are as follows: Lips; Vestibule of Mouth; Tongue and Floor of Mouth; Dentoalveolar Structures; Palate and Uvula; Salivary Gland and Ducts; Pharynx, Adenoids, and Tonsils; Esophagus; Stomach; Intestines (Except Rectum); Meckel's Diverticulum and the Mesentery; Appendix; Colon and Rectum; Anus; Liver; Biliary Tract; Pancreas; and Abdomen, Peritoneum, and Omentum.

Upper Alimentary Tract

Gastroenterologists focus on diagnosis and treatment of disorders of the esophagus, stomach, intestines, colon, and rectum/anus (see figure 19.2), even though additional anatomical structures are technically included in this body system.

Many of the anatomical structures located in the Digestive System subsection are outside of the realm of treatment for a gastroenterologist, which include those performed on the upper alimentary tract: lips; vestibule of mouth; tongue and floor of mouth; dentoalveolar structures; palate and uvula; salivary gland and ducts; and

Figure 19.1. Gastrointestinal system

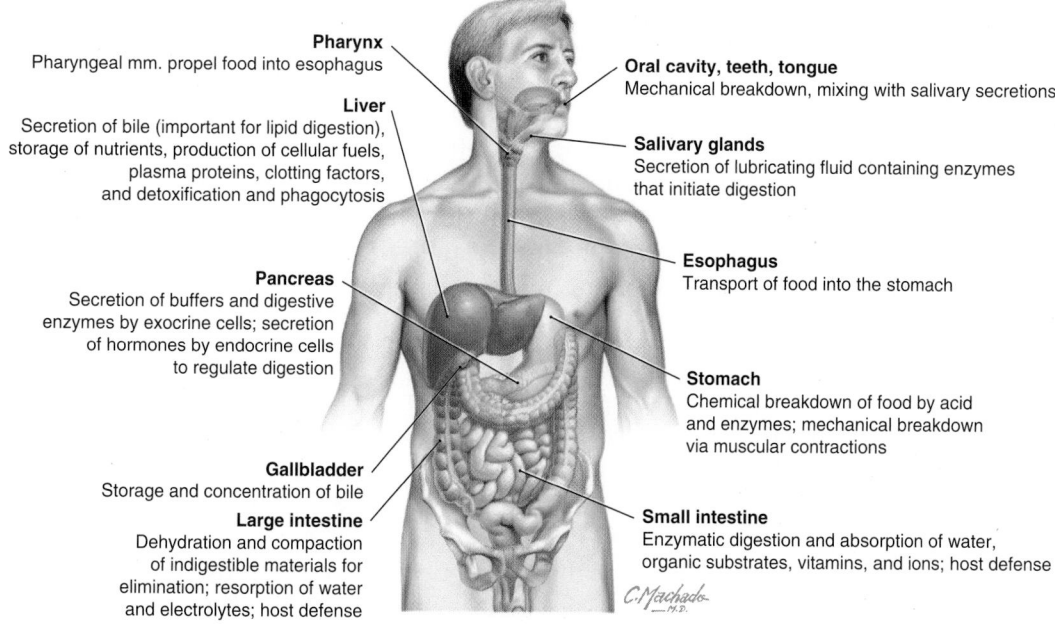

Pharynx
Pharyngeal mm. propel food into esophagus

Oral cavity, teeth, tongue
Mechanical breakdown, mixing with salivary secretions

Liver
Secretion of bile (important for lipid digestion), storage of nutrients, production of cellular fuels, plasma proteins, clotting factors, and detoxification and phagocytosis

Salivary glands
Secretion of lubricating fluid containing enzymes that initiate digestion

Pancreas
Secretion of buffers and digestive enzymes by exocrine cells; secretion of hormones by endocrine cells to regulate digestion

Esophagus
Transport of food into the stomach

Stomach
Chemical breakdown of food by acid and enzymes; mechanical breakdown via muscular contractions

Gallbladder
Storage and concentration of bile

Large intestine
Dehydration and compaction of indigestible materials for elimination; resorption of water and electrolytes; host defense

Small intestine
Enzymatic digestion and absorption of water, organic substrates, vitamins, and ions; host defense

Figure 19.2. Digestive system

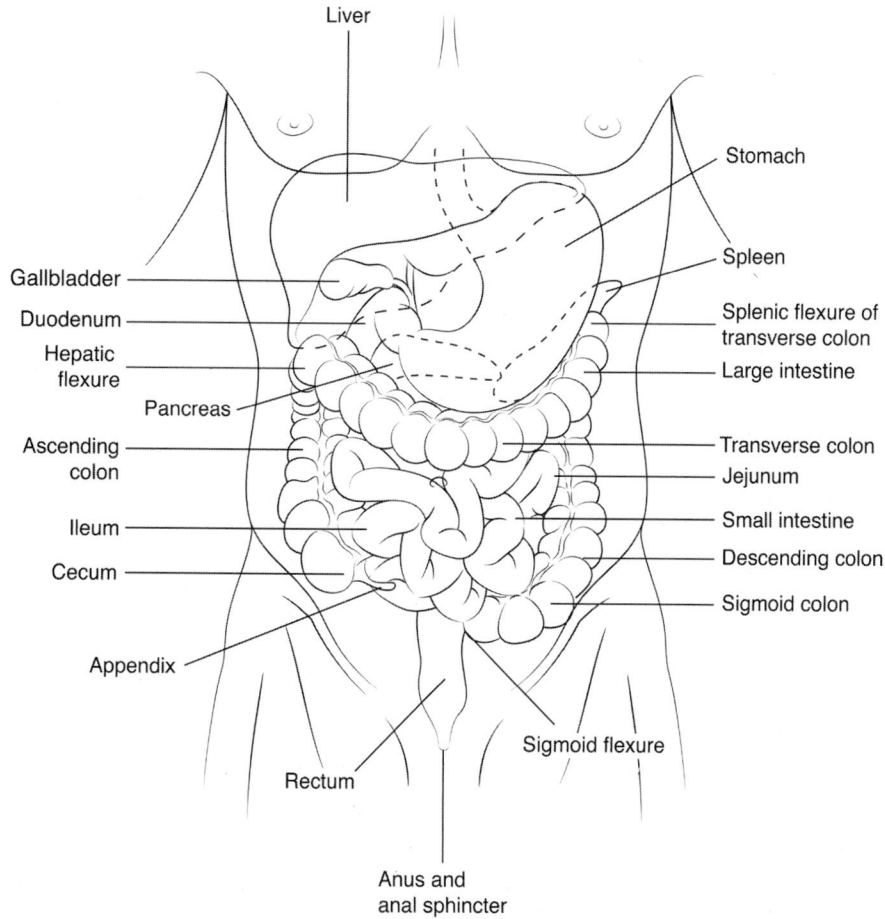

Liver

Stomach

Gallbladder

Spleen

Duodenum

Splenic flexure of transverse colon

Hepatic flexure

Large intestine

Pancreas

Ascending colon

Transverse colon

Jejunum

Ileum

Small intestine

Cecum

Descending colon

Sigmoid colon

Appendix

Sigmoid flexure

Rectum

Anus and anal sphincter

pharynx, adenoids, and tonsils. Procedures on the Lips (40490 to 40799) are likely to be performed by plastic or reconstructive surgeons who specialize in working with the soft tissues of the face. Procedures on the Vestibule of the Mouth (40800 to 40899), Tongue and Floor of Mouth (41000 to 41599), Dentoalveolar Structures (41800 to 41899), Palate and Uvula (42000 to 42299), and Salivary Gland and Ducts (42300 to 42699), are likely to be performed by oral/maxillofacial surgeons who focus on the surgical treatment of the mouth and jaw, such as cleft lip or cleft palate repair. Finally, procedures on the Pharynx, Adenoids, and Tonsils (42700 to 42999), are often performed by otorhinolaryngologists—ear, nose, and throat (ENT) doctors—who focus on the diagnosis and treatment of conditions in the throat, and who perform procedure on the tonsils and adenoids, like tonsillectomies (refer to chapter 11).

Esophagus

Procedures on the esophagus include Incision (43020 to 43045) and Excision (43100 to 43135), but by far the majority of procedures on the esophagus are Endoscopy (43180 to 43278). Because the esophagus is a large, natural opening that allows access to a large part of the gastrointestinal system, endoscopic examinations and procedures are a common procedure.

Remember that there are three components to endoscopy coding: approach, extent, and surgical versus diagnostic services (see chapter 11). These three components play a large part in coding for endoscopies. For example, an esophagoscopy is the examination of the esophagus. The term used to identify the endoscopy usually indicates where the endoscope stopped and did not proceed any further (an *esophagoscopy* stopped in the *esophagus*). An esophagogastrostomy is the examination of the esophagus and stomach, which does not extend to the duodenum. An **esophagogastroduodenoscopy (EGD)** is the examination of the esophagus and the stomach, and extends to the duodenum. EGDs are a common type of endoscopic examination of the digestive system, as they are a complete examination from the esophagus to the duodenum at the end of the stomach.

Once the endoscope is inserted, several different procedures may be performed. Be careful, though, as there are many bundled codes in this section, and one code may include procedures that are described by different codes. In this section, the coder must pay close attention to the parenthetical notes within the codes, as they describe when specific codes may or may not be used with each other, or when alternative codes may be appropriate in given situations. For example, under code 43235, Esophagogastroduodenoscopy, flexible, transoral; diagnostic, including collection of specimen(s) by brushing or washing, when performed, is the following parenthetical note: *Do not report 43235 in conjunction with 43197, 43198, 43210, 43236-43259, 43266, 43270, 44360, 44361, 44363, 44364, 44365, 44366, 44369, 44370, 44372, 44373, 44376, 44377, 44378, 44379.* In this example, the parenthetical notes identify specific codes that may not be reported with the previously -referenced code.

Key to Success

Codes for esophageal endoscopies can be challenging, as there are only one or two standalone parent codes for the endoscopy procedures and countless pages of indented codes. To help make sure you do not get lost, consider highlighting or underlining the parent codes, or using a straight edge or ruler when reviewing the pages, to ensure that you do not miss the next parent code and that you select the most appropriate code available.

Remaining procedural categories of codes in the Esophagus subheading include Laparoscopy (43279 to 43289), Repair (43300 to 43425), Manipulation (43450 to 434600), and Other Procedures (43496 to 43499).

Stomach

Codes for procedures on the stomach include Incision (43500 to 43520), Excision (43605 to 43641), and Introduction (43752 to 43761) procedures. Laparoscopy (43644 to 43659), Bariatric Surgery (43770 to 43775), and Other Procedures (43800 to 43999) codes report, among other things, bariatric surgeries as a treatment for morbid obesity. Bariatric surgery is a type of surgery that focuses on reducing the size of the stomach and the patient feeling full faster than he or she normally would. Ultimately the patient would then eat less and lose weight (ASMBS 2017).

One form of bariatric surgery is a **gastric bypass** procedure, also called a Roux-en-Y procedure, in which a small stomach pouch is created by separating the top of the stomach from the rest of the stomach and creating a small pouch. Then this pouch is attached to a part of the small intestine, in essence creating a small stomach out of the larger stomach. Codes for gastric bypass depend on whether the procedure was performed laparoscopically or via an open approach. For example, 43644, Laparoscopy, surgical, gastric restrictive procedure; with gastric bypass and Roux-en-Y gastroenterostomy (roux limb 150 cm or less), or 43846, Gastric restrictive procedure, with gastric bypass for morbid obesity; with short limb (150 cm or less) Roux-en-Y gastroenterostomy. See figure 19.3 for an illustration of different gastric surgery procedures.

Figure 19.3. Gastric surgeries for obesity

Gastric stapling (vertical banded gastroplasty)
Esophagus
Stomach pouch
Band

Gastric bypass (Roux-en-Y)
Stomach pouch
Oversewn staple lines
End-to-side type anastomosis between the gastric pouch and the Roux-en-Y limb
Duodenum
Bypassed portion of the stomach
Jejunum

Laparoscopic adjustable gastric banding
Adjustable band
Stomach
Skin
Subcutaneous port (reservoir)
Rectus abdominis muscle

C. Machado

Intestines

Procedures on the intestines include Incision (44005 to 44055), Excision (44100 to 44160) including codes for intestinal donation and transplantation, Laparoscopy (44180 to 44238), and Enterostomy (44300 to 44346). Codes for endoscopic examinations of the intestines specifically highlight one of the components of endoscopies—the coder should report the code according to the *approach* to the procedure. Endoscopy codes for the intestines are categorized depending on the approach to the procedure: Endoscopy, Small Intestine (44360 to 44379), and Endoscopy, Stomal (44380 to 44408). Endoscopies in the small intestine category are ones that have extended through the esophagus, stomach, and the duodenum into the first portion of the small intestine. Note the approach described in the code description (in italics): 44376, Small intestinal endoscopy, *enteroscopy beyond second portion of duodenum, including ileum;* diagnostic, with or without collection of specimen(s) by brushing or washing. Alternatively, read the approach for a Stomal endoscopy (in italics): 44382, Ileoscopy, *through stoma;* with biopsy, single or multiple. In the first example, the approach was through the duodenum, whereas in the second example, the approach was through a stoma.

Meckel's Diverticulum and the Mesentery

There are only four codes total for Meckel's Diverticulum, a rare bulge in the small intestine that is a remnant of the umbilical cord, and the Mesentery, the membrane that connects the intestines with the walls of the internal abdominal cavity. These codes report Excision (44800 to 44820), Suture (44850), and Other Procedures (44899).

Appendix

Procedures on the Appendix include Incision (44900), Excision (44950 to 44960), and Laparoscopy (44970 to 44979). The one incision procedure is coded with 44900, Incision and drainage of appendiceal abscess. The excision and laparoscopy procedure codes all describe different forms of appendectomies, described more in depth in chapter 11 (Surgical Services). When coding for appendectomies, identify whether the procedure was open or laparoscopic; and for open procedures, identify why the procedure was performed and if the appendix was ruptured.

Colon and Rectum

Procedures on the colon and rectum include Incision (45100 to 45020), Excision (45100 to 45172), and Destruction (45190). However, by far the most common procedures of the colon are Endoscopy (45300 to 45939, 45398).

The colon is divided into the ascending, transverse, descending, and sigmoid portions (see figure 19.4). The ascending portion is the most distal portion from the anus. The ascending colon extends to the transverse portion, which stretches lengthwise to form the descending colon that descends downward toward the anus. The sigmoid colon is the closest to the rectum and anus, and forms an S-shaped loop. To code for an endoscopic examination of the colon properly, coders should use all three components of endoscopy codes.

- *Extent*: Colonoscopy codes are divided based on how far the endoscope was inserted into the colon. A **proctosigmoidoscopy** is the examination of the rectum and may include a portion of the sigmoid colon. A **sigmoidoscopy** is the examination of the entire rectum and sigmoid colon, and may include an examination of the descending colon. A **colonoscopy** is the examination of the entire colon, from the rectum to the cecum at the end of the ascending colon, and may include an examination of the ileum.
- *Approach*: Colonoscopies may be performed through a stoma, an artificial opening from the colon to the outside of the body (such as a colostomy).
- *Surgical versus diagnostic*: Colonoscopy codes are divided based on whether the procedure was solely diagnostic or if a surgical procedure was performed during the colonoscopy, such as biopsy or destruction of colonic polyps.

Figure 19.4. Colon

The Large Intestine

Source: Blausen.com staff 2013c.

For example, a full diagnostic colonoscopy is extended through the entire colon (from the rectum to the cecum or terminal ileum), and no other procedures are performed during the procedure (such as a biopsy or destruction of a lesion). The diagnostic colonoscopy code is 45378, Colonoscopy, flexible; diagnostic, including collection of specimen(s) by brushing or washing, when performed. If any other procedures were performed during the colonoscopy, then code 45378 would be replaced by the code(s) that identify the surgical procedure(s). For example, if the doctor identified a colonic polyp during the diagnostic colonoscopy and then used a snare technique to remove the lesion, then the code reported would be 45385, Colonoscopy, flexible; with removal of tumor(s), polyp(s), or other lesion(s) by snare technique. Note that the CPT professional edition includes a flowchart that aids in the decision process for colonoscopies.

Anus

Procedures on the anus include Incision (46020 to 46083), Excision (46200 to 46320), Introduction (46500 to 46505), Endoscopy (46600 to 46615), Repair (46700 to 46762, 46947), Destruction (46900 to 46942), and Other Procedures (46999). The excision category includes codes for hemorrhoidectomy, the removal of hemorrhoids. These codes depend on whether the hemorrhoids are internal or external, as well as the number of columns or groups that were excised, and if the procedures were performed along with a fissurectomy (excision of anal fissure) or fistulectomy (removal of anal fistula).

Liver, Biliary Tract, Pancreas, Abdomen, Peritoneum, and Omentum

Procedures on the Liver (47000 to 47399), Biliary Tract (47400 to 47999), Pancreas (48000 to 48999), and Abdomen, Peritoneum, and Omentum (49000 to 49999) are likely to be performed by both gastroenterology surgeons and general surgeons (hernia repair, for example). Refer to chapter 11 (Surgical Services) for guidelines on coding for these procedures.

Complete the exercises in There's a Code for That 19.1 for practice reporting gastro-enterology procedures.

19.1

There's a Code for That

Gastroenterology procedures

Read the following documentation of the service and identify the CPT procedure code(s).

1. Endoscope was extended through the rectum and into sigmoid colon, and two polyps were removed via snare technique.

   CPT code: _____

2. Diagnostic proctosigmoidoscopy.

   CPT code: _____

3. Diagnostic EGD.

   CPT code: _____

4. Excision of esophageal lesion through cervical incision.

   CPT code: _____

5. Transoral esophagoscopy with band ligation of esophageal varices.

   CPT code: _____

6. Laparoscopic fundoplasty with repair of esophageal hernia and implantation of synthetic mesh.

   CPT code: _____

7. Surgical closure of gastrostomy opening.

   CPT code: _____

8. Laparoscopic resection of two separate sections of small intestine, with anastomosis.

   CPT code: _____, _____

9. Diagnostic colonoscopy through stoma with removal of foreign body.

   CPT code: _____

Gastroenterology Diagnoses

Diagnosis codes for gastroenterology conditions are found mostly in chapter 11: Diseases of the Digestive System, of the ICD-10-CM code book. There are no guidelines for this chapter, so appropriate code selection depends on provider documentation and careful reading of the notations in the Tabular List. Note that this chapter is similar to the Digestive System subsection of the CPT code book because it includes codes for conditions beginning with the lips, teeth, gums, and mouth, and includes codes for conditions through the alimentary tract to the anus and rectum. Common conditions include esophageal reflux, colonic polyps and screening colonoscopies, and diverticulitis and diverticulosis.

Esophageal Reflux

Gastro-esophageal reflux disease (GERD) is a common condition that causes heartburn, indigestion, and chest pain in affected individuals. There are only two codes for GERD, which differ depending on whether the condition presents with or without esophagitis (inflammation of the esophagus): K21.0, Gastro-esophageal reflux disease with esophagitis, and K21.9, Gastro-esophageal reflux disease without esophagitis.

Colon Screenings and Colonic Polyp

Routine colonoscopies are a regular part of preventive health procedures and are referred to as screening colonoscopies. When a patient presents for a routine screening colonoscopy, the primary diagnosis code should be Z12.11, Encounter for screening for malignant neoplasm of colon. If any abnormal findings, such as a polyp, are encountered, then an additional code should be reported to identify the polyp. See figure 19.5 for an illustration of colon screening techniques.

Figure 19.5. Colon cancer screening techniques

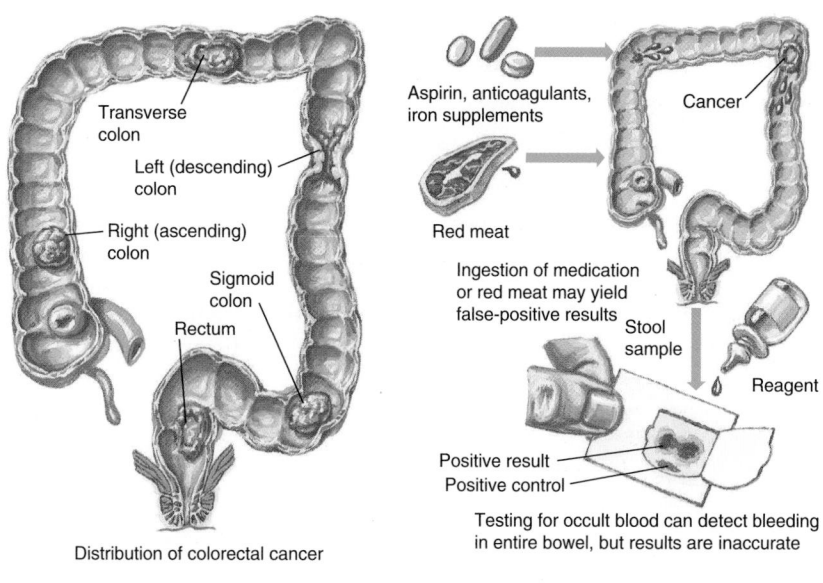

Colonic polyps are coded from a few different areas in the ICD-10-CM code set, including:

- K63.5, Polyp of colon. Use this code to report an unspecified polyp of the colon.
- K51.4-, Inflammatory polyps of colon. These codes identify polyps that are inflammatory in nature, and any additional complications like rectal bleeding, intestinal obstruction, fistula, abscess, or other specified complication.
- D12.6, Benign neoplasm of colon, unspecified. Use this code when a colonic polyp has been determined to be benign in nature.

Diverticulitis and Diverticulosis

Diverticulitis and diverticulosis are both coded from category K57, Diverticular disease of intestine. **Diverticulitis** is the inflammation of the diverticula small pockets lining the inside of the intestines (see figure 19.6). **Diverticulosis** is a condition in which diverticula begin forming within the intestines (see figure 19.7). Although these conditions are closely related, code selection depends on the ability to differentiate between the two.

Code selection depends on the identification of the condition as:

- Either diverticulitis or diverticulosis
- The location of the condition (small intestine, large intestine, or both large and small intestine)
- With or without perforation or abscess
- With or without bleeding.

For example, code K57.51, Diverticulosis of both small and large intestine without perforation or abscess with bleeding, identifies whether the condition is diverticulosis or

Figure 19.6. Diverticulitis

Figure 19.7. Diverticulosis

Diverticulum

Peritoneum
Circular muscle
Taenia coli
Epiploic appendix

Mucosa

Concentration
in diverticulum

Blood vessel
piercing musculature

Relationship of
diverticula to blood vessels
and taeniae (schematic)

diverticulitis (*diverticulosis*), the location of the condition (*both small and large intestine*), with or without perforation or abscess (*without perforation or abscess*), and with or without bleeding (*with bleeding*).

For practice assigning diagnosis codes to gastroenterology conditions, complete the exercises in There's a Code for That 19.2.

Gastroenterology diagnosis coding

19.2

There's a Code for That

Read the following documentation and assign the appropriate diagnosis code(s) for the patient's condition(s).

1. 45-year-old male presents with esophagitis and GERD. He has been dependent on daily alcohol consumption for the last 25 years.

   ICD-10-CM code: _____, _____

2. 65-year-old male presents for routine colonoscopy, which reveals five 1-2 mm polyps of the transverse colon.

   ICD-10-CM code: _____, _____

(Continued on next page)

19.2

Continued

3. Adenocarcinoma of the rectosigmoid junction.

ICD-10-CM code: _____

4. Acute ulcer of the stomach with hemorrhage and perforation.

ICD-10-CM code: _____

5. Crohn's disease of large intestine with intestinal obstruction.

ICD-10-CM code: _____

6. Patient presents with severe diarrhea in irritable bowel syndrome.

ICD-10-CM code: _____

7. Intestinal malabsorption following gastrointestinal surgery.

ICD-10-CM code: _____

Procedural and Diagnostic Coding for Cardiology

A cardiologist is a healthcare provider who specializes in the diagnosis and treatment of the diseases of the heart, coronary vessels, and cardiovascular system. There are numerous subspecialties in the field of cardiology, such as cardiologists who specialize in invasive or noninvasive cardiology, as well as cardiology treatment strategies and cardiac electrophysiology (the study of the electrical system of the heart). Surgical cardiology specialties include cardiac and cardiothoracic surgery, which focuses on the surgical treatment of the heart and organs in the thorax (such as the lungs). Because the cardiovascular system runs throughout the entire body, additional subspecialties may focus on peripheral vascular diseases that affect the extremities of the body.

Because cardiovascular services are so varied, codes for these services are located in various sections of the CPT code book. Just as in other specialties, evaluation and management (E/M) codes are used to identify services such as office visits and consultations. Surgical services are coded from the Cardiovascular System subsection of the CPT code book. Additional cardiology services are found in both the Radiology and Medicine sections. The Radiology section includes codes for diagnostic imaging of the cardiovascular system and imaging guidance for cardiovascular procedures; and the Medicine section includes noninvasive or minimally invasive procedures of the cardiovascular system, such as electrocardiograms (ECGs). When coding for cardiovascular services, codes from many different sections of the CPT code book may need to be reported, depending on the service that was performed. The coder must remain flexible and pay attention to parenthetical notes to determine accurate code selection.

Coding for cardiology requires an understanding of the numerous areas in which cardiovascular procedures are found in the CPT code book—cardiovascular surgery, cardiovascular radiology procedures, and cardiovascular medicine procedures. Diagnosis codes for cardiovascular services are found in chapter 9: Diseases of the Circulatory System, of the ICD-10-CM code book. Note that cardiology patients may present with additional conditions and comorbidities, so it is still important to use effectively all necessary chapters of the ICD-10-CM code book.

Cardiology Procedures

There are three areas of the CPT code book in which cardiovascular codes are found, depending on the type of procedure performed: cardiovascular surgery, cardiovascular radiology, and cardiovascular medicine procedures. Codes in the cardiovascular surgery section identify invasive procedures on the cardiovascular system, such as open-heart surgery or venipuncture. Cardiovascular radiology procedures are performed to produce images to help inform a provider about a patient's cardiovascular medical condition, and assist providers in performing cardiovascular surgical and medical procedures. Cardiovascular medicine procedures include all the noninvasive tests and procedures (such as ECGs and cardiovascular stress tests) that may be performed on the patient, as well as some minimally invasive procedures like insertions of cardiac catheters. Although these procedures are in different sections of the CPT code book, they may be reported together, as cardiovascular services sometimes entail all three surgical, radiological, and medical components.

Cardiovascular Surgery

Surgical procedures performed on the cardiovascular system are located in the Cardiovascular System subsection of the CPT code book. This subsection lists invasive surgical procedures on all areas of the cardiovascular system, including the heart and pericardium, and arteries and veins throughout the human body.

Note that there is some overlap between the services listed in the Surgery subsection, versus the services listed in both the Radiology and Medicine sections. For example, cardiac catheterizations are found in both the Surgery and Medicine sections. When coding for cardiology services, pay close attention to the guidelines, definitions, and parenthetical notes to ensure correct code selection. Parenthetical notes sometimes supply invaluable information, such as when or when not to use a specific code, which services may be bundled into a specific code or when they must be reported separately, and when to use an additional code or alternative code from a different section of the CPT code book.

Heart and Pericardium

The procedures listed in the Heart and Pericardium (33010 to 33999) subheading include surgical procedures on the heart, including the coronary valves and vessels, and the pericardium—the sac that holds the heart.

Among these procedures are codes for the reporting of Pacemaker and Implantable Defibrillator (33202 to 33273) services. A pacemaker is a small, battery-powered device that is implanted in the patient's chest or abdomen and helps maintain a normal heart rhythm (see figure 19.8). An implantable cardiac defibrillator (ICD) is a small device similar to a pacemaker that monitors the heart rate and delivers a small shock to the heart when it detects heart-threatening arrhythmias (see figure 19.9). Both devices send electrical impulses directly into the heart through a series of leads placed in certain areas within the heart, as needed by the patient's condition. Leads are made up of one or more electrodes, conductor wires, insulation, and a fixation mechanism. The leads are attached to a pulse generator and battery pack that provides the electrical stimulation. The pulse generator is placed in a small pocket of skin (subcutaneous pocket), either under the collarbone, above the heart, or above the abdominal muscles below the ribcage. Leads are either inserted into the heart via a vein (transvenous) or placed on the surface of the heart (epicardial).

Codes for pacemaker and ICDs differ, depending on the service performed, type of device, and type of system.

- A *single chamber* system includes a pulse generator and one electrode, which is inserted in either the atrium or the ventricle of the heart. This is also referred to as a single lead system.

- A *dual chamber* system includes a pulse generator and two leads, one of which is inserted into the right atrium, and the other is inserted into the right ventricle. This is also referred to as a dual lead system.

- A *bi-ventricular pacing* system is a dual chamber system in which an additional lead is inserted into the left ventricle. (This results in three leads—right atrium, left ventricle, and right ventricle). This is also referred to as a multiple lead system (NHLBI 2012).

Figure 19.8. Dual-chamber pacemaker

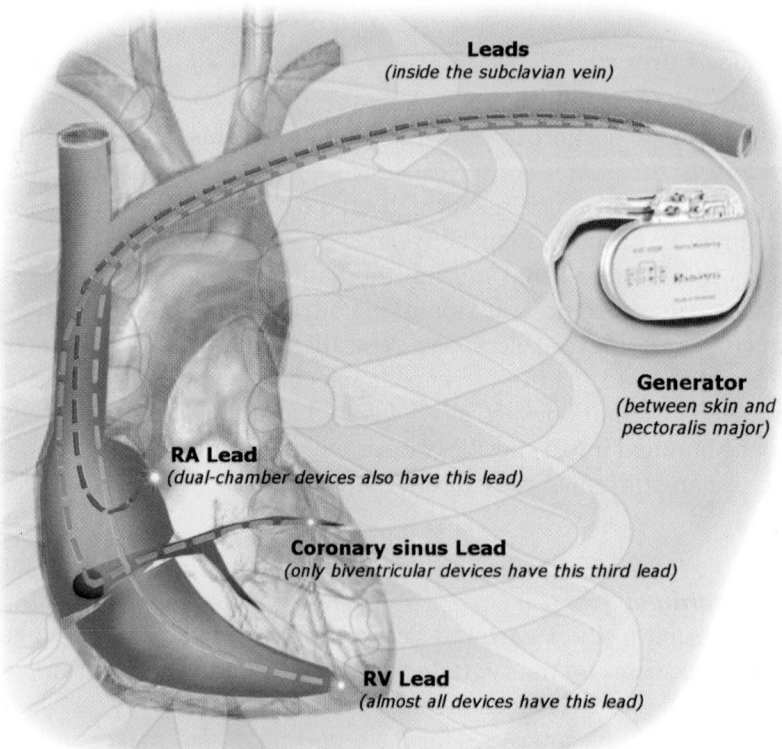

Source: Npatchett 2016.

Figure 19.9. Implantable cardiac defibrillator with dual leads

Implantable Cardioverter Defibrillator

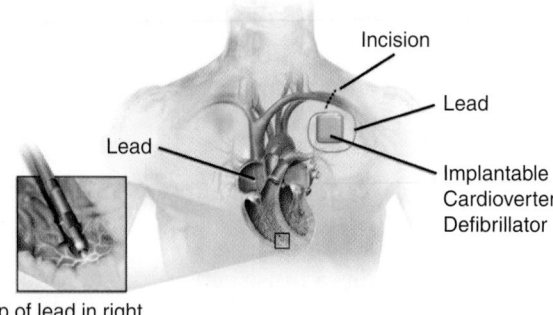

Source: Blausen.com staff 2013b.

Services provided include insertion of the system, leads, and components; replacement of the system or any component parts; upgrade of the system and components; removal of the system or components; removal and replacement of the system; and conversion of the existing system to a different system. For example, code 33234, Removal of transvenous pacemaker electrode(s); single lead system, atrial or ventricular, identifies the service (*removal of electrodes*), type of device (*pacemaker*), and type of system (*single lead system*).

Patient-Activated Event Recorder (33282 to 33284) codes identify the implantation or removal of a **patient-activated cardiac event recorder**. This is an implanted device that records the electrical rhythm of the heart when activated by the patient. When a patient has symptoms, he or she activates the device and records the heart rhythm. This device is used to obtain more information about hard-to-diagnose cardiac conditions.

An important component of several cardiovascular procedures is cardiopulmonary bypass, which may impact code selection. **Cardiopulmonary bypass (CPB)** is a technique in which a machine takes over the function of the heart and lungs during surgery, maintaining the circulation and oxygenation of the blood during the procedure. Many of the codes for procedures on the heart differ depending on whether or not cardiopulmonary bypass was used. For example, code 33300, Repair of cardiac wound; without bypass, reports the procedure performed *without* bypass, whereas code 33305, Repair of cardiac wound; with cardiopulmonary bypass, identifies the same procedure but performed *with* bypass.

Cardiac Valve (33361 to 33478) codes report services performed on the valves of the heart. Codes depend on the type of service performed, as well as the specific valve(s) involved in the procedure: Aortic Valve (33361 to 33417), Mitral Valve (33418 to 33430), Tricuspid Valve (33460 to 33468), or Pulmonary Valve (33470 to 33478). The guidelines in this section are lengthy, so it is especially important to read through all of them to ensure correct code selection.

Coronary artery bypass grafts (**CABG**—sounds like "cabbage") are procedures in which a small piece of vein or artery is used to bypass a coronary artery (see figure 19.10). CABGs are commonly performed for atherosclerosis and arteriosclerosis of the arteries, which reduce blood flow and can cause infarctions among other serious heart problems. Codes for coronary artery bypass grafts depend on the vessel used in the repair.

Figure 19.10. Coronary artery bypass graft (CABG)

| Single | Double | Triple | Quadruple |

Coronary Artery Bypass Graft (CABG)

Source: Blausen.com staff 2013a.

- A venous graft is one in which a vein is used for the procedure. Venous grafts are reported with codes from the subheading Venous Grafting Only for Coronary Artery Bypass (33510 to 33516). Codes identify the number of veins used in the CABG. For example, a CABG using three venous grafts would be coded with 33512, Coronary artery bypass, vein only; 3 coronary venous grafts.

- An arterial graft is one in which an artery is used for the procedure. Arterial grafts are reported with codes from the subheading Arterial Grafting for Coronary Artery Bypass (33533 to 33548). These codes identify the number of arteries used in the CABG. For example, CABG using two arterial grafts would be reported with code 33534, Coronary artery bypass, using arterial graft(s); 2 coronary arterial grafts.

- If both an artery and a vein are used in the CABG, the procedure is reported with at least two codes—one code to identify the arterial grafts and then an add-on code to report the venous grafting. These add-on codes are found under the subheading Combined Arterial-Venous Grafting for Coronary Bypass (33517 to 33523). Note that these are all add-on codes and cannot be used alone—they must be added to the code for the primary procedure, the arterial graft. For example, a CABG using two arterial grafts and three venous grafts would be reported with 33534, Coronary artery bypass, using arterial graft(s); 2 coronary arterial grafts, and 33519, Coronary artery bypass, using venous graft(s) and arterial graft(s); 3 venous grafts. Note that in this example, the number of arterial and venous grafts is the same in the previous two examples, but the code for the venous grafts changed. Instead of using 33512, Coronary artery bypass, vein only; 3 coronary venous grafts, the correct code is 33519, Coronary artery bypass, using venous graft(s) and arterial graft(s); 3 venous grafts, which identifies that the venous grafts were performed in addition to the arterial grafts.

The last component of CABGs is the procurement of the vessel used in the grafting procedure. The procurement (also called harvesting) of the vessel is the procedure performed to obtain the vessel (vein or artery) to be used in the procedure. Coding for the harvesting of the vessel depends on the vessel, as follows:

- Harvesting of the saphenous vein is included in the code for venous CABG, and should not be coded separately.

- Harvesting of an upper extremity vein should be reported with 35500, Harvest of upper extremity vein, 1 segment, for lower extremity or coronary artery bypass procedure.

- Harvesting of a femoropopliteal vein segment should be reported with 35572, Harvest of femoropopliteal vein, 1 segment, for vascular reconstruction procedure (e.g., aortic, vena caval, coronary, peripheral artery).

- Harvesting of an upper extremity artery should be reported with 35600, Harvest of upper extremity artery, 1 segment, for coronary artery bypass procedure.

Arteries and Veins

The Arteries and Veins (34001 to 37799) subheading of codes is large, as it identifies procedures on the vascular system throughout the body (with the exception of the heart, coronary vessels, and pericardium).

There are numerous endovascular procedures in this section of codes. An **endovascular procedure** is one in which a catheter is inserted into the body to perform a procedure. Literally, the procedure is performed "inside the vessel" (*endo-* meaning *inside*, and *vascular* pertaining to the vessel). A common endovascular procedure is the repair of aneurysms, such as the repairs listed in the subheading for Endovascular Repair Abdominal Aorta and/or Iliac Arteries (34701 to 34834), and Endovascular Repair of Iliac Aneurysm (34900).

Bypass grafts can be performed on areas other than the coronary arteries. Bypass grafts of the vascular system are reported with Bypass Graft (35500 to 35671) codes. These codes identify the beginning and ending site of the bypass graft. For example, a bypass graft from the subclavian to the brachial artery would be reported with code 35512, Bypass graft, with vein; subclavian-brachial. Once again, code selection depends on the vessel used for the graft—either Vein (35500 to 35587) or Other Than Vein (35600 to 35671). Grafts using arteries or synthetic grafts are reported with "Other Than Vein" codes.

An **angiography** is the x-ray examination of blood vessels after the administration of a contrast material (see figure 19.11). Codes for angiographies are found in two sections of the CPT code book: the Surgery section (discussed here) as well as the Radiology

Figure 19.11. Coronary angiography

Coronary Angiography

Angiogram of normal right coronary artery (RCA) and normal posterolateral (PL) and posterior descending (PDA) branches

Angiogram of normal left anterior descending coronary artery (LAD) and left circumflex (LC) artery

Angiographic demonstration of narrowing of RCA

Angiogram demonstrating filling of LAD by dye injected into RCA via collateral vessels section (discussed in chapter 13 of this text). Code for angiographies in the Cardio-vascular Surgery section report the catheterization of the vessel, the angiography pro-cedure, and the radiological supervision and interpretation of the procedure. Rather than having one code for the catheterization and one for the radiological supervision and interpretation (S&I), these codes are combination codes that combine the com-ponents and are reported with 36221 to 36228. It is important to read through these code descriptions carefully, as well as all parenthetical notes and guidelines, to ensure correct code selection.

Central venous access procedures (36555 to 36598) are performed on **central venous access devices (CVAD),** which are flexible tubes inserted in patients who require fre-quent access to the bloodstream; and can stay in place for up to a year. They can be used to deliver chemotherapy, parenteral nutrition, blood and blood products, antibiotics, and other medicinal substances (USNLM 2017). Procedures on central venous access devices include:

- Insertion (36555 to 36571). Codes identify the specific type of device (non-tunneled or tunneled, with or without subcutaneous port), and the age of the patient.
- Repair (36575 and 36576).
- Partial replacement (36578).
- Complete Replacement (36580 to 36585).
- Removal (36589 and 36590).
- Other Procedures (36591 to 36598).

Cardiovascular Radiology

Within the Radiology section, there are codes that report vascular procedures on the aorta and arteries and veins and lymphatics. There is also a selection of codes for trans-catheter procedures.

Procedures on the Aorta and Arteries (75600 to 75756, 75774) include aortography (imaging of the aorta) and angiography (imaging of the arteries). These procedures provide detailed images of the vascular structures that allow healthcare providers to diagnose and treat vascular conditions (see figure 19.12 for an example of a thoracic aortography). Note that the procedures listed in this subsection of codes are diag-nostic, and are used to provide an image to assist the provider in making a diagno-sis. Therapeutic procedures are reported with codes in the Transcatheter Procedures subheading.

Procedures on the Veins and Lymphatics (75801 to 75893) are similar in nature to those for the aorta and arteries, with the exception that the procedures reported are lymphangiography (imaging of the lymph system) and venography (imaging of the veins). Again, these codes identify diagnostic procedures. Therapeutic procedures on the veins and lymphatics are reported with transcatheter procedures codes.

Transcatheter Procedures (75894 to 75989) identify the radiological component of catheterizations, in which specific procedures were performed. These codes include the injection of contrast material, angiography and venography, roadmapping, fluoro-scopic guidance, and vessel measurement, so these components should not be reported separately. It is important to pay close attention to detail when reporting codes from this section, as parenthetical notes alert the coder to the appropriate code(s) for the sur-gical service performed in conjunction with the radiological procedure. For example, code 75901, Mechanical removal of pericatheter obstructive material (e.g., fibrin sheath) from central venous access device via separate venous access, radiologic supervision

Figure 19.12. Thoracic aortography

Thoracic Aortography

R. common carotid a.
R. vertebral a.

A. Retrograde transfemoral catheterization of the aortic arch

R. subclavian a.
Brachiocephalic trunk
Aorta
R. coronary a.

L. common carotid a.
L. vertebral a.
L. inferior thyroid a.
L. subclavian a.
L. internal thoracic a.
L. coronary a.
Catheter

Normal arteriogram

B. Retrograde transfemoral catheterization with selective injection of distal branches

R. common carotid a.

L. internal carotid a.
L. external carotid a.
L. common carotid a.
L. vertebral a.

R. subclavian a.
Brachiocephalic trunk
Catheter (three positions shown)
L. subclavian a.
Aorta

R. vertebral a. not seen; l. vertebral a. has anomalous origin from aortic arch, between and behind l. common carotid and subclavian aa.

and interpretation is followed by a parenthetical note: *For procedure, use 36595.* Code 36595, Mechanical removal of pericatheter obstructive material (e.g., fibrin sheath) from central venous device via separate venous access identifies the actual procedure to remove the obstructive material. Code 75901 reports the radiology imaging service that was performed with the surgical removal of the obstructive device, to provide imaging guidance during the procedure. In this case, if the provider performed both the imaging service as well as the removal of the device, then both codes should be reported.

Cardiovascular Medicine Procedures

Cardiovascular procedures in the Medicine section of the CPT code book include coronary therapeutic services and procedures, cardiovascular monitoring services, cardiac device evaluations, cardiac catheterizations, electrophysiologic evaluations, and noninvasive vascular diagnostic studies. The codes in the Medicine section for cardiovascular services are primarily noninvasive or minimally invasive. This means that they may invade the body cavity, but only percutaneously (through the skin). Although some of the procedures in the Medicine section sound similar to those in the Surgery section, as a whole they are less invasive than those in the Surgery section.

Coronary Therapeutic Services and Procedures (92920 to 92979) report an array of different procedures performed transluminally. A **transluminal** procedure is one that is performed within a vessel. One common procedure listed here is a **percutaneous transluminal coronary angioplasty (PTCA)**. In this procedure, a catheter is threaded into the body through an incision in the femoral artery in the groin, to the site of the angioplasty (usually an area clogged by atherosclerosis). Then a small balloon at the tip of the catheter is slowly inflated, stretching the sides of the vessel and creating a wider opening through which blood can flow (see figure 19.13). Code 92920, Percutaneous transluminal coronary angioplasty; single major coronary artery or branch is

Figure 19.13. Percutaneous transluminal coronary angioplasty (PTCA)

reported for the first site of balloon inflation. If additional branches of the same major coronary artery are also treated, then report code 92921, Percutaneous transluminal coronary angioplasty; each additional branch of a major coronary artery. Note that codes in this section report PTCA when performed with additional procedures, such as atherectomy (removal of fatty substance from the artery), or placement of intracoronary stent.

Implantable and Wearable Cardiac Device Evaluations (93279 to 93299) report the additional services performed with pacemaker and implantable defibrillators. In the Surgery section, pacemaker and implantable defibrillator codes identify the surgical services involved in the procedure, such as implantation or removal. However, the codes in the Medicine section identify the programming, evaluation, and management of the pacemaker or implantable defibrillator system. Codes identify the service performed and the patient's type of system.

Cardiac Catheterization (93451 to 93592) codes identify the direct catheterization of the heart. This procedure involves the introduction, positioning and repositioning (when necessary) of the catheter within the vascular system, recoding of intravascular pressures, and final evaluation and report of the catheterization procedure. When coding for heart catheterizations, it is important to identify three components, all of which impact code selection:

- Was the catheterization performed for congenital cardiac anomalies?
- Which area of the heart was accessed—right, left, coronary artery, bypass graft, or a combination thereof?
- Was there a definitive procedure, test, or vascular study performed during the catheterization? If so, then an additional code should be reported to identify the add-on procedure. Examples of additional procedures include transseptal or transapical puncture; pharmacological studies; exercise studies; injection procedures for selective right ventricular of right atrial angiography; injection procedures for supravalvular aortography; and injection procedures for pulmonary angiography.

For example, code 93455, Catheter placement in coronary artery(s) for coronary angiography, including intraprocedural injection(s) for coronary angiography, imaging supervision and interpretation, with catheter placement(s) in bypass graft(s), (internal mammary, free arterial, venous grafts) including intraprocedural injection(s) for bypass graft angiography identifies the area(s) of the heart that were accessed (*coronary artery and bypass grafts*). If an additional injection procedure was performed, then it would be reported in addition to the primary code for the procedure, such as code 93567, Injection procedure during cardiac catheterization including imaging supervision, interpretation, and report; for supravalvular aortography (in this case the additional procedure was an injection for supravalvular aortography performed in addition to the injection(s) for bypass graft angiography as described in the primary procedure code). The professional edition of the CPT code book includes a helpful decision-making chart that aids in the selection of the heart catheterization code(s) that include all necessary elements.

Additional procedures in the Medicine section of cardiovascular codes include electrophysiological studies (Intracardiac Electrophysiological Procedures/Studies 93600 to 93662), which study the electrical conduction system of the heart, as well as additional Noninvasive Vascular Diagnostic Studies (93880-93998) of the vascular system throughout the body.

For practice reporting codes for cardiology procedures, complete the exercises in There's a Code for That 19.3.

19.3

There's a Code for That

Cardiology procedures

Read the following documentation of the service and identify the CPT procedure code(s).

1. Patient underwent a pericardiocentesis on day 1 of admission and now on day 2 is receiving a subsequent pericardiocentesis.

   CPT code: _____

2. Valvuloplasty via leaflet reconstruction with transmyocardial laser revascularization.

   CPT codes: _____, _____

3. Open-heart valvotomy with CPB.

   CPT code: _____

4. CABG of three coronary vessels using femoropopliteal vein (harvested at same surgical session by surgical assistant).

   CPT codes: _____, _____-_____

5. Coronary artery bypass graft using 2 venous and 1 arterial grafts.

   CPT codes: _____, _____

6. Aortofemoral bypass graft, using upper extremity vein harvested at same surgical session.

   CPT codes: _____, _____

7. Routine venipuncture.

   CPT code: _____

8. Insertion of implantable defibrillator system with dual transvenous leads and insertion of pacing electrode for left ventricular pacing.

   CPT codes: _____, _____

9. CT angiography of abdominal aorta and bilateral iliofemoral runoff, with and without contrast.

   CPT code: _____

10. Injection of contrast material and venography of bilateral posterior tibial veins.

    CPT codes: _____, _____

11. Percutaneous transluminal balloon angioplasty of two pulmonary arteries.

    CPT codes: _____, _____

Cardiology Diagnoses

Diagnosis codes for cardiovascular conditions are located in chapter 9: Diseases of the Circulatory System, of the ICD-10-CM code book. In this chapter there are a number of guidelines that apply to hypertension, sequela of vascular diseases, and myocardial infarctions. Hypertension, myocardial infarction, and sequela of cerebrovascular disease are discussed in chapter 8 (Primary Care) and chapter 16 (Therapy Services), respectively. Additional important cardiovascular conditions include atherosclerosis and arteriosclerosis, cerebrovascular diseases, thrombosis, arrhythmias, aneurysms, and varicose veins and varices.

Atherosclerosis

Atherosclerosis (a form of arteriosclerosis, the hardening of the walls of the arteries), is the hardening of fatty substances within the blood vessels that leads to a buildup of plaque. This narrows the diameter of the blood vessel and reduces blood flow and causes the formation of blood clots that can travel through the vessels and cause further obstruction of blood flow (see figure 19.14). Atherosclerosis is one of the most common conditions affecting the arteries and is treated through a variety of surgically invasive and minimally invasive strategies (as described previously).

Figure 19.14. Atherosclerosis

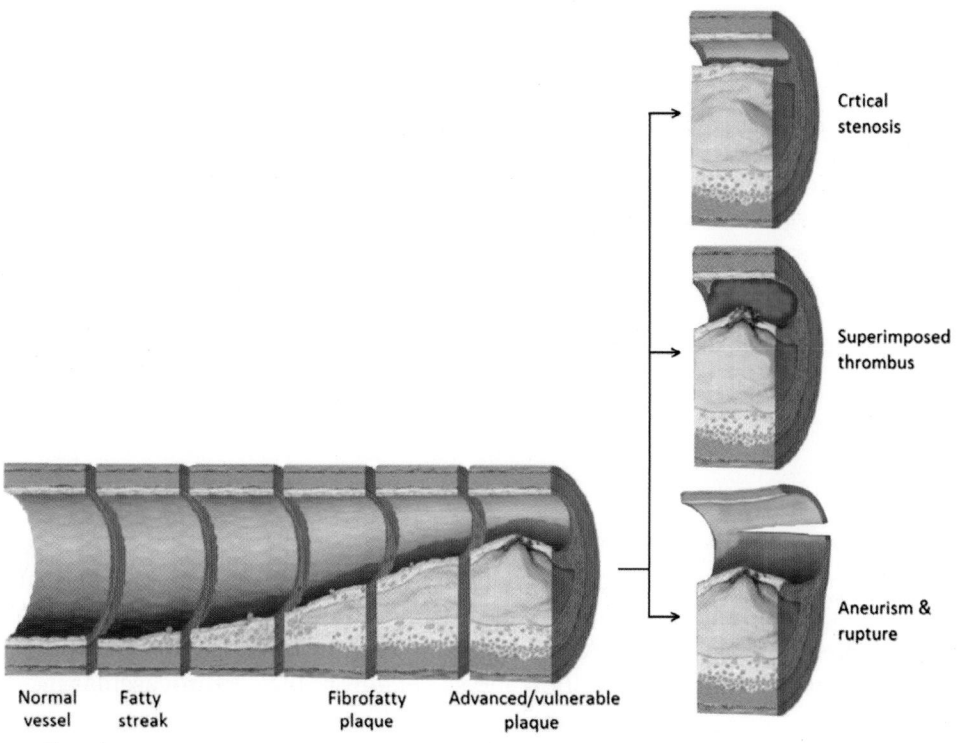

Source: Npatchett 2016.

Atherosclerosis is reported with codes from category I70, Atherosclerosis. Codes for atherosclerosis contain several components. First, the codes identify the blood vessel affected by the condition. Most codes identify the vessel as either native or a bypass graft. Atherosclerosis can occur in the vessel that had been used previously in a bypass procedure. If the atherosclerosis is in a bypass graft, codes differ depending on whether the graft is an autologous vein, nonautologous biological, nonbiological, or other type of bypass graft. Codes also specify the body area (such as leg, thigh calf, or such) and the laterality of the condition (right, left, or bilateral). Furthermore, the codes identify any complications that present with the atherosclerosis, such as intermittent claudication, rest pain, ulceration, or gangrene.

For example, code I70.421, Atherosclerosis of autologous vein bypass graft(s) of the extremities with rest pain, right leg, identifies the site of the atherosclerosis (*bypass graft*), type of bypass graft (*autologous vein*), specific body area (*leg*) and laterality (*left*), and any further complications (*rest pain*). Note also that atherosclerosis codes are included in HCCs, which means that these components must be identified clearly in the documentation with the most specific ICD-10-CM code.

Atherosclerosis of the coronary arteries is a commonly diagnosed condition and one of the leading causes of death of both men and women in the United States. This condition, often called coronary artery disease or CAD, is when atherosclerotic changes are detected in the arteries of the heart (coronary arteries) (Boudi 2016). Healthcare providers often document this condition as CAD, rather than coronary atherosclerosis, although these two conditions are essentially the same. To search for CAD in the ICD-10-CM code book, look up the term *Disease*, and then refer to the subterm *artery*, which should lead you to the subterm *coronary*. If the patient also presents with angina pectoris in addition to the CAD, then report the combination code for the CAD with angina. See the related OGCR in figure 19.15.

Figure 19.15. OGCR I.C.9.b

---

b. Atherosclerotic Coronary Artery Disease and Angina

ICD-10-CM has combination codes for atherosclerotic heart disease with angina pectoris. The subcategories for these codes are I25.11, Atherosclerotic heart disease of native coronary artery with angina pectoris and I25.7, Atherosclerosis of coronary artery bypass graft(s) and coronary artery of transplanted heart with angina pectoris.

When using one of these combination codes it is not necessary to use an additional code for angina pectoris. A causal relationship can be assumed in a patient with both atherosclerosis and angina pectoris, unless the documentation indicates the angina is due to something other than the atherosclerosis.

If a patient with coronary artery disease is admitted due to an acute myocardial infarction (AMI), the AMI should be sequenced before the coronary artery disease.

See Section I.C.9. Acute myocardial infarction (AMI)

Source: CMS 2018.

Cerebrovascular Diseases

Cerebrovascular diseases (I60 to I69) codes are reported for intracerebral and subdural incidents, including nontraumatic subarachnoid hemorrhage and cerebral infarction, also referred to as a stroke. As mentioned in chapter 16, codes for cerebrovascular diseases identify the current condition and sequela from the cerebrovascular incident. This is an important distinction to make, as a healthcare provider or surgeon treating the current infarction, hemorrhage, or other vascular condition would code for the current condition, such as I63.6, Cerebral infarction due to cerebral venous thrombosis, nonpyogenic. These codes identify the current condition only, and not any sequela from the condition such as dysphagia or hemiparesis.

Sequela from cerebrovascular diseases are reported with codes from category I69, Sequela of cerebrovascular disease and are reported when the healthcare provider is treating the sequela of the disease, such as partial paralysis or difficulty swallowing (refer to chapter 16). For example, I69.131, Monoplegia of upper limb following nontraumatic intracerebral hemorrhage affecting right dominant side. See figure 19.16 for the OGCR related to coding for cerebrovascular diseases.

Codes for cerebrovascular diseases fall into HCCs, so it is important to be careful when assigning these codes to patient cases and ensure the selection of each code is supported by clear documentation in the health record.

Thrombosis

A thrombosis, otherwise known as a blood clot, is a formation of blood cells, fatty deposits, or other particles that form a clot within the blood vessel. Thrombosis can form in either an artery or a vein, and codes differ depending on which vessel is

Figure 19.16. OGCR I.C.9.d

---

d. Sequelae of Cerebrovascular Disease

  1) Category I69, Sequelae of Cerebrovascular disease

   Category I69 is used to indicate conditions classifiable to categories I60-I67 as the causes of sequela (neurologic deficits), themselves classified elsewhere. These "late effects" include neurologic deficits that persist after initial onset of conditions classifiable to categories I60-I67. The neurologic deficits caused by cerebrovascular disease may be present from the onset or may arise at any time after the onset of the condition classifiable to categories I60-I67.

   Codes from category I69, Sequelae of cerebrovascular disease, that specify hemiplegia, hemiparesis and monoplegia identify whether the dominant or nondominant side is affected. Should the affected side be documented, but not specified as dominant or nondominant, and the classification system does not indicate a default, code selection is as follows:

   • For ambidextrous patients,the default should be dominant.

   • If the left side is affected, the default is non-dominant.

   • If the right side is affected, the default is dominant.

  2) Codes from category I69 with codes from I60-I67

   Codes from category I69 may be assigned on a health care record with codes from I60-I67, if the patient has a current cerebrovascular disease and deficits from an old cerebrovascular disease.

  3) Codes from category I69 and Personal history of transient ischemic attack (TIA) and cerebral infarction (Z86.73)

   Codes from category I69 should not be assigned if the patient does not have neurologic deficits.

   See Section I.C.21. 4. History (of) for use of personal history codes

---

Source: CMS 2018.

impacted by the clot. The most common type of thrombosis is a **deep vein thrombosis (DVT),** which forms in the deep veins of the lower extremities. If the thrombosis dislodges from the vessel and begins to travel through the blood, it is referred to as an **embolus.** This embolus can then travel through the blood vessel and get lodged in a smaller vessel, where it can obstruct blood flow. A **pulmonary embolism** is an embolus that may be the result of a DVT becoming dislodged and traveling into the lungs.

Codes for both emboli and thromboses differ depending on the type of vessel impacted by the clot (either a vein or artery), the specific vessel impacted, and the acuity of the condition. For example, code I82.513, Chronic embolism and thrombosis of femoral vein, bilateral identifies the type of vessel impacted (*vein*), the specific vessel impacted (*femoral*), and the acuity of the condition (*chronic*). For paired organs the code also identifies the laterality of the condition, as in the example code (*bilateral*). Note that these conditions also fall into HCCs, and so care must be taken to ensure they are coded to the utmost level of specificity.

Aneurysm

An **aneurysm** is the bulging or ballooning of a small portion of an artery, caused by weakening or degeneration of the wall of the vessel. Aneurysms are classified according to three characteristics: non-ruptured, ruptured, and dissecting. **Non-ruptured aneurysms** are often symptom-less and are usually found during a radiological imaging procedure. If the walls of the aneurysm burst, it is referred to as a **ruptured aneurysm.** This is a dangerous condition that causes hemorrhaging into the surrounding body cavity or tissues. A **dissecting aneurysm** is one that contains a small tear in the inner lining of the arterial walls, in which blood is beginning to accumulate. Dissecting aneurysms typically result in a rupture of the aneurysm. A common medical condition, an **abdominal aortic aneurysm (AAA)** is an aneurysm located in the abdominal aorta, which can be life-threatening if it bursts (see figure 19.17).

Figure 19.17. Abdominal aortic aneurysm (AAA)

Source: BruceBlaus 2016.

 Codes for aneurysms are located in categories I71, Aortic aneurysm and dissection, and I72, Other aneurysm. Category I71 codes identify the site of the aneurysm and if it is dissecting or ruptured. Aneurysm codes qualify as HCC codes and so care should be taken to ensure the code is reported to the highest level of specificity and supported by documentation in the health record.

Varicose Veins and Varicosities

Varicose veins are a result of an insufficiency in the valves of the lower veins to push blood upward toward the heart, causing a buildup of blood (see figure 19.18). Management of varicose veins ranges from wearing compression stockings to surgical intervention. Codes for varicose veins (located in category I83, Varicose veins of lower extremities) depend on the site of the varicosity (the affected vein), including the laterality, and any complications due to the varicose veins. Complications include ulcer, inflammation, both ulcer and inflammation, or other specified complication such as pain, edema, or swelling. For example, code I83.225 Varicose veins of left lower extremity with both ulcer other part of foot and inflammation, identifies the site, including laterality (*left lower extremity, other part of foot*), and complications (*ulcer and inflammation*).

Key to Success

Note that many cardiovascular conditions fall into HCC categories. This is because many of them identify chronic health conditions that require continuous healthcare treatment, follow-up, or observation. When coding for cardiovascular conditions, ensure that provider documentation is complete and all additional pertinent conditions are captured and reported.

Figure 19.18. Varicose veins

Source: NIH 2017.

For practice assigning diagnosis codes for cardiology conditions, complete the exercises in There's a Code for That 19.4.

Cardiology diagnosis coding

19.4

Read the following documentation and assign the appropriate diagnosis code(s) for the patient's condition(s).

There's a Code for That

1. Prinzmetal angina.

   ICD-10-CM code: _____

2. Persistent atrial fibrillation.

   ICD-10-CM code: _____

3. Cardiomegaly.

   ICD-10-CM code: _____

4. Cerebral infarction due to embolism of bilateral vertebral arteries.

   ICD-10-CM code: _____

(Continued on next page)

19.4

Continued

5. Atherosclerosis of autologous vein bypass graft of lower left extremity with ulceration of calf with exposure of fat layer.

   ICD-10-CM codes: _____, _____

6. Acute DVT of left calf.

   ICD-10-CM code: _____

7. Patient on long-term use of oral anticoagulants presents for evaluation of chronic pulmonary embolism.

   ICD-10-CM codes: _____, _____

8. Abdominal aortic aneurysm.

   ICD-10-CM code: _____

9. 82-year-old female presents complaining of pain and inflammation of bilateral varicose veins of the lower extremities.

   ICD-10-CM codes: _____, _____, _____

Putting It All Together: Coding for Healthcare Specialist Services, Part II

Coding for healthcare specialist services requires reading the documentation of the service provided carefully, then accessing each code book to find the procedure or service provided and the corresponding diagnosis or diagnoses to support the medical necessity for the service. Procedural and supply codes are found in the CPT and HCPCS code books, and diagnosis codes are found in the ICD-10-CM code book. Refer to chapter 18 for tips on how to determine the correct code(s) for medical specialist services, and study the following vignette that demonstrates how to select the appropriate diagnosis and procedure codes. Then complete the following practice exercises in There's a Code for That 19.5.

Maria is studying for her coding examination and she is currently coding the case for a 38-year-old female patient. This patient has been overweight most of her life, and is now weighing in at 348 pounds. Her current BMI is 49.9, making her morbidly obese (due to excess calories). Her clinical history is also significant for type 2 diabetes mellitus with neuropathy, controlled with daily use of insulin, and essential hypertension, controlled with daily use of ACE inhibitor. After careful consideration of her weight loss options, including non-surgical interventions, she has decided to undergo a gastric bypass procedure. Surgeon performed Roux-en-Y gastroenterostomy with small intestine reconstruction without complications.

First, Maria asks herself: What did the healthcare provider do? The physician performed a Roux-en-Y gastroenterostomy with a small intestine reconstruction. Maria checks to make sure that there were no complications or additional procedures noted on the documentation of the procedure, so no additional procedure codes or modifiers are necessary. She then reports the following procedure code:

• *43847, Gastric restrictive procedure, with gastric bypass for morbid obesity; with small intestine reconstruction to limit absorption*

Now that she has the procedure codes, Maria asks herself: Why did the healthcare provider do it? This female had multiple medical conditions in addition to the obesity. She has a current health history of both diabetes with mononeuropathy, which is controlled by insulin (each of which will be reported with diagnosis codes), and hypertension (which will be reported with another diagnosis code). Maria also needs to assign additional diagnosis codes for the patient's morbid obesity and her body mass index measurement (49.9). After accessing the Main Index to find her codes and verifying them in the Tabular List, she reports the following codes:

- *E11.41, Type 2 diabetes mellitus with diabetic mononeuropathy*
- *I10, Essential (primary) hypertension*
- *E66.01, Morbid (severe) obesity due to excess calories*
- *Z68.42, Body mass index (BMI) 45.0-49.9, adult*
- *Z79.4, Long-term (current) use of insulin*

She then rechecks the documentation to make sure she has coded everything for the encounter and reports the chosen codes on the claim for the service.

Diagnostic and procedural coding for medical specialist services

19.5

There's a Code for That

Read the following documentation and assign the appropriate CPT, HCPCS, and ICD-10 CM code(s) for the encounter.

1. Diagnostic flexible EGD performed on 45-year-old male revealed Barrett esophagus with low grade dysplasia.

   CPT code: _____

   ICD-10-CM code: _____

2. Dr. Hidalgo was called out to the emergency department to perform a gastric intubation on a patient who was experiencing severe generalized stomach pains, vomiting, and elevated blood pressure due to ingestion of noxious berries.

   CPT code: _____

   ICD-10-CM code: _____, _____, _____,

   _____

3. Cardiothoracic surgeon was called into the ER to perform an emergency surgery for a ruptured abdominal aortic aneurysm (AAA) on a 50-year-old male patient with stage 3 chronic kidney disease due to hypertension. Patient is a current cigarette smoker and smokes about one pack per day. Surgeon performed an endovascular repair of the infrarenal abdominal and visceral aorta with fenestrated visceral aortic endograft and two visceral artery endoprostheses of the superior mesenteric arteries.

   CPT code: _____

   ICD-10-CM code: _____, _____, _____,

   _____

End of Chapter Content

Instructions: Indicate whether the following statements are true or false (T or F). For false statements, rewrite the statement on the line below to make the statement true.

1. A gastroenterologist is a healthcare provider who specializes in the treatment and management of genitourinary diseases.

_____

_____

2. A bariatric surgeon performs surgeries on the genitourinary system.

_____

_____

3. The lips are included within the gastroenterology subsection of the CPT code book.

_____

_____

4. A Roux-en-Y procedure is performed for weight loss.

_____

_____

5. A cardiologist treats conditions of the heart and surrounding vessels.

_____

_____

6. A pacemaker helps to maintain normal heart rhythm.

_____

_____

7. CPB is a technique in which a machine takes over the function of the heart and lungs during surgery.

_____

_____

8. When only veins are used during CABG surgery, use a code from 33510 to33516.

_____

_____

9. Coronary artery bypass grafts that use both arteries and veins are coded from 33533 to 33548.

_____

_____

10. An angiography is the x-ray examination of only the aorta.

_____

_____

Instructions: Choose the best answer.

1. Which of the following types of healthcare providers performs surgeries meant to assist with weight loss?

a. Bariatric surgeon
b. Colorectal surgeon
c. Gastroenterologist
d. Surgical urologist

2. An EGD is the endoscopic examination of which of the following?

a. Esophagus, duodenum, and rectum
b. Esophagus, stomach, and duodenum
c. Stomach, duodenum, and small intestine
d. Anus, rectum, and colon

3. Which of the following is a rare bulge in the small intestine that is a remnant of the umbilical cord?

a. Bartholin's gland
b. Meckel's diverticulum
c. Seminal vesicle
d. Mesentery

4. Which of the following conditions causes heartburn and indigestion?

a. Vesicoureteral reflux
b. Angina
c. Esophageal varices
d. GERD

5. Which of the following types of colon polyps are inflammatory in nature?

a. K63.5
b. D12.6
c. K51.40
d. D37.4

6. Which of the following types of cardiovascular providers would treat cardiovascular conditions that affect the extremities of the body?

a. Cardiothoracic surgeon
b. Cardiac electrophysiologist
c. Interventional cardiologic specialist
d. Peripheral vascular surgeon

7. Noninvasive cardiovascular procedures and studies are found in which section of the CPT code book?

a. Surgery
b. Radiology
c. Medicine
d. Anesthesia

8. Which of the following is an ICD system in which two leads are placed into the heart, in the right atrium and right ventricle?

a. Dual chamber pacemaker
b. Single chamber implantable cardiac defibrillator
c. Bi-ventricular pacemaker
d. Dual chamber implantable cardiac defibrillator

9. Harvesting of which of the following vessels is included in a CABG procedure?

a. Upper extremity artery
b. Saphenous vein
c. Femoropopliteal vein
d. Brachial artery

10. Which of the following best describes cardio-vascular procedures found in the Radiology section?

    a. Injection of contrast material
    b. Imaging of peripheral vessels
    c. Noninvasive cardiovascular studies
    d. Cardiovascular surgery

11. Which of the following conditions is a harden-ing of the fatty substances within a vessel?

    a. Arteriosclerosis
    b. Deep vein thrombosis
    c. Pulmonary embolism
    d. Atherosclerosis

12. Which of the following is a blood clot that has dislodged and is moving through the blood stream?

    a. Peripheral vascular disease
    b. Deep vein thrombosis
    c. Pulmonary nodule
    d. Embolus

Instructions: Answer the following questions with the appropriate code(s) and modifier(s).

1. Percutaneous catheter inserted with imaging guidance for fluid collection from 40-year-old male with abscessed appendix.

    CPT codes: _____

    ICD-10 code: _____

2. 43-year-old new patient with severe GERD presents for surgical consultation. Comprehensive history and evaluation with moderate complexity MDM. Diagnos-tic transoral esophagoscopy performed in office revealed significant reflux esophagitis. Decision for surgery was made and patient scheduled for laparoscopic fundoplasty in two weeks.

    CPT codes: _____- ____, _____

    ICD-10 code: _____

3. Cardiopulmonary resuscitation performed on patient with acute cardiac arrest.

    CPT codes: _____

    ICD-10 code: _____

4. Endovascular repair of dissected aor-tic aneurysm using modular bifurcated prosthesis with two docking limbs, with radiological S&I.

    CPT codes: _____

    ICD-10 code: _____

5. Right heart catheterization for atrial septal defect.

    CPT codes: _____

    ICD-10 code: _____

6. Venipuncture of scalp vein in an 18-month-old female with severe dehydration.

    CPT codes: _____

    ICD-10 code: _____

References

American Society for Metabolic and Bariatric Surgery. 2017. Bariatric Surgery Procedures. https://asmbs.org /patients/bariatric-surgery-procedures.

Boudi, F.B. 2016 (April 25). Coronary Artery Atherosclerosis. https://emedicine.medscape.com/article/153647 -overview.

BruceBlaus. 2016. "Abdominal Aortic Aneurysm Location. png." Digital image. Wikimedia Commons. Accessed December, 2017. https://en.wikipedia.org/wiki /Abdominal_aortic_aneurysm#/media /File:Abdominal_Aortic_Aneurysm_Location.png.

Blausen.com staff. 2013a. "Blausen 0152 CABG All. png." Digital image. Wikimedia Commons. Accessed December, 2017. https://en.wikipedia.org/wiki /Coronary_artery_bypass_surgery#/media /File:Blausen_0152_CABG_All.png.

Blausen.com staff. 2013b. "Blausen 0543 ImplantableCardioverterDefibrillator InsideLeads. png." Digital image. Wikimedia Commons. Accessed December, 2017. https://en.wikipedia.org/wiki /Implantable_cardioverter-defibrillator#/media /File:Blausen_0543_ImplantableCardioverterDefibrillator _InsideLeads.png.

Blausen.com staff. 2013c. "Blausen 0604 LargeIntestine2. png." Digital image. Wikimedia Commons. Accessed December, 2017. https://en.wikipedia.org/wiki /Large_intestine#/media/File:Blausen_0604 _LargeIntestine2.png.

Centers for Medicare and Medicaid Services. 2018. ICD-10-CM Official Guidelines for Coding and Reporting FY 2018. https://www.cms.gov/Medicare/Coding/ICD10 /Downloads/2018-ICD-10-CM-Coding-Guidelines.pdf.

National Heart, Lung, and Blood Institute. 2012 (February 28). What Is a Pacemaker? https://www.nhlbi.nih.gov /health/health-topics/topics/pace.

National Heart Lung and Blood Institute. 2017. "Varicose veins-en.svg." Digital image. National Heart Lung and Blood Institute. Accessed December, 2017. https:// commons.wikimedia.org/wiki/File:Varicose_veins-en.svg.

Npatchett. 2016. "PPM.png." Digital image. Wikimedia Commons. Accessed December, 2017. https:// en.wikipedia.org/wiki/Artificial_cardiac_pacemaker# /media/File:PPM.png.

Npatchett. 2015. "Late complications of atherosclerosis. PNG." Digital image. Wikimedia Commons. Accessed December, 2017. https://en.wikipedia.org/wiki /Atherosclerosis#/media/File:Late_complications_of _atherosclerosis.PNG.

US National Library of Medicine. 2017 (August 16). Central Venous Catheters–Ports. https://medlineplus.gov /ency/patientinstructions/000491.htm.

Johns Hopkins Medicine. 2017. Percutaneous Transluminal Angioplasty. http://www.hopkinsmedicine.org /interventional-radiology/procedures/pta/.

Texas Heart Association. 2016 (August). Cardiovascular Glossary. http://www.texasheart.org/HIC/Gloss/.

University of California San Francisco. 2017. Endovascular Surgery. https://www.ucsfhealth.org/treatments /endovascular_surgery/.

US Department of Health and Human Services. 2014 (February 13). What Are Varicose Veins? https://www .nhlbi.nih.gov/health/health-topics/topics/vv.

US National Library of Medicine. 2017. Meckel Diverticulum. https://www.ncbi.nlm.nih.gov /pubmedhealth/PMHT0022924/.

US National Library of Medicine. 2017. Mesentery. https:// www.ncbi.nlm.nih.gov/pubmedhealth/PMHT0028174/.

US National Library of Medicine. 2017 (February 28). Pacemakers and Implantable Defibrillators. https://medlineplus.gov /pacemakersandimplantabledefibrillators.html.

Resources

American Heart Association. 2016 (December 21). Cardiac Event Recorder. http://www.heart.org /HEARTORG/Conditions/Arrhythmia /PreventionTreatmentofArrhythmia/Cardiac-Event -Recorder_UCM_447317_Article.jsp#.WVVY3GgrLb0.

DecisionHealth. 2013. *Advanced Anatomy and Physiology for ICD-10-CM/PCS*. Salt Lake City, UT: Contexo Media.

CHAPTER

Inpatient Hospital Services

Learning Objectives

- Identify ICD-10-PCS codes and explain their use in the healthcare setting.
- Examine the structure of ICD-10-PCS codes and code book.

- Use general ICD-10-PCS coding guidelines to create ICD-10-PCS codes.

Key Terms

Alteration
Bypass
Change
Code table
Control
Creation
Delivery
Destruction
Detachment
Device
Diagnosis-related groups (DRGs)
Dilation
Division

Drainage
Excision
Extirpation
Extraction
Fragmentation
Fusion
Insertion
Inspection
Map
Occlusion
Prospective payment system (PPS)
Qualifier
Reattachment

Release
Removal
Repair
Replacement
Reposition
Resection
Restriction
Revision
Root operation
Supplement
Transfer
Transplantation
UB-04

Inpatient hospital facility services are reported with ICD-10-PCS codes, which are seven-character alphanumeric codes used to identify services provided to patients in the inpatient facility setting. Depending on the facility, some outpatient facilities may also include ICD-10-PCS codes for reporting purposes. This depends on the organization and business affiliations of the facility doing the reporting. As previously discussed in chapter 3 (Basics of Coding), they represent procedures or services and are similar in nature to the services reported by CPT and HCPCS codes, as they identify the actual service that was provided to the patient. However, ICD-10-PCS codes (also referred to as PCS codes) identify services that were performed in the inpatient setting only. For example, if a patient received an appendectomy (removal of the appendix) in an inpatient hospital, then the hospital would use a PCS appendectomy code to report the procedure. As discussed in chapter 1, inpatient services are provided to patients who have been admitted to an acute-care facility where they receive around-the-clock healthcare services, in addition to medical and surgical procedures. Inpatient coding differs from outpatient coding in that the healthcare facility does not report the procedure codes (as identified by ICD-10-PCS codes) directly for reimbursement, as is the case in professional billing (in which CPT or HCPCS codes are directly tied to the services provided). In inpatient billing, PCS codes are reported to identify the service(s) the healthcare provider performed on the patient. The PCS code is added to the claim for the service, and compiled into a diagnostic-related group (DRG), discussed later, to determine the amount of payment that will be received for the services. Reimbursement for the services provided by the inpatient facility is therefore based on the diagnosis code(s)—the medical necessity—for the patient's stay, as well as the procedures performed and other factors (such as the patient's gender and discharge status). Refer to chapters 1 and 3 for more information on the difference between inpatient and outpatient coding.

ICD-10-PCS coding requires an in-depth understanding of the multiaxial structure of the codes themselves, which must be built according to the procedure that was performed. In the case of ICD-10-PCS coding, this multiaxial structure is based on coding tables, each of which contains options for each of the seven characters in the code (characters 1 through 7). To build the code, the coder must carefully select one character from the table for each of the seven required characters. This allows the coder to create a code that describes precisely the procedure performed. Rather than simply selecting a PCS code from the Tabular List (as in CPT or HCPCS coding), PCS codes must be built character by character, depending on what, where, and how each procedure was performed. Coders must be able to locate the tables for each procedure type and create the code based on the documentation of the procedure.

This chapter briefly discusses ICD-10-PCS coding in general, what it is used for, how to use the ICD-10-PCS code book to create a PCS code, and finally how to create a PCS code for the documented procedure.

ICD-10-PCS Coding

There are numerous differences between coding for services performed in the inpatient setting, as reported with ICD-10-PCS codes. Unlike CPT or HCPCS codes, PCS codes are not directly used for reimbursement. Furthermore, facility services are reported on the UB-04 form (as opposed to the CMS-1500 form used in professional billing). Payment for facility services is based on a prospective payment system, rather than fee-for-service.

Inpatient Facility Coding and Prospective Payment System

As previously mentioned, PCS codes are used only in the inpatient or facility setting to identify the services that were performed by the healthcare provider(s). This is in contrast to *professional* services, as most of these services are reported on a fee-for-service basis—the procedure codes(s) assigned for the procedure are attached to a fee for that service. For example, an evaluation and management (E/M) code for an office visit charge may be $100. However, *facility* procedures reported with PCS codes are *not* reported with specific charges per procedure. ICD-10-PCS coding is part of a prospective payment system (PPS), a type of reimbursement system based on preset payment levels rather than actual charges billed after the service has been provided. Payment is based on predetermined payment rates or periods and linked to the anticipated intensity of services delivered as well as the beneficiary's condition (as identified by the patient's diagnosis codes, procedures performed in the facility setting, and additional factors).

In inpatient prospective payment systems, IPPS—the prospective payment system used in the inpatient facility setting—the diagnosis code(s) and procedure code(s) are combined using diagnosis-related groups (DRGs) to identify the predetermined amount of payment for hospital services. DRG classification is a system that groups patients according to diagnosis, type of treatment, age, and other relevant criteria. Under the prospective payment system, hospitals are paid a set fee for treating patients in a single DRG category.

In inpatient facility coding, the coder is responsible for reporting the ICD-10-CM and ICD-10-PCS codes, which are linked to the appropriate DRG via the facility's practice management software program, to obtain a prospective payment amount for the services performed. This allows the hospital facility to bill for the services that were provided during the procedure (such as hospital bed, staff, nursing services, meals, the use of equipment such as x-rays and surgical supplies), but not actually bill for the procedure itself (the procedure is billed by the performing provider using the appropriate CPT or HCPCS codes).

Key to Success

The codes reported by the hospital are facility codes (ICD-10-CM and ICD-10-PCS), and the codes reported by the healthcare provider are the professional codes for the services performed (ICD-10-CM, CPT, and HCPCS).

Procedures represented by PCS codes must still be supported with medical necessity, which means that both ICD-10-CM and PCS codes may be reported on the same claim. Keep in mind that PCS codes are only used for *facility* billing—such as inpatient hospital services, skilled nursing facility services, or inpatient mental hospital services. They also may be used to report outpatient hospital services, if the outpatient hospital participates in facility reporting. See figure 20.1 for a refresher of the different types of codes.

UB-04 Claim Form

An additional difference between inpatient and outpatient coding is the form used for billing third-party insurance payers. In professional coding, the CMS-1500 form is used. In facility inpatient and outpatient reporting, the UB-04, also known as the

Figure 20.1. Healthcare codes and their uses

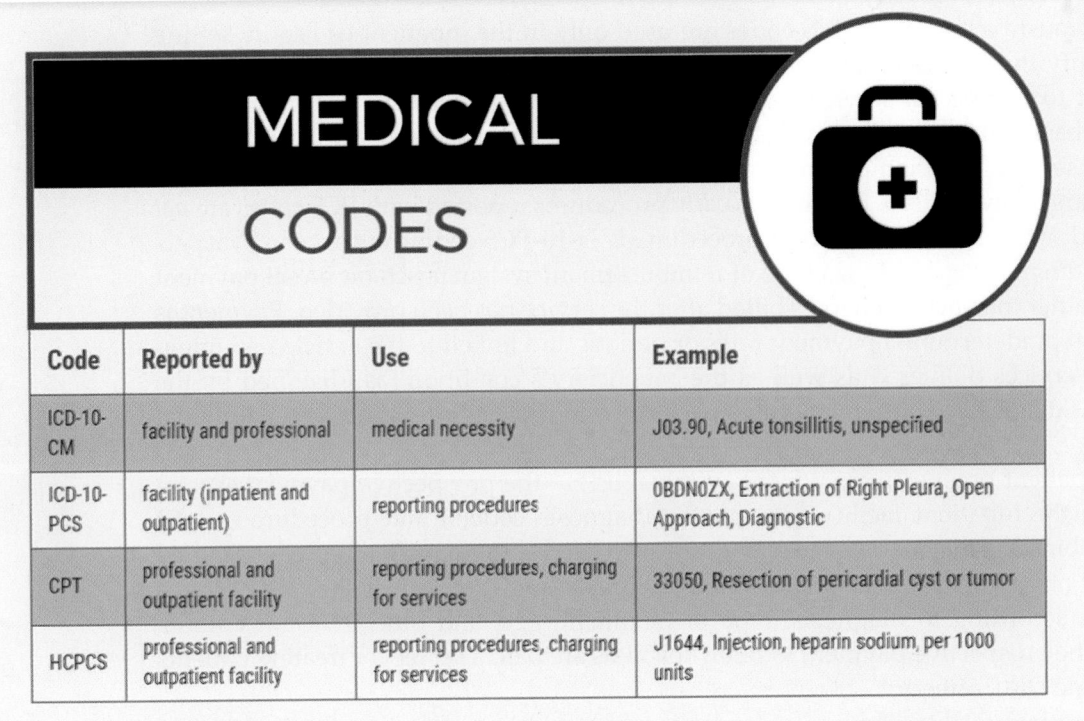

Code	Reported by	Use	Example
ICD-10-CM	facility and professional	medical necessity	J03.90, Acute tonsillitis, unspecified
ICD-10-PCS	facility (inpatient and outpatient)	reporting procedures	0BDN0ZX, Extraction of Right Pleura, Open Approach, Diagnostic
CPT	professional and outpatient facility	reporting procedures, charging for services	33050, Resection of pericardial cyst or tumor
HCPCS	professional and outpatient facility	reporting procedures, charging for services	J1644, Injection, heparin sodium, per 1000 units

CMS-1450, form is the hardcopy claim form used for billing services performed in the inpatient setting (see figure 20.2). Note that the UB-04 form includes more than twice as many informational fields than the CMS-1500 form used for outpatient billing; these fields are for information regarding the patient's inpatient services such as discharge information, information regarding the hospital services, and the providers that performed the services.

While the CMS-1500 form has 12 lines in which a coder may enter ICD-10-CM diagnosis codes, the UB-04 form has over 20 lines. ICD-10-CM codes are entered in form locator (FL) 67 through 67.Q, FL 69, and FLs 70.a, 70.b, and 70.c, as necessary (see figure 20.3). Furthermore, ICD-10-CM diagnosis coding guidelines for inpatient services may be different from those used in the outpatient setting. When reporting diagnosis codes for inpatient services, it is important to understand the OGCR related to inpatient coding and pay attention to notations in the Tabular List of the ICD-10-CM code book.

PCS codes identify the procedure(s) that were performed during the patient's admission, necessitated as indicated by the diagnosis code(s) (CM codes). There is room on the UB-04 form for up to six individual PCS codes, in FLs 74 through 74.e (see figure 20.4). One PCS code should be entered on the left under the word CODE, and the date the procedure was performed in the box under the word DATE. If more than six codes need to be reported, then an additional form or forms would be included.

These facility services include all the services that may be performed on the patient, such as surgical treatments, face-to-face encounters, maternal care and delivery, and chiropractic services. Due to the multiaxial structure of the codes, PCS codes are more variable than CPT codes, so coders can report an additional level of specificity by adjusting the code to report exactly what and how the procedure was performed. In PCS coding, the coder builds the code to report the specifics of how the procedure was performed.

Figure 20.2. UB-04 form

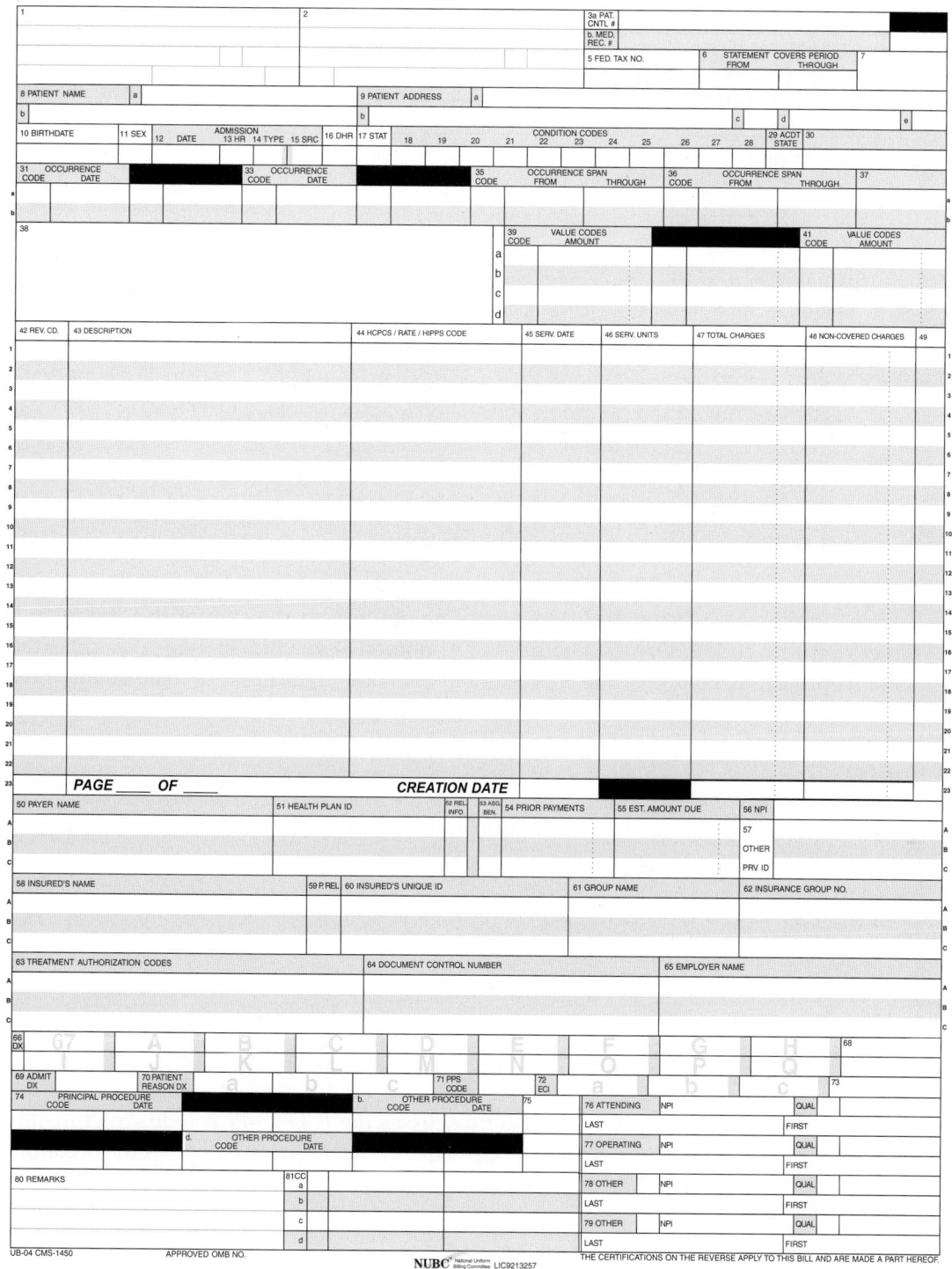

Source: CMS 2017.

Figure 20.3. UB-04 FL 67 through 67.Q, 69, 70.a through 70.c

Source: CMS 2017.

Figure 20.4. UB-04 FL 74 through 74.e

74 PRINCIPAL PROCEDURE CODE DATE	a. OTHER PROCEDURE CODE DATE	b. OTHER PROCEDURE CODE DATE
c. OTHER PROCEDURE CODE DATE	**d.** OTHER PROCEDURE CODE DATE	**e.** OTHER PROCEDURE CODE DATE

Source: CMS 2017.

Key to Success

Assigning codes for facility services (just as in professional services), requires an in-depth understanding of medical terminology, anatomy and physiology, and the various procedure types and treatment strategies for patient conditions. It is helpful to use as many resources as possible when learning PCS coding, like a medical dictionary, medical terminology, and anatomy and physiology texts.

ICD-10-PCS Code Structure and Code Book

PCS codes contain both numbers and letters that are seven characters in length. For example, the incision and drainage of an abscess on the skin of the abdomen is reported with code 0H97X0Z, Drainage of Abdomen Skin with Drainage Device, External Approach. Each one of the characters in the code identifies a specific detail of the procedure and must be selected by accessing the appropriate table in the PCS code set, depending on the specifics of the procedure. For example, in the characters of the code 0H97X0Z:

1. 0 identifies the procedure as medical and surgical in nature

2. H identifies the procedure on the skin and breast

3. 9 identifies the procedure as drainage

4. 7 identifies the area of the procedure as on the skin of the abdomen

5. X describes the approach to the procedure as external

6. 0 describes the device used as a drainage device

7. Z identifies that there are no further qualifying characteristics of this procedure

The following section of this chapter discusses the ICD-10-PCS code structure and how to use PCS code tables to build a PCS code. The last section discusses the organization of the ICD-10-PCS code book.

ICD-10-PCS Code Structure

PCS codes have seven characters, each of which depend on the section from which the code is being reported. Each character has a different meaning, based on the section from which it is selected. For example, the code for an open appendectomy is 0DTJ0ZZ, Resection of Appendix, Open Approach (see table 20.1). These characters are presented in a code table—a table of all of the character options (starting from character 4). Coders use the code table to build the additional characters into the code until all seven characters have been selected, according to how the procedure was performed.

Table 20.1. Open appendectomy PCS code

Character 1	Character 2	Character 3	Character 4	Character 5	Character 6	Character 7
0	D	T	J	0	Z	Z
Medical and Surgical	Gastro-intestinal	Resection	Appendix	Open	No Device	No Device

Each one of the characters in the code was selected carefully to identify a specific component of the procedure—such as that it was performed with an open approach or that the procedure was performed on the appendix. Coders must access the code tables in each section and carefully select the characters to build the code out to seven total characters. Review the following character components, their descriptions, and the code structure given (see also table 20.2).

Table 20.2. PCS characters and locations

Character 1	Character 2	Character 3	Character 4	Character 5	Character 6	Character 7
Section	Body System	Root Operation	Body Part	Approach	Device	Qualifier

1. The first character identifies the Section, which is the general type of procedure.
2. The second character identifies the Body System, which is the general physiological or anatomical region on which the procedure is performed.
3. The third character identifies the Root Operation or Type, which is the type and objective of the procedure.
4. The fourth character identifies the Body Part or Region, which is the specific organ or anatomical region involved in the procedure.
5. The fifth character identifies the Approach to the procedure, which is the technique used to gain access to the surgical site.
6. The sixth character identifies the Device that was used in the procedure, which is any material or appliance that remains after the procedure is performed.
7. The seventh character identifies the Qualifier for the procedure, which identifies any additional attributes of why or how the procedure was performed.

The sixth and seventh characters, device and qualifier, are not applicable for many procedures. As such, if no device or qualifier is applicable, use the character Z for no device or qualifier. This is noted in the code table.

The characters are listed in a set of tables, which are used by the coder to add each individual character and thus build a seven-character code. The sections that make up the great deal of the PCS code book are comprised of these tables. The table in the Medical and Surgical section for resection of the gastrointestinal system is in table 20.3.

The coder selects the appropriate component of the procedure and builds the code character-by-character, according to the table. To find the correct table, the coder must be able to locate the first three characters of a code, as all tables are listed by their first three codes. Note that in the previous example, the table lists the first three characters above the table. In this case, it is helpful to use the Index, as well as knowledge of the root operation definitions, to identify the first three characters of a code, then access that code table (using the first three characters) to build the rest of the code.

Table 20.3. 0DT table in the Medical and Surgical section

Section	0	**Medical and Surgical**
Body System	D	**Gastrointestinal System**
Operation	T	**Resection:** Cutting out or off, without replacement, all of a body part

Body Part (4th)	Approach (5th)	Device (6th)	Qualifier (7th)
1 Esophagus, Upper 2 Esophagus, Middle 3 Esophagus, Lower 4 Esophagogastric Junction 5 Esophagus 6 Stomach 7 Stomach, Pylorus 8 Small Intestine 9 Duodenum A Jejunum B Ileum C Ileocecal Valve E Large Intestine F Large Intestine, Right H Cecum J Appendix K Ascending Colon P Rectum Q Anus	0 Open 4 Percutaneous Endoscopic 7 Via Natural or Artificial Opening 8 Via Natural or Artificial Opening Endoscopic	Z No Device	Z No Qualifier
G Large Intestine, Left L Transverse Colon M Descending Colon N Sigmoid Colon	0 Open 4 Percutaneous Endoscopic 7 Via Natural or Artificial Opening 8 Via Natural or Artificial Opening Endoscopic F Via Natural or Artificial Opening With Percutaneous Endoscopic Assistance	Z No Device	Z No Qualifier
R Anal Sphincter U Omentum	0 Open 4 Percutaneous Endoscopic	Z No Device	Z No Qualifier

Source: Casto 2018, 618.

Review figure 20.5 to build the code for an open appendectomy.

The first three characters are located at the top of the table: 0DT. The fourth character is located in the first column on the left, under Body Part. Locate the word *Appendix* and select the character to which it corresponds: J. The fifth character is selected from the next column, under the heading Approach. Locate the word *Open* and assign the character to which it corresponds: 0. The last two characters are located in the last two columns. In this case, there is only one option for each: Z for no device and no qualifier. This builds the complete code 0DTJ0ZZ, Resection of Appendix, Open Approach.

Key to Success

To verify that the code that you have built is valid and complete, flip past the tables in each section to find the code listing for each code section. This is a list of the codes that can be created using the tables in that section. For example, if you want to verify that code 0DTJ0ZZ is valid, locate the code in the Gastrointestinal System Code Listing section at the end of the section to find: 0DJT0ZZ Resection of Appendix, Open Approach. Note that these lists are available in the AHIMA version of the ICD-10-PCS code book, and may not be available in all code books.

Figure 20.5. Building the code for open appendectomy

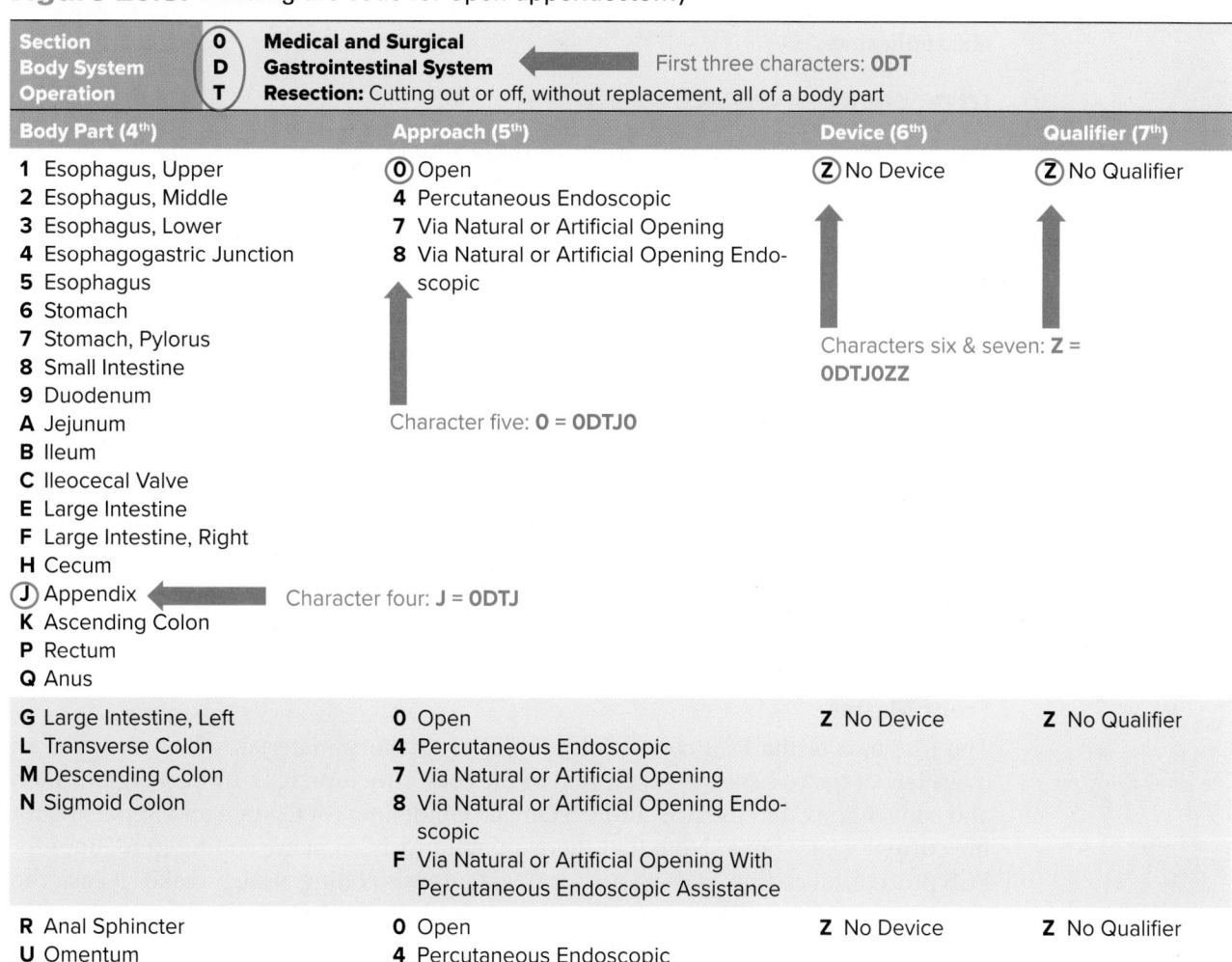

Section Body System Operation	**0** **D** **T**	**Medical and Surgical** **Gastrointestinal System** ← First three characters: **0DT** **Resection:** Cutting out or off, without replacement, all of a body part		
Body Part (4ᵗʰ)		**Approach (5ᵗʰ)**	**Device (6ᵗʰ)**	**Qualifier (7ᵗʰ)**
1 Esophagus, Upper 2 Esophagus, Middle 3 Esophagus, Lower 4 Esophagogastric Junction 5 Esophagus 6 Stomach 7 Stomach, Pylorus 8 Small Intestine 9 Duodenum A Jejunum B Ileum C Ileocecal Valve E Large Intestine F Large Intestine, Right H Cecum J Appendix ← Character four: **J = 0DTJ** K Ascending Colon P Rectum Q Anus		**0** Open 4 Percutaneous Endoscopic 7 Via Natural or Artificial Opening 8 Via Natural or Artificial Opening Endo- scopic Character five: **0 = 0DTJ0**	**Z** No Device Characters six & seven: **Z =** **0DTJ0ZZ**	**Z** No Qualifier
G Large Intestine, Left L Transverse Colon M Descending Colon N Sigmoid Colon		0 Open 4 Percutaneous Endoscopic 7 Via Natural or Artificial Opening 8 Via Natural or Artificial Opening Endo- scopic F Via Natural or Artificial Opening With Percutaneous Endoscopic Assistance	Z No Device	Z No Qualifier
R Anal Sphincter U Omentum		0 Open 4 Percutaneous Endoscopic	Z No Device	Z No Qualifier

Source: Casto 2018, 618.

Key to Success

When reporting PCS codes, be careful to differentiate between the letter O and the number 0 as they are very similar. The letter O is always listed as a capital letter, so it closely resembles the number 0. However, the letter O is rounder—more circular—than the number 0. The number 0 is more elongated—like an oval—than the letter O, and may sometimes have a line through it (Ø) to indicate that it is a number rather than a letter.

When using PCS tables, note that some tables are too large to be included in full on one page, so they may be continued on the next page. Some tables are so large that they may span multiple pages. It helps to look past the table referenced to ensure that it either has or has not been continued to the next page. Note that some publishers may include a "continued" note at the bottom of a table or a small arrow, to indicate that the table continues on the next page.

Note also that not all options are available for all procedures. For example, in the previous table, the Approach column (fifth character) does not include all seven approach types. In this case, the External (character X), Percutaneous (character 3), and Via Natural or Artificial Opening with Percutaneous Endoscopic Assistance (character F) are not listed. This is because none of the procedures in that section, body system, operation, and body area may be performed in that manner and, therefore, those approaches are not applicable.

ICD-10-PCS Code Book

The ICD-10-PCS code book is organized in a similar fashion to the ICD-10-CM code book. Coders should first access the Index at the beginning of the book to help find procedure codes, which are then verified in the Tabular List in the remainder of the book. However, there are striking differences between CM and PCS coding, and the organization of the book is really the only similarity. The major difference between ICD-10-CM and ICD-10-PCS code books is that instead of including a Tabular List that identifies individual codes, each with code descriptions (as in the CM code book), the PCS code book's Tabular List is comprised of tables that the coder must use to build a code.

In this sense, PCS coding is much more interactive and requires attention to details identified by each particular character in the code. Coders may find that the PCS code table includes body areas, organs, devices, or other details specific to only certain types of procedures. It is in these instances that using available reference materials—including medical terminology and anatomy and terminology resources—may become invaluable, especially as a beginning coder.

The following sections identify each of the respective sections of the ICD-10-PCS code book: front matter, index, sections and code tables, and appendices.

Front Matter

The first part of the PCS code book is the Introductory material, which includes an overview of the code set, a description of the code structure, ICD-10-PCS organization and conventions, and the ICD-10-PCS Official Guidelines for Coding and Reporting for the current year's book. Note that there are not nearly as many coding guidelines for PCS procedural coding as there are for CM diagnosis coding, which makes it easier to access appropriate guidelines for the procedures being coded. Depending on the publisher of the code book, these guidelines may also be included before each respective section in the code tables for easy reference. Note that the PCS code set is published by the Centers for Medicare and Medicaid Services (CMS) and all of the codes and code tables are accessible via the CMS website.

Note that as publishers of the code books differ, the front matter of each code book may also differ. It is always helpful to be familiar with this front matter, as it may include information regarding how to use the book, how to select the codes, or how to use the guidelines.

Index

After the introductory material is the ICD-10-PCS Index. This works in the same way as the indices to the other code books. Coders should reference the Index to find the procedural description, which refers the coder to a code or cross-reference. It is important to still verify the code in the code tables, and add all necessary characters to the code to create a seven-character code.

When searching the Index, locate the procedure type, such as *Destruction*, *Excision*, or *Replacement*. Once a procedural description is found, identify the body area or organ on which the procedure was performed, or follow all cross-references until the Index identifies a code or code beginning. For example, if coding an incision and drainage procedure on an abscess of the skin of the abdomen, the coder would first search for *Drainage*, then *skin*, and then *abdomen*, which leads the coder to the code beginning *0H97*. Note that this is not a valid PCS code, as PCS codes are all seven characters in length. Once the coder finds the beginning characters, he or she must then build the rest of the code based on the appropriate table (steps to complete the code will be discussed in the next section).

Sections and Code Tables

After the Index are the PCS code sections, which include the code tables used to build the codes. There are 17 different sections of codes, each of which begins with a different character. For example, all the codes in the Medical and Surgical section begin with the number 0, and all of the codes in the Mental Health section begin with the character G. The 17 sections are listed in table 20.4.

Table 20.4. ICD-10-PCS sections and characters

Character	Section	Definition
0	Medical and Surgical	This character identifies invasive and non-invasive procedures performed on patients and compiles the vast majority of procedures reported with PCS codes.
1	Obstetrics	This character identifies procedures performed on the products of conception only, including the fetus, amnion, umbilical cord, and placenta. Procedures performed on the pregnant female are identified with codes from the Medical and Surgical section (character "0").
2	Placement	This character identifies procedures that involve placing an external device in or on a body part in order to protect, immobilize, stretch, compress, or for packing purposes.
3	Administration	This character identifies procedures that involve putting in or on a substance used as a therapeutic, diagnostic, nutritional, physiological, or prophylactic.
4	Measurement and Monitoring	This character identifies procedures that determine the level of a physical or physiological function.
5	Extracorporeal or Systemic Assistance and Performance Section	This character identifies procedures that utilize equipment outside of the body to assist or perform a physiological function.
6	Extracorporeal Therapies	This character identifies procedures that utilize equipment outside of the body for therapeutic purposes that do not assist or perform a physiological function.
7	Osteopathic	This character identifies procedures that involve the manual treatment of alleviating somatic dysfunction and related disorders.
8	Other Procedures	This character identifies a miscellaneous range of procedures that do not fall into any other section, including acupuncture, in vitro fertilization, and suture removal.
9	Chiropractic	This character identifies procedures that involve a direct thrust to a joint for the purpose of moving it as a therapeutic treatment.
B	Imaging	This character identifies procedures that involve creating images of the patient's anatomical structures, including plain radiography (x-ray), fluoroscopy, CT, MRI, and ultrasound. This does not include nuclear imaging studies (reported with character "C") or radiation oncology procedures (reported with character "D").
C	Nuclear Medicine	This character identifies procedures that introduce radioactive material into the patient in order to create an image of the patient's anatomical structures, such as PET.
D	Radiation Therapy	This character identifies procedures that utilize radiation to treat cancerous disorders (radiation oncology).
F	Physical Rehabilitation and Diagnostic Audiology	This character identifies procedures that identify physical, occupational, and speech language pathology services.
G	Mental Health	This character identifies procedures that are focused on treating the emotional and behavioral health of the patient, and includes crisis intervention and educational and vocational counseling.

(Continued on next page)

Table 20.4. *(Continued)*

Character	Section	Definition
H	Substance Abuse	This character identifies procedures aimed at eliminating substance use, abuse, and dependence, and includes detoxification services and individual counseling.
X	New Technology	This character identifies procedures that are not classified elsewhere in the ICD-10-PCS code set, and identify procedures that utilize a new device substance, or technology.

Source: CMS 2018.

Each one of these sections includes the code tables for those specific types of procedures. Code tables are used to identify the remaining characters so that each code can be built and total seven characters. The section identifier is the first character of a code (see table 20.5).

Table 20.5. PCS code character 1

Character 1	Character 2	Character 3	Character 4	Character 5	Character 6	Character 7
0						
Medical and Surgical						

Key to Success

It is a good idea to place tabs in your PCS code book for easy access to sections in the book. For example, have one tab for the Obstetrics section, another for the Placement section, and so on. Depending on the publisher your PCS code book may already have a page of blank tabs at the beginning of the book that can be used for this purpose. Also, note that each individual section in the ICD-10-PCS code book may have a colored outer edge, which helps to differentiate sections of the book.

The largest section of PCS codes is the Medical and Surgical section, which includes 31 different body systems, each of which has a selection of tables that apply to that specific body system. The body systems in the Medical and Surgical section are listed in table 20.6.

Table 20.6. ICD-10-PCS Medical and Surgical section body systems and characters

Body System	Character
Central Nervous System	0
Peripheral Nervous System	1
Heart and Great Vessels	2
Upper Arteries	3
Lower Arteries	4
Upper Veins	5
Lower Veins	6

Body System	Character
Lymphatic and Hemic Systems	7
Eye	8
Ear, Nose, Sinus	9
Respiratory System	B
Mouth and Throat	C
Gastrointestinal System	D
Hepatobiliary System and Pancreas	F
Endocrine System	G
Skin and Breast	H
Subcutaneous Tissue and Fascia	J
Muscles	K
Tendons	L
Bursae and Ligaments	M
Head and Facial Bones	N
Upper Bones	P
Lower Bones	Q
Upper Joints	R
Lower Joints	S
Urinary System	T
Female Reproductive System	U
Male Reproductive System	V
Anatomical Regions, General	W
Anatomical Regions, Upper Extremities	X
Anatomical Regions, Lower Extremities	Y

Each body system is identified by the corresponding character (letter or number) as identified in table 20.6. This is a glimpse of how to build PCS codes. For example, an appendectomy—the surgical removal (resection) of the appendix—would be coded from the Medical and Surgical section because it is a surgery, so the code would start with the character 0. The next character would correspond to the body system, in this case the gastrointestinal system, so the next character in the code would be D. So, the PCS code for an appendectomy would begin with the characters 0D (see table 20.7). (The following sections discuss how to build the rest of this code).

Table 20.7. PCS code character 2: body system

Character 1	Character 2	Character 3	Character 4	Character 5	Character 6	Character 7
0	D					
Medical and Surgical	Gastro-intestinal					

Appendices

Appendices follow the PCS code sections and contain additional information on terminology definitions, body parts, medical and surgical devices, and substances. They may include the following: Root Operations; Type and Qualifier Definitions; Approach Definitions; Medical and Surgical Body Parts; Medical and Surgical Device Table (Device Key) and Device Aggregation Table; and Substance Qualifier Table. Note that these appendices differ among publishers.

Root Operations Definitions Appendix

The Root Operations Definitions lists the definitions for the root operations for the first 10 sections of the PCS code book (Medical and Surgical through Chiropractic). **Root operations** are the type of surgery, operation, or procedure that was performed.

It is important to read through and thoroughly study the definitions of the root operations in this section, especially after learning CPT and HCPCS coding. The terminology for some procedures in the CPT or HCPCS code books may differ from the procedural terminology used in PCS coding. For example, in the CPT code book, the term *excision* is sometimes used to report the complete removal of an organ or body part, such as excision of a kidney (nephrectomy). However, in PCS coding, the term *excision* is used only when a portion of an organ or body part is removed, and the term *resection* is used to identify the complete removal of an organ or body part. It is imperative to understand the root operation terms to ensure correct code selection, so this appendix is a useful tool when learning PCS coding.

There are 31 different root operations for codes in the Medical and Surgical section. Table 20.8 lists the root operation name, character value, definition, and an example of the procedure.

There are additional root operation terms unique to each particular section of the PCS code book. For example, the root operation **delivery**, which is assisting the passage of the products of conception from the genital canal, is unique to the obstetrics section. The definitions for these additional root operations are included with the Root Operations Definitions appendix, after the Medical and Surgical Root Operation Definitions (listed previously), as well as in the guidelines at the beginning of each section of code tables.

Table 20.8. Root operations in Medical and Surgical sections

Root Operation	Character	Definition	Example
Alteration	0	Modifying the anatomic structure of a body part without affecting the function of the body part	Face lift, breast augmentation
Bypass	1	Altering the route of passage of the contents of a tubular body part	CABG, formation of colostomy
Change	2	Taking out or off a device from a body part and putting back an identical or similar device in or on the same body part without cutting or puncturing the skin or a mucous membrane	Urinary catheter change, gastrostomy tube change
Control	3	Stopping, or attempting to stop, postprocedural or other acute bleeding	Control of subdural hemorrhage or bleeding ulcer
Creation	4	Putting in or on biological or synthetic material to form a new body part that to the extent possible replicates the anatomic structure or function of an absent body part	Creation of right and left atrioventricular (AV) valve from common AV valve
Destruction	5	Physical eradication of all or a portion of a body part by the direct use of energy, force, or a destructive agent	Fulguration of a polyp

Root Operation	Character	Definition	Example
Detachment	6	Cutting off all of a portion of the upper or lower extremities	Amputation of the leg below knee
Dilation	7	Expanding an orifice of the lumen of a tubular body part	PTCA
Division	8	Cutting into a body part, without draining fluids and/or gases from the body part, in order to separate or transect a body part	Spinal cordotomy, osteotomy
Drainage	9	Taking or letting out fluids and/or gases from a body part	Incision and drainage
Excision	B	Cutting out or off, without replacement, a portion of a body part	Liver biopsy
Extirpation	C	Taking or cutting out solid matter from a body part	Thrombectomy
Extraction	D	Pulling or stripping out or off all or a portion of a body part by the use of force	Dilation and curettage
Fragmentation	E	Breaking solid matter in a body part into pieces	Transurethral lithotripsy
Fusion	G	Joining together portions of an articular body part rendering the articular body part immobile	Ankle arthrodesis
Insertion	H	Putting a nonbiological appliance that monitors, assists, performs, or prevents a physiological function but does not physically take the place of a body part	Central line insertion
Inspection	J	Visually and/or manually exploring a body part	Exploratory laparotomy
Map	K	Locating the route of passage of electrical impulses and/or locating functional areas in a body part	Cardiac mapping
Occlusion	L	Completely closing an orifice or the lumen of a tubular body part	Fallopian tube ligation
Reattachment	M	Putting back in or on all or a portion of a separated body part to its normal location or other suitable location	Reattachment of hand
Release	N	Freeing a body part from an abnormal physical constraint by cutting or by the use of force	Carpal tunnel release
Removal	P	Taking out or off a device from a body part	Cardiac pacemaker removal
Repair	Q	Restoring, to the extent possible, a body part to its normal anatomic structure and function	Suture of laceration
Replacement	R	Putting in or on biological or synthetic material that physically takes the place and/or function of all or a portion of a body part	Total hip replacement
Reposition	S	Moving to its normal location or other suitable location, all or a portion of a body part.	Fracture reduction
Resection	T	Cutting out or off, without replacement, all of a body part	Total nephrectomy
Restriction	V	Partially closing an orifice of the lumen of a tubular body part	Cervical cerclage
Revision	W	Correcting, to the extent possible, a portion of a malfunctioning device or the position of a displaced device to the extent possible	Re-cementing of hip prosthesis
Supplement	U	Putting in or on biological or synthetic material that physically reinforces and/or augments the function of a portion of a body part	Herniorrhaphy using mesh
Transfer	X	Moving, without taking out, all or a portion of a body part to another location to take over the function of all or a portion of a body part	Skin flap transfer
Transplantation	Y	Putting in or on all or a portion of a living body part taken from another individual or animal to physically take the place and/or function of all or a portion of a similar body part	Kidney transplant, heart transplant

Source: CMS 2018.

Root operations are listed in the third character location of PCS codes. So, if the first two characters for the PCS for an appendectomy are 0D, then the root operation character is added as the third character. An appendectomy is the complete removal of the appendix, which is classified as the root operation *resection*, and represented with character T. Therefore, the first three characters for an appendectomy are 0DT (see table 20.9).

Table 20.9. PCS code character 3: root operation

Character 1	Character 2	Character 3	Character 4	Character 5	Character 6	Character 7
0	D	T				
Medical and Surgical	Gastro-intestinal	Resection				

Key to Success

Read through the root operation terms, definitions, explanations, and examples located in the appendix of the PCS code book. These are terms under which procedures are listed in the Index, and as mentioned before, they do differ from the way these same terms may be used in either CPT or HCPCS coding. Do not forget to access this appendix when you are coding with ICD-10-PCS, especially if you are confused about a specific type of operation and under which root operation term it would be classified.

Type and Qualifier Definitions Appendix

The Type and Qualifier Definitions appendix contains the definitions of the type and qualifier characters found in five of the last seven sections of the PCS code book: Imaging; Nuclear Medicine; Physical Rehabilitation and Diagnostic Audiology; Mental Health; and Substance Abuse Treatment. These lists include the terms and definitions for the third, fourth, or fifth characters found in the codes for these sections, as well as the character values. Note that these third characters take the place of the root operation characters for these specific procedure types because these procedure types, such as substance abuse treatment, do not include an operation per se. Instead, these procedures are nonsurgical, and so the third character identifies a different component of the procedure. For example, the term Computerized Tomography (CT scan) (in the Imaging section) is identified by the number 2 and defined as a computer reformatted digital display of multiplanar images developed from the capture of multiple exposures of external ionizing radiation. Just as with the previous appendix, these characters are located in the third character value of the PCS code.

Approach Definitions Appendix

The Approach Definitions appendix lists the descriptions for the different types of approaches to a procedure. The **approach** of a procedure identifies the manner in which the provider accessed the area in order to perform the procedure. Appendix C lists the different approaches and the definitions for each, within each respective section of the PCS code book. The approaches for the Medical and Surgical section are as follows in table 20.10.

Table 20.10. Approaches for the Medical and Surgical section

Approach	Character	Definition	Example
External	X	Procedures performed directly on the skin or mucous membrane and procedures performed indirectly by the application of external force through the skin or mucous membrane.	Excision of skin lesion, closed reduction of fracture
Open	0	Cutting through the skin or mucous membrane and any other body layers necessary to expose the site of the procedure.	Open CABG, open abdominal appendectomy
Percutaneous	3	Entry, by puncture or minor incision, of instrumentation through the skin or mucous membrane and any other body layers necessary to reach the site of the procedure.	Liposuction, needle biopsy
Percutaneous Endoscopic	4	Entry, by puncture or minor incision, of instrumentation through the skin or mucous membrane and any other body layers necessary to reach and visualize the site of the procedure.	Laparoscopic appendectomy, arthroscopy of knee
Via Natural or Artificial Opening	7	Entry of instrumentation through a natural or artificial external opening to reach the site of the procedure.	Placement of urinary catheter, endotracheal intubation
Via Natural or Artificial Opening Endoscopic	8	Entry of instrumentation through a natural of artificial opening to reach *and visualize* the site of the procedure.	Colonoscopy, EGD
Via Natural or Artificial Opening with Percutaneous Endoscopic Assistance	F	Entry of instrumentation through a natural or artificial external opening and entry, by puncture or minor incision, of instrumentation through the skin or mucous membrane and any other body layers necessary to aid in the performance of the procedure.	Laparoscopic-assisted bariatric surgery

Source: CMS 2018.

Key to Success

When looking at the different types of approaches for surgical procedures, pay attention to those used with the aid of an endoscope versus those used without the aid of an endoscope, as the definitions are similar. For example, the only difference between the approaches Percutaneous and Percutaneous Endoscopic is the addition of "and visualize" in the definition of the approach. This is because an endoscope is used for visualization during the procedure.

Again, the first three characters of an appendectomy code are 0DT to identify the procedure as Medical and Surgical (0), on the Gastrointestinal System (D), and the procedure type as Resection (T). Once the coder has located the first three characters in a code, he or she can turn to that specific code table in the ICD-10-PCS code book to find the rest of the characters and complete the code. In the code table for 0DT, the first column identifies the characters for each specific body part within the gastrointestinal system. It is here that the coder would find the character J is used to identify the body part that was removed as the appendix.

The character for the approach to a surgical procedure is placed in the fifth location of a PCS code. For example, if the procedure was performed via an open incision, then the fifth character 0 should be selected to identify the procedure as open. All five of these characters are added together to create the code 0DTJ0. Note that this is only a five-character code, and so it is not yet complete. To complete the code, two more characters are still needed (see table 20.11).

Table 20.11. PCS code character 4 and 5: body part and approach

Character 1	Character 2	Character 3	Character 4	Character 5	Character 6	Character 7
0	D	T	J	0		
Medical and Surgical	Gastro-intestinal	Resection	Appendix	Open		

Medical and Surgical Body Parts Appendix

The Medical and Surgical Body Parts appendix includes tables that list the specific body parts identified by the fourth character for medical and surgical codes. These tables are helpful when trying to determine which specific body part belongs to which character. For example, if the description of the procedure was identified as being on the body part *hallux,* then the coder could refer to this table in the appendix of the ICD-10-PCS code book to make sure that the hallux is included in the character for first toe, left, or first toe, right (see figure 20.6).

Figure 20.6. Medical and Surgical Body Parts appendix

Section 0 - Medical and Surgical — Character 4 - Body Part	
1st Toe, Left **1st** Toe, Right	**Includes:** Hallux
Abdomen Muscle, Left **Abdomen** Muscle, Right	**Includes:** External oblique muscle Internal oblique muscle Pyramidalis muscle Rectus abdominis muscle Transversus abdominis muscle
Abdominal Aorta	**Includes:** Inferior phrenic artery Lumbar artery Median sacral artery Middle suprarenal artery Ovarian artery Testicular artery

Source: Casto 2018, 1472; Adapted from CMS 2018.

Medical and Surgical Device Table (Device Key) and Device Aggregation Table Appendix

The Medical and Surgical Device Table (Device Key) and Device Aggregation Table appendix lists the devices that may be used in medical and surgical codes, as well as additional devices and where they may be identified by a specific PCS character. This list also includes brand-name devices, and to which device character they should apply. For example, a feeding device in gastrointestinal system includes a PEG/J (percutaneous endoscopic gastrojejunostomy tube) (see figure 20.7).

Figure 20.7. Medical and Surgical Device table

Section 0 - Medical and Surgical — Character 6 - Device	
Extraluminal Device	**Includes:** AtriClip LAA Exclusion System LAP-BAND® adjustable gastric banding system REALIZE® Adjustable Gastric Band

Feeding Device in Gastrointestinal System	**Includes:**
	Percutaneous endoscopic
	    gastrojejunostomy (PEG/J) tube
	Percutaneous endoscopic gastrostomy
	    (PEG) tube

Hearing Device in Ear, Nose, Sinus	**Includes:** Esteem® implantable hearing system

Source: Casto 2018, 1486; Adapted from CMS 2018.

The character for device is located in the sixth character location of a PCS code. For example, in the code table for 0DT, there are no options for the sixth character other than Z for *No Device*. An open appendectomy does not use any type of device, so the letter Z is used in the sixth character location to identify that no device was placed during the procedure. This results in expanding the code to six characters: 0DTJ0Z. Note that at this point, this code still requires one additional character to reach seven characters and make it valid (see table 20.12).

Table 20.12. PCS code character 6: device

Character 1	Character 2	Character 3	Character 4	Character 5	Character 6	Character 7
0	D	T	J	0	Z	
Medical and Surgical	Gastro-intestinal	Resection	Appendix	Open	No Device	

Key to Success

The PCS code set uses the character Z when no other character is applicable for the procedure being reported. For example, if a procedure does not involve a device, or if no qualifier (as reported by character 7) is applicable, then the character Z is added for *No Device* or *No Qualifier*.

Substance Qualifier Table Appendix

The Substance Qualifier Table appendix lists the substances that are included in the substance character descriptions for two sections: Administration (section 3) and New Technology (section X). This appendix is used in the same manner as the previous two appendices, except it lists the substances that are included with the character descriptions for the code table. Coders can use this information to help identify specific substances used in procedures, and which character(s) identify those substances.

For example, if the description of the procedure described a substance used or administered as Seprafilm, then the coder could access this appendix and know what the character is for Adhesion Barrier (see figure 20.8).

Figure 20.8. Substance Qualifier table

Section 3 – Administration Character 6 – Substance	
4-Factor Prothrombin Complex Concentrate	**Includes:** Kcentra
Adhesion Barrier	**Includes:** Seprafilm
Anti-Infective Envelope	**Includes:** AIGISRx Antibacterial Envelope Antimicrobial envelope
Clofarabine	**Includes:** Clolar

Source: Casto 2018, 1494; Adapted from CMS 2018.

Putting It All Together: Building PCS Codes

Study the following vignette that demonstrates how to select the appropriate procedure codes. Then complete the practice exercises in There's a Code for That 20.1.

Helen is a new coder at a 200-bed inpatient hospital in a Midwestern town. She just graduated from a coding program at a local vocational college and after receiving brief training in ICD-10-PCS coding, she is practicing coding facility inpatient charts. She is coding the following case: 50-year-old female patient presented to the operating room with a herniated disc of the T4 level. Surgeon performed a partial discectomy via open incision.

To find the codes for the surgical service, Helen asks herself: What did the doctor do? In this case, the doctor removed part of a herniated disc from the patient. She has to build the PCS code for the service according to the specifics of how the procedure was performed. First, she must determine the first three characters of the code so she can locate the code table and build the rest of the code. She knows that the procedure was a partial removal of a vertebral disc, which is classified in PCS as an excision procedure. She searches for Excision in the PCS Index, and then locates the subterm Disc. Under the subterm Disc she locates the term Thoracic Vertebral, which gives her the first four characters for her code: 0RB9.

Now that she has the first four characters for her code, Helen accesses the Tabular List to find the code table for her first three characters. See figure 20.9 to view the code table.

Helen verifies the character 9 for the fourth character, as the procedure was performed on the disc of a thoracic vertebra, which brings her to the following: 0RB9. For the fifth character, she selects 0 as the approach, because the procedure was performed via an open

Figure 20.9 0RB code table

Section	0	Medical and Surgical
Body System	R	Upper Joints
Operation	B	Excision: Cutting out or off, without replacement, a portion of a body part

Body Part (4th)	Approach (5th)	Device (6th)	Qualifier (7th)
0 Occipital-cervical Joint 1 Cervical Vertebral Joint 3 Cervical Vertebral Disc 4 Cervicothoracic Vertebral Joint 5 Cervicothoracic Vertebral Disc 6 Thoracic Vertebral Joint 9 Thoracic Vertebral Disc A Thoracolumbar Vertebral Joint B Thoracolumbar Vertebral Disc C Temporomandibular Joint, Right D Temporomandibular Joint, Left E Sternoclavicular Joint, Right F Sternoclavicular Joint, Left G Acromioclavicular Joint, Right H Acromioclavicular Joint, Left J Shoulder Joint, Right K Shoulder Joint, Left L Elbow Joint, Right M Elbow Joint, Left N Wrist Joint, Right P Wrist Joint, Left Q Carpal Joint, Right R Carpal Joint, Left S Carpometacarpal Joint, Right T Carpometacarpal Joint, Left U Metacarpophalangeal Joint, Right V Metacarpophalangeal Joint, Left W Finger Phalangeal Joint, Right X Finger Phalangeal Joint, Left	0 Open 3 Percutaneous 4 Percutaneous Endoscopic	Z No Device	X Diagnostic Z No Qualifier

Source: Casto 2018, 1078; Adapted from CMS 2018.

incision. This brings her to the following: 0RB90. For the sixth character, she selects the character Z for no device. Not only is this the only option according to the code table, but there was no device left in place after the surgery (remember that a device is any material or appliance that remains after the procedure is performed). This leads her to the code 0RB90Z, which still needs one more character before it is complete. The last character she selects is Z for no qualifier, as the only other option is diagnostic and this was not a diagnostic procedure. This leads her to the following complete code:

- 0RB90ZZ, Excision of Thoracic Vertebral Disc, Open Approach.

Now that she has her PCS code, she needs to find the CM code for the service. According to the documentation, the procedure was performed because of a herniated T4 disc. She selects the following code:

- M51.24, Other intervertebral disc displacement, thoracic region.

She then rechecks the documentation to make sure she has coded everything for the encounter and reports the chosen codes.

20.1 Coding for inpatient services

There's a Code for That

Read the following documentation and select the appropriate ICD-10-CM and ICD-10-PCS code(s) for the procedure.

1. 45-year-old female underwent an open left kidney allotransplantation due to ESRD.

   ICD-10-PCS code: _____

   ICD-10-CM code: _____

2. Chest tube for drainage was changed in a patient with left primary spontaneous pneumothorax.

   ICD-10-PCS code: _____

   ICD-10-CM code: _____

3. Esophagogastroduodenoscopy performed on patient with dyspepsia and dysphagia.

   ICD-10-PCS code: _____

   ICD-10-CM code: _____, _____

4. 8-year-old male underwent a repair of umbilical hernia. The contents of the hernia were reduced into the abdominal cavity and the abdominal wall was sutured.

   ICD-10-PCS code: _____

   ICD-10-CM code: _____

End of Chapter Content

Instructions: Indicate whether the following statements are true or false (T or F). For false statements, rewrite the statement on the line below to make the statement true.

1. ICD-10-CM codes are reported for inpatient services in addition to ICD-10-PCS codes.

   _____

   _____

2. Facility inpatient services are reported on the CMS-1500 paper claim form.

   _____

   _____

3. Facility inpatient services are paid on a fee-for-service basis.

   _____

   _____

4. ICD-10-PCS codes have seven alphabetical characters.

_____

_____

5. A device is any material or appliance that remains after the procedure is performed.

_____

_____

6. The Medical and Surgical section is identified by the character 0.

_____

_____

7. The PCS code book does not include an index; coders must rely only on their knowledge of the procedure performed to find the code.

_____

_____

8. The procedure qualifier is the type of surgery, operation, or procedure performed.

_____

_____

9. A percutaneous endoscopic procedure is performed by cutting into the skin or mucous membrane in order to gain entrance into the body area.

_____

_____

Instructions: Choose the best answer.

1. Which of the following codes would an inpatient facility report to identify an appendectomy procedure?

a. ICD-10-PCS
b. ICD-10-CM
c. CPT
d. HCPCS

2. Which of the following codes would the healthcare provider report to identify an appendectomy procedure?

a. ICD-10-PCS
b. ICD-10-CM
c. CPT
d. HCPCS

3. In prospective payment, what is used to identify the predetermined amount of payment?

a. PPS
b. Fee-for-service
c. PCS codes
d. DRGs

4. How many ICD-10-CM codes can be reported on the UB-04 form?

a. 4
b. 12
c. Over 20
d. Over 30

5. A valid ICD-10-PCS code is how many characters?

a. 5

b. 3

c. 3 to 7

d. 7

6. The first character of a PCS identifies which of the following?

a. Section

b. Body system

c. Root operation

d. Body part or region

7. Which of the following identifies any additional attributes of why or how the procedure was performed?

a. Qualifier

b. Device

c. Root operation

d. Body system

8. Which of the following characters is used for the Chiropractic section?

a. A

b. X

c. 9

d. 7

9. Which of the following root operations is altering the route of passage of the contents of a tubular body part?

a. Alteration

b. Restriction

c. Transfer

d. Bypass

10. Which of the following root operations is cutting out or off, without replacement, all of a body part?

a. Excision

b. Resection

c. Transplantation

d. Extirpation

11. Which of the following root operations is breaking solid matter in a body part into pieces?

a. Extirpation

b. Extraction

c. Fragmentation

d. Occlusion

12. Which of the following types of approaches to a procedure is an incisional abdominal appendectomy?

a. External

b. Open

c. Percutaneous

d. Via natural opening

Instructions: Answer the following questions with the appropriate code(s) and modifier(s).

1. 60-year-old male with primary malignant neoplasm of the prostate underwent total prostatectomy via open approach.

ICD-10-PCS code: _____

ICD-10-CM code: _____

2. Amputation of right lower leg at the mid-calf-level of an 83-year-old female with DMII, with ulcer of the calf with necrosis of bone.

ICD-10-PCS code: _____

ICD-10-CM code: _____

References

Casto, A.B. 2018. *ICD-10-PCS Code Book*. Chicago: AHIMA.

Centers for Medicare and Medicaid Services. 2018. ICD-10-PCS Official Guidelines for Coding and Reporting FY 2018. https://www.cms.gov/Medicare /Coding/ICD10/Downloads/2018-PCS-Guidelines.pdf.

Centers for Medicare and Medicaid Services. 2017. Details for title: CMS 1450. https://www.cms.gov/Medicare /CMS-Forms/CMS-Forms/CMS-Forms-Items /CMS1196256.html.

Centers for Medicare and Medicaid Services. 2016. Development of the ICD-10 Procedure Coding System (ICD-10-PCS). https://www.cms.gov/Medicare /Coding/ICD10/Downloads/2016-Developmentofthe -ICD-10-Procedure-Coding-System.pdf.

Resources

Barta, A., K. DeVault, and M. Endicott. 2014. *2014 ICD-10-PCS Coder Training Manual*. Chicago: AHIMA.

Centers for Medicare and Medicaid Services. 2017. 2018 ICD-10 PCS and GEMs. https://www.cms.gov /Medicare/Coding/ICD10/2018-ICD-10-PCS-and -GEMs.html.

Centers for Medicare and Medicaid Services. 2006 (November 3). Pub 100-04 Medicare Claims Processing. https://www.cms.gov/Regulations-and Guidance /Guidance/Transmittals/downloads/r1104cp.pdf.

Centers for Medicare and Medicaid Services. 2016. Using the ICD-10-PCS New Technology Section Codes. https://www.cms.gov/Medicare/Coding/ICD10 /Downloads/2016-Section-X-New-Technology-.pdf.

DecisionHealth. 2013. *Advanced Anatomy and Physiology for ICD-10-CM/PCS*. Salt Lake City, UT: Contexo Media.

Appendix A: Coding Certifications and Professional Coding Organizations

Professional certifications are one of the best measures of one's ability, and as such are highly regarded within the world of health information management (HIM), billing, and coding. Going through the rigorous demands of the certification process is a great way to prove your coding prowess to potential employers and as a way to move up the career ladder.

There are dozens of different healthcare certifications, including specialty-specific coding, general billing practices, compliance, auditing, and other special topics. It is helpful to become familiar with a few of the more prominent certifications you may encounter as a professional coder. In addition, many educational coding and billing programs require students to take a certification exam to complete the course. Certain certifications may also be a requirement for employment at healthcare coding or billing organizations.

The following is a list of some of the certifications you can obtain after completing your coding education, as well as a selection of certifications that you can obtain after you gain more professional experience in medical billing and a number of additional areas within HIM.

Coding Certifications

The following are the more prominent coding certifications and are commonly the focus of medical coding programs. As you can see, there are general coding certifications that cover all areas of coding as well as other certifications that are very specific to certain areas of coding. Many HIM employers require one of the following coding certifications as a requirement for hire.

- **Certified Coding Associate (CCA):** The CCA credential offered by the American Health Information Management Association (AHIMA) is a nationally recognized HIM certification that focuses on inpatient and outpatient settings. CCA-certified individuals are committed, competent, and qualified to be professionals within the field of HIM and have basic ICD diagnostic and procedural and CPT coding knowledge (AHIMA 2017a).

- **Certified Coding Specialist (CCS):** The CCS credential, offered by AHIMA, is a highly regarded credential across both hospital and physician office settings. It indicates that a coder is proficient in ICD-10-CM, CPT, medical terminology, disease processes, pharmacology, and is familiar with the relationship between codes and their impact on practice revenues and patient health outcomes (AHIMA 2017b).

- **Certified Professional Coder (CPC):** The CPC credential is offered by the American Academy of Professional Coders (AAPC) for coders reporting professional services performed in both outpatient and inpatient settings. Individuals who obtain this certification demonstrate proficiency in ICD-10-CM, CPT, and HCPCS codes across a wide range of services and comprehend coding guidelines and regulations, including compliance and reimbursement for medical services. For coders interested in inpatient coding, the AAPC also offers the Certified Inpatient Coder (CIC) certification (AAPC 2017b).

- **Certified Billing and Coding Specialist (CBCS):** The CBCS, offered by the National Healthcareer Association (NHA), demonstrates a basic knowledge of billing and coding in the outpatient setting only. This includes the gathering and verification of patient demographics, a working knowledge of fraud and abuse in the medical setting, assigning ICD-10-CM, CPT, and HCPCS codes, and working with healthcare providers to receive optimal reimbursement for services provided (NHA 2017b).

Additional Certifications

Additional certifications in the field of HIM and health information technology are plentiful, to say the least. From medical billing to clinical documentation, informatics, and electronic health records, there are many career avenues that you can explore by obtaining a certification in a healthcare field other than coding. It is a good idea to start with a basic coding or billing certification, work in the industry for a few years to get experience, and then find a niche in which you can excel. Once you find this niche, you can pursue a certification in this field to prove to your employer, or to potential employers, that you are an expert in that area.

There is no glass ceiling with medical billing and coding. You can truly go as far as you want to go, and one of the best ways to move up is to get an additional certification. Figure A.1 shows many common and desirable certifications in multiple areas of billing, coding, and HIM, and the professional organization that offers each.

Figure A.1. Additional professional certifications

Professional Organization	Coding	Billing & Health Information Management	Practice Management & Administration	Health Information Technology	Other
American Health Information Management Association (AHIMA)	Certified Coding Associate (CCA), Certified Coding Specialist (CCS)	Registered Health Information Associate (RHIA), Registered Health Information Technician (RHIT)	Registered Health Information Associate (RHIA)	Certified Healthcare Technology Specialist (CHTS), Certified Professional in Health Informatics (CPHI)	Certified Health Data Analyst (CHDA), Certified in Healthcare Privacy and Security (CHPS), Certified Documentation Improvement Practitioner (CDIP)
American Academy of Professional Coders (AAPC)	Certified Professional Coder (CPC), Specialty Coding Certifications	Certified Professional Biller (CPB)	Certified Professional Practice Manager (CPPM)		Certified Professional Medical Auditor (CPMA), Certified Risk Adjustment Coder (CRC)
National Healthcareer Association (NHA)	Certified Billing and Coding Specialist (CBCS)	Certified Billing and Coding Specialist (CBCS)		Certified Electronic Health Records Specialist (CEHRS)	
Association of Clinical Documentation Improvement Specialists (ACDIS)					Certified Clinical Documentation Specialist (CCDS)
Medical Group Management Association (MGMA)			Certified Medical Practice Executive (CMPE)		

Professional Organizations

Certifications within the fields of billing, coding, and HIM are offered by professional organizations such as those listed below. Whether you obtain a certification from one of these organizations or not, it pays to be a member of the corresponding organization as you typically receive a number of benefits, such as monthly or quarterly publications with insights from the field, and access to networking forums where you can discuss important topics with others in the industry. As a student of medical billing and coding, there are three main professional organizations of which you need to be aware:

- **American Health Information Management Association (AHIMA).** AHIMA is an organization for HIM professionals and is a respected leader in the management of health data, heath records, and delivery of quality healthcare. They offer cutting-edge programs, professional development opportunities, continuing education, textbooks, credentials, online education, newsletters, monthly publications, and more. AHIMA is also significant as it is one of the four cooperating parties that collaborates to create and revise ICD-10 guidelines (AHIMA 2017c).

- **American Academy of Professional Coders (AAPC).** The AAPC was originally founded with the purpose of providing education and certifications to medical coders, but has expanded to elevate the entire profession of medical coding. It now provides training, 32 different certifications, networking opportunities, job opportunities, and monthly publications. Training and certifications provided by the AAPC cover not only medical coding, but also billing, medical auditing, clinical documentation, medical compliance, and practice management (AAPC 2017a).

- **National Healthcareer Association (NHA).** The NHA provides training and certifications for eight allied health careers including medical assistants, medical administrative assistants; phlebotomy, EKG, pharmacy, and patient care technicians; and medical billing, coding, and HIM professionals. The NHA's entry-level billing and coding credential, the CBCS, is an entry-level credential of choice for medical billing, coding, and HIM programs at vocational colleges (NHA 2017a).

Once you enter the world of healthcare, you might encounter additional professional organizations, such as the Association of Clinical Documentation Improvement Specialists (ACDIS) or the Medical Group Management Association (MGMA), to which you may become a member, depending on your job title and responsibilities. No matter which organization you choose, it is a good idea to become a member of at least one of these organizations to remain up to date in your field of expertise, as well as to improve your chances of career success.

Membership in a professional organization typically requires an annual membership fee, and if you have a certification, you must maintain continuing education units (CEUs). As discussed in chapter 1, a CEU is a unit of measurement used in continuing education programs, and a certified coder must attain a certain number of CEUs each year to maintain his or her certification. CEUs are earned by engaging in educational training, webinars, or in-field activities that show that you are keeping up to date with your profession. Depending on your type and number of certifications, you may need to complete more or less CEUs. It pays to do your research, determine the medical setting in which you want to work, join the right professional organization for you, and set your sights toward the future!

References

AAPC. 2017a. About Us. https://www.aapc.com/aboutus/.

AAPC. 2017b. Certified Professional Coder (CPC®). https://aapc.com/certification/cpc/.

AHIMA. 2017a. Overview of Certified Coding Associate (CCA®). http://www.ahima.org/certification/CCA.

AHIMA. 2017b. Overview Certified Coding Specialist (CCS®). http://www.ahima.org/certification/CCS.

AHIMA. 2017c. Who We Are. http://www.ahima.org/about/aboutahima.

NHA. 2017a. About NHA. https://www.nhanow.com/about-nha.

NHA. 2017b. Certified Billing & Coding Specialist (CBCS). https://www.nhanow.com/certifications/billing-coding.

Appendix B: Answer Key to There's a Code for That Exercises

Chapter 3 Basics of Coding

There's a Code for That 3.1

1. Procedure: Psychoanalysis and physical examination
Diagnosis: Depression

2. Procedure: Appendectomy
Diagnosis: Ruptured appendix (includes the diagnosis of severe abdominal pain, fever, and vomiting)

3. Procedure: Evaluation and management service
Diagnosis: Asthma

4. Procedure: Extended evaluation and management service
Diagnosis: Asthma with acute exacerbation (includes the diagnosis of wheezing and trouble breathing)

5. Procedure: Chest x-ray
Diagnosis: Pneumonia, left lower lobe

Chapter 4 Learning the ICD-10-CM Code Book

There's a Code for That 4.1

1. Pain
2. Disease
3. Difficulty
4. Degeneration
5. Hernia

There's a Code for That 4.2

1. Nonessential
2. Essential
3. Nonessential
4. Nonessential
5. Essential

There's a Code for That 4.3

1. ICD-10 Code: J13
2. ICD-10 Code: L22
3. ICD-10 Code: R13.12
4. ICD-10 Code: R48.8
5. ICD-10 Code: M04.2
6. ICD-10 Code: Q45.9

There's a Code for That 4.4

1. ICD-10 Code: D12.2
2. ICD-10 Code: C44.41
3. ICD-10 Code: C00.0
4. ICD-10 Code: C78.7
5. ICD-10 Code: D01.7
6. ICD-10 Code: C68.0

There's a Code for That 4.5

1. ICD-10 Code: T59.891
2. ICD-10 Code: T43.1X5
3. ICD-10 Code: T62.0X2
4. ICD-10 Code: T60.1X1
5. ICD-10 Code: T62.2X3
6. ICD-10 Code: T40.2X4

There's a Code for That 4.6

1. Injury mechanism: Struck by soccer ball
ICD-10 Code: W21.02

2. Place of occurrence: soccer field
ICD-10 Code: Y92.322

3. Activity: Soccer
ICD-10 Code: Y93.66

4. Patient status: Recreational or sport, not for income
ICD-10 Code: Y99.8

There's a Code for That 4.7

1. A-initial
D-subsequent
S-sequela

2. A-initial encounter for closed fracture
B-initial encounter for open fracture
D-subsequent encounter for fracture with routine healing
G-subsequent encounter for fracture with delayed healing
K-subsequent encounter for fracture with nonunion
S-sequela

3. 0-not applicable or unspecified
1-mild stage
2-moderate stage
3-severe stage
4-indeterminate stage

4. 0-not applicable or unspecified
1-fetus 1
2-fetus 2
3-fetus 3
4-fetus 4
5-fetus 5
9-other fetus

There's a Code for That 4.8

1. A-initial
2. D-subsequent
3. S-sequela
4. A-initial (patient is still in active treatment phase for the injury)

There's a Code for That 4.9

1. C
2. ICD-10 code: W54.0XXA
3. ICD-10 code: S60.00XD
4. ICD-10 code: W35.XXXA

Chapter 5 Learning the CPT and HCPCS Code Books

There's a Code for That 5.1

1. C. Category III
2. A. Category I
3. A. Category I
4. B. Category II
5. B. Category II

There's a Code for That 5.2

1. Appendix F
2. Appendix E
3. Appendix C
4. Appendix D
5. Appendix P

There's a Code for That 5.3

1. Index entry: 47544
2. Index entry: 96101
3. Index entry: 58262, 58263, 58291, 58292

4. Index entry: 58552, 58554
5. Index entry: 27598, 27880-27882

There's a Code for That 5.4

1. No, 20605
2. No, 61538
3. Yes
4. Yes
5. No, 58956

There's a Code for That 5.5

1. Index entry: G8417-G8422
2. Index entry: G0009
3. Index entry: A4650-A4927
4. Index entry: V5254-V5261
5. Index entry: G0127
6. Index entry: Q0481

There's a Code for That 5.6

1. No, E1615
2. Yes
3. Yes
4. No, Q0112
5. No, K0007

Chapter 6 Supplies and Services

There's a Code for That 6.1

1. HCPCS code: A0431
2. HCPCS modifier: SH
3. HCPCS code: A0431-SI
   HCPCS code: A0436 x 15
4. HCPCS code: A0431-SH
   HCPCS code: A0436 x 13
   Transportation Indicator: D2
   ICD-10 code: S41.111A
5. HCPCS code: A0130-RN
   HCPCS code: A0380 x 7
   ICD-10 code: G82.50
   ICD-10 code: Z99.11

There's a Code for That 6.2

1. HCPCS modifier: A5
2. HCPCS modifier: T3

3. HCPCS modifier: RT
4. HCPCS modifier: NU
5. HCPCS modifier: KL
6. HCPCS modifier: LM
7. HCPCS modifier: JA
8. HCPCS modifier: E2

There's a Code for That 6.3

1. HCPCS code: A4620
   HCPCS code: A4616 x 2
   ICD-10 code: J43.9
2. HCPCS code: K0019 x 2
3. HCPCS code: A4376
4. HCPCS code: A6412 x 5
5. HCPCS code: S8451

There's a Code for That 6.4

1. HCPCS code: J0135
2. HCPCS code: J0400 x 2
   ICD-10 code: F31.9
3. HCPCS code: J1650
   ICD-10 code: D68.2
4. HCPCS code: J7610 x 2
   ICD-10 code: J45.21

Chapter 7 Behavioral Health

There's a Code for That 7.1

1. Type of service: office visit
   Patient status: new
   Place of service: outpatient office
   E/M codes: 99201-99205
2. Type of service: subsequent care
   Patient status: N/A
   Place of service: nursing facility
   E/M codes: 99307-99310
3. Type of service: behavior change intervention (individual)
   Patient status: new
   Place of service: N/A
   E/M codes: 99406-99409

4. Type of service: initial care
   Patient status: inpatient
   Place of service: hospital
   E/M codes: 99221-99223

5. Type of service: emergency department visit
   Patient status: N/A (in the emergency department setting, patients are not identified as either new or established, see CPT guidelines)
   Place of service: emergency department
   E/M codes: 99281-99285

There's a Code for That 7.2

1. E/M Code: 99202
2. E/M Code: 99215
3. E/M Code: 99212
4. E/M Code: 99222
5. E/M Code: 99231
6. E/M Code: 99243
7. E/M Code: 99308
8. E/M Code: 99284

There's a Code for That 7.3

1. CPT Code: 90839
2. CPT Code: 90876
3. CPT Code: 90832-95
4. CPT Code: G0397
5. CPT Code: 90837, 90785
6. CPT Code: 90867

There's a Code for That 7.4

1. ICD-10 Code: F32.0
2. ICD-10 Code: F41.1, F33.1 Z62.819
3. ICD-10 Code: F50.02
4. ICD-10 Code: F91.3
5. ICD-10 Code: F11.21
6. ICD-10 Code: F43.12, Z65.5

There's a Code for That 7.5

1. CPT Code: 90867
   ICD-10 Code: F33.2

2. CPT Code: 90865
   ICD-10 Code: F10.24

3. CPT Code: 99205
   ICD-10 Code: F10.150

4. CPT Code: 99223
   ICD-10 Code: F20.0

5. CPT Code: 90832, 90863
   ICD-10 Code: F31.12, F40.11

Chapter 8 Primary Care

There's a Code for That 8.1

1. **8 elements** (location, right knee; quality, aching; severity, 4/10; duration, three days ago; timing, constant; modifying factors, when he lifts his leg; associated signs and symptoms, numbness, tingling, or redness of skin), level of HPI is **extended**

2. **5 systems** (constitutional, generally fine; allergic/immunologic, no problems; integumentary, no rash/no bruising; musculoskeletal, muscle cramps pain in knee joint; neurological; no tingling), level of ROS is **extended**

3. **Established, 1 element from each type of history** (past medical, no known drug allergies, no joint or immunologic problems or past injuries; family history, no history of osteoarthritis; social history, patient is active in football), level of PFSH is **complete**

4. **Detailed** (extended HPI, extended ROS, and complete PFSH bring the level of history to detailed. If the ROS was complete, then the level of history would be comprehensive, but because the level of ROS was extended,

then it is the lowest common denominator, and it brings down the levels of HPI and PFSH to detailed.)

Level of History	HPI	ROS	PFSH
Problem focused	Brief	N/A	N/A
Expanded problem focused	Brief	Problem pertinent	N/A
Detailed	Extended	Extended	Pertinent
Comprehensive	Extended	Complete	Complete

There's a Code for That 8.2

1. **5 body areas/organ systems** (cardiovascular, respiratory, lymphatic, musculoskeletal, integumentary), level of exam is **expanded problem focused** (limited exam of affected area and other related/symptomatic organ systems)

There's a Code for That 8.3

1. **4 points**, level of this element is **extensive**
2. **1 point**, level of this element is **minimal**
3. Level of this element is **low**
4. **Low**

There's a Code for That 8.4

1. **99213** (comprehensive history, expanded problem focused exam, low complexity MDM)

There's a Code for That 8.5

1. CPT Code: 99381
2. CPT Code: 99396
3. CPT Codes: 99392, 99212-25
4. CPT Code: 99396-32
5. Modifier: -57

There's a Code for That 8.6

1. CPT Codes: 90471, 90657

2. CPT Codes (DTaP admin): 90460, 90461 X 2
   CPT Code (DTaP): 90700
   CPT Code (Varicella admin): 90460
   CPT Code (Varicella): 90716

3. CPT Codes (HPV admin and serum): 90471, 90649
   CPT Codes (Meningococcal admin and serum): 90472, 90734

4. CPT Code (E/M service): 99392
   CPT Codes (rotavirus admin and serum): 90471, 90680
   CPT Codes (Hep B admin and serum): 90472, 90744
   CPT Codes (IPV admin and serum): 90474, 90713
   CPT Codes (influenza admin and serum): 90474, 90660

There's a Code for That 8.7

1. CPT Code (E/M service): 99203-25
   CPT Code (urinalysis): 81005
   CPT Code (catheterization): 51701

2. CPT Code: 17110

3. CPT Codes: 99392, 99173

There's a Code for That 8.8

1. ICD-10 Code: J11.1

2. ICD-10 Codes: R50.9, R51, J02.9

3. ICD-10 Codes: R10.31, R11.2

4. ICD-10 Codes: Z00.110

5. ICD-10 Codes: Z00.00, Z23, Z85.3, Z90.11

There's a Code for That 8.9

1. ICD-10 Code: E11.9

2. ICD-10 Codes: E11.3293, E11.36, Z79.84

3. ICD-10 Codes: E24.9, E08.9

4. ICD-10 Codes: E11.9, I10, E78.5, E66.09, Z68.34

5. ICD-10 Code: E10.9

6. ICD-10 Codes: I11.0, I50.21

7. ICD-10 Codes: I12.9, N18.3, E11.40, I50.9

8. ICD-10 Codes: J44.0, J20.9

9. ICD-10 Codes: J45.41, Z77.22

There's a Code for That 8.10

1. CPT Codes: 99213-25, 69210
   ICD-10 Codes: H61.22, H66.011

2. CPT Code: 99212
   ICD-10 Codes: N39.0, B95.62

3. CPT Codes: 99214, 85025
   ICD-10 Codes: N18.3, D63.1

4. CPT Codes: 99215, 99173
   ICD-10 Codes: E11.321, E11.36, Z79.4

5. CPT Codes: 99396, 90471, 90658
   ICD-10 Codes: Z00.00, Z23

Chapter 9 Eye and Vision Services

There's a Code for That 9.1

1. CPT Codes: 92014, 92015

2. CPT Codes: 92004, 76514, 92132, 92083

3. CPT Codes: S0621, V2020, V2100-RT, V2100-LT, V2750

4. CPT Codes: 99213-57, 65222

There's a Code for That 9.2

1. CPT Code: 67210-RT

2. HCPCS Code: S0800

3. CPT Code: 65820, 66990

4. CPT Code: 66984

5. CPT Code: 67801-E4

There's a Code for That 9.3

1. ICD-10 Code: Z01.00

2. ICD-10 Codes: Z01.01, H52.221

3. ICD-10 Codes: E11.3511, E11.3592

4. ICD-10 Code: Q12.0

5. ICD-10 Code: H40.1131

6. ICD-10 Codes: H26.122, W21.210S

7. ICD-10 Code: H35.30

There's a Code for That 9.4

1. CPT Code: 92225
   ICD-10 Codes: H53.149, H53.19, H43.392

2. CPT Codes: 67312-LT, 67314-LT, 67334-LT
   ICD-10 Code: H50.012

3. CPT Code: 67105-RT
   ICD-10 Code: H33.011

Chapter 10 Urgent Care and Emergency Department Services

There's a Code for That 10.1

1. CPT Codes: 99202, 73110, S9088

2. CPT Codes: 99214, 87880, 85025, 99051

3. CPT Codes: 12032, 12052-59, 12004-59, S9088

4. CPT Codes: 99214, 87850, 99051, S9088

There's a Code for That 10.2

1. CPT Codes: 99283-25, 30320, 99151

2. CPT Codes: 31500

3. CPT Code: 30901

4. CPT Code: 20103

5. CPT Code: 99285-25, 62270

There's a Code for That 10.3

1. ICD-10 Code: M25.562, Y93.72

2. ICD-10 Codes: S71.111A, S71.011A, S31.119A, S51.811A, S41.011A, S01.81XA

3. ICD-10 Codes: B27.90

4. ICD-10 Code: J13

5. ICD-10 Codes: S20.219A, W52.XXXA, Y93.66, Y92.322, Y99.8

There's a Code for That 10.4

1. ICD-10 Code: I21.21

2. ICD-10 Codes: I21.02, I25.2

3. ICD-10 Codes: A41.02, R65.21, N17.9

4. ICD-10 Code: T22.692A, T22.691A, T23.691A, T23.692A, T31.30

There's a Code for That 10.5

1. CPT Codes: 99285, 74176
   ICD-10 Code: K35.80

2. CPT Codes: 99213-25, 94760, 94640, 90471, 90658, S9088, 99051
   ICD-10 Codes: J45.41

3. CPT Code: 32551
   ICD-10 Codes: S27.0XXA, V57.0XXA

Chapter 11 Surgical Procedures

There's a Code for That 11.1

1. Code range: 61000-61070

2. Code range: 24800-24802

3. Code range: 55000

4. Code range: 53400-53520

5. Code range: 57452-57461

There's a Code for That 11.2

1. Modifier: -53

2. Modifier: -51

3. Modifier: -55

4. Modifier: -74

5. Modifier: -PB

6. Modifier: -66

There's a Code for That 11.3

1. CPT Code: 11643
   ICD-10 Code: C44.321

2. CPT Code: 11200
   ICD-10 Code: L91.8

3. CPT Code: 17110
   ICD-10 Code: B07.8

4. CPT Codes: 17263, 17262 -51, 17261 -51, 17260 -51
   ICD-10 Codes: C43.61, C43.62 (Each lesion destruction should be listed separately, with modifier -51 to indicate that they were multiple procedures all performed in the same surgical session. Diagnosis code C43.61 supports the medical necessity for all three of the procedures performed on the right arm/shoulder, and it should only be reported once.)

5. CPT Code: 17311
   ICD-10 Code: C44.319

There's a Code for That 11.4

1. CPT Code: 14000 (Note that lesion excision is included within the skin advancement code and is not coded separately)
   ICD-10 Code: D23.5

2. CPT Code: 16025
   ICD-10 Code: T24.202

3. CPT Code: 15935 (Note that the skin flap closure is included within the code description and is not coded separately)
   ICD-10 Code: L89.154

There's a Code for That 11.5

1. CPT Code: 49500
   ICD-10 Code: K42.9

2. CPT Code: 47562
   ICD-10 Code: K80.00

3. CPT Code: 44970
   ICC-10 Code: K35.3

Chapter 12 Anesthesia and Pain Management Services

There's a Code for That 12.1

1. 00402

2. 00406

3. CPT Code: 00211 (the base units for 00211 are 10, and the base units for 00215 are 9, so code 00211 would be reported, as it represents the most work-the highest number of base units)

4. CPT Code: 00520

There's a Code for That 12.2

1. CPT Code: 01382 -AA, -P1

2. CPT Code: 01742 -P2, -QX

3. CPT Code: 01990 -P6, QZ

4. CPT Codes: 00567 -AA, -P3, 99100

There's a Code for That 12.3

1. CPT Code: 95869

2. CPT Code: 62321

3. CPT Codes: 64615, 95873

4. CPT Code: 63655

There's a Code for That 12.4

1. ICD-10 Codes: T88.3XXA, T41.0X5A

2. ICD-10 Code: S72.301B

3. ICD-10 Codes: G89.29, M45.5

4. ICD-10 Code: M51.14

5. ICD-10 Code: M60.112

There's a Code for That 12.5

1. CPT Codes: 22513, 22515
   ICD-10 Code: S22.050A (chronic pain is not coded because the encounter is to treat the underlying condition

2. CPT Codes: 00620 -P2-QZ, 99100
   ICD-10 Code: S22.050A

3. CPT Code: 00580 -P4
   ICD-10 Code: D15.1, I50.9, I42

4. CPT Codes: 64490 -50, 64491 -50, 64492 -50

ICD-10 Codes: G89.29, M54.2, M25.511, M25.512, M79.601, M79.602

Chapter 13
Radiology and Imaging Services

There's a Code for That 13.1

1. a. Technical
2. b. Professional
3. c. Global
4. b. Professional
5. c. Global

There's a Code for That 13.2

1. CPT Code: 74150 (the contrast material is not coded because it was not administered intravenously, intrathecally, or intra-articularly)
2. CPT Code: 74176
3. CPT Code: 71046
4. CPT Code: 72050
5. CPT Code: 73222 HCPCS Code: Q9966 x 100
6. CPT Codes: 73610 -26, 73630-26

There's a Code for That 13.3

1. CPT Code: 76770
2. CPT Code: 78071
3. CPT Code: 76857
4. CPT Code: 77075
5. CPT Code: 77059
6. CPT Code: 78206

There's a Code for That 13.4

1. ICD-10 Code: R10.9
2. ICD-10 Code: E83.52
3. ICD-10 Codes: Z12.31, N63.20, Z80.3
4. ICD-10 Code: N20.2
5. ICD-10 Code: J81.0, I50.9

There's a Code for That 13.5

1. CPT Code: 73630 -LT ICD-10 Code: M79.672
2. CPT Codes: 70553, A9585 x 500 ICD-10 Codes: C72.41, H91.91
3. CPT Code: 74178 ICD-10 Codes: R10.9, Z90.49

Chapter 14
Laboratory and Pathology Services

There's a Code for That 14.1

1. B. Quantitative (this information is contained in the guidelines paragraph directly above the code)
2. B. Quantitative (this code is within the same subsection of codes as the previous one, and so the guidelines still apply)
3. A. Qualitative
4. A. Qualitative
5. B. Quantitative

There's a Code for That 14.2

1. CPT Code: 80053
2. CPT Codes: 82040, 84075, 84155, 84460, 84450
3. CPT Codes: 80053, 80061, 80074
4. CPT Code: 82009
5. CPT Code: 82128
6. CPT Codes: 83718, 83719, 83721

There's a Code for That 14.3

1. CPT Code: 80305
2. CPT Code: 80307
3. CPT Code: 80325
4. CPT Code: 82075
5. CPT Code: 80186

6. CPT Code: 80171
7. CPT Code: 80346

There's a Code for That 14.4

1. CPT Code: 81211
2. CPT Code: 80415
3. CPT Code: 81025
4. CPT Code: 87086
5. CPT Code: 87660

There's a Code for That 14.5

1. CPT Code: 88304 x 2
2. CPT Codes: 88305
3. CPT Code: 88307, 88305 x 2

There's a Code for That 14.6

1. ICD-10 Codes: Z11.4, Z20.6, Z71.7, Z72.51
2. ICD-10 Code: A49.02
3. ICD-10 Code: A40.0
4. ICD-10 Codes: B20, C46.51
5. ICD-10 Code: J09.X2
6. ICD-10 Code: A56.19
7. ICD-10 Code: A02.0

There's a Code for That 14.7

1. CPT Codes: 88175, 87624 ICD-10 Codes: R87.619
2. CPT Codes: 87077, 87181 ICD-10 Codes: L02.31, B95.62

Chapter 15
Orthopedic Services

There's a Code for That 15.1

1. CPT Codes: 27356, 27358
2. CPT Code: 24073
3. CPT Codes: 21045, 21215
4. CPT Code: 28041

There's a Code for That 15.2

1. CPT Code: 20606 -50
2. CPT Code: 20610-RT
3. CPT Code: 20612, 20612 -59

There's a Code for That 15.3

1. CPT Code: 24505-RT

2. CPT Code: 28420

3. CPT Codes: 26605, 26605 -59, 26605 -59

4. CPT Codes: 26605, 26608
   CPT Codes: 73110, 29075
   (Reporting the evaluation and management procedure for this encounter would be considered unbundling. The CPT code book states that additional E/M services should be reported only if they identify significant, further services, other than the application of the cast or strapping.)

There's a Code for That 15.4

1. CPT Codes: 22610, 22614 x 3

2. CPT Codes: 29827, 29824 -51, 29828 -59, 29826

There's a Code for That 15.5

1. ICD-10 Code: S82.852A

2. ICD-10 Code: S82.852K

3. ICD-10 Code: S52.351B

4. ICD-10 Codes: S02.0XXA, S06.5X0A

5. ICD-10 Codes: S22.41XA, S62.101A

6. ICD-10 Codes: M13.152, S72.002S

7. ICD-10 Code: S42.432D

8. ICD-10 Code: M84.374G

9. ICD-10 Code: M84.521K, C79.51

There's a Code for That 15.6

1. ICD-10 Code: M25.361, S83.271S

2. ICD-10 Code: S83.222A

3. ICD-10 Code: S86.011A

4. ICD-10 Codes: S83.512A

There's a Code for That 15.7

1. CPT Codes: 20610-RT, 73562-RT
   ICD-10 Codes: M65.161, E66.01, E11.9, F17.220

2. CPT Code: 27236-RT
   ICD-10 Codes: S72.031A, W01.0XXA, Y92.010

Chapter 16
Physical, Speech, and Occupational Therapy Services

There's a Code for That 16.1

1. CPT Code: 97010

2. CPT Code: 97018

3. CPT Code: 97110 x 2

4. CPT Code: 96001 (Gait training is bundled into the code for comprehensive gait and motion analysis procedures, and should not be reported separately)

5. CPT Code: 97140 x 3

6. CPT Codes: 97167, 97535

There's a Code for That 16.2

1. CPT Code: 92507

2. CPT Code: 92523

3. CPT Code: 97127 x 2

4. CPT Code: 92606

5. HCPCS Code: V5336

There's a Code for That 16.3

1. ICD-10 Code: G80.1

2. ICD-10 Code: G10

3. ICD-10 Code: M25.661, M17.11, Z96.651

4. ICD-10 Codes: M54.2, G89.29

There's a Code for That 16.4

1. CPT Code: 97542 x 3
   ICD-10 Codes: G82.21, S24.114D

2. CPT Code: 92610
   ICD-10 Codes: I69.091, R13.12, I69.051, I69.020

3. CPT Code: 97537
   ICD-10 Code: Q90

Chapter 17
Obstetrics and Gynecology Services

There's a Code for That 17.1

1. CPT codes: 99212, 81025

2. CPT code: 56634-LT

3. CPT code: 56810

4. CPT code: 58544

5. CPT codes: 99213, 58300, J7298

6. CPT codes: 57455, 58110

7. CPT code: 99214

There's a Code for That 17.2

1. CPT code: 59320

2. CPT code: 59514

3. CPT code: A. 59425
              B. 59515

4. CPT code: 59400

5. CPT code: 59001

6. CPT code: 59830

There's a Code for That 17.3

1. ICD-10-CM Code: N92.2

2. ICD-10-CM Codes: Z31.69, E28.2

3. ICD-10-CM Code: R87.619

4. ICD-10-CM Code: N95.1, G47.00, R51

5. ICD-10-CM Code: N76.0

There's a Code for That 17.4

1. ICD-10-CM Codes: Z34.82, Z3A.16

2. ICD-10-CM Codes: T22.212A, Z33.1, Z3A.32

3. ICD-10-CM Codes: O98.712, Z21, Z3A.22

4. ICD-10-CM Codes: O24.415, Z79.84

5. ICD-10-CM Codes: O99.332, Z71.6, F17.210, Z3A.20

There's a Code for That 17.5

1. CPT Code: 58120
   ICD-10 Code: N80.0

2. CPT Code: 59612
   ICD-10 Code: O34.219, O70.1, Z37.0, Z3A.38

3. CPT Code: 99214
   ICD-10 Code: N83.201, N83.202

Chapter 18 Medical Specialist's Services, Part I

There's a Code for That 18.1

1. CPT codes: 57156, 77332

2. CPT code: 77290

3. CPT code: 77762

4. CPT code: 77261

5. CPT code: 77412

6. CPT codes: 96360, 96361

7. CPT code: 96402

8. CPT code: 96450

There's a Code for That 18.2

1. ICD-10-CM Code: D50.9

2. ICD-10-CM Codes: C25.9, D63.0

3. ICD-10-CM Code: C02.2

4. ICD-10-CM Codes: N63.11, Z80.3, Z15.01

5. ICD-10-CM Code: C78.02

6. ICD-10-CM Codes: Z51.11, C22.3

There's a Code for That 18.3

1. CPT code: 61253

2. CPT code: 61519

3. CPT code: 61690

4. CPT code: 62192

5. CPT code: 63015

6. CPT codes: 63077, 63078 X 2

There's a Code for That 18.4

1. ICD-10 Codes: G20, F02.81

2. ICD-10 Code: G11.0

3. ICD-10 Code: G21.4

4. ICD-10 Codes: G31.83, F02.80

5. ICD-10 Code: G35

6. ICD-10 Code: G40.A19

There's a Code for That 18.5

1. CPT code: 50070

2. CPT code: 50400

3. CPT code: 50590

4. CPT codes: 51728-51, 51741

5. CPT code: 54115

6. CPT code: 55650-50

7. CPT code: 55866

8. CPT code: 90961

9. CPT code: 90945

There's a Code for That 18.6

1. ICD-10 Codes: N18.6, Z99.2

2. ICD-10 Code: N32.81

3. ICD-10 Codes: E29.1, N52.1

4. ICD-10 Codes: N40.1, R39.16

5. ICD-10 Code: C61

6. ICD-10 Code: N39.46

There's a Code for That 18.7

1. CPT code: 99245
   ICD-10-CM Codes: C50.412, Z17.0, Z80.3

2. CPT Code: 27365
   ICD-10-CM Code: C40.22

3. CPT Code: 64858
   ICD-10-CM Code: S74.02XA

4. CPT Code: 99253
   ICD-10-CM Code: G40.301

Chapter 19 Medical Specialist's Services, Part II

There's a Code for That 19.1

1. CPT code: 45338

2. CPT code: 45300

3. CPT code: 43235

4. CPT code: 43100

5. CPT code: 43205

6. CPT code: 43282

7. CPT code: 43870

8. CPT codes: 44202, 44203

9. CPT code: 44390

There's a Code for That 19.2

1. ICD-10-CM Codes: K21.0, F10.20

2. ICD-10-CM Codes: Z12.11, K63.5

3. ICD-10-CM Code: C19

4. ICD-10-CM Code: K25.2

5. ICD-10-CM Code: K50.112

6. ICD-10-CM Code: K58.0

7. ICD-10-CM Code: K91.2

There's a Code for That 19.3

1. CPT code: 33011

2. CPT code: 33391, 33141

3. CPT code: 33422

4. CPT codes: 33512, 35572-80

5. CPT codes: 33533, 33518

6. CPT codes: 35539, 35500

7. CPT code: 36415

8. CPT codes: 33249, 33225

9. CPT code: 75635

10. CPT codes: 75822, 36005

11. CPT codes: 92997, 92998

There's a Code for That 19.4

1. ICD-10 Code: I20.1

2. ICD-10 Code: I48.1

3. ICD-10 Code: I51.7

4. ICD-10 Code: I63.112

5. ICD-10 Codes: I70.442, L97.222

6. ICD-10 Code: I82.4Z2

7. ICD-10 Cods: I27.82, Z79.01

8. ICD-10 Code: I71.4

9. ICD-10 Codes: I83.11, I83.12, I83.813

There's a Code for That 19.5

1. CPT code: 43235
   ICD-10-CM Code: K22.710

2. CPT code: 43753
   ICD-10-CM Codes: R10.84, R11.10, R03.0, T62.1X1A

3. CPT code: 34846
   ICD-10-CM Codes: I71.3, I13.10, N18.3, F17.210

Chapter 20 Inpatient Hospital Services

There's a Code for That 20.1

1. ICD-10-PCS Code: 0TY10Z0, Transplantation of Left Kidney, Allogeneic, Open Approach
   ICD-10-CM Code: N18.6, End stage renal disease

2. ICD-10-PCS Code: 0W2BX0Z, Change Drainage Device in Left Pleural Cavity, External Approach

ICD-10-CM Code: J93.11, Primary spontaneous pneumothorax

3. ICD-10-PCS Code: 0DJ08ZZ, Inspection of Upper Intestinal Tract, Via Natural or Artificial Opening Endoscopic
   ICD-10-CM Code: R10.13, Epigastric pain, R13.10, Dysphagia, unspecified

4. ICD-10-PCS Code: 0WQF0ZZ, Repair Abdominal Wall, Open Approach
   ICD-10-CM Code: K42.9, Umbilical hernia without obstruction or gangrene

Glossary

8-minute rule: When reporting time-based codes, for any time over 15 minutes, the additional time must be at least 8 minutes over the 15-minute unit to report an additional unit of the service; each additional 8 minutes over the last 15-minute mark equals one additional unit

Abdominal aortic aneurysm (AAA): An aneurysm located in the abdominal aorta, which can be life-threatening if it bursts

Ablation: A procedure that destroys tissue performed in several different ways including laser surgery, electrosurgery, cryosurgery, chemosurgery, surgical curettement, radiocautery, radiofrequency ablation, or tissue volume reduction; also called *destruction*

Abortion: Procedure performed to evacuate the uterus of the products of conception, or the remaining fetal and placental tissues after either a spontaneous miscarriage or elective pregnancy termination

Accidental intent: An unintentional effect of a substance that was either taken on accident or in excess

Accountable Care Organization (ACO): A legal entity that is recognized and authorized under applicable state, federal, or tribal law, is identified by a Taxpayer Identification Number (TIN), and is formed by one or more ACO participant(s) that is (are) defined at 425.102(a) and may also include any other ACO participants described at 425.102(b) (42 CFR 425.20 2011)

Accreditation: 1. An evaluative process in which a healthcare organization undergoes an examination of its policies, procedures, and performance by an external organization ("accrediting body") to ensure that it is meeting predetermined criteria. It usually involves both on- and off-site surveys (CMS 2017a) **2.** The act of granting approval to a healthcare organization based on whether the organization has met a set of voluntary standards developed by an accreditation agency

Acquired condition: Condition that develops over the course of a person's life

Activity: What the patient was doing when the injury occurs

Acupuncture: An ancient method of treating a variety of medical ailments, that consists of inserting thin, flexible needles into specific areas of the body, to restore the body's balance and relieve discomfort

Acute conditions: Severe and sudden onset of conditions

Add-on code: A CPT/HCPCS code that describes a service that, excluding codes associated with the National Correct Coding Initiative (NCCI), is always performed in conjunction with another primary service (CMS 2017b)

Administrative personnel: Individuals who handle the daily functions of the business side of the healthcare practice, such as sending claims and billing patients, as well as non-clinical patient services such as healthcare records requests, registering patients, scheduling appointments, and sending referrals to healthcare specialists

Administrative safeguards: Under HIPAA, administrative actions and policies and procedures to manage the selection, development, implementation, and maintenance of security measures to protect electronic protected health information and to manage the conduct of the covered entity's or business associate's workforce in relation to the protection of that information (45 CFR 164.304 2013)

Admitting provider: The provider that admitted the patient to the hospital

Advanced beneficiary notice (ABN): A notice that a doctor or supplier should give a Medicare beneficiary when furnishing an item or service for which Medicare is expected to deny payment. If you do not get an ABN before you get the service

(Continued on next page)

from your doctor or supplier, and Medicare does not pay for it, then you probably do not have to pay for it (CMS 2017a)

Advanced life support (ALS): A higher level of care used for patients with life-threatening illnesses, injuries, or other severe conditions, during transport to a facility that can provide them with full medical care that includes life-saving protocols to further support airway, breathing, and circulation

Adverse effect: An unintended effect caused by a substance that is correctly prescribed and correctly administered

Allograft: A skin graft from tissue from a donor

Alteration: Modifying the anatomic structure of a body part without affecting the function of the body part

Alzheimer's disease: A progressive form of dementia that causes loss of memories and cognitive abilities that interfere with activities of daily living

Ambulance modifier: Modifiers required on ambulance claims that identify the origin and destination for each transportation

Ambulance supplier: Those tasked with transporting a patient with a healthcare need to a provider or facility capable of treating that need usually in an emergency or urgent situation; the emergency responders must stabilize and provide a certain level of healthcare services to the patient until he or she can receive care from a healthcare provider

Ambulatory surgical center (ASC): Under Medicare, an outpatient surgical facility that has its own national identifier; is a separate entity with respect to its licensure, accreditation, governance, professional supervision, administrative functions, clinical services, recordkeeping, and financial and accounting systems; has as its sole purpose the provision of services in connection with surgical procedures that do not require inpatient hospitalization; and meets the conditions and requirements set forth in the Medicare Conditions of Participation; Also called ambulatory surgical center

American Health Information Management Association (AHIMA): The professional membership organization for managers of health record services and healthcare information systems as well as coding services; provides accreditation, advocacy, certification, and educational services

Amputation: The complete removal of a body part, performed to remove dead, diseased, or damaged tissue, leaving only healthy and functional tissue behind

Amputee: The patient who has undergone an amputation

Amyotrophic lateral sclerosis (ALS): Also known as Lou Gehrig's Disease, a degenerative disease in which motor neurons slowly die, causing muscle weakness, stiffness, and twitching; and for which there is no cure

Analgesia: The inability to feel pain

Anemia: Occurs when a person has abnormally low red blood cells or hemoglobin in the blood

Anesthesia section: Section of the CPT code book that lists services performed by anesthesiologists, anesthesia assistants, or other healthcare providers

Anesthesia services: Procedures that create analgesia, the absence of pain, and are provided for a brief amount of time to facilitate a medical procedure, such as a surgery

Anesthesiology: The healthcare specialty of relieving patient pain before, during, and after surgery

Aneurysm: The bulging or ballooning of a small portion of an artery, caused by weakening or degeneration of the wall of the vessel

Angiography: The x-ray examination of blood vessels after the administration of a contrast material

Antepartum: The period of pregnancy before childbirth

Anterior: Situated toward the front of the body (such as the face or the breasts)

Antero-posterior: Two projections during an imaging service consisting of two views that pass through the front to the back of the body

Anxiety disorders: Mental disorders that result in constant feelings of worry, fear, and panic when faced with everyday situations

Aphonia: Loss of voice

Appendectomy: Removal of the appendix

Appendicitis: A noninfectious process, such as heatstroke or a traumatic injury

Arthritis: An inflammation of the joints

Arthrocentesis: The aspiration of a joint, a process that involves inserting a hollow needle into a joint or bursa to allow for the removal of fluid

Arthrodesis: The surgical fixation of a joint, performed to treat deformities of the bones and pain

Arthropathy: Any disease of the joints

Arthroplasty: Surgical repair of a joint

Arthroscopy: An endoscopically-assisted procedure of a joint

ASA crosswalk: A book that crosswalks all applicable CPT surgical and therapeutic procedure codes to the appropriate anesthesia codes

Assault: A toxic effect that occurs due to assault is one that was purposefully inflicted upon one person by another person, with the intent of hurting the recipient of the substance

Atherosclerosis: The hardening of fatty substances within the blood vessels, which leads to a buildup of plaque; this narrows the diameter of the blood vessel and reduces blood flow, and causes the formation of blood clots that can travel through the vessels and cause further obstruction of blood flow

Attention-deficit hyperactivity disorder: Disorder that typically appears in school-age children and impact a child's school and social functioning; symptoms include impulsivity, inattention, difficulty concentrating and following directions, difficulty completing tasks, too much energy and restlessness

Augmentative and alternative communication (AAC): Method used to communicate with other people that does not include oral communication; for example, hand gestures or facial expressions when speaking

Autograft: A skin graft from a different site from the patient's own body

Axial plane: A horizontal line, perpendicular to the long axis of the body that divides the body into superior and inferior portions (the top and the bottom halves); also known as the transverse plane

Bacteriology: The study of bacteria

Bariatric surgery: Surgery performed on the stomach or intestines to induce weight loss

Bartholin's glands: Greater vestibular glands that secrete mucus to lubricate the vagina

Base units: A set of numerical values created and maintained by the American Society of Anesthesiologists (ASA), that give each anesthesiology service a numerical relative value in relation to how complicated or risky a procedure is, and are used to set the relative cost of each procedures

Basic life support (BLS): A basic level of care that is used for patients with life-threatening illnesses, injuries, or other severe conditions, while they are being transported to a facility that can provide them with full medical care

Behavioral health services: A broad array of psychiatric services provided in acute, long-term, and ambulatory care settings; includes treatment of mental disorders, chemical dependency, mental retardation, and developmental disabilities, as well as cognitive rehabilitation services

Benign neoplasm: Non-cancerous growths of tissue that are not invasive and will not spread to other tissues

Benign prostatic hyperplasia (BPH): A condition in which the prostate gland is enlarged, which causes urinary frequency and urgency, nocturia (urinating at night), and urinary retention (among other symptoms)

Bilateral: Affecting both right and left sides

Billable code: A code that has been extended out to the full amount of required characters

Bipolar disorder: A mental disorder that affects a person's mood and behavior by switching from extreme highs (called mania) to extreme lows (called depression)

Birthing center: A facility that specializes in providing a comfortable setting for labor, delivery, postpartum care, and immediate newborn care

Block: Frozen specimen being examined by the surgeon

Body area: General area of the body, rather than specific organ systems, which may be examined during an evaluation and management encounter

Brachytherapy: A cancer treatment method in which small radioactive seeds, capsules, or elements are placed within or near a cancer or cancerous organ

Burn codes: Codes for thermal burns that come from a heat source such as fire or hot appliance

Business associates (BAs): 1. A person or organization other than a member of a covered entity's workforce that performs functions or activities on behalf of or affecting a covered entity that involve the use or disclosure of individually identifiable health information **2.** As amended by HITECH, with respect to a covered entity, a person who creates, receives, maintains, or transmits PHI for a function or activity regulated by HIPAA, including claims processing or administration, data analysis, processing or administration, utilization review, quality assurance, patient safety activities, billing, benefit management, practice management, and repricing or provides legal, actuarial, accounting, consulting, data aggregation, management, administrative, accreditation, or financial services (45 CFR 160.103 2013)

Bypass: Altering the route of passage of the contents of a tubular body part

Cadaver donor: Brain dead patient from whom organs are being harvested

Capitation: A specified amount of money paid to a health plan or doctor. This is used to cover the cost of a health plan member's healthcare services for a certain length of time (CMS 2017a)

Carcinoma in situ: Neoplasms that are potentially cancerous growths of tissue

Cardiac electrophysiology: The study of the electrical system of the heart

Cardiologist: A healthcare provider who specializes in the diagnosis and treatment of the diseases of the heart, coronary vessels, and cardiovascular system

Cardiopulmonary bypass (CPB): A technique in which a machine takes over the function of the heart and lungs during surgery

Cardiopulmonary resuscitation (CPR): A medical procedure that involves the healthcare provider repeatedly compressing a patient's chest in an attempt to circulate the blood and restore breathing to a patient who has suffered cardiac arrest (a stopping of the heart)

Cardiothoracic surgery: Surgery that focuses on the surgical treatment of the heart and organs within the thorax (such as the lungs)

Category I code: The largest set of codes within the CPT code book, commonly referred to as simply CPT codes; these procedures have been approved by the Food and Drug Administration (FDA), are performed by physicians or other healthcare practitioners throughout the United States at a frequency consistent with their intended clinical use, are consistent with current clinical practice, and have a documented clinical efficacy for treating healthcare conditions

Category II code: Codes intended to facilitate data collection for performance measurement purposes; category II codes are supplemental tracking codes that report the performance of a test, evaluation, counseling service, or other procedure that is part of a facility's performance measurement program

Category III code: A set of temporary codes used to report emerging technology, services, procedures, and service paradigms, and the use of these codes is integral to the identification and establishment of new healthcare procedures and treatments

Catheterization: Procedure that involves the insertion of a catheter tube in through the urethra and into the bladder to drain urine

Centers for Medicare and Medicaid Services (CMS): The Department of Health and Human Services agency responsible for Medicare and parts of Medicaid. Historically, CMS has maintained the UB-92 institutional EMC format specifications, the professional EMC NSF specifications, and specifications for various certifications and authorizations used by the Medicare and Medicaid programs. CMS is responsible for the oversight of HIPAA administrative simplification transaction and code sets, health identifiers, and security standards. CMS also maintains the HCPCS medical code set and the Medicare Remittance Advice Remark Codes administrative code set (CMS 2017a)

Central venous access devices (CVAD): Flexible tubes inserted in patients who require frequent access to the bloodstream; they can stay in place for up to a year

Cerclage: A stitch or band device that helps the cervix remain closed at the external os

Cerebrospinal fluid (CSF) shunt: A small one-way valve that is inserted within the ventricles of a patient's brain to allow for the drainage of cerebrospinal fluid from the brain and into the peritoneal cavity

Certificate of Medical Necessity (CMN): An official document completed by the physician and the DME supplier that details the patient's diagnosis, necessity for the DME supply, and other important patient demographics and information

Certified Coding Associate (CCA): The CCA credential offered by the American Health Information Management Association (AHIMA) is a nationally recognized HIM certification that focuses on inpatient and outpatient settings. CCA-certified individuals are committed, competent, and qualified to be professionals within the field of HIM and have basic ICD diagnostic and procedural and CPT coding knowledge (AHIMA 2017a)

Certified Coding Specialist (CCS): An AHIMA credential awarded to individuals who have demonstrated skill in classifying medical data from patient records, generally in the hospital setting, by passing a certification examination

Certified nurse midwife (CNM): A mid-level practitioner (as discussed in chapter 1) with an advanced degree as a registered nurse in midwifery, the study of assisting pregnant females in obstetric care and childbirth, including the postpartum period, female care, and birth control

Cervicalgia: Neck pain

Cervix uteri: Also known as the cervix, is the lowest part of the uterus, about two to three centimeters long and round in shape, and forms a canal from the upper portion of the vagina to the uterus

Change: Removing a device from a body part and replacing it with an identical or similar device in or on the same body part without cutting or puncturing the skin or a mucous membrane

Charge amount: A price assigned to a unit of medical or health service, such as a visit to a physician or a day in a hospital; may be unrelated to the actual cost of providing the service

Chemodenervation: The injection of botulinum toxin, a potent neurotoxin, to an affected nerve for

Chemotherapy: The use of a drug to treat a medical condition

Chief complaint (C/C): The principal problem a patient reports to a healthcare provider

Children's Health Insurance Program (CHIP): A program similar to Medicaid that covers children in low-income families but whose income is not low enough to qualify for Medicaid coverage

Cholangiography: An examination of the bile ducts, used to identify an obstruction

Cholangitis: Inflammation of the bile ducts

Cholecystectomy: Removal of the gallbladder

Cholecystitis: Inflammation of the gallbladder

Choledocholithiasis: The presence of one of more gallstones within the common bile duct

Cholelithiasis: The presence of gallstones

Chronic condition: A syndrome or condition that has been in development for a long period of time, and is a constant disease state

Chronic Obstructive Pulmonary Disease (COPD): A lung disease characterized by chronically poor airflow; symptoms include shortness of breath, chronic cough, and sputum production

Chronic pain: Constant or long-term sensation of pain that may be due to postoperative complications, past injuries, or nerve conditions

Circumcision: The surgical removal of the foreskin at the tip of the penis

Classification system: A clinical vocabulary, terminology, or nomenclature that lists words or phrases with their meanings, provides for the proper use of clinical words as names or symbols, and facilitates mapping standardized terms to broader classifications for administrative, regulatory, oversight, and fiscal requirements

CLIA-waived: Status that allows performance of certain in-office laboratory procedures, such as blood counts and bacterial cultures; CLIA-waived laboratory tests are simple and have low risk

Clinical modification (CM): The compilation of ICD codes used to report diagnoses

Clinical personnel: Individuals who are trained as healthcare providers or practitioners, such as doctors, nurse practitioners, and physician assistants, as well as personnel who are trained and qualified to provide assistive healthcare services, such as registered nurses, healthcare assistants, and clinical nursing assistants

Closed fracture: Fracture in which the broken bone does not penetrate the skin

Closed procedure: Procedure in which the skin is not opened to perform the procedure

Closed treatment: The site of the fracture is not surgically opened to perform the repair

CMS-1500: The uniform professional claim form (CMS 2017a)

Code edit: An accuracy checkpoint in the claims-processing software that ensures all codes are valid and may be reported in conjunction with each other, and if any modifiers are necessary

Code first: Instructions that list conditions that should be coded *before* the code identified

Code linkage: Linking the diagnosis and procedure code together to identify the medical necessity for specific procedures

Code table: A table of all of the character options for PCS codes

Coding certification: Professional document of achievement given only to those coders who can demonstrate proficiency on a coding examination

Coding guidelines: The rules that specify what codes to use in which situations, how to sequence them, which modifiers to use, and how to combine them with other codes

Cognitive communication disorder: Disorder that includes difficulties for patients when organizing thoughts, remembering, paying attention, planning, and problem-solving

Coinsurance: Cost sharing in which the policy or certificate holder pays a preestablished percentage of eligible expenses after the deductible has been met; the percentage may vary by type or site of service

Colonoscopy: The examination of the entire colon, from the rectum to the cecum at the end of the ascending colon, and may include an examination of the ileum

Colorectal surgery: Surgery of the colon, rectum, and anus

Combination code: Includes both the etiology and manifestation in one code

Commercial insurance: Insurance plans run by for-profit companies that are not government entities and require a monthly premium in return for healthcare coverage

Comminuted fracture: Fracture with more than two parts, usually with multiple broken pieces

Comorbid condition: 1. A medical condition that coexists with the primary cause for hospitalization and affects the patient's treatment and length of stay (IHS 2017) 2. Pre-existing condition that, because of its presence with a specific diagnosis, causes an increase in length of stay by at least one day in approximately 75 percent of the cases (as in complication and comorbidity [CC]) (HHS 2010, 23905)

Complication of care: A condition that occurs as a result of the medical care or surgery

Complication: 1. A medical condition that arises during an inpatient hospitalization (for example, a postoperative wound infection) (IHS 2017) 2. Condition that arises during the hospital stay that prolongs the length of stay at least one day in approximately 75 percent of the cases (as in complication and comorbidity [CC]) (HHS 2010, 23905)

Compound fracture: Fracture in which the bone penetrates the skin; otherwise known as an open fracture

Comprehensive ophthalmological services: Ophthalmological services that include a general evaluation of the complete ophthalmological system

Compression fracture: Fracture found in the spine that occurs when one or more vertebrae collapse under their own pressure

Computed tomography (CT): An imaging study that combines a number of x-ray images from different angles to produce a virtual cross-section of the area being studied; also known as computed axial tomography (CAT) scan

Computerized physician order entry (CPOE): Electronic systems that allow physicians to record medication or treatment orders, access electronic health records (EHR), and radiology, laboratory, and pharmacy applications electronically. These systems usually contain error prevention software that provides the user with prompts that warn against the possibility of drug interaction, allergy, or overdose and other relevant information condition; always reported as a secondary diagnosis conditions

Confidentiality agreement: A legal document signed by the employee after HIPAA training, which indicates that the employee has been trained in aspects of HIPAA compliance and agrees to abide by the healthcare facility's measures taken to ensure HIPAA compliance

Congenital condition: Condition that was present at or before birth

Conization: A procedure that uses either an electrical wire (LEEP), cold knife, or laser to remove a cone of tissue from the cervix, either for diagnostic purposes (biopsy) or to remove cancerous or precancerous cells

Constant attendance code: Code reported according the length of time that the provider spent performing the service

Consultation: An evaluation and management encounter that is provided by one healthcare professional, often a healthcare specialist, at the request of another healthcare professional, such as a primary care practitioner

Continuing education unit (CEU): Unit of measurement used in continuing education programs—any type of industry-specific training that offers specific instruction on a topic within the professional's field of expertise; a certified coder must attain a certain number of CEUs each year in order to maintain his or her certification

Contralateral: The opposite side of the body (the right arm and the left arm)

Contrast material: A substance that is injected into the patient to enhance the contrast of certain structures within the body while performing x-rays and imaging procedures

Contributory factors: Counseling, coordination of care, and the nature of the presenting problem, which are used to help determine the level of the E/M service

Control: Stopping, or attempting to stop, postprocedural or other acute bleeding

Conversion factor (CF): The dollar amount per unit for the reimbursement of anesthesia services

Coordination of care: The cooperation between at least two healthcare practitioners to provide care to a patient

Copayment: Cost-sharing measure in which the policy or certificate holder pays a fixed dollar amount (flat fee) per service, supply, or procedure that is owed to the healthcare facility by the patient. The fixed amount that the policyholder pays may vary by type of service, such as $20 per prescription or $15 per physician office visit

Coronal plane: A vertical line that divides the body into anterior and posterior halves (front and back)

Coronary artery bypass grafts (CABG): Procedures in which a small piece of vein or artery is used to bypass a coronary artery

Coronary artery disease: Occurs when atherosclerotic changes are detected in the arteries of the heart

Corpora cavernosa: Erectile tissue

Corpora spongiosum: Tissue that lies under the corpora cavernosa and forms the internal shape of the penis, with a bulbous shape at the end of the penis, and helps to prevent urethral compression during erection

Corpus uteri: Also known as the uterus, is the body of the uterus above the internal os of the cervix and connects to the fallopian tubes at the fundus at the top of the uterus

Corrosion codes: Codes for burns due to chemicals

Cortical cataract: Cataracts that begin on the peripheral edges of the lens and work their way inward toward the center

Counseling: The discussion between a healthcare provider and a patient and/or patient's family

Coverage limitations: The services that an insurance plan will pay for (cover) when they are provided by a healthcare practitioner, as well as what services will not be covered and classified as the patient's out-of-pocket charges

Covered entity: As amended by HITECH, (1) a health plan, (2) a healthcare clearinghouse, (3) a healthcare provider who transmits any health information in electronic form in connection with a transaction covered by this subchapter (45 CFR 160.103 2013)

Craniectomy: The removal of a portion of the skull

Craniotomy: An incision into the skull

Creation: Inserting biological or synthetic material to form a new body part that to the extent possible replicates the anatomic structure or function of an absent body part

Cross-reference: Instructs the coder to look elsewhere for a code

Current Procedural Terminology (CPT): A comprehensive, descriptive list of terms and associated numeric and alphanumeric codes used for reporting diagnostic and therapeutic procedures and other medical services performed by physicians; published and updated annually by the American Medical Association (AMA 2017)

Cytopathology: Study that examines cells from a specimen to determine a cause or nature of a disease

Data analytics: The science of examining raw data with the purpose of drawing conclusions about that information. It includes data mining, machine language, development of models, and statistical measurements. Analytics can be descriptive, predictive, or prescriptive

Date of service: The date a test, procedure, or service was rendered

Debridement: The removal of dead, diseased, infected, or otherwise nonviable tissue from a wound to improve the healing ability of the area

Deductible: 1. The amount of cost, usually annual, that the policyholder must incur (and pay) before the insurance plan will assume liability for remaining covered expenses. 2. Under Medicare, the amount a beneficiary must pay for healthcare before Medicare begins to pay, either for each benefit period for Part A, or each year for Part B, these amounts can change every year (CMS 2017a)

Deep vein thrombosis (DVT): Blood clot that forms in the deep veins of the lower extremities

Definitive diagnosis: The condition or disease that has been confirmed to be the cause of the signs exhibited or symptoms experienced

De-identified documentation: 1. The act of removing from a health record or data set any information that could be used to identify the individual to whom the data apply in order to protect his or her confidentiality 2. To remove the names of the principal investigator (PI), co-investigators, and affiliated organizations to allow reviewers to maintain objectivity

Delivery: Assisting the passage of the products of conception from the genital canal

Dementia: Loss of memory and mental abilities due to an underlying physical change in the brain Dentofacial anomaly

Depression: A mental disorder that affects a person's mood, thoughts, and actions

Destination: Location where the patient is taken by ambulance service

Destruction: 1. A procedure that destroys tissue performed in several different ways including laser surgery, electrosurgery, cryosurgery, chemosurgery, surgical curettement, radiocautery, radiofrequency ablation, or tissue volume reduction; also called *ablation;* 2. Physical eradication of all or a portion of a body part by the direct use of energy, force, or a destructive agent

Detachment: Cutting off all of a portion of the upper or lower extremities

Device: Any material or appliance that remains after a procedure is performed

Diabetes mellitus: A condition in which the body does not control the amount of glucose (sugar) in the blood, and the kidneys excrete large amounts of urine

Diagnosis: A word or phrase used by a physician to identify a disease from which an individual patient suffers or a condition for which the patient needs, seeks, or receives medical care

Diagnosis-related group (DRGs): 1. A unit of case-mix classification adopted by the federal government and some other payers as a prospective payment mechanism for hospital inpatients in which diseases are placed into groups because related diseases and treatments tend to consume similar amounts of healthcare resources and incur similar amounts of cost; in the Medicare and Medicaid programs, one of more than 500 diagnostic classifications in which cases demonstrate similar resource consumption and length-of-stay patterns. Under the prospective payment system (PPS), hospitals are paid a set fee for treating patients in a single DRG category, regardless of the actual cost of care for the individual. **2.** A classification system that groups patients according to diagnosis, type of treatment, age, and other relevant criteria. Under the prospective payment system, hospitals are paid a set fee for treating patients in a single DRG category, regardless of the actual cost of care for the individual (CMS 2017a)

Diagnostic and Statistical Manual of Mental Disorders (DSM-5): A nomenclature developed by the American Psychiatric Association to standardize the diagnostic process for patients with psychiatric disorders; the fifth edition is the product of more than 10 years of effort by hundreds of international experts in all aspects of mental health (APA 2017)

Diagnostic procedure: Procedure that is performed to determine a diagnosis

Dialysis: The process of filtering waste products from the blood, which replaces the function of the kidneys for patients with end-stage renal disease or renal failure

Diaphragm: 1. A barrier birth control method in which a small, cup-like device is placed over the cervix during intercourse, along with spermicide that is later removed; **2.** A muscle that lies underneath the thoracic cavity, separating the heart and lungs from the abdominal contents

Dilation: Expanding an orifice of the lumen of a tubular body part

Dislocation reduction: The act of relocating a joint to its original location, in the case of joint dislocation or subluxation (partial dislocation) dislodged and traveling into the lungs

Displaced fracture: Fracture in which the bone moves so the two ends of the bones are misaligned

Dissecting aneurysm: Aneurysm that contains a small tear in the inner lining of the arterial walls, in which blood is beginning to accumulate

Distal: Away from the body (the fingertips)

Diverticulitis: The inflammation of the diverticula small pockets lining the inside of the intestines

Diverticulosis: A condition in which diverticula begin forming within the intestines

Division: Cutting into a body part, without draining fluids or gases from the body part, to separate or transect a body part

Dominant side: The side of the body that the patient prefers when performing daily functions, such as writing with the right hand

Doppler ultrasound: A special technique that uses color-coded mapping during the ultrasound procedure, which allows the viewer to see oxygenated and de-oxygenated blood flow through body organs in real time

Dosimetry: Process performed to calculate the exact radiation dose amount

Drainage: Taking or letting out fluids or gases from a body part

Durable Medical Equipment (DME): Medical equipment designed for long-term use in the home, including eyeglasses, hearing aids, surgical appliances and supplies, orthotics and prostheses, and bulk and cylinder oxygen (CMS 2017a)

Durable Medical Equipment, Prosthetics, Orthotics, and Supplies (DMEPOS): A category of durable medical equipment supplies that includes prosthetics and orthotics

Dyslexia: Difficulty reading

Dysphagia: Difficulty swallowing

Eating disorders: Disorders that affect the way a person eats or processes food and nutrition; there are two types of eating disorders, anorexia nervosa and bulimia

Electrical stimulation: Therapeutic modality that causes one muscle or a group of muscles to contract, which helps to increase muscle strength and blood supply to the muscle, and decrease pain

Electrocardiogram (ECG/EKG): Procedure that records the heart's electrical activity as a line tracing on paper and can be used to evaluate heart rhythm and function

Electroconvulsive therapy (ECT): Involves the application of an electric current to a patient's brain to produce a seizure or series of seizures to alleviate mental illness

Electrodiagnostic studies: A way of measuring the electrical activity in muscles and nerves that can help diagnose the cause or specific area from which pain is originating

Electroencephalogram (EEG): A diagnostic study of the electrical impulses of the brain

Electromyography (EMG): Evaluates the condition of muscle and nerves to determine the cause of pain, such as a pinched nerve or a diseased muscle (Mount Sinai Hospital 2017a)

Electronic brachytherapy: The use of a small, high-dose x-ray source, applied directly to the malignancy

Electronic Protected Health Information (e-PHI): Protected health information (PHI) that is stored in an electronic format. As amended by HITECH, means information that comes within paragraphs (1)(i) or (1)(ii) of this definition of protected health information as specified in this section which is (1)(i) information transmitted by electronic media, and (1)(ii) information maintained in electronic media (45 CFR 160.103)

Embolus: Thrombosis that dislodges from the vessel and begins to travel through the blood

Emergency department: Facility that provides same-day care for patients with healthcare emergencies or urgent healthcare needs and may be either a standalone facility or attached to a larger facility, such as a hospital

Emergency services: Services provided to patients in a life-threatening situation, when loss of life or limb is imminent

Emergency transportation: Ambulance service that responds immediately to the scene of an accident or incident to provide medical assistance and transport to a healthcare facility if necessary

Emergent: Life-threatening medical issues

Employer-sponsored insurance: An umbrella term used to describe health plans that are funded directly by employers to provide coverage for their employees exclusively in which employers establish accounts to cover their employees' medical expenses and retain control over the funds but bear the risk of paying claims greater than their estimates

Encounter: The face-to-face contact between a patient and a provider who has primary responsibility for assessing and treating the condition of the patient at a given time and who exercises independent judgment in the care of the patient

Encryption: The process of transforming text into an unintelligible string of characters that can be transmitted via communications media with a high degree of security and then decrypted when it reaches a secure destination

Endocervical curettage (ECC): Cervical tissue removal in which a curette is used to scrape cells off of the cervical canal

Endoscopy: A procedure performed with the aid of an endoscope—a device with a small camera attached

Endotracheal intubation: Procedure performed to maintain an open airway, or to allow the administration of certain drugs, such as anesthesia (also called intubation)

Endovascular procedure: Procedure in which a catheter is inserted into the body to perform a procedure; literally, the procedure is performed "inside the vessel"

Enforcement Rule: Part of HIPAA that contains provisions that cover compliance to HIPAA rules and regulations, investigations into breaches in privacy, and the imposition of monetary penalties for HIPAA violations

Enthesopathy: An inflammation of the tendon or ligament at the site of attachment to the bone, which causes pain, tenderness, stiffness, and swelling

Entitlement health insurance: A type of insurance coverage for which individuals must be eligible, based on differing criteria

Enucleation: Removing the eyeball while leaving the orbital structures intact, including the extraocular muscles

Epididymis: A duct behind the testes, in which newly created sperm cells mature and then move into the vas deferens

Epidural steroid injection: A minimally invasive procedure that can treat pain in the neck, shoulders, arms, back, buttocks, and legs, resulting from irritation of spinal nerves due to conditions such as herniated discs, degenerative disc disease, and arthritis; it is an injection of long-lasting

(Continued on next page)

corticosteroid, which is an anti-inflammatory agent, and not an anesthetic substance

Epilepsy: A neurological condition that manifests in sensory disturbances, loss of consciousness, and seizures (convulsions) as a result of abnormal electrical activity in the brain

Episode of care: 1. In home health, all home care services and nonroutine medical supplies delivered to a patient during a 60-day period; the episode of care is the unit of payment under the home health prospective payment system (HHPPS) 2. The healthcare services given during a certain period of time, usually during a hospital stay (CMS 2017a)

Eponym: Coding convention in ICD-10-CM codes assigned to diseases or syndromes named for a person; listed in the alphabetic index as main terms in the index

Esophagogastroduodenoscopy (EGD): A common type of endoscopic examination of the digestive system that is a complete examination from the esophagus to the duodenum at the end of the stomach

Essential modifier: In ICD-10-CM and ICD-10-PCS, they qualify the main term by listing alternative sites, etiology or clinical status. It is indented two spaces under the main term; also called subterms

Established patient: A patient who has received professional services from the physician or another physician of the same specialty in the same practice group within the past three years

Etiology: The cause of a disease

Evaluation and management (E/M) service: A patient encounter with a healthcare professional in which the patient receives assessment, counseling, or routine health services

Evaluation and management services section: The first section of Category I codes in the CPT code book; these codes describe patient encounters with healthcare and make up the majority of all codes reported for professional services in either the inpatient or outpatient setting

Evisceration: The removal of the contents of the globe of the eye, while leaving the remaining structures intact

Examination: The act of evaluating the body to determine the presence or absence of disease

Excised diameter: The size of the lesion in addition to the margins around the lesion that were removed

Excision: Cutting out or off a portion of a body part without replacement

Excludes 1: Under ICD-10-CM, a type 1 Excludes note is a pure excludes note. It means "not coded here." An Excludes 1 note indicates that the code excluded should never be used at the same time as the code above the note (NCHS 2017)

Excludes 2: A type 2 Excludes note represents "not included here." An Excludes 2 note indicates that the condition excluded is not a part of the condition represented by the code, but a patient may have both conditions at the same time (NCHS 2017)

Excludes notes: Identify conditions that are similar but independent of each other

Exenteration: [Of the orbit] the removal of the eye and ocular adnexa

External cause codes: Codes used to identify the circumstances surrounding an injury, poisoning, or adverse event, such as the activity that the patient was engaged in when the injury occurred, where the patient was when the injury took place, and the injury mechanism (how the injury happened)

External Causes of Injury Index: Location where codes identifying the external cause of an injury or illness are listed

External os: Lower end of the cervix

Extirpation: Taking or cutting out solid matter from a body part

Extracapsular cataract extraction (ECCE): In this procedure the lens is either broken up via phacoemulsification or it is surgically removed in one piece, leaving the lens capsule intact

Extracorporeal shock wave lithotripsy (ESWL): A procedure in which shock waves are sent through the patient's body to break up a nephrolithiasis into tiny fragments

Extraction: Pulling or stripping out or off all or a portion of a body part by the use of force

Facet joint injection: Injections made into the facet joint of the vertebra, used to treat pain coming from the small joints of the spine

Fallopian tubes: Oviducts resembling long tubes that are attached to the fundus of the uterus and end with small finger-like fimbriae, through which eggs releases from the ovaries travel

Fee schedule: A complete listing of fees used by health plans to pay doctors or other providers (CMS 2017a)

Fee-for-service: A method of reimbursement through which providers retrospectively receive payment based on either billed charges for services provided or on annually updated fee schedules

Fibromyalgia: A myalgia characterized by chronic, full-body pain, with a sensitivity to pressure; also causes fatigue, problems sleeping, memory problems, restless leg syndrome, numbness or tingling, and other psychological factors, such as depression and anxiety

First-listed diagnosis: In outpatient coding, this is the first diagnosis code that is listed on a claim when more than one diagnosis code is applicable

Foreign body (FB): Any unnatural object that is present inside the body or organ structure

Fragmentation: Breaking solid matter in a body part into pieces

Frozen block: A frozen piece of a specimen

Frozen section: For procedures that need a pathological examination quickly, the specimen may be frozen rapidly into a frozen block (a frozen piece of a specimen), which is cut into small slices of the tissue (a frozen section), and visualized under a microscope

Fusion: Joining together portions of an articular body part rendering the articular body part immobile

Gastric bypass: Also called a Roux-en-Y procedure, a procedure in which a small stomach pouch is created by dividing the top of the stomach from the rest of the stomach; the first portion of the small intestine is separated and attached to the top stomach pouch, in essence creating a small stomach out of the larger stomach

Gastroenterologist: A healthcare provider who specializes in the diagnosis and treatment of disorders of the digestive system, including but not limited to disorders of the esophagus, stomach, intestines, colon, and rectum and anus

Gastro-esophageal reflux disease (GERD): A common condition that causes heartburn, indigestion, and chest pain in affected individuals

General anesthesia: The administration of a substance that results in a complete loss of consciousness in order to produce analgesia to facilitate a surgical or other healthcare procedure (Palmetto 2013)

Gestation: The time period between conception (the moment at which the egg is fertilized) and birth (when the fetus is delivered)

Gestational condition: Condition that is a direct result from pregnancy

Glaucoma: A buildup of intraocular pressure that causes damage to the eye's optic nerve over time, and may eventually lead to irreversible vision loss

Global period: Amount of time included in the surgical package

Global radiology service: The performance of both components of the procedure—professional and technical—by the same facility

Global surgical package: A set of services that are included within a single code that identify the surgery performed, other services that are integral to the procedure, and a certain amount of time after the surgery

Goniolens: An ophthalmic endoscope

Government-sponsored insurance: A type of entitlement health insurance coverage that is provided by the government and managed at either the state or the federal level or a combination thereof, depending on the type of insurance

Gravida: Pregnant female

Greenstick fracture: Fracture that occurs when a bone bends and cracks on one side

Gross examination: An examination of the physical characteristics of the specimen, including the size, weight, consistency, and visual features such as discoloring

Gustilo-Anderson classification: Classification used to identify the type of open fracture, which is included as part of the code description for open fractures

Gynecologists: Medical providers who specialize in the health of the female reproductive system including the vagina, uterus, and ovaries, as well as the breasts

HCC coding: Coding that is specially focused on capturing all patient conditions that impact the hierarchical condition category, and which are fully supported by documentation in the health record

HCPCS Level I codes: Commonly referred to as CPT and developed, maintained, and copyrighted by the AMA, these codes represent the healthcare procedure, treatment, or service provided at the healthcare encounter

HCPCS Level II codes: Commonly referred to as CPT as simply HCPCS or Level II codes, are codes developed, maintained, and published by CMS that represent the supply, service, or other treatment provided to the patient; they also include ambulance services

Health insurance exchange: Government-run health insurance exchange that allows insurance companies to offer health insurance plans to individuals, who must pay premiums for coverage

Health Insurance Marketplace: The federal online health insurance exchange that allows individuals to purchase insurance plans offered by commercial companies

Health Insurance Portability and Accountability Act (HIPAA): The federal legislation enacted to provide continuity of health coverage, control fraud and abuse in healthcare, reduce healthcare costs, and guarantee the security and privacy of health information; limits exclusion for pre-existing medical conditions, prohibits discrimination against employees and dependents based on health status, guarantees availability of health insurance to small employers, and guarantees renewability of insurance to all employees regardless of size; requires covered entities (most healthcare providers and organizations) to transmit healthcare claims in a specific format and to develop, implement, and comply with the standards of the Privacy Rule and the Security Rule; and mandates that covered entities apply for and utilize national identifiers in HIPAA transactions (Public Law 104-191 1996)

Healthcare billing: The practice of sending a coded healthcare claim to a third-party payer or insurance company for payment, described in full in Chapter 2, and then following that claim until it is paid in full

Healthcare codes: The numeric or alphanumeric translations of all the services, supplies, treatments, diagnoses, conditions, and other reasons for medical treatments

Healthcare coding: The practice of assigning numeric or alphanumerical codes to identify the treatment, services, or supplies provided to a patient during a healthcare encounter, also known as the procedure

Healthcare Common Procedure Coding System (HCPCS): A medical code set that identifies healthcare procedures, equipment, and supplies for claim submission purposes. It has been selected for use in the HIPAA transactions. HCPCS Level I contains numeric CPT codes which are maintained by the AMA. HCPCS Level II contains alphanumeric codes used to identify various items and services that are not included in the CPT medical code set (CMS 2017a)

Healthcare operations: Includes various services provided by healthcare practitioners during which patient PHI may be accessed and used

Healthcare provider: Physician or other qualified healthcare professional who is qualified by education, training, licensure/regulation (when applicable), and facility privileging (when applicable) who performs a professional service within his/her scope of practice and independently reports that professional service (AMA 2018, p. xii)

Healthcare specialty: A branch of healthcare practice in which a provider specializes after completing his or her residency after medical school, typically divided among four possible characteristics—surgical or internal technique, body or organ system, diagnostic or therapeutic services, or the age of patients treated

Heart failure: A condition in which the heart cannot pump enough blood to meet the body's needs

Hematologist: A healthcare provider who specializes in the diagnosis, treatment, and prevention of diseases of the blood (hematology)

Hemodialysis: The process of filtering the blood of waste products, through the use of a dialyzer machine, which removes the waste products from the blood

Hemothorax: Blood in the pleural cavity

Hierarchical Condition Category (HCC): The practice of placing all patient diagnosis claims into groups of conditions, which are positioned strategically in order of risk from least to most risky

Histologic type: The specific type of microscopic structure of the growth such as carcinoma, myeloma, or sarcoma

History of present illness (HPI): A chronological description of the development of the patient's present illness from the first sign or symptom or from the previous encounter to the present

History: The pertinent information about the patient, including chief complaint, past and present illnesses, family history, social history, and review of body systems

Homograft: A skin graft taken from a donor of the same species

Hospital: A healthcare entity that has an organized medical staff and permanent facilities that include inpatient beds and continuous medical or nursing services and that provides diagnostic and therapeutic services for patients as well as overnight accommodations and nutritional services

Hubbard tank: A large tub in which the patient can be fully immersed, to allow patients to perform exercises while in the water

Hydration: The administration of fluids or electrolytes without the presence of drugs

Hydrocele: A fluid-filled sac that can cause pain and discomfort

Hypercholesterolemia: A condition in which there are high levels of cholesterol in the blood

Hyperlipidemia: A condition in which there are high levels of lipids, or fats, in the blood

Hypernasality: Excessive nasal tone to the voice

Hypertension: High blood pressure

Imaging services: An inclusive term used for the wide array of different types of techniques used to produce images of the inside of the body, including radiology services, ultrasounds, fluoroscopy, and nuclear imaging

Immune globulin: Serum globulins that are extracted from human blood, or recombinant immune globulin products created in a laboratory through genetic modification of human and/or animal proteins

Impacted fracture: Fracture in which the ends of a bone are pushed into each other

Implantable cardiac defibrillator (ICD): A small device similar to a pacemaker that monitors the heart rate and delivers a small shock to the heart when it detects heart-threatening arrhythmias

Incidental appendectomy: Performed in addition to a primary procedure within the abdomen

Incidental pregnancy: Pregnancy that in no way complicates the reason for the medical encounter

Incision and drainage (I&D): A procedure performed on an abscess or cyst that requires drainage and consists of cutting into the skin above the cyst or abscess to allow for drainage of the pustular material; a treatment performed for soft tissue abscesses, for which medical treatment alone is insufficient; the abscess is incised with a sharp blade and drained of material

Incision: A cut made on a body part or organ

Includes notes: Coding convention in ICD-10-CM; a note listed below certain tabular list categories to further define, clarify or provide examples

Inclusion terms: These terms work similarly to includes notes, but instead pertain to specific codes, rather than a category of codes; they may be synonyms for the condition, or may be a list of various conditions that are assigned to a specific code

Indented code: Codes indented beneath a standalone code that depend on the explanation of the procedure within the standalone (or parent) code to complete the description of the indented code

Independent laboratory: A facility that is recognized and accredited to test and evaluate patient specimens as an independent entity free from a hospital or private practice

Independent radiology and imaging center: An office that specializes in only radiology and imaging techniques

Index to Diseases and Injury: The main index to the ICD-10-CM code book, often referred to as the Main Index

Individual insurance: Insurance plan that is purchased by a single individual, who does not go through an employer to attain coverage

Inferior: Toward the bottom of the body (the feet)

Infusion: The administration of a diagnostic, prophylactic, or therapeutic fluid or drug, given over a period of time longer than 15 minutes

Initial encounter: This episode of care is used during the active treatment phase of a condition, or when the patient is still receiving active treatment for a condition

Injection: Administration of a therapeutic substance given intramuscularly

Injury mechanism: The way an injury happens

Inpatient: A patient who is provided with room, board, and continuous general nursing services in an area of an acute care facility where patients generally stay at least overnight

Inpatient: A patient who is provided with room, board, and continuous general nursing services in an area of an acute care facility where patients generally stay at least overnight

Insertion: Putting a nonbiological appliance that monitors, assists, performs, or prevents a physiological function but does not physically take the place of a body part

Inspection: Visually or manually exploring a body part

Insurance policy: 1. A purchased contract (policy) according to which the purchaser (insured) is protected from loss by the insurer's agreeing to reimburse for such loss 2. Reduction of a person's (insured's) exposure to risk by having another party (insurer) assume the risk

Insured party: A holder of a health insurance policy

Integrative medicine: Consists of complementary and alternative therapies that may be used to treat chronic pain

Intensity Modulated Radiation Treatment Delivery (IMRT): A radiation treatment method that uses computer-based mapping to create dosing distributions delivered by a radiotherapy treatment machine

Intent: Intent of the toxic effect is the reason why the toxic effect happened

Intentional self-harm: A toxic effect resulting from intentional self-harm is due to a substance that is taken deliberately as an act of hurting one's self

Interactive complexity: A psychotherapy service that is provided to a patient with specific communication factors that complicate delivery of psychiatric procedures

Intermediate ophthalmological services: Ophthalmological services that include an evaluation of a new or existing condition complicated with a new diagnosis

Internal fixation device: A device that is inserted into or across a bone or set of bones to fix it into place

Internal medicine provider: Provider who establishes the diagnosis and treatment of patients without using surgical techniques

Internal os: The upper end of the cervix, which opens into the uterus

International Classification of Disease (ICD): Code set developed by the World Health Organization and revised for usage in the United States through a development committee composed of CMS, NCHS, AHA, and AHIMA

International Classification of Diseases, Eleventh Revision, ICD-11: Coding classification system currently in development, and is expected to be implemented after 2018

International Classification of Diseases, Ninth Revision, ICD-9: Code set composed of three volumes, all published in the same code book: Volumes one and two are the index and tabular listings for diagnosis codes, and volume three contains procedure codes and was replaced by the ICD-10-PCS code set, which is used in essentially the same manner, but has greatly expanded the specificity for reporting inpatient procedures

International Classification of Diseases, Tenth Revision, Clinical Modification ICD-10-CM: The coding classification system that replaced ICD-9-CM, Volumes 1 and 2, on October 1, 2015. ICD-10-CM is the United States' clinical modification of the WHO's ICD-10. ICD-10-CM has a total of 21 chapters and contains significantly more codes than ICD-9-CM, providing the ability to code with a greater level of specificity (CDC 2017)

International Classification of Diseases, Tenth Revision, Procedure Coding System ICD-10-PCS: The coding classification system that replaced ICD-9-CM, Volume 3, on October 1, 2015. ICD-10-PCS has 16 sections and contains significantly more procedure codes than ICD-9-CM, providing the ability to code procedures with a greater level of specificity (CDC 2017)

Interspace: The space between two vertebrae

Interstitial brachytherapy: Brachytherapy that involves placing the radioactive elements into a body cavity, such as the vagina or the bladder

Interventional pain procedures: A range of different procedures that utilize invasive interventions to treat the patient's pain, that include epidural injections, medial branch blocks and facet joint injections, radiofrequency nerve ablations, joint injections, occipital nerve blocks, and kyphoplasty

Intracapsular cataract extraction (ICCE): This procedure removes both the lens and the lens capsule, and is performed only in rare cases

Intracavitary brachytherapy: Brachytherapy that involves placing the radioactive elements directly into the tumor or organ

Intractable condition: Condition that does not respond to medical treatment

Intraocular pressure: The pressure inside the eyeball

Intrauterine device (IUD): A small, T-shaped device inserted into the uterus for birth control purposes

Introduction: The insertion of a device, object, or substance into a body part or organ

Introitus: The vagina orifice

Invalid code: A code that is not extended out to seven characters and may not be used for coding or billing purposes

Iontophoresis: A form of electrical stimulation that is used to push medication through the skin to the affected body area, muscle, tendon, or ligament

Ipsilateral: The same side of the body (the right upper and lower extremities)

Kidney: Bean-shaped organ that functions to filter waste products from the blood and to control electrolyte balance and the body's balance of fluid

Kyphoplasty: A treatment for vertebral compression fractures and the pain they cause where a balloon is threaded through an incision in the back, to the site of the compression fracture, and slowly inflated to push the compressed bone back into place; once in place, cement is injected into the area to hold the bone in the proper position (Mount Sinai Hospital 2017b)

Kyphosis: A condition in which the back rounds forward

Labia majora: The tissue that surrounds the labia minora and the clitoris

Labia minora: Skin that surrounds the vaginal vestibule and the external urethra

Laboratory and pathology services: Diagnostic analyses of bodily tissue samples, such as urine, blood, or tissue

Language disorder: Difficulty with understanding or producing oral speech

Laparoscopy: Procedure that uses a fiber-optic laparoscope inserted into the body through several small incisions to perform a diagnostic or therapeutic procedure

Large group practice: A practice that may have anywhere from six to dozens of providers

Last menstrual period (LMP): The first day of the patient's last period (start of menstruation)

Lateral (view): Two projections during an imaging service consisting of two views that pass from one side of the body to the other (for example, from the right to the left)

Lateral: Away from the midline of the body (the sides)

Laterality: Refers to the side on which a condition appears

Legacy system: A type of computer system that uses older technology but may still perform optimally

Lifestyle impairments: Descriptions of how the patient's eye condition has negatively impacted his or her lifestyle

Living donor: The organ being donated is one that can be harvested from a living patient

Local anesthesia: Anesthesia blocks a small amount of nerves using an injection or a topical cream or spray that numbs a specific amount of the body

Loop electrosurgical excision procedure (LEEP): Procedure in which a fine wire with an electrical charge is used to remove cervical tissue

Lower urinary tract symptoms (LUTS): The different symptoms that can be present with benign prostatic hyperplasia, such as urinary frequency, urinary retention, or urinary urgency

Lumbago: Low back pain

Lumbar puncture: A diagnostic procedure used to evaluate cerebrospinal fluid that surrounds the brain and spinal cord (also called a spinal tap)

Lund-Browder classification: Chart that divides the body's surface into differing percentages, depending on the age of the patient

Macular degeneration: A deterioration of the central portion of the retina, called the macula

Magnetic resonance imaging (MRI): A form of imaging that utilizes strong magnetic fields and radio waves to produce detailed images of the anatomy and physiology of the internal structures of a patient's body, and can be used to diagnose a range of medical conditions

Main term: The noun that describes the patient's diagnosis or reason for encounter

Malignant neoplasm: Commonly referred to as cancer, these neoplasms invade surrounding tissues and destroy them, and can be fatal

Malunion: Occurs when the bones have fused back together in the wrong position after a fracture

Mammography: An x-ray image of the breast used to diagnose breast conditions such as tumors or fibrocystic diseases

Manifestation: Coding convention in ICD-10-CM; a condition that occurs as the result of another

Manipulation: Manually moving one body part into its original location or into another location; the attempt to return a fractured bone to its original location with manually applied forces

Map: Locating the route of passage of electrical impulses or locating functional areas in a body part

Margin: The area around a lesion that is excised in addition to the lesion

Marsupialization: A procedure in which a cyst is incised along one edge to form an open pouch, and then sutured open to allow for continuous drainage

Maternal fetal medicine (MFM) specialist: A medical doctor who specializes in high-risk pregnancies and focuses on the health of the mother and fetus before, during, and after pregnancy

Maternity services: Procedure or condition is one that is performed on a pregnant woman or related to a woman's pregnancy, such as a delivery or complication of pregnancy

Medial: Toward the midline of the body (the belly button

Mediastinum: The area within the thorax in-between the lungs

Medicaid: A joint federal and state program that helps with medical costs for some people with low incomes and limited resources. Medicaid programs vary from state to state, but most healthcare costs are covered if a patient qualifies for both Medicare and Medicaid (CMS 2017a)

Medical decision making (MDM): The portion of the evaluation and management encounter in which the healthcare provider makes a decision about the patient's diagnosis and care or treatment plan

Medical necessity: 1. The likelihood that a proposed healthcare service will have a reasonable beneficial effect on the patient's physical condition and quality of life at a specific point in his or her illness

(Continued on next page)

or lifetime 2. The concept that procedures are only eligible for reimbursement as a covered benefit when they are performed for a specific diagnosis or specified frequency (42 CFR 405.500 1995)

Medicare: A federally funded health program established in 1965 to assist with the medical care costs of Americans 65 years of age and older as well as other individuals entitled to Social Security benefits owing to their disabilities (CMS 2017a)

Medicine section: The last section of the Category I codes in the CPT code book; it is a miscellaneous grouping of all of the procedures, treatments, studies, and tests that can be performed on patients, which do not belong elsewhere in the book

Medigap: A supplemental insurance policy that is specifically for Medicare beneficiaries designed to "fill the gap" left by patient out-of-pocket expenses such as copayments, deductibles, and coinsurance amounts

Mental health: A person's emotional, psychological, and social well-being

Mental illness: A condition that affects a person's thinking, feeling, or mood, and affects a person's ability to perform major life activities and functions each day

Metastasis: Offshoots (spreading) of the original cancer

Methicillin-resistant Staphylococcus aureus (MRSA): A bacterium that can cause infections throughout the human body; it is resistant to certain antibiotics, making it especially hard to treat and cure

Methicillin-susceptible Staphylococcus aureus (MSSA): A strain of the same Staphylococcus aureus bacteria that is susceptible to antibiotics, rather than resistant to them like methicillin-resistant Staphylococcus aureus

Microscopic examination: The examination of the specimen at a microscopic level, which allows the pathologist to visualize the cells of a specimen

Mid-level provider: Additional healthcare providers who are also trained, qualified, and licensed to provide healthcare services

Minimum necessary: States that only the least amount of information needed for treatment, payment, and healthcare operations may be released from a patient's health record

Minor surgical procedure: Minimally invasive (meaning that they only break the skin or mucous membranes and connective tissues) procedures that do not require any general anesthesia or respiratory assistance during the procedure

Moderate (conscious) sedation: A drug-induced depression of consciousness that allows a patient to respond to commands and tactile stimulation during a medical or surgical procedure; a type of anesthesia given either orally or via an injection that allows the patient to be sedated but awake, so he or she can respond to commands if necessary

Modifier: A two-digit numeric code listed after a procedure code that indicates that a service was altered in some way from the stated CPT descriptor without changing the definition; also used to enhance a code narrative to describe the circumstances of each procedure or service and how it individually applies to a patient

Modifying factors: Factors similar to CPT modifiers, that add additional information to the anesthesia procedure description and describe an anesthesia procedure that was more complex than it would have been had it been performed on a normal, healthy patient, or that required additional skill to complete

Modifying term: Term that alters (or modifies) the main term; it is indented below the main term, and present different versions of the procedure

Mohs micrographic surgery: Surgery used for the removal of complex and ill-defined skin malignancies, and includes the examination of all the excised margins; the surgeon acts as both the surgeon and the pathologist

Monitored anesthesia care (MAC): An anesthesia service that is made up of a conscious sedation, control of patient anxiety, and pain control

Monoarthritis: Arthritis in a localized joint

Morphology: The science of structure and form of organisms without regard to function

Motor vehicle accident (MVA): Any type of accident that involves any type of motor vehicle

Multiple sclerosis (MS): A disease that affects the central nervous system and causes nerve deterioration and damage

Musculoskeletal system: The body system comprised of all the bones, joints, muscles, cartilage, tendons, and ligaments in the human body

Myalgia: Muscle pain, which may be a symptom of many medical conditions including overuse of the muscle, overstretching, infection, or disease process

Mycology: The study of fungi

Myocardial infarction: The death of a portion of the heart muscle due to lack of oxygen supply; otherwise known as a heart attack

Myositis: An inflammation of the muscle that can be caused by an infection, injury, medicine, or a chronic disease, and causes muscle weakness and pain, along with other symptoms

Narcosynthesis for psychiatric purposes: The administration of sodium amobarbitol, otherwise known as a truth serum, which hinders inhibitions so that a psychiatric interview can be conducted

Nasal packing: Procedure performed for uncontrollable hemorrhage from the nose (epistaxis or bloody nose)

National Correct Coding Initiative (NCCI): Program developed to promote national correct coding methodologies and to control improper coding leading to inappropriate payment in Part B claims (CMS 2017b)

Nature of the presenting problem: The type of condition for which the patient is receiving the evaluation and management service

Neoplasm of uncertain behavior: Neoplasms that have not yet been confirmed as any of the other three types (benign, malignant, or ca in situ) and require further evaluation and testing before their behavior can be determined

Neoplasm: An abnormal growth of tissue that can be fast-growing and invasive, such as malignant cancer, or a benign mass or tumor

Nephrolithiasis: Kidney stones

Nephrolithotomy: Incision into the kidney for the removal of a kidney stone

Nephrologist: A medical doctor who focuses on the diagnosis and treatment of conditions of the kidneys

Nerve condition study (NCS): A test that activates nerves and gauges their responses as a way of determining if there is a problem with the functioning of the nerve

Neurologist: A medical doctor who specializes in the diagnosis and treatment of neurological disorders, including disorders of the nerves and the nervous system

Neuropsychiatry: The treatment of mental or behavioral disturbances as a result of neurological

Neurosurgery: Surgical treatment of disorders of the nerves and nervous system

Never events: A term coined in 2001 by Ken Kizer of the National Quality Forum (NCF) to identify serious errors in medical treatment that should never happen (AHRQ 2017)

New patient: An individual who has not received professional services from the physician, or any other physician of the same specialty in the same practice group before or within three years; an individual who has not received professional services from any provider of a organization/ healthcare facility before or within three years

Non-ambulatory: Unable to walk about independently

Noncovered services: Services not reimbursable under a managed care plan

Non-displaced fracture: Fracture in which the bone itself is fractured, but the bone has not moved and is still properly aligned

Nonemergency transportation: Ambulance services typically scheduled in advance for patient transfers from one facility to another, or to transport non-ambulatory patients for healthcare

Nonessential modifier: Words located in parentheses next to the main term or a subterm within the Index that offer more information, but do not impact code selection

Non-obstetric: Refers to a procedure performed to treat or manage signs and symptoms, or other medical encounter for gynecological or genitourinary services, such as reproductive, urinary, and breast health

Non-pressure ulcer: An ulcer on the skin that was caused by anything other than pressure, such as one caused by atherosclerosis of the extremities (and loss of blood circulation), chronic venous hypertension, diabetes mellitus, postthrombotic syndrome, postphlebitic syndrome, or varicose veins

Non-ruptured aneurysms: Often symptom-less aneurysms that are typically found during a radiological imaging procedure

Nonspecific test: Tests for a quality, such as whether or not any type of drug from a drug class is present

Nonunion: Occurs when the bones have not fused back together after a fracture

Not elsewhere classifiable (NEC): In ICD-10-CM this abbreviation in the Alphabetic Index represents "other specified" when a specific code is not available for a condition (NCHS 2017)

Not otherwise specified (NOS): In ICD-10-CM this abbreviation is the equivalent of unspecified (NCHS 2017)

Notice of Privacy Practices: As amended by HITECH, a statement (mandated by the HIPAA Privacy Rule) issued by a healthcare organization that informs individuals of the uses and disclosures of patient-identifiable health information that may be made

(Continued on next page)

by the organization, as well as the individual's rights and the organization's legal duties with respect to that information (45 CFR 164.520 2013)

Nuchal cord: Umbilical cord around the neck

Nuclear cataract: Cataracts that form in the nucleus of the lens and are often associated with aging

Nuclear medicine: The practice of using small radioactive elements designed to travel to a specific organ or type of tissue, which are introduced into the patient through an intravenous injection

Nulligravida: Female who has never been pregnant

Nulliparous: Female who has never carried a pregnancy longer than 20 weeks

Oblique fracture: Travels diagonally across the bone

Oblique: Two projections during an imaging service consisting of two views that pass through the body at a diagonal angle

Obstetric: Refers to a procedure performed on a pregnant woman or condition related to a woman's pregnancy, such as a delivery or complication of pregnancy

Obstetricians: Medical providers who specialize in the health of a patient during pregnancy, childbirth, and the postpartum period

Obstetrics and gynecology services: Services focused on the gynecological and reproductive health of female patients, as well as providing services for pregnant patients and performing deliveries

Occipital nerve block: An injection directly into the greater and lesser occipital nerves, used to treat headaches and migraines (Mount Sinai Hospital 2017b)

Occlusion: Completely closing an orifice or the lumen of a tubular body part

Occupational therapist (OT): A healthcare professional who uses constructive activities to help restore a patient's ability to perform essential activities of daily living (occupations) and improve or maintain functional ability

Occupational therapy services: Noninvasive procedures aimed at improving fine motor skills and functions

Ocular adnexa: The accessory structures of the eye, including the extraocular muscles, eyelids, lacrimal system, orbit, and optic nerve and pathways

Official Guidelines for Coding and Reporting (OGCR): The set of official guidelines for the use of the ICD-10-CM code set, published by the set of four organizations that make up the Cooperating Parties for ICD-10: AHA, AHIMA, CMS, and NCHS

Oncologist: A healthcare provider who specializes in the development, diagnosis, and treatment of malignant neoplasms and tumors (oncology)

Open fracture: Fracture in which the bone penetrates the skin

Open procedure: Procedure in which the skin is incised (or cut into) to perform the procedure

Open treatment: The fracture site has been surgically opened to visualize the fracture site or apply internal fixation devices

Ophthalmologist: Healthcare provider who specializes in pathology and diseases of the eyeball, and performs surgeries to correct eye problems

Ophthalmology: Practitioners in this field specialize in the anatomy, physiology, and pathology of diseases of the eyeball, and perform medical and surgical procedures on the ey

Optometrist: Healthcare specialist who examines the eyes for visual defects, such as myopia (nearsightedness), and prescribes lenses to correct the defect (either glasses or contact lenses)

Optometry: Practitioners in this field perform examinations of the ophthalmological system, as well as medical treatment and management of eye conditions

Orchiopexy: Surgical fixation of undescended testes in the scrotal sac

Organ system: Specific group of organs that may be examined during an evaluation and management encounter

Origin: Location where a patient is picked up for transportation service

Orthopedic services: Services that focus on the management and treatment of conditions affecting the musculoskeletal system, such as fractures, arthritis, joint sprains and strains, and osteoporosis

Orthopedist: A medical doctor who specializes in correcting congenital or acquired abnormalities of the bones and musculoskeletal system through the use of casting, bracing, and surgical techniques

Orthotics: Instruments used on the outside of the body to support, align, or correct deformities, or to improve the movements of joints, the spine, or the limbs (CMS 2017)

Osteoarthritis: A degenerative condition of the joints that results from wear and tear of the cartilage between joints, and causes pain, swelling, and problems with range of motion of the joint

Osteoarthritis: A type of arthritis that results from wear and tear on the joints over a period of time

Otitis: Ear infection

Outcome of delivery code: Code that identifies the number of births and if they were live or stillborn

Out-of-pocket expense: Healthcare costs that a patient must pay out of pocket because they are not covered by Medicare or other insurance (CMS 2017a)

Outpatient hospital: A part of the hospital facility that is designed to treat patients who do not need a bed or to be admitted as an inpatient for overnight care

Outpatient: A hospital patient who receives services in one or more of a hospital's facilities when he or she is not currently an inpatient or a home care patient

Outpatient: A patient who receives ambulatory care services in a hospital-based clinic or department

Ovaries: The glands found on either side of the uterus, below and behind the fallopian tubes, anchored to the uterus with suspensory ligaments

Overcoding: The practice of assigning more codes than needed to describe a patient's condition. Some instances of overcoding may be contrary to the guidance provided in the Official Coding Guidelines

Oviducts: The ducts through which the ovaries travel; also known as the fallopian tubes

Oximetry: A noninvasive test that measures a patient's oxygen saturation level

Pacemaker: A small, battery-powered device that is implanted in the patient's chest or abdomen and helps maintain a normal heart rhythm

Pain management services: Services performed as a treatment for chronic pain in patients who are not undergoing any type of surgical procedure

Panel: A group of specific tests (from the chemistry section) that are commonly performed together, such as a lipid or comprehensive metabolic panel

Parasitology: The study of parasites

Parenthetical note: instructions for use of the codes, presented in parenthesis throughout the tabular list that are intended to prevent errors and help coders report codes appropriately

Paring: The process of cutting or trimming away the outer edges of a skin growth to make it smaller, remove pressure points, or remove it completely

Parity (or para): The number of previous pregnancies

Parkinson's disease: A progressive disorder of the central nervous system that causes tremors rigidity, and postural problems

Partial hospitalization: A structured program of active treatment for psychiatric care that is more intense than the care a patient receives in a doctor or therapist's office (CMS 2017a)

Pass-through billing: Occurs when a laboratory performs an ordered lab test and sends the ordering provider a bill for the services (instead of billing the insurance company themselves), and the ordering provider bills the patient's insurance on the lab's behalf

Past, family, social history (PFSH): The patient's past experience with illnesses, hospitalizations, operations, injuries, and treatments; a review of medical events in the patient's family, including diseases that may be hereditary or place the patient at risk; age-appropriate review of past and current activities

Pathological fracture: Fracture that occurs in a diseased bone, such as osteoporosis or neoplastic disease (bone cancer)

Pathology and Laboratory section: Section of the CPT code book that lists codes that represent diagnostic studies on human specimens and tissue samples

Patient status: Identifies the patient's status during an accident, and identifies if the patient's injury was related to employment, volunteer work, or military status

Patient-activated cardiac event recorder: An implanted device that records the electrical rhythm of the heart when activated by the patient

Patient-Centered Medical Home (PCMH): A program to provide comprehensive primary care that partners physicians with the patient and their family to allow better access to healthcare and improved outcomes

Payment: 1. The money that a healthcare practice or facility receives in return for providing a healthcare service to a patient. 2. As amended by HITECH, the activities undertaken by a health plan to obtain premiums or to determine or fulfill its responsibility for coverage and provision of benefits under the health plan; or a healthcare provider or health plan to obtain or provide reimbursement for the provision of healthcare (45 CFR 164.501 2013)

Penetrating wound: Wound that results from a trauma that pierces the skin and goes into the body's deeper structures, such as a stab wound or gunshot wound

Penis: The main male reproductive organ

Per member per month (PMPM): Amount of money paid monthly for each individual enrolled in a capitation-based health insurance plan

Percutaneous: Through the skin

Percutaneous skeletal fixation: A type of fracture treatment in which fixation devices are placed across the fracture site, typically under x-ray imaging guidance

Percutaneous transluminal coronary angioplasty (PTCA): Procedure where a catheter is threaded into the body through an incision in the femoral artery in the groin, to the site of the angioplasty (usually an area clogged by atherosclerosis); then a small balloon at the tip of the catheter is slowly inflated, stretching the sides of the vessel and creating a wider opening through which blood can flow

Performance measures: A gauge used to assess the performance of a process or function of any organization (CMS 2017a)

Performing provider: The provider performing the surgery or other service

Pericardium: The sac that holds the heart

Perinatal: Period that extends before and after childbirth and pertains to the health and medical services for the fetus (and later newborn); extends from 20 to 28 weeks before childbirth to up to six weeks post-delivery

Perinatologist: A medical doctor who specializes in high-risk pregnancies and focuses on the health of the mother and fetus before, during, and after pregnancy

Perineum: The area between the vagina and the anus

Peripartum: Period that pertains to the mother's health and medical services, and extends from about one month before childbirth to up to five months after childbirth

Peripheral nerve stimulation: Pain treatment procedure performed by placing small electrodes next to peripheral nerves to ensure that the correct nerves have been identified; once the nerves causing the pain are found, the trial leads are removed and a neurostimulator is placed, with permanent leads and a small battery pack, to continuously stimulate the nerves and relieve pain (Mount Sinai Hospital 2017c)

Peritoneal dialysis: Dialysis that involves the placement of a dialyzing solution into the peritoneal cavity in the abdomen, where it removes waste products from the body and is then drained, removing extra fluid and waste products

Peritonitis: Infection within the peritoneal cavity

Permanent block: A specimen contained in a small mold and surrounded with paraffin wax and cooled

Permanent section: A permanent section procedure is similar to a frozen section, except that instead of freezing the block, it is placed in a fixative agent, which makes the cells fixed so that they will not change; it is then placed in a small mold and surrounded with paraffin wax and cooled so the specimen is contained within a permanent block that may be stored indefinitely for future evaluations

Pessary: A small device placed inside the vagina to support the internal structures of the female reproductive system such as the uterus, vagina, bladder, or rectum

Phacoemulsification: A technique used during extracapsular cataract excision that uses ultrasound vibrations to break up the cloudy lens and extract it through a small hollow tube

Physeal fracture: Fractures of the growth plate in long bones in children

Physical safeguards: As amended by HITECH, security rule measures such as locking doors to safeguard data and various media from unauthorized access and exposures; including facility access controls, workstation use, workstation security, and device and media controls (45 CFR 164.310 2013)

Physical status modifier: Modifiers that should be appended to the code for the anesthesia service

Physical therapist (PT): A licensed healthcare professional who focuses on noninvasive procedures that alleviate pain and improve and restore mobility

Physical therapy services: Noninvasive procedures and treatments that alleviate pain and improve and restore mobility to limbs and areas of the body

Physician: A medical doctor who has completed post-doctoral medical training in his or her chosen specialty

Physician's Desk Reference (PDR): A compilation of information for prescription drugs to ensure that the correct drug is selected for the service

Place of occurrence: Where the patient was when the injury occurred

Place of service (POS): Place of service or point of service

Placeholder X: In ICD-10-CM "X" is used to extend a code to the required number of characters so that a seventh character extension may be placed

Plan of care (POC): A doctor's written plan saying what kind of services and care the patient needs for their health problems (CMS 2017a)

Pleural effusion: A collection of fluid in the pleural space between the pleural sac, which lines the lung, and the lung itself; this fluid places pressure on the lung and does not allow it to expand completely, causing shortness of breath or chest pain

Pneumothorax: Collapsed lung

Polyarthritis: Arthritis that occurs in many different areas

Posterior: Situated toward the back of the body (such as the buttocks or heels)

Postero-anterior: Two projections during an imaging service consisting of two views that pass through the back to the front of the body

Postoperative diagnosis: The definitive medical condition of the patient either diagnosed or treated during the procedure

Postpartum: Post-pregnancy period that extends after childbirth to six weeks post-delivery

Premium: Amount of money that a policyholder or certificate holder must periodically pay an insurer in return for healthcare coverage

Preoperative diagnosis: The diagnosis that is given to the patient at the beginning of a procedure

Pressure ulcer: An ulcer that has occurred on the skin as a result of prolonged pressure on the skin; also known as a bedsore or decubitus ulcer

Preventive medicine services: Comprehensive health evaluations that involve a physical examination, including an age and gender appropriate history, counseling and anticipatory guidance and health risk factor reduction interventions, and the ordering of laboratory and diagnostic procedures

Primary care provider (PCP): 1. Physician who provides, supervises, and coordinates the healthcare of a member and who manages referrals to other healthcare providers and utilization of healthcare services both inside and outside a managed care plan (CMS 2017a) **2.** The physician who makes the initial diagnosis of a patient's medication condition

Primary care: A basic level of care usually given by doctors who work with general and family medicine, internal medicare, pregnant women, and children (CMS 2017a)

Primary neoplasm: Location where the growth originated

Prior authorization (PA): Process of obtaining approval from a healthcare insurance company before receiving healthcare services

Privacy Rule: The federal regulations created to implement the privacy requirements of the simplification subtitle of the Health Insurance Portability and Accountability Act of 1996; effective in 2002; afforded patients certain rights to and about their protected health information

Procedural coding system (PCS): Compilation of ICD codes used to report hospital inpatient procedures

Procedure: An action of diagnosis or treatment of a medical condition by a medical professional

Proctosigmoidoscopy: The examination of the rectum and may include a portion of the sigmoid colon

Products of conception (POC): The remaining fetal and placental tissues after either a spontaneous miscarriage or elective pregnancy termination

Professional component (PC): 1. The portion of a healthcare procedure performed by a physician **2.** A term generally used in reference to the elements of radiological procedures performed by a physician, which may include the supervision and interpretation of a technical service

Professional organization: An association of individuals that is committed to furthering the interests of a particular profession

Projection: The direction in which the imaging rays pass through the body

Prospective payment system (PPS): A type of reimbursement system that is based on preset payment levels rather than actual charges billed after the service has been provided; specifically, one of several Medicare reimbursement systems based on predetermined payment rates or periods and linked to the anticipated intensity of services delivered as well as the beneficiary's condition

Prostate: A gland only found in males that stores and assists in making seminal fluid, and sits under the urinary bladder surrounding part of the urethra

Prosthetics: Designed to replace all or part of an internal body organ (such as an artificial hip or knee replacement) or to replace an external appendage as an artificial limb (such as a lower leg prosthesis for an amputee)

Protected Health Information (PHI): 1. Health information that is individually identifiable, such as health records, laboratory reports, and patient healthcare history forms. PHI can be held on any type of media including paper, electronic, and orally transmitted information. **2.** As amended by HITECH, individually identifiable health information: (1) Except as provided in paragraph (2) of this definition, that is: (i) transmitted by electronic media; (ii) maintained in electronic media; or (iii) transmitted or maintained in any other form or medium. (2) Protected health

(Continued on next page)

information excludes individually identifiable health information: (i) in education records covered by the Family Educational Rights and Privacy Act, as amended, 20 U.S.C. 1232g; (ii) in records described at 20 U.S.C. 1232g(a)(4)(B)(iv); (iii) in employment records held by a covered entity in its role as employer; and (iv) regarding a person who has been deceased for more than 50 years (45 CFR 160.103 2013)

Provider contracting: Occurs iwhen the insurance company and the healthcare provider come into an agreement so that when the healthcare provider delivers healthcare services to patients, the insurance company will provide reimbursement for the healthcare services provided

Proximal: Toward the center of the body (the upper arm)

Psychotherapy: The treatment of mental illness and behavioral disturbance in which the healthcare provider attempts to alleviate the emotional disturbances, reverse or change patterns of behavior, and encourage personality growth and development through discourse with the patient

Puerperium: From birth to six weeks after birth

Pulmonary edema: Afluid collection within the lungs themselves caused by heart failure, myocardial infarction, cardiac ischemia, and other heart problems, as well as sepsis and severe anemia

Pulmonary embolism: An embolus that has traveled to the lungs, and can be a result of a DVT becoming

Push: The administration of a therapeutic, prophylactic, or diagnostic substance via an IV line

Qualifier: Identifies any additional attributes of why or how the procedure was performed

Qualifying circumstances CPT codes: Add-on codes that should be used in addition to the code for the anesthesia service (as well as any applicable physical status modifier)

Qualitative examination: An examination that studies the quality of a specimen

Quality improvement (QI): A set of activities that measures the quality of a service or product through systems or process evaluation and then implements revised processes that result in better healthcare outcomes for patients, based on standards of care

Quantitative examination: An examination that identifies the quantity of a specific substance found in a specimen

Radiation oncologist: Oncologists who specialize in the treatment of cancers via radiation treatments, also known as an interventional radiologist

Radiculopathy: A nerve-related pain

Radiofrequency nerve ablation: A procedure used to treat back and neck pain by using a controlled heat source to disable nerves that are responsible for causing pain; it is performed using a small needle with a heated tip placed near the nerve causing the pain, to disrupt the nerve's ability to send a pain signal (Mount Sinai Hospital 2017b)

Radiologic guidance: Procedure performed along with an invasive or minimally invasive procedure, to help guide the provider performing the procedure to the correct anatomical location

Radiological supervision and interpretation (S&I): The professional component of the study and includes the supervision of the radiology service as well as interpretation of the results

Radiologist: A medical doctor who specializes in the diagnosis and treatment of medical conditions using radiology and imaging techniques

Radiology section: Section of the CPT code book that lists all of the procedures that use radiant energy to diagnose and treat medical conditions, such as x-rays, MRIs, and ultrasounds

Radiology services: Services that use radiation to produce images of the inside of the body, such as bones and organs

Reattachment: All or a portion of a separated body part is put back in its normal location or other suitable location

Referral: A written approval from the primary care doctor for the patient to see a specialist or get certain services. In many Medicare Managed Care Plans, a patient needs a referral before he or she can get care from anyone except a primary care doctor. If a referral is not obtained first, the plan may not pay for the patient's care (CMS 2017a)

Refraction: A test performed to determine if a patient has any abnormalities with his or her vision, and used to identify the appropriate prescription for eyeglasses or contact lenses

Refractive surgery: Surgery performed to reshape the cornea of the eye and improve eye sight

Regional anesthesia: Anesthesia that employs an injection to block a large amount of nerves to numb a more extensive body area and prepare the patient for a more extensive surgery or procedure

Reimbursement: Compensation or repayment for healthcare services

Release: Freeing a body part from an abnormal physical constraint by cutting or by the use of force

Remote coding: Position in which the coder is not required to actually be present in the office or facility setting while completing his or her work

Removal: Taking out a device, object, or substance from a body part or area

Repair: A procedure performed to return an organ or body part to its original function, or to improve functioning or improve a cosmetic outcome; restoring a body part to its normal anatomic structure and function to the extent possible

Replacement: Inserting biological or synthetic material that physically takes the place or function of all or a portion of a body part

Reposition: Moving all or a portion of a body part to its normal location or other suitable location

Reproductive endocrinology and infertility (REI) specialist: A medical doctor with additional training and expertise in human reproduction, including the function of hormones in reproduction

Reproductive surgery: Specialty that focuses on surgical treatments to treat infertility

Resection: The removal of all or part of an organ, body tissue, or body part without replacement

Resequenced code: Codes that are not placed numerically within the tabular list and are out of numerical sequence; they are identified with the # symbol

Restriction: Partially closing an orifice of the lumen of a tubular body part

Retinal detachment: Occurs when the retina, which is a layer of tissue at the back of the eye, detaches from the eye tissues

Review of systems (ROS): A uniform system of performing an inventory of body systems through a series of questions seeking to identify signs or symptoms the patient may be experiencing or has experienced

Revision: Correcting a portion of a malfunctioning device or the position of a displaced device to the extent possible

Rhinoplasty: The surgical repair or revision of the nose, either for cosmetic or functional or medical purposes

Risk adjustment: The way that payments to health plans are changed to take into account a person's health status (CMS 2017a)

Risk analysis: The first step to risk management, includes assessing security threats, security vulnerabilities, and the likely impact should the system expose a vulnerability

Robot-assisted surgery: A type of laparoscopic surgery that is performed with the aid of a robot with miniature instruments controlled by the surgeon

Root operation: The type of surgery, operation, or procedure that was performed

Route of administration: The way in which the drug is administered to the patient

Rule of nines: Divides the body's surface into percentages based on the number nine, with the groin area making up the remaining one percent of body surface

Ruptured aneurysm: Aneurysm whose walls have burst causing hemorrhaging into the surrounding body cavity or tissues

Sagittal plane: A vertical line that divides the body into right and left halves

Salter-Harris classification: Classification that identifies the type of physeal fracture

Schizophrenia: A mental disorder which manifests in the symptoms of delusions, hallucinations, paranoia, confused speech, isolation, outbursts of anger, and catatonic behavior that persist for at least one month

Sciatica: A combination of pain, numbness, and weakness along the sciatic nerve from the lower back area, radiating to the buttocks and the leg; typically caused by a lower back problem putting pressure on the sciatic nerve

Scoliosis: A condition in which the spine curves sideways

Screening, Brief Intervention and Referral to Treatment (SBIRT): Behavior change interventions administered to patients with suspected alcohol or substance abuse

Scrotum: A pouch of skin where the testes are located

Secondary neoplasm: The site of the metastatic growth of a neoplasm

Security Rule: The federal regulations created to implement the security requirements of HIPAA

See also: Instructs the coder to look elsewhere for a code if the precise condition cannot be found in the current index entry

See condition: Instructs the coder to search for the code by looking up the condition, rather than the term that is currently located

Segment: Two vertebrae with the space between it

Segmental fracture: Fracture made up of at least two fracture lines, which isolate a larger section of bone

Seminal vesicles: Small male accessory sex glands that help to form the lubricating fluid of semen

Separate procedure: A procedure that is commonly part of another, more complex procedure, but which may be performed independently or be otherwise unrelated to the procedure

Sepsis: A complication of an infection outside of the bloodstream, such as a tooth abscess or skin infection; once a patient is deemed septic, the infectious organism has invaded the bloodstream and has been carried throughout the blood to other sites of the body (also referred to as septicemia or bacteremia)

Septic shock: A severe drop in blood pressure, caused by sepsis, that can lead to organ failure or death

Sequela: A condition that is the consequence of a previous disease or injury Sequencing priority

Sequencing: Placing multiple diagnoses codes in the correct order

Service-based code: A code that describes a full service, such as a physical therapy evaluation, application of hot or cold packs, or the performance of electrical stimulation; these codes are untimed, and one code should be reported no matter how long the provider spent performing the service

Services: Identified by HCPCS codes, miscellaneous services that may be provided to patients in the healthcare setting; some of these services are also identified by CPT codes, whereas other services are only identified by codes found in the HCPCS code book

Seventh character extension: The last possible character in a code, which is in the seventh location

Shaving: The act of sharp removal by transverse incision or horizontal slicing

Sigmoidoscopy: The examination of the entire rectum and sigmoid colon, and may include an examination of the descending colon

Signs: objective evidence of a disease that can be observed or detected by someone other than the individual affected by the condition

Skeletal traction: An invasive form of traction, in which a screw, pin, or wire is inserted into the bone, after which weights, ropes, and pulleys are used to pull the bone into the correct position

Skin lesion: Any abnormality in the skin; includes freckles and moles, precancerous and malignant areas, skin tags, and scrapes or cuts

Skin traction: Traction that employs straps, ropes, pulleys, and weights are applied externally to the skin to slowly stretch and realign bones into place until they can be set and casted until fully healed

Skin ulcer: An open wound on the skin that may be caused by infection, pressure, or venous problems

Slit lamp: A high-intensity light that can be focused into a thin sheet to shine into the eye

Small group practice: A practice that has from two to five healthcare providers, all of whom see patients each day

Smear: If the specimen is a liquid or submerged in a fluid substance, then it may be smeared onto the surface of a slide, then allowed to dry; it is then fixed with a fixative agent, and then stained to allow for the visualization of certain cells

Social communication disorder: Disorder that occurs when a patient has difficulty understanding social cues in verbal and nonverbal communication

Solo practice: A practice in which the physician is self-employed and legally the sole owner

Special report: Included with the reporting of an unlisted procedure or other procedure that is rarely provided, unusual, variable, or new, and should include a complete description of the procedure, including the nature of the procedure; extent of the procedure performed; need for the procedure (the medical necessity for the procedure); amount of time spent on the procedure; effort needed to complete the procedure; and equipment necessary to provide the service

Specific test: Test that evaluates a specimen for an identified substance

Specificity: Ability to detect the absence of a characteristic when the characteristic is absent

Specimen: A bodily tissue sample from the patient

Speech therapy services: Services that help adults and children improve their speech, advance social and cognitive communication skills, and treat swallowing disorders

Speech-language pathologist (SLP): A healthcare professional who provides speech therapy services

Spermatic cord: A cord-like structure made up of the vas deferens and surrounding tissues

Spinal cord stimulation (SCS): Pain treatment procedure that identifies the exact spinal nerves causing the paint and places a battery and lead wires on these nerves to alleviate pain; similar to peripheral nerve stimulation

Spiral fracture: Fracture that spirals around and extends down the length of the bone

Sprain: The stretching or tearing of a ligament

Stage: Each layer excised

Staghorn calculus: Large kidney stones that are too big to pass naturally through the urinary system and may require surgical treatment

Standalone code: Codes that include a full description and do not depend on a parent code to provide more information

Status asthmaticus: An extreme form of asthma exacerbation that does not respond to treatment and can result in hypoxia and ultimately respiratory failure

Status epilepticus: A type of epilepsy in which the seizures occur too close together for the patient to fully recover in-between seizures, or when a seizure lasts for a long period of time

Stereotactic body radiation treatment (SBRT): Whole-body stereotactic radiosurgery (SRS) treatment used on body tumors

Stereotactic radiosurgery (SRS): A type of radiation treatment used for intracranial lesions that delivers a precision dose of radiation

Strabismus: A misalignment of the eye muscles that can be surgically corrected by repositioning and strengthening the muscles of the eye

Strain: An injury to a muscle or tendon, which ranges from a simple stretching of the muscle or tendon to complete tear of the muscle and tendon

Subcapsular cataract: Cataracts that form at the back of the lens and are more common in individuals with diabetes mellitus or patients on high doses of steroids

Subsequent encounter: This episode of care is used when the patient is seen during the healing phase of the encounter and is no longer under active treatment for the condition

Substance abuse: The misuse of alcohol or drugs, which impairs a person's ability to meet daily responsibilities

Subterm: Terms that are indented under the main term to indicate that they pertain to the main term, and to identify different variations of the main term

Superior: Toward the top of the body (the head)

Supplement: Inserting biological or synthetic material that physically reinforces or augments the function of a portion of a body part

Supplemental insurance: Insurance policies that help patients pay the out-of-pocket expenses related to healthcare. Supplemental insurance policies differ depending on the type of insurance offered and the specifics of coverage, ranging from accident coverage, coverage for cancer treatments, coverage for disabilities only, or for coverage of a specific set of healthcare services or treatments. Supplemental insurance plans are typically low cost, and patients can pick and choose which type of coverage they prefer and tailor coverage to their specific needs. These plans act as an umbrella, in that they help cover the patient from the financial burdens for which he or she may be responsible in the case of a healthcare emergency or unplanned treatment

Supplies: Items provided to the patient in the healthcare setting, typically designed for long-term or multiple uses

Surgery section: The largest of all sections within the CPT code book; it lists all of the invasive procedures that may be performed to treat patients

Surgical procedure: Any single, separate, systematic process upon or within the body that can be complete in itself; is normally performed by a physician, dentist, or other licensed practitioner; can be performed either with or without instruments; and is performed to restore disunited or deficient parts, remove diseased or injured tissues, extract foreign matter, assist in obstetrical delivery, or aid in diagnosis

Surgical specialist: Provider who treats and diagnoses patients through major surgical techniques

Symptoms: Subjective evidence of a disease or a disease process experienced

Synonym: Word or phrase that means the same thing as another word or phrase

Systemic inflammatory response syndrome (SIRS): A noninfectious process, such as heatstroke or a traumatic injury

Table of Drugs and Chemicals: The third section of the ICD-10-CM book that lists the toxic effects of drugs, chemicals, and other substances

Table of Drugs: A reference tool in the HCPCS code book that helps coders find the appropriate HCPCS code for drugs and medications administered in the healthcare setting, organized by the name of the drug or medicinal, dosage or unit amount given, and the method of administration of the drug

Table of Neoplasms: An index that allows coders to identify codes for neoplastic conditions, such as malignant tumors and diseases, and benign growths

Tabular List: The structured list of ICD-10-CM codes, organized alphanumerically, and divided into chapters based on body system or condition

Technical component (TC): The portion of radiological and other procedures that is facility based or nonphysician based (for example, radiology films, equipment, overhead, endoscopic suites, and so on)

Technical safeguards: As amended by HITECH, the Security Rule means the technology and the policy and procedures for its use that protect electronic protected health information and control access to it (45 CFR 164.304 2013)

Telemedicine service: 1. Professional services given to a patient through an interactive telecommunications system by a practitioner at a distant site (CMS 2017a) **2.** A telecommunications system that links healthcare organizations and patients from diverse geographic locations and transmits text and images for (medical) consultation and treatment

Testes: Glands of the reproductive and endocrine systems that produce and store sperm and male sex hormones

Therapeutic procedure: Procedure that is performed to treat a diagnosis

Therapy services: Treatments aimed at rehabilitating the patient to optimal bodily function

Third-party payer: An insurance company (for example, Blue Cross/Blue Shield) or healthcare program (for example, Medicare) that pays or reimburses healthcare providers (second party) or patients (first party) for the delivery of medical services

Thoracostomy: An opening created in the thoracic cavity, otherwise known as a chest tube that acts as a drain for the thoracic cavity to drain blood, fluid, or air from around your lungs, heart, or esophagus

Thrombosis: A formation of blood cells, fatty deposits, or other particles that form a clot within the blood vessel, otherwise known as a blood clot

Time units: Values for anesthesia services that take into account the duration of the procedure, from the beginning of the anesthesia service until the patient is released to a postoperative or post-anesthesia care unit

Time-based code: Code reported according the length of time that the provider spent performing the service to the end of a long, thin, lighted tube, inserted through a natural opening or stoma; the healthcare provider can maneuver the endoscope through a body passage, such as the gastrointestinal tract, to see inside the organ for diagnostic or therapeutic services

Torus fracture: Fracture that occurs in children, when only one part of the bone buckles

Toxic effect: The result of a toxin, such as a chemical, medicinal, or other substance on the body

Trabeculectomy: Procedure used as a treatment for glaucoma by lowering the intraocular pressure (the pressure inside the eyeball)

Tracheostomy: Connection that is established by the insertion of the tracheostomy tube

Tracheotomy: Procedure that cuts through the trachea to allow for the insertion of a tracheostomy tube, or trach tube

Traction: The use of mechanical devices and mechanisms to straighten bones or relieve pressure

Transcranial magnetic stimulation (TMS): A non-invasive procedure that utilizes magnetic fields to stimulate areas of the brain

Transfer: Moving, without taking out, all or a portion of a body part to another location to take over the function of all or a portion of a body part

Transluminal procedure: Procedure that is performed within a vessel

Transplantation: Inserting all or a portion of a living body part taken from another individual or animal to physically take the place or function of all or a portion of a similar body part; procedure that removes a damaged, diseased, or otherwise nonfunctioning organ from the body and replaces it with a donated organ in its place

Transportation indicator: A two-character code used to identify why the transportation service was medically necessary

Transurethral resection of the prostate (TURP): Procedure that involves the insertion of a resectoscope through the male urethra, which is threaded to the area of the prostate tissue to be removed; an electrocautery knife is then used to cut away at the enlarged prostatic tissue

Transverse fracture: Fracture that travels horizontally across the bone

Transverse plane: A horizontal line, perpendicular to the long axis of the body that divides the body into superior and inferior portions (the top and the bottom halves); also known as the axial plane

Traumatic brain injury (TBI): Brain injury that requires invasive surgery and a lifetime of medical treatment and rehabilitative services

Traumatic fracture: Fracture that occurs as a result of some sort of traumatic injury

Treatment modality: A method of therapeutic treatment designed to treat or rehabilitate a specific patient condition

Treatment, payment, and healthcare operations (TPO): Standard of the Privacy Rule that allows the use of protected health information for the following: treatment or the provision, coordination, and management of a patient's healthcare and related services by that patient's healthcare providers; payment or the activities of the patient's health insurance plan to obtain premiums for health insurance, to determine coverage benefits, and to furnish payment for healthcare services delivered to a covered beneficiary; and healthcare operations including various services provided by healthcare practitioners

Treatment: As amended by HITECH, the provision, coordination, or management of healthcare and related services by one or more healthcare providers, including the coordination or management of healthcare by a healthcare provider with a third party; consultation between healthcare providers relating to a patient; or the referral of a patient for healthcare from one healthcare provider to another (45 CFR 164.501 2013)

TRICARE: A healthcare program for active duty and retired uniformed services members and their families, formerly referred to as CHAMPUS (CMS 2017a)

Trimesters: Three, roughly three-month periods of time, into which the 40 weeks of pregnancy are grouped

Tunica vaginalis: A layer of tissue covering the testes in the shape of a pouch

UB-04: A uniform institutional provider hardcopy claim form suitable for use in billing multiple third-party payers. The UB-04 is the only hardcopy claim form that CMS accepts from institutional providers (CMS 2017a)

Ultrasound: Imaging that uses high-frequency sound waves applied to the body via a transducer on a specific area of the body; the sound waves bounce off internal structures within the body, creating an image on a computer screen

Unbundling: The practice of using multiple codes to bill for the various individual steps in a single procedure rather than using a single code that includes all the steps of the comprehensive procedure

Undercoding: A form of incomplete documentation that results when diagnoses or procedures that should be coded are not assigned

Underdose: Occurs when a patient does not take the correctly prescribed amount of a medication

Underdosing: An underdosing occurs when a patient takes too little or a prescribed substance and suffers an unintended consequence

Undetermined intent: An undetermined intent of a toxic effect is used only when the intention of the toxic effect cannot be determined to be any of the other types: accidental, intentional, assault, adverse effect, or underdosing

Unlisted procedure codes: Codes available in each section of CPT to describe procedures that have no specific procedure code assigned because the procedure is new or unusual

Ureters: Two thin tubes that connect the kidneys to the urinary bladder

Urethra: Part of the urinary system through which urine passes during elimination from the bladder

Urgent care facility: Facility that provides same-day care for patients with healthcare emergencies or urgent healthcare needs and may be either a stand-alone facility or attached to a larger facility, such as a hospital

Urgent care: Services provided to patients who need healthcare for non–life-threatening situations, illnesses, or injuries

Urinary bladder: A hollow muscular organ that holds urine until it is emptied from the body through the urethra

Urodynamics: The study of the motion and flow of urine

Urologist: A medical doctor who specializes in the diagnosis and treatment of conditions of the urinary system and the male and female genital systems

Use additional code: Instructions that list conditions that should be coded *after* the code identified

Uterus: Organ in the female reproductive system where the fetus develops during gestation

Vaccine administration: The act of giving the patient a vaccine

Vaccine toxoid: The actual substance that is injected or given to a patient and that creates an immune response from the patient

Vagina: The lower portion of the birth canal, which serves as the conduit for the birth of a fetus, uterine secretions and menstrual flow, and as the receptacle for semen from a male during intercourse

Vaginectomy: Removal of all or part of the vagina

Vagus nerve stimulation: The stimulation of implanted electrodes in the vagus nerve in the cranium as a treatment for depression that is resistant to medication

Varicose vein: Vein that is a result of an insufficiency in the valves of the lower veins to push blood upward toward the heart, causing a buildup of blood various reasons including pain management and to reduce muscle spasticity

Vas deferens: Duct made of smooth muscle located within the spermatic cord that transport sperm from the epididymis to the urethra, which is later ejaculated through the urethral orifice

Vasectomy: An outpatient procedure that is performed commonly for elective sterilization where a small section of the vas deferens are cut and removed, so that semen does not flow through the vas to the urethra during ejaculation

Vasopneumatic device: Device used on the external extremities (like the arms and legs) that applies external pressure to the soft tissues and decreases swelling

Virology: The study of viruses

Vision insurance: Insurance similar to health insurance, but that only covers services that are related to visual acuity assessments, refractions, and corrective lenses

Vulva: Female genitalia that consists of the labia (both labia majora and labia minora), the bulb of the vestibule, vestibule of the vagina, the greater vestibular glands (known as Bartholin's glands, they secrete mucus to lubricate the vagina), the lesser vestibular gland, and the vagina orifice, also known as the introitus

Workers' compensation insurance: Insurance that employers are required to have to cover employees who get sick or injured on the job (CMS 2017a)

Xenograft: A skin graft made from a different species (commonly pig skin)

X-ray: A form of imaging that produces a beam of x-rays, a form of electromagnetic radiation, that pass through the body

References

42 CFR 405.500. 60 FR 63175, Dec. 9, 1995. http://www.ecfr .gov.

42 CFR 425.20. 76 FR 67973, Nov. 2, 2011. http://www.ecfr .gov.

45 CFR 160.103. 65 FR 82798, Dec. 28, 2000, as amended at 78 FR 5687, Jan. 25, 2013. http://www.ecfr.gov.

45 CFR 164.304. 68 FR 8376, Feb. 20, 2003, as amended at 78 FR 5693, Jan. 25, 2013. http://www.ecfr.gov.

45 CFR 164.310. 68 FR 8376, Feb. 20, 2003, as amended at 78 FR 5694, Jan. 25, 2013. http://www.ecfr.gov.

45 CFR 164.501. 65 FR 82802, Dec. 28, 2000, as amended at 78 FR 5695, Jan. 25, 2013. http://www.ecfr.gov.

45 CFR 164.502. 65 FR 82802, Dec. 28, 2000, as amended at 78 FR 5696, Jan. 25, 2013. http://www.ecfr.gov.

Agency for Healthcare Research and Quality. 2017 (June). Never Events. https://psnet.ahrq.gov/primers /primer/3/never-events.

American Health Information Management Association. 2017. Pocket Glossary of Health Information Management and Technology, 5th ed. Chicago: AHIMA.

American Health Information Management Association. 2017a. Overview of Certified Coding Associate (CCA®). http://www.ahima.org/certification/CCA.

American Medical Association. 2018. *CPT 2018 Professional Edition*. Chicago: AMA.

American Medical Association (AMA). 2017. http://www .ama-assn.org.

American Psychiatric Association. 2017. https://www .psychiatry.org/psychiatrists/practice/dsm.

Centers for Disease Control and Prevention (CDC). 2017. http://www.cdc.gov.

Centers for Medicare and Medicaid Services (CMS) Glossary. 2017a. https://www.cms.gov/apps/glossary /default.asp?Letter=ALL&Language=English.

Center for Medicare and Medicaid Services. 2017b. National Correct Coding Initiative. https://www.cms.gov /Medicare/Coding/NationalCorrectCodInitEd/index .html.

Center for Medicare and Medicaid Services. 2017c. 2017-PCS-Code-Tables. https://www.cms .gov /Medicare/Coding/ICD10/2017-ICD-10-PCS-and -GEMs.html.

Department of Health and Human Services (HHS). 2010. Medicare Program: Proposed Changes to the Hospital Inpatient Prospective Payment Systems for Acute Care Hospitals and the Long-Term Care Hospital Prospective Payment System and Proposed Fiscal Year 2011 Rates. Federal Register 75(88): 23851–24362.

Indian Health Service (IHS). 2017. Indian Health Manual. https://www.ihs.gov/ihm/index.cfm/dsp_folder/doa /progdel/documents/org_charts/dsp_folder/pc/p6c1 /documents/functionalstmts/index.cfm.

Mount Sinai Hospital. 2017a. Electromyography. http:// www.mountsinai.org/patient-care/service-areas /pain-management/pain-management-services /electrodiagnostic-studies.

Mount Sinai Hospital. 2017b. Interventional Pain Procedures Under X-Ray Guidance. http:// www.mountsinai.org/patient-care/service-areas /pain-management/pain-management-services /interventional-spinal-procedures-under-x-ray -guidance.

Mount Sinai Hospital. 2017c. Peripheral Nerve Stimulation. http://www.mountsinai.org/patient-care/service -areas/pain-management/pain-management-services /peripheral-nerve-stimulation.

National Centers for Health Statistics (NCHS). 2017. https://www.cdc.gov/nchs/.

Palmetto GBA. 2013 (July). Anesthesia Billing Guide. https://engage.ahima.org/HigherLogic/System /DownloadDocumentFile.ashx?DocumentFileKey =9af2a07d-26e1-4694-b1de-a4c59d0dbc30.

Public Law 104-191. 1996. 110 Stat. 1936. Short title see 42 U.S.C. 201 note. http://uscode.house.gov/.

Index

Trust AHIMA for Your Coding Education and Training

IMA is widely recognized and highly
garded as a leader in coding education
d training. AHIMA has been at the
refront of providing coding expertise
over 85 years and served as one of
ur cooperating parties responsible for
e ICD-10 Coding Guidelines.

AHIMA HAS A VARIETY OF CODING PRODUCTS AND RESOURCES TO ASSIST YOU AND YOUR TEAM:

- Professional Books and Textbooks
- Meetings
  - In-Person
  - Virtual
- Online Courses
- Toolkits and Practice Briefs
- Webinars

or a complete list of all AHIMA coding
roducts and resources, visit ahimastore.org.

AHIMA
American Health Information
Management Association®

PREPARE FOR YOUR FUTURE WITH AHIMA MEMBERSHIP

Are you ready for a job
health information (H
Seeking to take steps towa
a successful career pat
Get started with an AHIM
student membersh
Join AHIMA today and ga
multiple professional benefi
Our resources will prepare y
to find one of the thousan
of projected new HIM jo

EXCEL IN SCHOOL AND PLAN FOR YOUR FUTURE WITH AHIMA MEMBER BENEFITS!

- Follow industry news in the digital edition of the *Journal of AHIMA*, *CareerMinded*, and other e-newsletters

- Explore the job market through Career Assist: Job Bank

- Find someone to listen and look up to through AHIMA's mentor program

- Discounts on books, events, webinars, credentials, and more

- Get ready to enter the job market with AHIMA's career prep resources, including free webinars, a toolkit, and the HIM Career Map

- Build your resume with volunteer opportunities

- Network locally with component state association (CSA) membership

- AHIMA's new Body of Knowledge (BoK), an onlin HIM library, makes study a research a breeze

- Interact with HIM professio and fellow students on AHIMA's Engage Online Communities

- Free admission to the AHIM Convention Student Acade

- AHIMA Foundation Merit Scholarships available

JOIN TODAY AT AHIMA.ORG/JOIN.